PORTABLE

Signs
&
Symptoms

 Wolters Kluwer | Lippincott Williams & Wilkins
Health

Philadelphia • Baltimore • New York • London
Buenos Aires • Hong Kong • Sydney • Tokyo

STAFF

Executive Publisher
Judith A. Schilling McCann, RN, MSN

Editorial Director
David Moreau

Clinical Director
Joan M. Robinson, RN, MSN

Art Director
Mary Ludwicki

Senior Managing Editor
Jaime Stockslager Buss, MSPH, ELS

Clinical Manager
Collette Bishop Hendler, RN, BS, CCRN

Clinical Editor
Dorothy P. Terry, RN

Editors
Julie Munden, Liz Schaeffer

Copy Editors
Kimberly Bilotta (supervisor),
Amy Furman, Shana Harrington,
Pamela Wingrod

Designer
Arlene Putterman

Digital Composition Services
Diane Paluba (manager),
Joyce Rossi Biletz, Donna S. Morris

Associate Manufacturing Manager
Beth J. Welsh

Editorial Assistants
Megan L. Aldinger, Karen J. Kirk,
Jeri O'Shea, Linda K. Ruhf

Design Assistant
Georg W. Purvis IV

Indexer
Barbara Hodgson

PortSS010607

Library of Congress
Cataloging-in Publication Data

Portable signs and symptoms.
        p. ; cm.
    Includes bibliographical references and index.
    1. Nursing assessment—Handbooks, manuals, etc. 2. Nursing diagnosis—Handbooks, manuals, etc. 3. Symptoms—Handbooks, manuals, etc.   I. Lippincott Williams & Wilkins.
    [DNLM: 1. Nursing Assessment—Handbooks. 2. Diagnostic Techniques and Procedures—Handbooks. 3. Physical Examination—Handbooks. 4. Signs and Symptoms—Handbooks. WY 49 P8395 2008]
    RT48.P65 2008
    616.07′5—dc22
ISBN-13: 978-1-58255-679-6 (alk. paper)
ISBN-10: 1-58255-679-2 (alk. paper)   2007010117

Contents

Contributors and consultants

Helen C. Ballestas, RN, MSN, CRRN
Nursing Instructor; New York Institute of Technology;
Old Westbury

Julie A. Calvery, RN, MSN
Instructor; University of Arkansas; Fort Smith

Kim Cooper, RN, MSN
Nursing Department Program Chair; Ivy Tech Community College;
Terre Haute, Ind.

Vivian C. Gamblian, RN, MSN
Professor of Nursing; Collin County Community College;
McKinney, Tex.

Dana Reeves, RN, MSN
Assistant Professor; University of Arkansas; Fort Smith

Kendra S. Seiler, RN, MSN
Nursing Instructor; Rio Hondo Community College; Whittier, Calif.

Fernisa Sison, RN, MSN, FNP-BC
Medical/Surgical Instructor; San Joaquin Delta College; Stockton, Calif.
Registered Nurse; St. Josephs Medical Center; Stockton, Calif.
Family Nurse Practitioner; Lodi (Calif.) Memorial Hospital

PART

I

Assessment

Reviewing assessment techniques

Performing a 10-minute assessment

You won't always want or need to assess a patient in 10 minutes. However, rapid assessment is crucial when you must intervene quickly—such as when a hospitalized patient has a change in his physical, mental, or emotional status.

You may also perform a rapid assessment to confirm a diagnostic finding. For example, if arterial blood gas analysis indicates a low oxygen content, you'll quickly assess the patient for other signs of oxygen deprivation, such as increased respiratory rate and cyanosis.

General guidelines

Try to assess the patient quickly but systematically. To save time, cover some of the assessment components simultaneously. For example, make your general observations while checking the patient's vital signs or asking history questions.

Be flexible. You won't necessarily use the same sequence each time. Let the patient's chief complaint and your initial observations guide your assessment. Sometimes, you may be unable to obtain a quick history and instead will need to rely on your observations and the information on the patient's chart.

Keep the patient calm and cooperative. If you don't know him, first introduce yourself by name and title. Remain calm, and reassure him that you can help. If your demeanor can reduce his anxiety, he'll be more likely to give you accurate information.

Avoid drawing quick conclusions. In particular, don't assume that the patient's current symptom is related to his admitting diagnosis.

When every minute counts, follow these steps.

Assess airway, breathing, and circulation

As your first priority, this assessment may consist of just a momentary observation. However, when a patient appears to be unconscious or has difficulty breathing, you'll assess him more thoroughly to detect the problem and allow immediate intervention.

Make general observations

Note the patient's mental status, general appearance, and level of consciousness (LOC) for clues about the nature and severity of his condition.

Assess vital signs

Take the patient's body temperature, pulse, respiratory rate, and blood pressure. They provide a quick overview of his physiologic condition as well as valuable information about the heart, lungs, and blood vessels. The seriousness of the patient's chief complaint and your general observations of his condition will determine how frequently you measure vital signs. A patient's age, activity level, and physical and emotional condition may affect his vital signs. Compare with the patient's baseline, if available.

Conduct the health history

Use pointed questions to explore the patient's perception of his chief complaint. Find out what's bothering him the most. Ask him to quantify the problem. For instance, does he feel worse today than he did yesterday? Such questions will help you to focus your assessment. If you're in a hurry or if the patient can't respond, obtain information from other sources, such as family members, admission forms, the medical history, and the patient's chart.

Perform the physical examination

Begin by concentrating on areas related to the patient's chief complaint—the abdomen, for example, if the patient complains of abdominal pain. Compare the results with baseline data, if available.

Sometimes, you may have to perform a complete head-to-toe or body systems assessment—for instance, if a patient is unresponsive (yet has no breathing or circulatory problems) or is confused and, thus, unreliable. However, in most cases, the patient's chief complaint, your general observations, and your findings about the patient's vital signs will guide your assessment.

Guidelines for an effective interview

When you have time for a full assessment, begin by interviewing the patient. Developing an effective interviewing technique will help you to collect pertinent health history information efficiently. Use these guidelines to enhance your interviewing skills.

Be prepared

◆ Before the interview, review all available information. Read the current clinical records and, if applicable, previous records. Doing so will focus the interview, prevent the patient from tiring, and save you time.
◆ Review with the patient what you've learned to ensure that the information is correct. Keep in mind that the patient's current complaint may be unrelated to his history.

Create a pleasant interviewing atmosphere

◆ Select a quiet, well-lit, and relaxing setting. Keep in mind that extraneous noise and activity can interfere with concentration, as can excessive or insufficient light. A relaxing atmosphere eases the patient's anxiety, promotes comfort, and conveys your willingness to listen.
◆ Ensure privacy. Some patients won't share personal information if they suspect that others can overhear. You may, however, let friends or family members remain if the patient requests it or if he needs their help.
◆ Make sure that the patient feels as comfortable as possible. If the patient is tired, short of breath, or frightened, provide care and reschedule the history taking.
◆ Take your time. If you appear rushed, you may distract the patient. Give him your undivided attention. If you have little time, focus on specific areas of interest and return later instead of hurrying through the entire interview.

Establish a good rapport

◆ Sit and chat with the patient for a few minutes before the interview. Standing may suggest that you're in a hurry, leading the patient to rush and omit important information.
◆ Explain the purpose of the interview. Emphasize how the patient benefits when the health care team has the information needed to diagnose and treat a disorder.
◆ Show your concern for the patient's story. Maintain eye contact, and occasionally repeat what he tells you. If you seem preoccupied or uninterested, he may choose not to confide in you.
◆ Encourage the patient to help you to develop a realistic care plan that will serve his perceived needs.

Set the tone and focus
◆ Encourage the patient to talk about his chief complaint. Doing so helps you to focus on his most troublesome signs and symptoms and provides an opportunity to assess the patient's emotional state and level of understanding.
◆ Keep the interview informal but professional. Allow the patient time to answer questions fully and to discuss his perceptions.
◆ Speak clearly and simply. Avoid using medical terms. Make sure the patient understands you, especially if he's elderly. If you think he doesn't, ask him to restate what you've discussed.
◆ Pay close attention to the patient's words and actions, interpreting not only what he says but also what he doesn't say. If the patient is a child, direct as many questions as possible to him. Rely on the parents for information if the child is very young.

Choose your words carefully
◆ Ask open-ended questions to encourage the patient to provide complete and pertinent information. Avoid yes-or-no questions.
◆ Listen carefully to the patient's answers. Use his words in your subsequent questions to encourage him to elaborate on his signs, symptoms, and other problems.

Take notes
◆ Avoid documenting everything during the interview, but make sure to jot down important information, such as dates, times, and key words or phrases. Use these to help you recall the complete history for the medical record.
◆ If you're tape-recording the interview, obtain written consent from the patient.

Assessing overall health

For a quick look at the patient's overall health, ask these questions.
◆ Has your weight changed? Do your clothes, rings, and shoes fit?
◆ Do you have nonspecific signs and symptoms, such as weakness, fatigue, night sweats, or fever?
◆ Can you keep up with your normal daily activities?
◆ Have you had any unusual symptoms or problems recently?
◆ How many colds or other minor illnesses have you had in the last year?
◆ What prescription and over-the-counter drugs or herbal remedies do you take?

Assessing activities of daily living

For a comprehensive look at the patient's health and health history, ask these questions.

Diet and elimination
◆ How would you describe your appetite?
◆ What do you normally eat in a 24-hour period?
◆ What foods do you like and dislike? Is your diet restricted at all?
◆ How much fluid do you drink during an average day?
◆ Are you allergic to any food?
◆ Do you prepare your meals, or does someone prepare them for you?
◆ Do you go to the grocery store, or does someone else shop for you?
◆ Do you snack and, if so, on what?
◆ Do you eat a variety of foods?
◆ Do you have enough money to purchase the groceries you need?
◆ How is your digestion?
◆ Do you have trouble with your bowels?

◆ Do you take foods, fluids, drugs, or herbal remedies to maintain your normal elimination patterns?

Exercise and sleep

◆ Do you have a special exercise program? What is it? How long have you been following it? How do you feel after exercising?
◆ How many hours do you sleep each day? When? Do you feel rested afterward?
◆ Do you fall asleep easily?
◆ Do you take drugs or do anything special to help you to fall asleep?
◆ What do you do when you can't sleep?
◆ Do you wake up during the night?
◆ Do you have sleepy spells during the day? When?
◆ Do you routinely take naps?
◆ Do you have recurrent, disturbing dreams?
◆ Have you ever been diagnosed with a sleep disorder, such as narcolepsy or sleep apnea?

Recreation

◆ What do you do when you aren't working?
◆ What kind of unpaid work do you do for enjoyment?
◆ How much leisure time do you have?
◆ Are you satisfied with what you can do in your leisure time?
◆ Do you and your family share leisure time?
◆ How do your weekends differ from your weekdays?

Tobacco, alcohol, and drugs

◆ Do you use tobacco? If so, what kind? How much do you use each day? Each week? When did you start using it? Have you ever tried to stop?
◆ Do you drink alcoholic beverages? If so, what kind (beer, wine, whiskey)?

◆ How much alcohol do you drink each day? Each week? What time of day do you usually drink?
◆ Do you usually drink alone or with others?
◆ Do you drink more when you're under stress?
◆ Has drinking ever hampered your job performance?
◆ Do you or does anyone in your family worry about your drinking?
◆ Do you feel dependent on alcohol?
◆ Do you feel dependent on coffee, tea, or soft drinks? How much of these beverages do you drink in an average day?
◆ Do you use drugs that aren't prescribed by a physician (marijuana, cocaine, heroin, steroids, sleeping pills, tranquilizers)?

Assessing the family

When assessing how and to what extent the patient's family fulfills its functions, remember to assess both the family into which the patient was born (family of origin) and, if different, the patient's current family.

Because the following questions target a nuclear family—that is, mother, father, and children—you may need to modify them somewhat for other types of families, such as single-parent families, families that include grandparents, patients who live alone, or unrelated individuals who live as a family. Remember, you're assessing the *patient's perception* of family function.

Affective function

To assess how family members regard each other, ask these questions.
◆ How do the members of your family treat one another?
◆ How do they feel about one another?
◆ How do they regard one another's needs and wants?

◆ How are feelings expressed in your family?

◆ Can family members safely express both positive and negative feelings?

◆ What happens when family members disagree?

◆ How do family members deal with conflict?

◆ Do you feel safe in your environment?

Socialization and social placement

To assess the flexibility of family responsibilities, which aids discharge planning, ask these questions.

◆ How satisfied are you and your partner with your roles as a couple?

◆ Do you and your partner agree about how to bring up the children? If not, how do you work out differences?

◆ Who's responsible for taking care of the children? Is this arrangement mutually satisfactory?

◆ How well do you feel your children are growing up?

◆ Are family roles negotiable within the limits of age and ability?

◆ Do you share cultural values and beliefs with your children?

Health care function

To identify the family caregiver and thus facilitate discharge planning, ask these questions.

◆ Who takes care of family members

Performing palpation

Palpation uses pressure to assess structure size, placement, pulsation, and tenderness. Ballottement, a variation, involves bouncing tissues against the hand to assess rebound of floating structures. Ballottement can be used to assess a mass in a patient with ascites.

Light palpation

To perform light palpation, press gently on the skin, indenting it ½″ to ¾″ (1 to 2 cm). Use the lightest touch possible; too much pressure blunts your sensitivity. Close your eyes to concentrate on feeling.

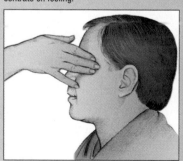

Deep palpation

To perform deep palpation, indent the skin about 1½″ (4 cm). Place your other hand on top of the palpating hand to control and guide your movements. To perform a variation of deep palpation that allows you to pinpoint an inflamed area, push down slowly and deeply, and then lift your hand away quickly. If the patient complains of increased pain as you release the pressure, you have identified rebound tenderness.

when they're sick? Who makes physician appointments?

◆ Are your children learning about personal hygiene, healthful eating, and the importance of adequate exercise, sleep, and rest?

◆ How does your family adjust when a member is ill and unable to fulfill expected roles?

Family and social structure

To assess the value the patient places on family and other social structures, ask these questions.

◆ How important is your family to you?

◆ Do you have friends whom you consider family?

◆ Does anyone other than your immediate family (for example, grandparents) live with you?

◆ Are you involved in community affairs? Do you enjoy the activities?

Economic function

To explore money issues and their relation to power roles within the family, ask these questions.

◆ Does your family income meet the family's basic needs?

◆ Who makes decisions about family money allocation?

◆ If you take prescription drugs, do you have enough money to pay for them?

(Text continues on page 10.)

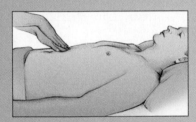

Use both hands (bimanual palpation) to trap a deep, hard-to-palpate organ (such as the kidney or spleen) or to fix or stabilize an organ (such as the uterus) while palpating with the other hand.

Light ballottement

To perform light ballottement, apply light, rapid pressure from quadrant to quadrant of the patient's abdomen (top right). Keep your hand on the surface of the skin to detect tissue rebound.

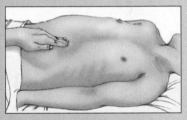

Deep ballottement

To perform deep ballottement, apply abrupt, deep pressure; then release, but maintain contact.

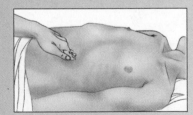

Performing percussion

Percussion has two basic purposes: to produce percussion sounds and to elicit tenderness. It involves three types: indirect, direct, and blunt percussion.

Indirect percussion

The most commonly used method, indirect percussion, produces clear, crisp sounds when performed correctly. To perform indirect percussion, use the second finger of your non-dominant hand as the pleximeter (the mediating device used to receive the taps) and the middle finger of your dominant hand as the plexor (the device used to tap the pleximeter). Place the pleximeter finger firmly against a body surface, such as the upper back or abdomen. With your wrist flexed loosely, use the tip of your plexor finger to deliver a crisp blow just beneath the distal joint of the pleximeter. Make sure you hold the plexor perpendicular to the pleximeter. Tap lightly and quickly, removing the plexor as soon as you have delivered each blow.

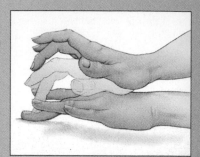

Identifying percussion sounds

Percussion produces sounds that vary according to the tissue being percussed. This chart shows important percussion sounds along with their characteristics and typical locations.

SOUND	INTENSITY	PITCH	DURATION
Resonance	Moderate to loud	Low	Moderate to long
Tympany	Loud	High	Moderate
Dullness	Soft to moderate	High	Long
Hyperresonance	Very loud	Very low	Long
Flatness	Soft	High	Short

Direct percussion

To perform direct percussion, tap your hand or fingertip directly against the body surface as shown. This method helps assess an adult's sinuses for tenderness.

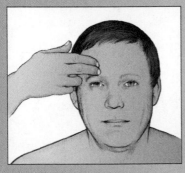

Blunt percussion

To perform blunt percussion, strike the ulnar surface of your fist against the body surface. Alternatively, you may use both hands by placing the palm of one hand over the area to be percussed and then making a fist with the other hand and using it to strike the back of the first hand. Both techniques aim to elicit tenderness—not to create a sound—over organs such as the kidneys.

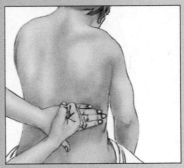

QUALITY	SOURCE
Hollow	Normal lung
Drumlike	Gastric air bubble or intestinal air
Thudlike	Liver, full bladder, pregnant uterus, or spleen
Booming	Hyperinflated lung (as in emphysema)
Flat	Muscle, bone, or tumor

Performing auscultation

Auscultation of body sounds—particularly those produced by the heart, lungs, blood vessels, stomach, and intestines—detects both high-pitched and low-pitched sounds. Auscultation is performed using a stethoscope. To prevent the spread of infection among patients, clean the chest piece and end pieces of the stethoscope with alcohol or a disinfectant before each use.

Assessing high-pitched sounds

To assess high-pitched sounds properly, such as breath sounds and first and second heart sounds, use the diaphragm of the stethoscope. Make sure you place the entire surface of the diaphragm firmly on the patient's skin. Hair on the patient's chest may cause friction on the diaphragm or bell of the stethoscope, which can mimic abnormal breath sounds, such as crackles. You can minimize this problem by lightly wetting the hair before auscultating.

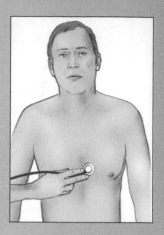

Assessing the cardiovascular system

Initial questions

◆ Ask the patient about cardiac problems, such as palpitations, tachycardia or other irregular rhythms, chest pain, dyspnea on exertion, paroxysmal nocturnal dyspnea, and cough.
◆ Explore vascular problems. Does the patient experience cyanosis, edema, ascites, intermittent claudication, cold extremities, or phlebitis?
◆ Ask about orthostatic hypotension, hypertension, rheumatic fever, varicose veins, and peripheral vascular diseases.
◆ Ask when, if ever, the patient had his last electrocardiogram.

Inspecting the precordium

◆ First, place the patient in a supine position, with his head flat or elevated for his respiratory comfort. If you're examining an obese patient or a patient with large breasts, have the patient sit upright. This position will bring the heart closer to the anterior chest wall and make pulsations more visible. If time allows, you can use tangential lighting to cast shadows across the chest. Doing so makes it easier to see abnormalities.
◆ Standing to the patient's right (unless you're left-handed), remove the clothing covering his chest wall. Quickly identify the following anatomic sites, named for their underlying structures: sternoclavicular, pulmonary, aortic, right ventricular, epigastric, and left ventricular areas.

Assessing low-pitched sounds

To assess low-pitched sounds, such as heart murmurs and third and fourth heart sounds, lightly place the bell of the stethoscope on the appropriate area. Don't exert pressure. If you do, the patient's chest will act as a diaphragm and you will miss low-pitched sounds. If the patient is extremely thin or emaciated, use a stethoscope with a pediatric chest piece.

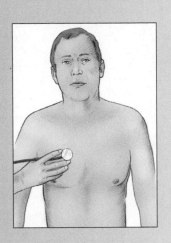

◆ Make a visual sweep of the chest wall, watching for movement, pulsations, and exaggerated lifts or heaves (strong outward thrusts seen at the sternal border or apex during systole).

Measuring blood pressure

When you assess the patient's blood pressure, you're measuring the fluctuating force that blood exerts against arterial walls as the heart contracts and relaxes. To measure blood pressure accurately, follow these steps.

Preparing the patient

◆ Before beginning, make sure that the patient is relaxed and hasn't eaten or exercised in the last 30 minutes.
◆ The patient can sit, stand, or lie down during blood pressure measurement.

Applying the cuff and stethoscope

◆ To obtain a reading in an arm (the most common measurement site), wrap the sphygmomanometer cuff snugly around the upper arm, above the antecubital area (the inner aspect of the elbow). Center the cuff bladder over the brachial artery. When measuring blood pressure in an infant, child, thin patient, or obese patient, use an appropriate-sized cuff. Because blood pressure may be inaudible in children younger than age 2, consider using an electronic stethoscope or Doppler to obtain a more accurate measurement.
◆ Most cuffs have arrows that should be placed over the brachial artery.
◆ Keep the mercury manometer at eye level. If your sphygmomanometer has an aneroid gauge, place it level with the patient's arm. Keep the patient's

arm level with the heart by placing it on a table or a chair arm or by supporting it with your hand. Rest a recumbent patient's arm at his side. Don't use the patient's muscle strength to hold up the arm; tension from muscle contraction can elevate systolic pressure and distort the findings.

◆ Palpate the brachial pulse, just below and slightly medial to the antecubital area. Place the earpieces of the stethoscope in your ears, and position the stethoscope head over the brachial artery, just distal to the cuff or slightly beneath it.

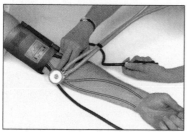

◆ Generally, you'll use the flat diaphragm to auscultate the pulse. However, if the patient has a diminished or hard-to-locate pulse, you may need to use the bell to detect the low-pitched sound of arterial blood flow more effectively.

Obtaining the blood pressure reading

◆ Watch the manometer while you pump the bulb until the mercury column or aneroid gauge reaches about 20 to 30 mm Hg above the point at which the pulse disappears.

◆ Slowly open the air valve and watch the mercury drop or the gauge needle descend. Release the pressure at a rate of about 3 mm Hg/second, and listen for pulse sounds (Korotkoff's sounds). These sounds, which determine the blood pressure measurement, are classified as follows.

Phase I
A clear, faint tapping starts and increases in intensity to a thud or a louder tap.

Phase II
The tapping changes to a soft, swishing sound.

Phase III
A clear, crisp tapping sound returns.

Phase IV (first diastolic sound)
The sound becomes muffled and takes on a blowing quality.

Phase V
The sound disappears.

◆ As soon as you hear blood begin to pulse through the brachial artery, note the reading on the aneroid dial or mercury column. This sound reflects phase I (the first Korotkoff's sound) and coincides with the patient's systolic pressure. Continue to deflate the cuff, noting the point at which pulsations diminish or become muffled—phase IV (the fourth Korotkoff's sound)—and the point at which they disappear—phase V (the fifth Korotkoff's sound). For children and highly active adults, many authorities consider phase IV the most accurate reflection of blood pressure. For children younger than age 13, pregnant women, and highly active adults, record phases I, IV, and V.

◆ The American Heart Association and the World Health Organization recommend documenting phases I and V in most adults. To avoid confusion and to make your measurements more useful, follow this format for recording blood pressure: systolic/disappearance (for example, 120/76 mm Hg).

(Text continues on page 18.)

Positioning the patient for cardiac auscultation

During auscultation, you will typically stand to the right of the patient, who's in a supine position. The patient may lie flat or at a comfortable elevation.

If the heart sounds seem faint or undetectable, try repositioning the patient. Alternate positioning may enhance the sounds or make them seem louder by bringing the heart closer to the surface of the chest. Common alternate positions include the seated, forward-leaning position and the left-lateral decubitus position. If these positions don't enhance the heart sounds, try auscultating with the patient standing or squatting.

Forward-leaning position

The forward-leaning position is best for hearing high-pitched sounds related to semilunar valve problems, such as aortic and pulmonic valve murmurs. Aortic insufficiency is sometimes heard only in the forward-leaning position. To auscultate these sounds, help the patient into the forward-leaning position and place the diaphragm of the stethoscope over the aortic and pulmonic areas in the right and left second intercostal spaces.

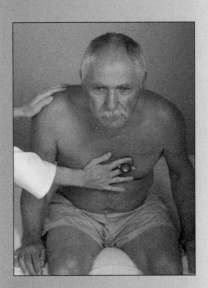

Left-lateral decubitus position

The left-lateral decubitus position is best for hearing low-pitched sounds related to atrioventricular valve problems, such as mitral valve murmurs and extra heart sounds. A mitral stenosis murmur is sometimes heard only in the left-lateral position. A pericardial rub (an abnormal finding) can be heard in this position as well. To auscultate these sounds, help the patient into the left-lateral decubitus position and place the bell of the stethoscope over the apical area.

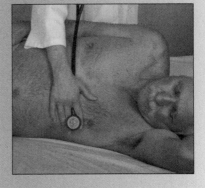

Auscultating heart sounds

Using a stethoscope with 10″ to 12″ (25- to 30-cm) tubing, follow these steps to auscultate heart sounds.

◆ Locate the four different auscultation sites, as illustrated. In the aortic area, blood moves from the left ventricle during systole, crossing the aortic valve and flowing through the aortic arch. In the pulmonic area, blood ejected from the right ventricle during systole crosses the pulmonic valve and flows through the main pulmonary artery. In the tricuspid area, sounds reflect the movement of blood from the right atrium across the tricuspid valve, filling the right ventricle during diastole. In the mitral, or apical, area, sounds represent blood flow across the mitral valve and left ventricular filling during diastole.

◆ Begin auscultation in the aortic area (1), placing the stethoscope in the second intercostal space along the right sternal border.
◆ Move to the pulmonic area (2), located in the second intercostal space at the left sternal border.
◆ Next, assess the tricuspid area (3), which lies in the fifth intercostal space along the left sternal border.
◆ Finally, listen in the mitral area (4), located in the fifth intercostal space near the midclavicular line.
Note: If the patient's heart is enlarged, the mitral area may be closer to the anterior axillary line.

Palpating arterial pulses

To palpate the arterial pulses, you'll apply pressure with your index and middle fingers positioned as shown here.

Carotid pulse
Lightly place your fingers just medial to the trachea and below the angle of the jaw.

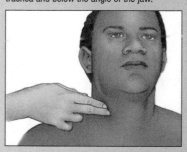

Brachial pulse
Position your fingers medial to the biceps tendon.

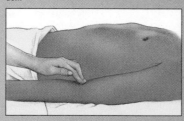

Radial pulse
Apply gentle pressure to the medial and ventral side of the wrist, just below the thumb.

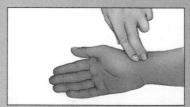

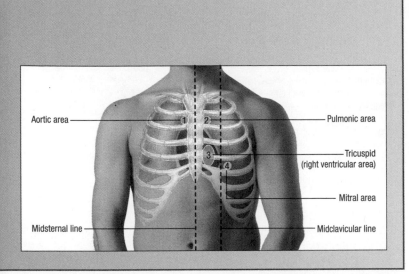

Aortic area

Pulmonic area

Tricuspid
(right ventricular area)

Mitral area

Midsternal line

Midclavicular line

Femoral pulse

Press relatively hard at a point inferior to the inguinal ligament. For an obese patient, palpate in the crease of the groin, halfway between the pubic bone and the hip bone.

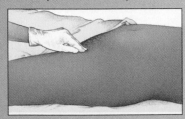

Popliteal pulse

Press firmly against the popliteal fossa at the back of the knee.

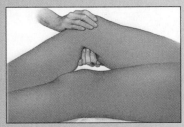

Posterior tibial pulse

Curve your fingers around the medial malleolus, and feel the pulse in the groove between the Achilles tendon and the malleolus.

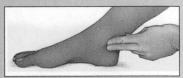

(continued)

Palpating arterial pulses *(continued)*

Dorsalis pedis pulse

Lightly touch the medial dorsum of the foot while the patient points the toes down. In this site, the pulse is difficult to palpate. If you can't palpate a pulse in this location, palpate the dorsum of the foot more laterally. Decreased or absent pedal pulses suggest occlusive disease in the lower popliteal artery, when normal femoral and popliteal pulses are present.

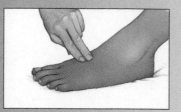

Evaluating edema

To assess pitting edema, press firmly for 5 to 10 seconds over a bony surface, such as the tibia, fibula, sacrum, or sternum. Then remove your finger and note how long the depression remains. Document your observation on a scale of +1 (barely detectable depression) to +4 (persistent pit as deep as 1″ [2.5 cm]).

In severe edema, also referred to as *brawny edema*, tissue swells so much that fluid can't be displaced, making pitting impossible. The surface feels rock-hard, and subcutaneous tissue becomes fibrotic.

+1 PITTING EDEMA

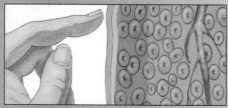

+4 PITTING EDEMA

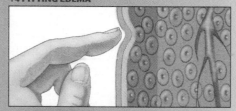

BRAWNY EDEMA

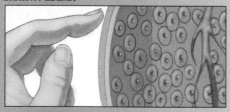

Palpating the thorax

Palpation of the anterior and posterior thorax can detect structural and skin abnormalities, areas of pain, and chest asymmetry. To perform this technique, use the fingertips and palmar surfaces of one or both hands to palpate systematically and in a circular motion. Alternate palpation from one side of the thorax to the other.

Anterior thorax

Begin palpation in the supraclavicular area (#1 in the diagram at right). Then palpate the anterior thorax in the following sequence: infraclavicular, sternal, xiphoid, rib, and axillary areas.

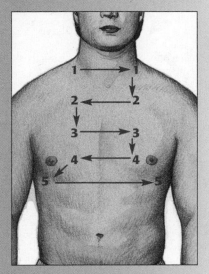

Posterior thorax

Begin palpation in the supraclavicular area. Then move to the area between the scapulae (interscapular), then to the area below the scapulae (infrascapular), and finally down to the lateral walls of the thorax.

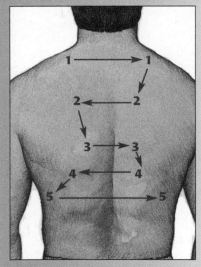

Assessing the respiratory system

Initial questions

◆ Inquire about dyspnea or shortness of breath. Does your patient have breathing problems after physical exertion? Also ask him about pain, wheezing, paroxysmal nocturnal dyspnea, and orthopnea (for example, number of pillows used).

◆ Ask whether the patient has a cough, sputum production, hemoptysis, or night sweats.

◆ Find out whether he has emphysema, pleurisy, bronchitis, tuberculosis, pneumonia, asthma, sleep apnea, or frequent respiratory tract infections.

Inspecting the chest

◆ Position the patient to allow access to his posterior and anterior chest. If his condition permits, have him sit on the edge of a bed or examining table or on a chair, leaning forward with his arms folded across his chest. If this isn't possible, place him in semi-Fowler's position for the anterior chest examination. Then ask him to lean forward slightly and use the side rails or mattress for support while you quickly examine his posterior chest. If he can't lean forward, place him in a lateral position or ask another staff member to help him to sit up.

◆ Systematically compare one side of the chest with the other.

◆ First, inspect the patient's chest for obvious problems, such as draining, open wounds, bruises, abrasions, scars, and cuts. Also look for less obvious problems, such as rib deformities, fractures, lesions, or masses.

◆ Examine the shape of the patient's chest wall. Observe the anteroposterior and transverse diameters.

◆ To find the patient's respiratory rate, count for a full minute—longer if you note abnormalities. Don't tell the patient what you're doing or he might alter his breathing pattern. Adults normally breathe at a rate of 12 to 20 breaths/minute; children in early childhood, 20 to 40 breaths/minute; and children in late childhood, 15 to 25 breaths/minute.

◆ Note the patient's respiratory pattern, watching for such abnormal patterns as tachypnea, bradypnea, apnea, Cheyne-Stokes respirations, Kussmaul's respirations, and Biot's respirations. Also look for such characteristics as pursed-lip breathing.

◆ Observe the movement of the chest during respirations. The chest should move upward and outward symmetrically on inspiration. Factors that may affect movement include pain, poor positioning, and abdominal distention. Watch for paradoxical movement (possibly resulting from fractured ribs or flail chest) and asymmetrical expansion (indicating atelectasis or underlying pulmonary disease).

◆ Check for use of the accessory muscles and retraction of the intercostal spaces during inspiration (possibly indicating respiratory distress). You may notice sudden, violent intercostal retraction (airway obstruction or tension pneumothorax); retraction of the abdominal muscles during expiration (chronic obstructive pulmonary disease and other obstructive disorders); inspiratory intercostal bulging (cardiac enlargement or aneurysm); or localized expiratory bulging (rib fracture or flail chest).

Palpating for tactile fremitus

Because sound travels more easily through solid structures than through air, assessing for tactile fremitus— which involves palpating for voice vibrations—provides valuable information about the contents of the lungs. Follow this procedure.

◆ Place your open palm flat against the patient's chest without touching the chest with your fingers.

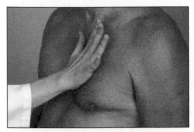

◆ Ask the patient to repeat a resonant phrase, such as "ninety-nine" or "blue moon," as you systematically move your hands over his chest from the central airways to the lung periphery and back. Always proceed systematically from the top of the suprascapular area to the interscapular, infrascapular, and hypochondriac areas (found at the levels of the fifth and tenth intercostal spaces to the right and left of the midline).

◆ Repeat this procedure on the posterior thorax. You should feel fremitus (vibrations) of equal intensity on either side of the chest. Fremitus normally occurs in the upper chest, close to the bronchi, and feels strongest at the second intercostal space on either side of the sternum. Little or no fremitus should occur in the lower chest. The intensity of the vibrations varies according to the thickness and structure of the patient's chest wall as well as the intensity and pitch of his voice.

Percussing the thorax

Percussion of the thorax helps to determine the boundaries of the lungs and the amount of gas, liquid, or solid in the lungs. Percussion can effectively assess structures as deep as $1^3/4''$ to $3''$ (4.5 to 7.5 cm).

To percuss a patient's thorax, always use indirect percussion, which involves striking one finger with another. Proceed systematically, percussing the anterior, lateral, and posterior chest over the intercostal spaces.

Avoid percussing over bones, such as the manubrium, sternum, xiphoid, clavicles, ribs, vertebrae, or scapulae. Because of their denseness, bones produce a dull sound on percussion and, therefore, yield no useful information.

Always follow the same sequence when performing percussion, comparing variations in sound from one side to the other. Doing so helps to ensure consistency and prevents you from overlooking important findings.

Anterior thorax

◆ Place your hands over the lung apices in the supraclavicular area.
◆ Proceed downward, moving from side to side at intervals of $1^1/2''$ to $2''$ (4 to 5 cm).

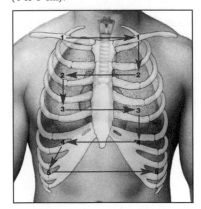

◆ Anterior chest percussion should produce resonance from below the clavicle to the fifth intercostal space on the right (where dullness occurs close to the liver) and to the third intercostal space on the left (where dullness occurs near the heart).

Posterior thorax
◆ Progress in a zigzag fashion from the suprascapular to the interscapular to the infrascapular areas, avoiding the vertebral column and the scapulae, as shown below.

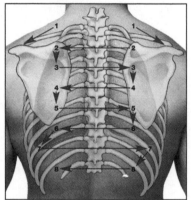

◆ Posterior percussion should sound resonant to the level of T10.

Auscultating breath sounds

Auscultating breath sounds helps you to detect abnormal accumulation of fluid or mucus and obstructed air passages. Breath sounds may be normal, abnormal, or absent. Classify breath sounds by their location, intensity, pitch, and duration during the inspiratory and expiratory phases. To detect breath sounds, follow these steps.
◆ Auscultate the anterior, lateral, and posterior thorax, following the same sequence that you used for percussion of the thorax. Begin at the upper lobes, and move from side to side and down, comparing findings.
◆ If the patient is a child, begin just below the right clavicle, moving to the midsternum, left clavicle, left nipple, and right nipple.
◆ Assess one full breath (inspiration and expiration) at each point.

Assessing the neurologic system

Initial questions

◆ Ask the patient to state his full name and the date, time, and place where he is now.
◆ Investigate the character of any headaches (frequency, intensity, location, and duration).
◆ Determine whether your patient has vertigo or syncope.
◆ Ask whether he has a history of seizures or use of anticonvulsants.
◆ Explore cognitive disturbances, including recent or remote memory loss, hallucinations, disorientation, speech and language dysfunction, or inability to concentrate.
◆ Ask whether the patient has a history of sensory disturbances, including tingling, numbness, and sensory loss.
◆ Explore motor problems, including problems with gait, balance, coordination, tremor, spasm, or paralysis.
◆ Ask the patient whether cognitive, sensory, or motor symptoms have interfered with his activities of daily living.

Assessing neurologic vital signs

Neurologic vital signs are used to evaluate the patient's LOC, pupillary activity, and level of orientation to time, place, and person. These assessment findings supplement routine measurements of temperature, blood pressure, pulse, and respirations.

LOC reflects brain stem function and usually provides the first sign of central nervous system deterioration. Changes in pupillary activity may signal increased intracranial pressure (ICP). Level of orientation evaluates higher cerebral functions. Evaluating muscle strength and tone, reflexes, and posture may also help to identify nervous system damage. Finally, evaluating the respiratory rate and pattern can help to locate brain lesions and determine their size.

Equipment
Penlight ◆ thermometer ◆ stethoscope ◆ sphygmomanometer ◆ pupil size chart

Implementation
◆ Explain the procedure to the patient, even if he's unresponsive.
◆ Assess the patient's LOC.
◆ Ask the patient to state his full name. If he responds appropriately, then he's oriented to person. Then assess his orientation to time and place. Assess the quality of his replies.
◆ Assess the patient's ability to understand and follow one-step commands that require a motor response. For example, ask him to open and close his eyes. Note whether he can maintain his LOC.
◆ If the patient doesn't respond to commands, squeeze the nail beds on his fingers and toes with moderate pressure and note his response. Alternately, rub the upper portion of his sternum between the second and third intercostal spaces with your knuckles.

Check the motor responses bilaterally to rule out monoplegia and hemiplegia.

Examine pupils and eye movement
◆ Ask the patient to open his eyes. If he's unresponsive, lift his upper eyelids. Inspect the pupils for size and shape, and compare them for equality. To evaluate them more precisely, use a chart showing the various pupil sizes.
◆ Test the patient's direct light response. First, darken the room. Hold each eyelid open in turn, keeping the other eye covered. Swing the penlight from the patient's ear toward the midline of the face. Shine the light directly into the eye. Normally, the pupil constricts immediately when exposed to light and then dilates immediately when the light is removed. Wait 20 seconds before testing the other pupil to allow it to recover from reflex stimulation.
◆ Test consensual light response. Hold both eyelids open, but shine the light into one eye only. Watch for constriction in the other pupil, which indicates proper nerve function.
◆ Brighten the room, and ask the conscious patient to open his eyes. Observe the eyelids for ptosis or drooping. Then check the extraocular movements. Hold up one finger and ask the patient to follow it with his eyes as you move your finger up, down, laterally, and obliquely. See whether the patient's eyes track together to follow your finger (conjugate gaze). Watch for involuntary jerking or oscillating movements (nystagmus).
◆ Check accommodation. Hold up one finger midline to the patient's face and several feet away. Ask the patient to focus on your finger as you move it toward his nose. His eyes should converge, and his pupils should constrict equally.

Assessing the pupils

Pupillary changes can signal different conditions. Use these illustrations and lists of causes to help you detect problems.

Bilaterally equal and reactive

◆ Normal

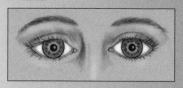

Unilateral, dilated (4 mm), fixed, and nonreactive

◆ Uncal herniation with oculomotor nerve damage
◆ Brain stem compression by an expanding lesion or an aneurysm
◆ Increased intracranial pressure
◆ Tentorial herniation
◆ Head trauma with subsequent subdural or epidural hematoma
◆ Normal in some people

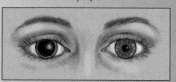

Bilateral, dilated (4 mm), fixed, and nonreactive

◆ Severe midbrain damage
◆ Cardiopulmonary arrest (hypoxia)
◆ Anticholinergic poisoning
◆ Deep anesthesia
◆ Dilating drops

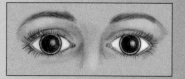

Bilateral, midsized (2 mm), fixed, and nonreactive

◆ Midbrain involvement caused by edema, hemorrhage, infarction, laceration, or contusion

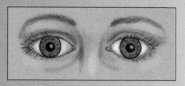

Unilateral, small (1.5 mm), and nonreactive

◆ Disruption of the sympathetic nerve supply to the head caused by a spinal cord lesion above T1

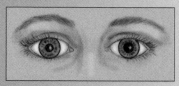

Bilateral, pinpoint (less than 1 mm), and usually nonreactive

◆ Lesion of the pons, usually after hemorrhage, leading to blocked sympathetic impulses
◆ Opiates such as morphine (pupils may be reactive)
◆ Iritis
◆ Pilocarpine drugs

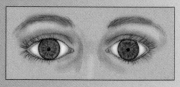

◆ Test the corneal reflex with a wisp of cotton. Have the patient look straight ahead. Bring the cotton wisp in from the side to lightly touch the cornea. Observe the patient for bilateral blinking. Tearing will occur in the eye that's touched.

◆ If the patient is unconscious, test the oculocephalic (doll's eye) reflex. Hold the patient's eyelids open. Quickly but gently turn the patient's head to one side and then to the other. If the patient's eyes move in the opposite direction from the side to which you turn the head, the reflex is intact, indicating that the brain stem is functioning.

◆ **ALERT** Never test this reflex if you know or suspect that the patient has a cervical spine injury.

Evaluate motor function

◆ If the patient is conscious, test his grip strength in both hands at the same time. Extend your hands, ask the patient to squeeze your fingers as hard as he can, and compare the strength of each hand. Grip strength is usually slightly stronger in the dominant hand.

◆ Test arm strength by having the patient close his eyes and hold his arms straight out in front of him, with the palms up. See whether either arm drifts downward or pronates, which indicates weakness.

◆ Test leg strength by having the patient raise his legs, one at a time, against gentle downward pressure from your hand.

◆ If the patient is unconscious, exert pressure on each fingernail bed. If the patient withdraws, compare the strength of each limb. If decorticate or decerebrate posturing develops in response to painful stimuli, notify the physician immediately.

◆ Flex and extend the extremities on both sides to evaluate muscle tone.

◆ Test the plantar reflex in all patients. Stroke the lateral aspect of the sole of the patient's foot with your thumbnail. Normally, this elicits flexion of all toes. Watch for a positive Babinski's sign—dorsiflexion of the great toe with fanning of the other toes—which indicates an upper motor neuron lesion.

◆ Test for Brudzinski's and Kernig's signs in patients suspected of having meningitis.

Complete the neurologic examination

◆ Take the patient's temperature, pulse rate, respiratory rate, and blood pressure. Especially check pulse pressure—the difference between systolic and diastolic pressure—because widening pulse pressure can indicate increasing ICP.

◆ **ALERT** If a patient's status was previously stable and he has a sudden change in neurologic or routine vital signs, assess his condition further and notify the physician immediately.

Assessing cerebellar function

To evaluate cerebellar function, you'll test the patient's whole-body coordination and extremity coordination.

Heel-to-toe walking
◆ To assess balance, ask the patient to walk heel to toe.
◆ Although the patient may be slightly unsteady, he should be able to walk and maintain his balance.

Romberg's test
◆ Ask the patient to stand with his feet together, his eyes open, and his arms at his side. Hold your outstretched arms on either side of him

(Text continues on page 26.)

Comparing delirium, dementia, and depression

This table highlights the distinguishing characteristics of delirium, dementia, and depression.

CLINICAL FEATURE	DELIRIUM
Onset	Acute, sudden
Course	Short, with diurnal fluctuations in symptoms; symptoms worse at night, in darkness, and on awakening
Progression	Abrupt
Duration	Hours to less than 1 month; seldom longer
Awareness	Reduced
Alertness	Fluctuates; lethargic or hypervigilant
Attention	Decreased
Orientation	Generally impaired but reversible
Memory	Recent and immediate memory impaired
Thinking	Disorganized, distorted, and fragmented; incoherent speech, either slow or accelerated
Perception	Distorted, with illusions, delusions, and hallucinations; difficulty distinguishing between reality and misperceptions
Speech	Incoherent
Psychomotor behavior	Variable; hypokinetic, hyperkinetic, and mixed
Sleep and wake cycle	Altered
Affect	Variable affective anxiety, restlessness, and irritability; reversible
Findings on mental status testing	Distracted from task; numerous errors

DEMENTIA	DEPRESSION
Gradual	Sudden or brief
Lifelong; symptoms progressive and irreversible	Diurnal effects, with symptoms typically worse in the morning; situational fluctuations but less than with acute confusion
Slow but uneven	Variable, rapid, or slow, but even
Months to years	At least 2 weeks but can be several months to years (Note: *Diagnostic and Statistical Manual of Mental Disorders,* Fourth Edition, Text Revision, specifies duration of at least 2 weeks for diagnosis.)
Clear	Clear
Generally normal	Normal
Generally normal	May decrease temporarily
May be impaired as disease progresses	May be disoriented
Recent and remote memory impaired	Selective or patchy impairment
Difficulty with abstraction; impoverished thoughts and impaired judgment; words difficult to find	Intact, with themes of hopelessness, helplessness, or self-deprecation
Misperceptions usually absent	Intact, without delusions or hallucinations, except in severe cases
Dysphasia as disease progresses; aphasia	Normal, slow, or rapid
Normal; may have apraxia	Variable, with psychomotor retardation or agitation
Fragmented	Insomnia or somnolence
Superficial, inappropriate, and labile; attempts to conceal deficits in intellect; may show personality changes, aphasia, and agnosia; lacks insight	Depressed, dysphoric mood, with exaggerated and detailed symptoms; preoccupied with personal thoughts; insight present; verbal elaboration
Failings highlighted by family; struggles with test, with frequent "near miss" answers; exerts great effort to find an appropriate reply; commonly requests feedback on performance	Failings highlighted by patient; commonly responds "don't know"; exerts little effort; commonly gives up; appears indifferent toward examination and doesn't care or attempt to find answer

so you can support him if he sways to one side or the other.

◆ Observe his balance; then ask him to close his eyes. Note whether he loses his balance or sways.

◆ If he falls to one side, Romberg's test result is abnormal. Patients with cerebellar dysfunction have difficulty maintaining their balance with their eyes closed because they can't use the visual cues that orient them to the upright position.

Finger-to-finger movements

◆ To evaluate the patient's extremity coordination, have the patient sit about 2′ (0.5 m) away from you.

◆ Hold your index finger up, and ask him to touch the tip of his index finger to the tip of yours and then to touch his nose.

◆ Move your finger and ask him to repeat the maneuver. Gradually, have him increase his speed as you repeat the test.

◆ Test his other hand. Expect the patient to be more accurate with his dominant hand.

◆ A patient with cerebellar dysfunction will overshoot his target, and his movements will be jerky.

Rapid skilled movements

◆ To further evaluate the patient's extremity coordination, ask the patient to touch the thumb of his right hand to his right index finger and then to each of his remaining fingers.

◆ Instruct him to increase his speed.

◆ Observe his movements for smoothness and accuracy.

◆ Repeat the test on his left hand.

Assessing reflexes

Assessment of the deep tendon and superficial reflexes provides information about the intactness of the sensory receptor organ. It also evaluates how well the afferent nerve relays the sensory message to the spinal cord, the spinal cord or brain stem segment mediates the reflex, the lower motor neurons transmit messages to the muscles, and the muscles respond to motor messages.

To evaluate the patient's reflexes, test deep tendon and superficial reflexes and observe the patient for primitive reflexes.

Deep tendon reflexes

Before you test a deep tendon reflex, make sure that the limb is relaxed and the joint is in midposition; for instance, the knee or elbow should be flexed at a 45-degree angle. Then distract the patient by asking him to focus on an object across the room. If he focuses on his performance, the cerebral cortex may dampen his response. Simply instruct him to clench his teeth or to squeeze his thigh. If needed, you can distract the patient by using Jendrassik's maneuver to enhance the patellar reflex. Have the patient lock his fingers together and pull against them with all possible strength. Document which technique you used to distract the patient.

Always move from head to toe in testing deep tendon reflexes, and compare contralateral reflexes. To elicit the reflex, tap the tendon lightly but firmly with the reflex hammer. Then grade the briskness of the response: 0 (no response), 1+ (diminished), 2+ (normal), 3+ (brisker than average), or 4+ (hyperactive).

Biceps reflex

◆ Position the patient's arm so that his elbow is flexed at a 45-degree angle and his arm is relaxed.

◆ Place your thumb or index finger over the biceps tendon and your remaining fingers loosely over the triceps muscle.

◆ Strike your thumb or index finger with the pointed tip of the reflex hammer, and watch and feel for contraction of the biceps muscle and flexion of the forearm.

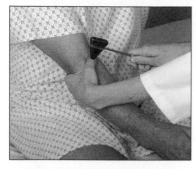

Triceps reflex

◆ Have the patient abduct his arm and place his forearm across his chest.

◆ Strike the triceps tendon about 2″ (5 cm) above the olecranon process on the extensor surface of the upper arm, as shown below.

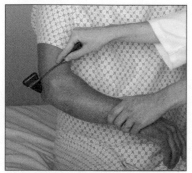

◆ Watch for contraction of the triceps muscle and extension of the forearm.

Brachioradialis reflex

◆ Instruct the patient to rest the ulnar surface of his hand on his knee and to partially flex his elbow.

◆ With the flat end of the hammer, strike the radius about 2″ proximal to the radial styloid, as shown below.

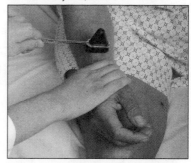

◆ Watch for supination of the hand and flexion of the forearm at the elbow.

Patellar reflex

◆ Have the patient sit on the side of the bed with his legs dangling freely. If he can't sit up, flex his knee at a 45-degree angle and place your nondominant hand behind it for support.

◆ Strike the patellar tendon just below the patella, as shown below.

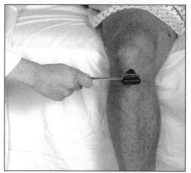

◆ Look for contraction of the quadriceps muscle in the anterior thigh and for extension of the leg.

Achilles reflex

◆ Slightly flex the foot and support the plantar surface.

◆ Using the flat end of the reflex hammer, strike the Achilles tendon.

◆ Watch for plantar flexion of the foot and ankle.

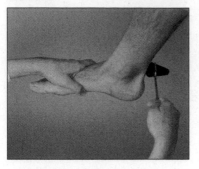

Superficial reflexes

Superficial reflexes include the abdominal, cremasteric, and plantar reflexes. To elicit these reflexes, stimulate the skin or mucous membranes. To document your findings, use a plus sign (+) to indicate that a reflex is present and a minus sign (−) to indicate that it's absent.

Abdominal reflex

◆ Place the patient in the supine position, with his arms at his sides and his knees slightly flexed.

◆ Using the tip of the reflex hammer, a key, or an applicator stick, briskly stroke both sides of the abdomen above and below the umbilicus, moving from the periphery toward the midline, as shown below.

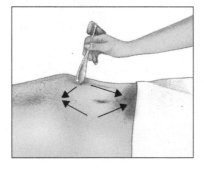

◆ After each stroke, watch for contraction of the abdominal muscles and movement of the umbilicus toward the stimulus. If you're evaluating an obese patient, retract the umbilicus to the side opposite the stimulus and note whether it pulls toward the stimulus.

◆ Aging and disease of the upper and lower motor neurons cause an absent abdominal reflex.

Cremasteric reflex

◆ With a male patient, use an applicator stick to lightly stimulate the inner thigh. Watch for contraction of the cremaster muscle in the scrotum and prompt elevation of the testicle on the side of the stimulus.

◆ This reflex may be absent in patients with upper or lower motor neuron disease.

Plantar reflex

◆ Using an applicator stick, a pen, a tongue blade, or a key, slowly stroke the lateral side of the patient's sole, from the heel to the great toe and across the ball of the foot, forming an upside-down "J."

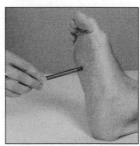

◆ The normal response is plantar flexion of the toes. In an elderly patient, this normal response may be diminished because of arthritic deformities of the toe or foot.

(Text continues on page 32.)

Assessing the cranial nerves

Assessment of the cranial nerves (CNs) provides valuable information about the condition of the central nervous system, particularly the brain stem. Because a disorder can affect any cranial nerve, knowing how to test each nerve is important. The techniques vary according to the nerve being tested.

CRANIAL NERVE AND ASSESSMENT TECHNIQUE	NORMAL FINDINGS
Olfactory (CN I)	
Check the patency of the patient's nostrils, and ask him to close both eyes. Occlude one nostril, and hold a familiar, pungent substance—such as coffee, tobacco, soap, or peppermint—under the patient's nose. Ask him to identify the substance. Repeat this technique with the other nostril.	The patient should be able to detect the smell and identify it correctly. If he says that he detects the smell but can't name it, offer a choice, such as, "Do you smell lemon, coffee, or peppermint?"
Optic (CN II)	
To assess the optic nerve, check visual acuity, visual fields, and the retinal structures.	Visual field intact.
Oculomotor (CN III), trochlear (CN IV), and abducens (CN VI)	
To assess the oculomotor nerve, check pupil size, pupil shape, and pupillary response to light.	The pupils should be equal, round, and reactive to light. When assessing pupil size, look for trends. For example, watch for a gradual increase in the size of one pupil or the appearance of unequal pupils in a patient whose pupils previously were equal.
To test the coordinated function of these three nerves, assess them simultaneously by evaluating the patient's extraocular eye movement.	The eyes should move smoothly and in a coordinated manner through all six directions of eye movement. Observe each eye for rapid oscillation (nystagmus), movement not in unison with that of the other eye, or inability to move in certain directions (ophthalmoplegia). Also note any mention of double vision (diplopia).

(continued)

Assessing the cranial nerves (continued)

CRANIAL NERVE AND ASSESSMENT TECHNIQUE	NORMAL FINDINGS

Trigeminal (CN V)

To assess the sensory portion of the trigeminal nerve, gently touch the right and then the left side of the patient's forehead with a cotton ball while his eyes are closed. Instruct him to indicate when the cotton touches the area. Compare right and then the left cheek and on the right and then the left jaw. Next, repeat the entire procedure using a sharp object. The cap of a disposable ballpoint pen can be used to test light touch (dull end) and sharp stimuli (sharp end). If you detect an abnormality, also test for temperature sensation by touching the patient's skin with test tubes filled with hot and cold water and asking him to differentiate between them.

A patient with a normal trigeminal nerve should report feeling both light touch and sharp stimuli in all three areas (forehead, cheek, and jaw) on both sides of his face.

To assess the motor portion of the trigeminal nerve, ask the patient to clench his jaws. Palpate the temporal and masseter muscles bilaterally, checking for symmetry. Try to open the patient's clenched jaws. Next, watch for symmetry as the patient opens and closes his mouth.

The jaws should clench symmetrically and remain closed against resistance.

Assess the corneal reflex.

The lids of both eyes should close when a wisp of cotton is lightly stroked across a cornea.

Facial (CN VII)

To test the motor portion of the facial nerve, ask the patient to wrinkle his forehead, raise and lower his eyebrows, smile to show his teeth, and puff out his cheeks. Also, with the patient's eyes closed tightly, attempt to open the eyelids. With each of these movements, observe closely for symmetry.

Normal facial movements and strength are symmetrical.

To test the sensory portion of the facial nerve, which supplies taste sensation to the anterior two-thirds of the tongue, first prepare four marked, closed containers: one containing salt; another, sugar; a third, vinegar (or lemon); and a fourth, quinine (or bitters). Then, with the patient's eyes closed, place salt on the anterior two-thirds of his tongue using a cotton-tipped applicator or dropper. Ask him to identify the

Normal taste sensations are symmetrical.

Assessing the cranial nerves (continued)

CRANIAL NERVE AND ASSESSMENT TECHNIQUE	NORMAL FINDINGS

Facial (CN VII) (continued)

taste as sweet, salty, sour, or bitter. Rinse the patient's mouth with water. Repeat this procedure, alternating flavors and sides of the tongue until all four flavors have been tested on both sides. The glossopharyngeal nerve (CN IX) supplies taste sensations to the posterior one-third of the tongue; these are usually tested at the same time.

Acoustic (CN VIII)

To assess the acoustic portion of this nerve, test the patient's hearing acuity.

The patient should be able to hear a whispered voice or the ticking of a watch.

Romberg's test is one way to test the vestibular nerve. Observing for nystagmus during extraocular movements is another test of the vestibular nerve.

The patient should display normal eye movement and balance, with no dizziness or vertigo.

Glossopharyngeal (CN IX) and vagus (CN X)

To assess these nerves, which have overlapping functions, first listen to the patient's voice for indications of a hoarse or nasal quality. Then watch the patient's soft palate when he says "ah." Next, test the gag reflex after warning the patient. To evoke this reflex, rough the posterior wall of the pharynx with a cotton-tipped applicator or tongue blade.

The patient's voice should sound strong and clear. The soft palate and uvula should rise when he says "ah," and the uvula should remain midline. The palatine arches should remain symmetrical during movement and at rest. The gag reflex should be intact. If it appears decreased or if the pharynx moves asymmetrically, evaluate each side of the posterior wall of the pharynx to confirm the integrity of both cranial nerves.

Spinal accessory (CN XI)

To assess this nerve, press down on the patient's shoulders as he attempts to shrug against this resistance. Note shoulder strength and symmetry while inspecting and palpating his trapezius muscle. Then apply resistance to his turned head while he attempts to return it to a midline position. Note neck strength while inspecting and palpating the sternocleidomastoid muscle. Repeat for the opposite side.

Normally, both shoulders should overcome resistance equally well. The neck should overcome resistance in both directions.

(continued)

Assessing the cranial nerves *(continued)*

CRANIAL NERVE AND ASSESSMENT TECHNIQUE	NORMAL FINDINGS
Hypoglossal (CN XII)	
To assess this nerve, observe the patient's protruded tongue for deviation from midline, atrophy, or fasciculations (very fine muscle flickerings indicative of lower motor neuron disease). Next, ask him to move his tongue rapidly from side to side with his mouth open, then to curl his tongue up toward his nose, and then down toward his chin. Then use a tongue blade to apply resistance to his protruded tongue, and ask him to try to push it to one side. Repeat on the other side, and note tongue strength. Listen to the patient's speech for the sounds d, l, n, and t. If general speech suggests a problem, ask the patient to repeat a phrase or series of words containing these sounds.	Normally, the tongue should be midline and the patient should be able to move it right to left equally as well as up and down. The pressure that the tongue exerts on the tongue blade should be equal on both sides. Speech should be clear.

◆ In patients with disorders of the pyramidal tract (such as stroke), Babinski's reflex, an abnormal response, is elicited. The patient responds to the stimulus with dorsiflexion of his great toe. You may also see a more pronounced response in which the other toes extend and abduct. In some cases, you may even see dorsiflexion of the ankle, knee, and hip.

Primitive reflexes
Although normal in infants, primitive reflexes are pathologic in adults.

Snout reflex
◆ Tap lightly on the patient's upper lip.
◆ Lip pursing indicates frontal lobe damage. Cerebral degenerative disease may be the cause.

Sucking reflex
◆ If the patient begins sucking while you're feeding him or suctioning his mouth, you've elicited the sucking reflex.
◆ This reflex indicates cortical damage characteristic of advanced dementia.

Grasp reflex
◆ Apply gentle pressure to the patient's palm with your fingers.
◆ If the patient grasps your fingers between his thumb and index finger, he may have cortical (premotor cortex) damage. This is the last of the reflexes to appear.

Glabellar reflex
◆ Repeatedly tap the bridge of the patient's nose.
◆ A persistent blinking response indicates diffuse cortical dysfunction.

Comparing decerebrate and decorticate postures

Decerebrate posture results from damage to the upper brain stem. In this posture, the arms are adducted and extended, with the wrists pronated and the fingers flexed. The teeth are clenched. The legs are stiffly extended, with plantar flexion of the feet.

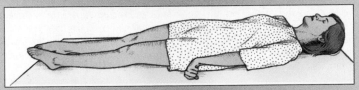

Decorticate posture results from damage to one or both corticospinal tracts. In this posture, the arms are adducted and flexed, with the wrists and fingers flexed on the chest. The legs are stiffly extended and rotated internally, with plantar flexion of the feet.

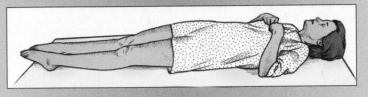

Using the Glasgow Coma Scale

The Glasgow Coma Scale provides an objective way to evaluate a patient's LOC and to detect changes from the baseline. To use this scale, evaluate and score your patient's best eye-opening response, verbal response, and motor response. A total score of 15 indicates that he's alert; is oriented to time, place, and person; and can follow simple commands. A comatose patient will score 7 points or less. A score of 3 indicates a deep coma and a poor prognosis.

Eye-opening response
◆ Open spontaneously (Score: 4)
◆ Open to verbal command (Score: 3)
◆ Open to pain (Score: 2)
◆ No response (Score: 1)

Verbal response
◆ Oriented and converses (Score: 5)
◆ Disoriented and converses (Score: 4)
◆ Uses inappropriate words (Score: 3)
◆ Makes incomprehensible sounds (Score: 2)
◆ No response (Score: 1)

Motor response
◆ Obeys verbal command (Score: 6)
◆ Localizes painful stimulus (Score: 5)
◆ Flexion, withdrawal (Score: 4)
◆ Flexion, abnormal—decorticate rigidity (Score: 3)
◆ Extension—decerebrate rigidity (Score: 2)
◆ No response (Score: 1)

Assessing the GI system

Initial questions

◆ Explore signs and symptoms, such as appetite and weight changes, dysphagia, nausea, vomiting, heartburn, stomach or abdominal pain, frequent belching or flatulence, hematemesis, and jaundice. Has the patient had ulcers?

◆ Determine whether the patient frequently uses laxatives. Ask about hemorrhoids, rectal bleeding, character of stools (color, odor, and consistency), and changes in bowel habits. Does he have a history of diarrhea, constipation, irritable bowel syndrome, Crohn's disease, colitis, diverticulitis, or cancer?

◆ Ask whether he has had hernias, gallbladder disease, or liver disease, such as hepatitis or cirrhosis.

◆ Find out whether he has had abdominal swelling or ascites.

◆ If the patient is older than age 50, ask about the date and results of his last Hemoccult test, fecal immunochemical test, or colonoscopy.

Inspecting the abdomen

◆ Place the patient in the supine position, with his arms at his sides and his head on a pillow to help relax the abdominal muscles.

◆ Mentally divide the abdomen into quadrants or regions. Systematically inspect all areas, if time and the patient's condition permit, concluding with the symptomatic area.

◆ Examine the patient's entire abdomen, observing the overall contour, color, and skin integrity. Look for rashes, scars, or incisions from past surgeries. Observe the umbilicus for protrusions or discoloration.

◆ Note visible abdominal asymmetry, masses, pulsations, or peristalsis. You can detect masses—especially hepatic and splenic masses—more easily by inspecting the areas while the patient takes a deep breath and holds it. This action forces the diaphragm downward, increasing intra-abdominal pressure and reducing the size of the abdominal cavity.

◆ Finally, examine the rectal area for redness, irritation, or hemorrhoids.

◆ **ALERT** If the patient is pregnant, vary the position used for assessment depending on the stage of pregnancy. For example, if the patient is in her final weeks, avoid the supine position because it may impair respiratory excursion and blood flow. To enhance comfort, have the patient lie on her side or assume semi-Fowler's position. Also, during the assessment, remember the normal variations associated with pregnancy: increased pigmentation of the abdominal midline, purplish striae, and upward displacement of the abdominal organs and umbilicus.

Auscultating bowel sounds

Bowel sounds result from the movement of air and fluid through the bowel. Auscultation detects sounds that provide information about bowel motility and the condition of the abdominal vessels and organs. To auscultate bowel sounds, follow these steps.

◆ Press the diaphragm of the stethoscope against the abdomen, and listen carefully. Auscultate the four quadrants systematically.

◆ The movement of air and fluid through the bowel by peristalsis normally creates soft, bubbling sounds with no regular pattern, commonly with soft clicks and gurgles interspersed. Loud, rapid, high-pitched, gurgling bowel sounds are hyperactive and may occur normally in a hungry patient. Sounds occurring at a rate of one every minute or longer are hypoactive and normally occur after bowel surgery or after the colon has filled with feces.

◆ When describing bowel sounds, be specific. For example, indicate whether sounds are quiet or loud gurgles, occasional gurgles, fine tinkles, or loud tinkles.

◆ In some cases, you may need to auscultate for a full 5 minutes before you hear sounds. Be sure to allow enough time in each quadrant before deciding that bowel sounds are absent.

◆ Before you report absent bowel sounds, make sure that the patient's bladder is empty. A full bladder may obscure the sounds. Gently pressing on the abdominal surface may initiate peristalsis and audible bowel sounds, as will having the patient eat or drink something.

◆ Next, lightly apply the bell of the stethoscope to each quadrant to auscultate for vascular sounds, such as bruits and venous hums, and for friction rubs. Normally, you shouldn't hear vascular sounds.

Percussing the abdomen

Abdominal percussion helps to determine the size and location of abdominal organs and helps you identify areas of tenderness, gaseous distention, ascites, or solid masses.

Percussion sounds vary depending on the density of underlying structures; usually, you'll detect dull notes over solids and tympanic notes over air. The predominant abdominal percussion sound is tympany, which is created by percussion over an air-filled stomach or intestine. Dull sounds normally occur over the liver and spleen, a lower intestine filled with feces, and a bladder filled with urine. Distinguishing ab-

dominal percussion notes may be difficult in obese patients.

To percuss the abdomen, use this technique.

◆ Percuss in all four quadrants, moving clockwise to the percussion sites in each quadrant, as shown below. When tapping, move your right finger away quickly to avoid inhibiting vibrations. Keep appropriate organ locations in mind as you progress.

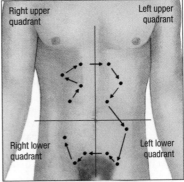

◆ If the patient has pain in a particular quadrant, adjust the percussion sequence to percuss that quadrant last.

◆ When assessing a tender abdomen, have the patient cough; then lightly percuss the area where the cough produced the pain to localize the involved area. As you percuss, note areas of dullness, tympany, and flatness as well as patient complaints of tenderness.

◆ **ALERT** Abdominal percussion or palpation is contraindicated in patients with abdominal organ transplants or suspected abdominal aortic aneurysm. Perform these assessments cautiously in patients with suspected appendicitis.

Palpating the abdomen

Abdominal palpation provides useful clues about the character of the abdominal wall; the size, condition, and consistency of the abdominal organs;

the presence and nature of abdominal masses; and the presence, degree, and location of abdominal pain.

Use light palpation to detect tenderness, areas of muscle spasm or rigidity, and superficial masses in the abdominal wall. If time permits, perform deep abdominal palpation to detect deep tenderness or masses and to evaluate organ size. For a rapid assessment, palpate primarily to detect areas of pain and tenderness, guarding, rebound tenderness, and costovertebral angle tenderness.

An abdominal mass in a child may be a nephroblastoma, commonly known as *Wilms' tumor.* Don't palpate it, to avoid spreading tumor cells.

Light palpation

◆ Have the patient raise his head and shoulders to tighten the abdominal muscles. Tension obscures a deep mass, but a wall mass remains palpable.
◆ Palpate using the finger pads or palmar surface of three to four fingers. Depress $1/2''$ to $1''$ (1 to 2.5 cm) using circular motions. This technique may also help you to determine whether pain originates from the abdominal muscles or from deeper structures.
◆ As the patient exhales, palpate the abdominal rectus muscles. Normally, they soften and relax on exhalation. Note abnormal muscle tension or inflexibility. If you detect tenderness, check for involuntary guarding or abdominal rigidity. In generalized peritonitis, rigidity is severe and diffuse, commonly described as a "boardlike" abdomen. Involuntary guarding points to peritoneal irritation.
◆ If the patient's abdomen is rigid, don't palpate it. Palpation could rupture an inflamed organ if the patient has peritoneal irritation.

◆ A tense or ticklish patient may exhibit voluntary guarding. Help him to relax with deep breathing. He should inhale through his nose and exhale through his mouth.
◆ If a patient has abdominal pain, check for rebound tenderness. Because this maneuver can be painful, perform it near the end of the abdominal assessment. Press your fingertips into the site where the patient reports pain or tenderness. As you quickly release the pressure, the abdominal tissue will rebound. If the patient reports pain as the tissue springs back, you've elicited rebound tenderness.

Deep palpation

◆ Press $1''$ to $3''$ (2.5 to 7.5 cm), assessing for tenderness and masses.
◆ If you feel a mass, note its size, shape, consistency, and location.
◆ If the patient has pain or tenderness, note whether the location is generalized or localized.
◆ Note guarding that the patient exhibits during deep palpation. You may feel tensing of a small or large area of abdominal musculature directly below your fingers.

Eliciting abdominal pain

Rebound tenderness and the psoas and obturator signs can indicate conditions consistent with an acute abdomen. These include appendicitis, cholecystitis, acute pancreatitis, diverticulitis, pelvic inflammatory disease, ruptured cyst, ruptured ectopic pregnancy, and peritoneal injury.

Rebound tenderness

◆ Place the patient in the supine position with the knees flexed to relax the abdominal muscles.

◆ Place your hands gently on the right lower quadrant at McBurney's point, located about midway between the umbilicus and the anterior superior iliac spine.

◆ Slowly and deeply dip your fingers into the area.

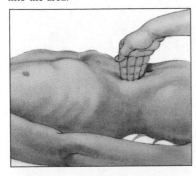

◆ Now release the pressure quickly in a smooth motion. Pain on release—rebound tenderness—is a positive sign. The pain may radiate to the umbilicus.

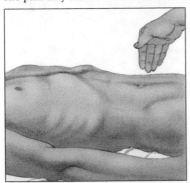

◆ **ALERT** Don't repeat this maneuver, to minimize the risk of rupturing an inflamed appendix.

Psoas sign

◆ Place the patient in the supine position with the legs straight.

◆ Instruct the patient to raise his right leg upward as you exert slight down-

ward pressure with your hand. Repeat the maneuver with the left leg.

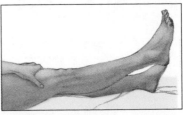

◆ Increased abdominal pain with testing on either leg is a positive result, indicating irritation of the psoas muscle.

Obturator sign

◆ Place the patient in the supine position with the right leg flexed 90 degrees at the hip and knee.

◆ Hold the leg just above the knee and at the ankle; then rotate the leg laterally and medially, as shown below.

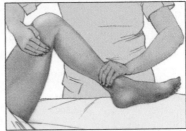

◆ Increased pain is a positive sign, indicating irritation of the obturator muscle.

Percussing, palpating, and hooking the liver

You can estimate the size and position of the liver through percussion and palpation. If liver palpation is unsuccessful, try hooking the liver.

Liver percussion

◆ Begin by percussing the abdomen along the right midclavicular line, starting below the level of the umbilicus.

◆ Move upward until the percussion notes change from tympany to dullness, usually at or slightly below the costal margin. Mark the point of change with a felt-tip pen.

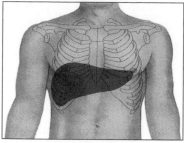

◆ Percuss along the right midclavicular line, starting above the nipple.
◆ Move downward until the percussion notes change from normal lung resonance to dullness, usually at the fifth to seventh intercostal space (as shown below). Again, mark the point of change with a felt-tip pen.

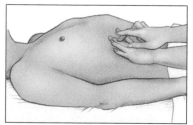

◆ Estimate the size of the liver by measuring the distance between the two marks.

Liver palpation

◆ Place one hand on the patient's back at the approximate height of the liver.
◆ Place your other hand below your mark of liver fullness on the right lateral abdomen.
◆ Point your fingers toward the right costal margin, and press gently in and up as the patient inhales deeply. This maneuver may bring the liver edge down to a palpable position.

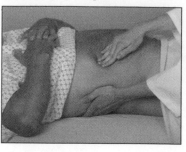

Liver hooking

◆ Stand on the patient's right side, below the area of liver dullness.
◆ As the patient inhales deeply, press your fingers inward and upward, attempting to feel the liver with the fingertips of both hands, as shown below.

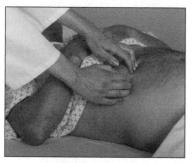

Palpating for indirect inguinal hernia

To check for an indirect inguinal hernia, examine the patient while he stands, using these steps. Then examine him in a supine position.
◆ Place your gloved index finger on the neck of his scrotum, and gently push upward into the inguinal canal, as shown on the next page.
◆ If you meet resistance or if the patient complains of pain, stop the examination.

◆ When you've inserted your finger as far as possible, ask him to bear down and cough. A hernia will feel like a mass of tissue that withdraws when met by the finger.

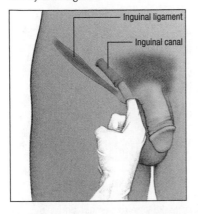

Inguinal ligament

Inguinal canal

Assessing the urinary system

Initial questions

◆ Ask about urine color, oliguria, and nocturia. Does your patient experience incontinence, dysuria, frequency, urgency, or difficulty with the urinary stream (such as reduced flow or dribbling)?
◆ Ask about pyuria, urine retention, and passage of calculi.
◆ Ask the patient whether he has a history of bladder, kidney, or urinary tract infections.
◆ If your patient is a child, ask his parents whether they've had problems with his toilet training or bed-wetting.

Evaluating urine color

For important clues about your patient's health, ask about changes in urine color. Such changes can result from fluid intake, medications, and dietary factors as well as from various disorders.

APPEARANCE	INDICATION
Amber or straw color	Normal
Cloudy	Infection, inflammation, glomerulonephritis, vegetarian diet
Colorless or pale straw color (dilute urine)	Excess fluid intake, anxiety, chronic renal disease, diabetes insipidus, diuretic therapy
Dark brown or black	Acute glomerulonephritis, drugs (such as nitrofurantoin, chlorpromazine, and antimalarials)
Dark yellow or amber (concentrated urine)	Low fluid intake, acute febrile disease, vomiting or diarrhea causing fluid loss
Green-brown	Bile duct obstruction
Orange-red to orange-brown	Urobilinuria, drugs (such as phenazopyridine and rifampin), obstructive jaundice (tea-colored urine)
Red or red-brown	Porphyria, hemorrhage, drugs (such as doxorubicin)

Inspecting
the urethral meatus

Put on gloves before examining the urethral meatus.

Male patients
◆ Have the patient lie in the supine position and drape him, exposing only his penis.
◆ Compress the tip of the glans to open the urethral meatus, which should be located in the center of the glans.
◆ Check for swelling, discharge, signs of urethral infection, and ulcerations, which can signal a sexually transmitted disease (STD).

Female patients
◆ Help the patient into the dorsal lithotomy position and drape her, exposing only the area to be assessed.
◆ Spread the labia and look for the urethral meatus. It should be a pink, irregular, slitlike opening located at the midline, just above the vagina.
◆ Check for swelling, discharge, signs of urethral infection, cystocele, and ulcerations, which may signal an STD.

Percussing
the urinary organs

Percuss the kidneys to elicit pain or tenderness, and percuss the bladder to elicit percussion sounds. Before you start, tell the patient what you're going to do. Otherwise, he may be startled and you could mistake his reaction for a feeling of acute tenderness.

Kidney percussion
◆ With the patient sitting upright, percuss each costovertebral angle (the angle over each kidney whose borders are formed by the lateral and downward curve of the lowest rib and the spinal column).

◆ To perform direct percussion, place your left palm over the costovertebral angle and gently strike it with your right fist, as shown below. Use just enough force to cause a painless but perceptible thud.

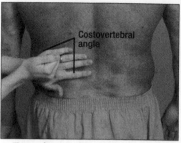

◆ To perform indirect percussion, gently strike your fist over each costovertebral angle.
◆ Make sure to percuss both sides of the body to assess both kidneys.
◆ A patient normally feels a thudding sensation or pressure during percussion. Pain or tenderness suggests a kidney infection.

Bladder percussion
◆ Have the patient urinate.
◆ Ask the patient to lie in the supine position.
◆ Directly percuss the area over the bladder, beginning 2″ (5.1 cm) above the symphysis pubis, as shown below.

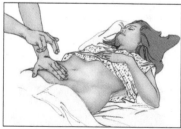

◆ To detect differences in sound, percuss toward the base of the bladder.
◆ Percussion normally produces a tympanic sound. Over a urine-filled bladder, it produces a dull sound.

Palpating the urinary organs

Bimanual palpation of the kidneys and bladder may detect tenderness, lumps, and masses. In the normal adult, the kidneys usually can't be palpated because of their location deep within the abdomen. However, they may be palpable in a thin patient or in a patient with reduced abdominal muscle mass. (The right kidney is slightly lower, so it may be easier to palpate.) Both kidneys descend with deep inhalation.

If palpable, the bladder normally feels firm and relatively smooth. However, an adult's bladder may not be palpable.

Kidney palpation
◆ Help the patient into the supine position, and expose the abdomen from the xiphoid process to the symphysis pubis.
◆ Standing at the patient's right side, place your left hand under the back, midway between the lower costal margin and the iliac crest.
◆ Place your right hand on the patient's abdomen, directly above your left hand. Angle your right hand slightly toward the costal margin.
◆ To palpate the right lower edge of the right kidney, press your right fingertips about 1½" (4 cm) above the right iliac crest at the midinguinal line; press your left fingertips upward into the right costovertebral angle, as shown below.

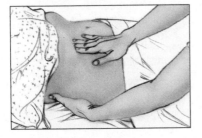

◆ Instruct the patient to inhale deeply so that the lower portion of the right kidney can move down between your hands. If it does, note the shape and size of the kidney. Normally, it feels smooth, solid, and firm, yet elastic.
◆ Ask the patient whether palpation causes tenderness.

◆ **ALERT** Avoid using excessive pressure to palpate the kidney because this may cause intense pain.
◆ To assess the left kidney, move to the patient's left side and position your hands as described earlier, but with this change: Place your right hand 2" (5.1 cm) above the left iliac crest.
◆ Apply pressure with both hands as the patient inhales.
◆ If the left kidney can be palpated, compare it with the right kidney; it should be the same size.

Bladder palpation
◆ Make sure that the patient has voided.
◆ Locate the edge of the bladder by pressing deeply in the midline about 1" to 2" (2.5 to 5 cm) above the symphysis pubis, as shown below.

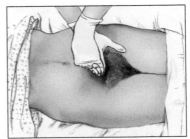

◆ As you palpate the bladder, note its size and location and check for lumps, masses, and tenderness. The bladder normally feels firm and relatively smooth. (Keep in mind that an adult's bladder may not be palpable.)
◆ During deep palpation, the patient may report the urge to urinate—a normal response.

Assessing the male reproductive system

Initial questions

◆ Ask the patient whether he has noticed sores, lumps, or ulcers on his penis. These signs can signal an STD. Ask whether he has experienced penile discharge or bleeding.

◆ Ask if he has scrotal swelling, which can indicate an inguinal hernia, a hematocele, epididymitis, or a testicular tumor.

◆ Ask whether the patient performs testicular self-examinations. Has he had a vasectomy?

◆ Ask about the patient's sexual history, including sexual orientation, type of activity, frequency, number of partners, safer sex practices, and condom use.

◆ Ask about STDs and other infections. Assess the patient's knowledge of how to prevent STDs, including acquired immunodeficiency syndrome.

◆ Find out whether the patient has a history of prostate problems.

◆ Ask whether he's satisfied with his sexual function. Does he have concerns about impotence or sterility? Also inquire about his contraceptive practices.

Inspecting and palpating the male genitalia

Ask the patient to disrobe from the waist down and to cover himself with a drape. Then put on gloves and examine his penis, scrotum, and testicles, inguinal and femoral areas, and prostate gland.

Usually, a physician performs prostate palpation as part of a rectal examination. However, if the patient hasn't scheduled a separate rectal examination, you may palpate the prostate during the reproductive system assessment.

Penis

◆ Observe the penis. Its size will depend on the patient's age and overall development. The penile skin should be slightly wrinkled and pink to light brown in a white patient, and light brown to dark brown in a black patient.

◆ Check the penile shaft and glans for lesions, nodules, inflammation, and swelling. Also check the glans for smegma, a cheesy secretion.

◆ Gently compress the glans, and inspect the urethral meatus for discharge, inflammation, and lesions, specifically genital warts. If you note a discharge, obtain a culture specimen for gonorrhea and chlamydia.

◆ Using your thumb and forefinger, palpate the entire penile shaft. It should be somewhat firm, and the skin should be smooth and movable. Note swelling, nodules, or indurations.

Scrotum and testicles

◆ Have the patient hold his penis away from his scrotum so that you can observe the general size and appearance of the scrotum. The skin will be darker than the rest of the body.

◆ Spread the surface of the scrotum, and examine the skin for swelling, nodules, redness, ulceration, and distended veins. You'll probably see some sebaceous cysts—firm, white to yellow, nontender cutaneous lesions. Also check for pitting edema, a sign of cardiovascular disease.

◆ Spread the pubic hair, and check the skin for lesions and parasites.

◆ Gently palpate both testicles between your thumb and first two fingers. Assess their size, shape, and response to pressure (typically, deep visceral pain). The testicles should be equal in size. They should feel firm, smooth, and rubbery, and they should move freely in the scrotal sac.

◆ If you note hard, irregular areas or lumps, transilluminate the testicle by darkening the room and pressing the head of a flashlight against the scrotum, behind the lump. The testicle will appear as an opaque shadow, as will lumps, masses, warts, or blood-filled areas. Transilluminate the other testicle to compare your findings.

◆ Palpate the epididymis, which is normally located in the posterolateral area of the testicle. It should be smooth, discrete, nontender, and free from swelling or induration.

◆ Palpate each spermatic cord, located above each testicle. Begin palpating at the base of the epididymis, and continue to the inguinal canal. The vas deferens is a smooth, movable cord inside the spermatic cord.

◆ If you feel swelling, irregularity, or nodules, transilluminate the problem area, as described earlier. If serous fluid is present, you'll see a red glow; if tissue and blood are present, you won't see this glow.

Prostate gland

◆ Because palpation of the prostate usually is uncomfortable and may embarrass the patient, begin by explaining the procedure and reassuring the patient that the procedure shouldn't be painful.

◆ Have the patient urinate to empty the bladder and reduce discomfort during the examination.

◆ Ask the patient to stand at the end of the examination table, with his elbows flexed and his upper body resting on the table. If he can't assume this position because he's unable to stand, have him lie on his left side with his right knee and hip flexed or with both knees drawn up toward his chest.

◆ Inspect the skin of the perineal, anal, and posterior scrotal surfaces. The skin should appear smooth and unbroken, with no protruding masses.

◆ Apply water-soluble lubricant to your gloved index finger. Then introduce the finger, pad down, into the patient's rectum. Instruct the patient to relax to ease passage of the finger through the anal sphincter.

◆ Using the pad of your index finger, gently palpate the prostate on the anterior rectal wall, located just past the anorectal ring. The prostate should feel smooth and rubbery. Normal size varies but usually is about that of a walnut. The prostate shouldn't protrude into the rectum lumen.

◆ Identify the median sulcus, which normally can be felt between the two lateral lobes.

Assessing the female reproductive system

Initial questions

◆ Ask your patient about her menstrual cycle. Ask how old she was when she began to menstruate. Ask how long her menses usually last, the date of her last menses, and whether she usually has cramps, spotting, or an unusually light or heavy flow. Ask if she has a history of menorrhagia, metrorrhagia, or amenorrhea. If she's postmenopausal, find out the date of menopause.

◆ Ask about her sexual practices, number of partners she currently has, whether she experiences pain during intercourse, if she's ever had an STD, and her human immunodeficiency virus status.

◆ Ask about her obstetric history, including the total number of pregnancies (G), number of births (P), number of premature births, number of abortions, and number of living children. Has she had problems with fertility?

◆ Ask the patient if she has experienced sexual assault or abuse.

◆ Inquire about the patient's birth control method, if any. Talk about the importance of safer sex and STD prevention.

◆ Determine the dates of her last gynecologic examination and Papanicolaou (Pap) test and what the result was.

◆ Ask the patient if she has questions or concerns.

Palpating the breasts and axillae

Before starting the breast examination, provide privacy and have the patient put on a gown. Ask the patient if she's had a mammogram, a biopsy, or breast surgery. If the patient has had breast cancer, fibroadenoma, or fibrocystic disease, ask for more information. Also ask about lumps, pain, breast changes, and discharge. Then follow these steps.

◆ Have the patient sit with her arms at her sides. Note breast size and symmetry. Closely inspect the skin. Breast skin should be smooth, without dimples, and the same color as the rest of the skin. Inspect the nipples, noting their size and shape.

◆ Inspect the breasts with the patient's arms over her head and then when she's leaning forward with her hands pressed into her hips. Visually note any abnormalities.

◆ Palpate each breast using the pads of your fingers. Use a specific pattern, such as spiraling outward, a circular motion, or moving vertically across the breast. Include the tail of Spence and axilla.

◆ Examine the breast with the patient supine. Place a pillow under the side you're examining, and have the patient raise her arm above her head and place her hand behind her head. Proceed to palpate each breast as described earlier.

◆ Note the consistency of the breast tissue. Check for nodules or unusual tenderness. Nodularity may increase before menstruation, and tenderness may result from premenstrual fullness, cysts, or cancer. A lump or mass that feels different from the rest of the breast may represent a pathologic change.

◆ Palpate the areola and nipple, and gently compress the nipple between your thumb and index finger to detect discharge. If you see discharge, note the color, consistency, and quantity.

◆ With the patient seated, palpate the axillae. Palpate the right axilla with the middle three fingers of one hand while supporting the patient's arm with your other hand. You can usually palpate one or more soft, small, nontender central nodes.

◆ If the central nodes feel large or hard or are tender, or if the patient has a suspicious-looking lesion, palpate the other groups of lymph nodes.

Inspecting the female genitalia

Before you begin the examination, ask the patient to urinate. Next, help her into the dorsal lithotomy position and drape her. After putting on gloves, examine the patient's external genitalia. If you're in advanced practice, examine the internal genitalia, as appropriate.

Inspecting the external genitalia

◆ Observe the skin and hair distribution of the mons pubis. Spread the hair with your fingers to check for lesions and parasites.

◆ Spread the labia and locate the urethral meatus. It should be a pink, irregular, slitlike opening at the midline, just above the vagina. Note the presence of discharge (a sign of urethral infection) or ulceration (a sign of an STD).

◆ Examine the vestibule, especially around the area of Bartholin's and Skene's glands and ducts, for swelling, erythema, enlargement, or discharge. If you detect any of these conditions, notify the practitioner and obtain a specimen for culture.

◆ Using your index finger and thumb, gently spread the labia majora and minora. They should be moist and free from lesions. You may detect a normal discharge that varies from clear and stretchy before ovulation to white and opaque after ovulation.

Inspecting the internal genitalia

◆ Select a speculum that's appropriate for the patient. In most cases, you'll use a Graves' speculum. However, if the patient is a virgin or nulliparous or has a contracted introitus as a result of menopause, you should use a Pedersen speculum.

◆ Hold the blades of the speculum under warm running water. This warms the blades and helps to lubricate them, making insertion easier and more comfortable for the patient. Don't use commercial lubricants—they're bacteriostatic and will distort cells on Pap tests.

◆ Sit or stand at the foot of the examination table. Tell the patient that she'll feel some pressure.

◆ Separate the labia with the fingers, and gently pull down on the posterior aspect to open the introitus.

◆ Place the index and middle fingers of your nondominant hand about 1" (2.5 cm) into the vagina and spread the fingers.

◆ Hold the speculum in your dominant hand, and insert the blades between your fingers.

◆ Point the speculum slightly downward, and insert the blades until the base of the speculum touches your fingers, inside the vagina.

◆ Rotate the speculum in the same plane as the vagina, and withdraw your fingers.

◆ Open the blades as far as possible and lock the blades.

◆ While inserting and withdrawing the speculum, note the color, texture, and mucosal integrity of the vagina and vaginal secretions. A thin, white, odorless discharge is normal.

◆ With the speculum in place, examine the cervix for color, position, size, shape, mucosal integrity, and discharge. The cervix should be smooth, round, rosy pink, and free from ulcerations and nodules. A clear, watery discharge is normal during ovulation; a slightly bloody discharge is normal just before menstruation. Obtain a culture specimen of any other discharge.

◆ After you inspect the cervix, obtain a specimen for a Pap test.

◆ When you've completed your examination, unlock the speculum blades and close them slowly while you begin to withdraw the instrument. Close the blades completely before they reach the introitus, and withdraw the speculum from the vagina.

Palpating the uterus

To palpate the uterus bimanually, follow these steps.

◆ Insert the index and middle fingers of one gloved hand into the patient's vagina, and place your other hand on the abdomen between the umbilicus and symphysis pubis.

◆ Press the abdomen in and down while you elevate the cervix and uterus with your two fingers, as shown below.

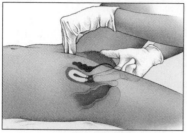

◆ Try to grasp the uterus between your hands. Note cervical motion tenderness. Palpate over the right and left ovaries. These will be small and almond-shaped.
◆ Slide your fingers farther into the anterior fornix, and palpate the body of the uterus between your hands. Note its size, shape, surface characteristics, consistency, and mobility.
◆ Note tenderness of the uterine body and fundus. Also note fundal position.

Assessing the musculoskeletal system

Initial questions

◆ Ask whether the patient has muscle pain, joint pain, swelling, tenderness, or difficulty with balance or gait. Does he have joint stiffness? If so, find out when it occurs and how long it lasts.
◆ Ask whether the patient has noticed noise with joint movement.
◆ Find out whether he has arthritis or gout.
◆ Ask about a history of fractures, injuries, back problems, or deformities. Also ask about weakness and paralysis.
◆ Explore limitations on walking, running, or participation in sports. Do muscle or joint problems interfere with activities of daily living?
◆ If the patient is an infant or a toddler, ask the parents whether the child has achieved developmental milestones, such as crawling and walking.

Assessing range of motion

After assessing the patient's posture, gait, and stance, test joint function by assessing joint range of motion (ROM). Ask the patient to move specific joints through the normal ROM. If he can't do so, move the joints through passive ROM.

The following pages show each joint and illustrate the tests for ROM, including the expected degree of motion for each joint.

Shoulders

◆ To assess forward flexion and backward extension, have the patient bring his straightened arm forward and up and then behind him.

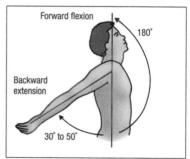

Forward flexion
180°
Backward extension
30° to 50°

◆ Assess abduction and adduction by asking the patient to bring his straightened arm to the side and up and then in front of him.

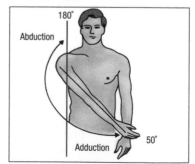

180°
Abduction
Adduction
50°

◆ To assess external and internal rotation, have the patient abduct his arm with his elbow bent. Then ask him to place his hand first behind his head and then behind the small of his back.

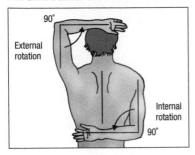

Elbows
◆ Assess flexion by having the patient bend his arm and attempt to touch his shoulder.
◆ Assess extension by having him straighten his arm.

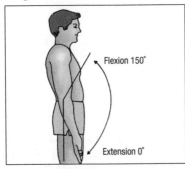

◆ To assess pronation and supination, hold the patient's elbow in a flexed position, and ask him to rotate his arm until his palm faces the floor. Then rotate his hand back until his palm faces upward.

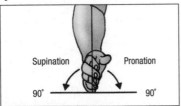

Wrists
◆ To assess flexion, ask the patient to bend his wrist downward; assess extension by having him straighten his wrist.
◆ To assess hyperextension, ask him to bend his wrist upward.

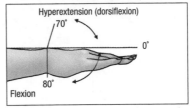

◆ Assess radial and ulnar deviation by asking the patient to move his hand first toward the radial side and then toward the ulnar side.

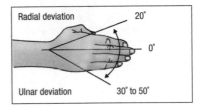

Fingers
◆ To assess abduction and adduction, have the patient first spread his fingers and then bring them together. In abduction, there should be 20 degrees between the fingers; in adduction, the fingers should touch.

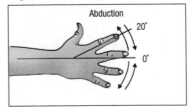

◆ To assess extension and flexion, ask the patient first to straighten his fingers and then to make a fist with his thumb remaining straight.

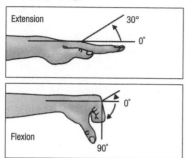

Thumbs

◆ Assess extension by having the patient straighten his thumb.
◆ To assess flexion, have the patient bend his thumb at the top joint and then at the bottom.

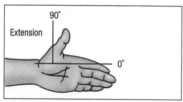

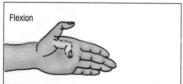

◆ Assess adduction by having the patient extend his hand, bringing his thumb first to the index finger and then to the little finger.

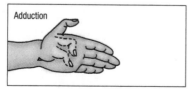

Hips

◆ Assess flexion by asking the patient to bend his knee to his chest while keeping his back straight. If he has undergone total hip replacement, don't ask him to perform this movement because doing so can dislocate the prosthesis.

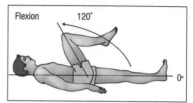

◆ Assess extension by having the patient straighten his knee.
◆ To assess hyperextension, ask the patient to extend his leg straight back. This motion can be performed with the patient in the prone or standing position.

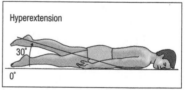

◆ To assess abduction, have the patient move his straightened leg away from the midline.
◆ To assess adduction, instruct the patient to move his straightened leg from the midline toward the opposite leg.

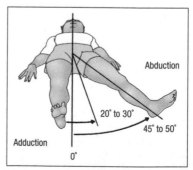

◆ To assess internal and external rotation, ask the patient to bend his knee and turn his leg inward. Then have him turn his leg outward.

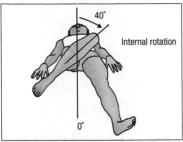

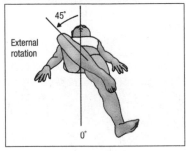

Knees
◆ Ask the patient to straighten his leg at the knee to show extension.
◆ Ask him to bend his knee and bring his foot up to touch his buttock to show flexion.

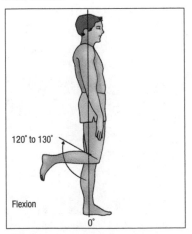

Toes
◆ Assess extension and flexion by asking the patient to straighten and then curl his toes.
◆ Check hyperextension by asking him to straighten his toes and point them upward.

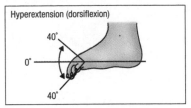

Ankles and feet
◆ Have the patient show plantar flexion by bending his foot downward.
◆ Have the patient show hyperextension by bending his foot upward.

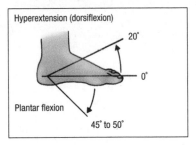

◆ To assess eversion and inversion, ask the patient to point his toes. Have him turn his foot inward and then outward.

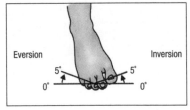

◆ To assess forefoot adduction and abduction, stabilize the patient's heel while he turns his foot first inward and then outward.

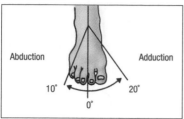

Testing muscle strength

Assess motor function by testing the patient's muscle strength. Before you begin these tests, find out whether the patient is right- or left-handed. The dominant arm is usually stronger. Have the patient attempt normal ROM movements against your resistance. Note the strength that the patient exerts. If the muscle group is weak, lessen your resistance to permit an accurate assessment. If necessary, position the patient so that his limb doesn't have to resist gravity, and repeat the test.

To minimize subjective interpretations of the test findings, rate muscle strength on a scale of 0 to 5, as follows:

0 = No visible or palpable contraction felt; paralysis
1 = Slight palpable contraction felt
2 = Passive ROM maneuvers when gravity is removed
3 = Active ROM against gravity
4 = Active ROM against gravity and light resistance
5 = Active ROM against full resistance; normal strength.

Deltoid
◆ With your patient's arm fully extended, place one hand over his deltoid muscle and the other hand on his wrist.

◆ Have the patient abduct his arm to a horizontal position against your resistance; as he does, palpate for deltoid contraction.

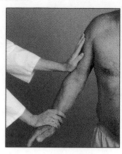

Biceps
◆ With your hand on the flexor surface of the patient's forearm, have him flex against your resistance, as shown below.

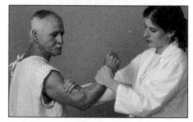

◆ Observe for biceps contraction.

Triceps
◆ Have the patient abduct and hold his arm midway between flexion and extension.
◆ Hold and support his arm at the wrist, and ask him to extend it against your resistance, as shown below.

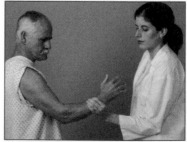

◆ Observe for triceps contraction.

Dorsal interosseous

◆ Have the patient extend and spread his fingers and then resist your attempt to squeeze them together.

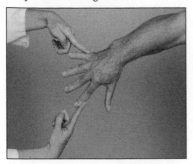

Forearm and hand (grip)

◆ Have the patient grasp your middle and index fingers and squeeze them as hard as he can.

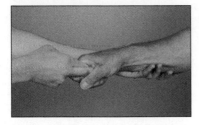

Psoas

◆ Support the patient's leg, and have him raise his knee and flex his hip against your resistance, as shown below.

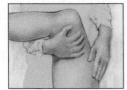

◆ Observe for psoas contraction.

Quadriceps

◆ Have the patient bend his knee slightly while you support his lower leg.

◆ Ask him to extend his knee against your resistance; as he's doing so, palpate for quadriceps contraction.

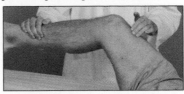

Gastrocnemius

◆ With the patient in the prone position, support his foot and ask him to plantarflex his ankle against your resistance, as shown below.

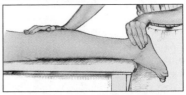

◆ Palpate for gastrocnemius contraction.

Anterior tibialis

◆ With the patient sitting on the side of the examination table with his legs dangling, place your hand on his foot.
◆ Ask him to dorsiflex his ankle against your resistance.

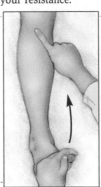

Extensor hallucis longus

◆ With your fingers on the patient's great toe, have him dorsiflex the toe against your resistance, as shown below.

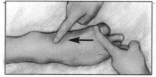

◆ Palpate for extensor hallucis contraction.

Assessing the skin

Initial questions

◆ Determine whether your patient has a known skin disease, such as psoriasis, eczema, or hives.
◆ Ask him to describe changes in skin pigmentation, temperature, moisture, or hair distribution.
◆ Explore skin signs and symptoms, such as itching, rashes, or scaling. Is his skin excessively dry or oily?
◆ Find out if the skin reacts to hot or cold weather. If so, how?
◆ Ask the patient about skin care, sun exposure, use of SPF products and SPF number used, and use of protective clothing.
◆ Ask whether your patient has noticed easy bruising or bleeding, changes in warts or moles, or lumps.
◆ Ask about the presence and location of scars, sores, and ulcers.

Inspecting and palpating the skin

Before you begin your examination, make sure that the lighting is adequate for inspection. Put on a pair of gloves.

To examine the patient's skin, you'll use both inspection and palpation—sometimes simultaneously. During your examination, focus on such skin tissue characteristics as color, texture, turgor, moisture, and temperature. Evaluate skin lesions, edema, hair distribution, and fingernails and toenails.

Color

◆ Begin by systematically inspecting the skin's overall appearance. Remember, skin color reflects the patient's nutritional, hematologic, cardiovascular, and pulmonary status.
◆ Observe the patient's general coloring and pigmentation, keeping in mind racial differences as well as normal variations from one part of the body to another.
◆ Examine all exposed areas of the skin, including the face, ears, back of the neck, axillae, and backs of the hands and arms.
◆ Note the location of bruising, discoloration, or erythema. Look for pallor, jaundice, and cyanosis.

Texture

◆ Inspect and palpate the texture of the skin, noting thickness and mobility. Does the skin feel rough, smooth, thick, fragile, or thin? Changes can indicate local irritation or trauma, or they may be a result of problems in other body systems. For example, rough, dry skin is common in hypothyroidism; soft, smooth skin is common in hyperthyroidism.
◆ To determine if the skin over a joint is supple or taut, have the patient bend the joint as you palpate.

Turgor

◆ Assessing the turgor, or elasticity, of the patient's skin helps you to evaluate

Evaluating skin color variations

COLOR	DISTRIBUTION	POSSIBLE CAUSE
Absent	Small, circumscribed areas	Vitiligo
	Generalized	Albinism
Blue	Around lips (circumoral pallor) or generalized	Cyanosis (*Note:* In black patients, bluish gingivae are normal.)
Deep red	Generalized	Polycythemia vera (increased red blood cell count)
Pink	Local or generalized	Erythema (superficial capillary dilation and congestion)
Tan to brown	Facial patches	Chloasma of pregnancy or butterfly rash of lupus erythematosus
Tan to brown-bronze	Generalized (not related to sun exposure)	Addison's disease
Yellow	Sclera or generalized	Jaundice from liver dysfunction (*Note:* In black patients, yellow-brown pigmentation of the sclera is normal.)
Yellow-orange	Palms, soles, and face; not sclera	Carotenemia (carotene in the blood)

hydration. To assess turgor, gently squeeze the skin on the forearm.
◆ If the skin quickly returns to its original shape, the patient has normal turgor. If it resumes its original shape slowly or maintains a tented shape, the skin has poor turgor.
◆ Decreased turgor occurs with dehydration as well as with aging. Increased turgor is associated with progressive systemic sclerosis.
◆ To accurately assess skin turgor in an elderly patient, try squeezing the skin of the sternum or forehead instead of the forearm. In an elderly patient, the skin of the forearm tends to be paper-thin, dry, and wrinkled, so it doesn't accurately represent the patient's hydration status.

Moisture
◆ Observe the skin for excessive dryness or moisture. If the patient's skin is too dry, you may see reddened or flaking areas. Elderly patients commonly have dry, itchy skin. Moisture that appears shiny may result from oiliness.
◆ If the patient is overhydrated, the skin may be edematous and spongy.
◆ Localized edema can occur in response to trauma or skin abnormalities such as ulcers.

◆ If you palpate local edema, document associated discoloration or lesions.

Temperature

◆ Touch the surface of the skin with the back of your hand.

◆ Inflamed skin will feel warm because of increased blood flow.

◆ Cool skin results from vasoconstriction. With hypovolemic shock, for instance, the skin feels cool and clammy.

◆ Make sure to distinguish between generalized and localized warmth or coolness.

◆ Generalized warmth, or hyperthermia, is associated with fever stemming from a systemic infection or viral illness.

◆ Localized warmth occurs with a burn or localized infection.

◆ Generalized coolness occurs with hypothermia.

◆ Localized coolness occurs with arteriosclerosis.

Skin lesions

◆ During your inspection, you may note vascular changes in the form of red, pigmented lesions.

◆ Among the most common lesions are hemangiomas, telangiectases, petechiae, purpura, and ecchymoses. These lesions may indicate disease. For instance, you'll see telangiectases in patients with hepatic cirrhosis.

Assessing dark skin

Be prepared for certain color variations when assessing dark-skinned patients. For example, some dark-skinned patients have a pigmented line, called *Futcher's line*, extending diagonally and symmetrically from the shoulder to the elbow on the lateral edge of the biceps muscle. This line is normal. Also normal are deeply pigmented ridges in the palms.

To detect color variations in dark-skinned and black patients, examine the sclerae, conjunctivae, buccal mucosa, tongue, lips, nail beds, palms, and soles. A yellow-brown color in dark-skinned patients or an ash gray color in black patients indicates pallor, which results from a lack of the underlying pink and red tones normally present in dark skin.

Among dark-skinned black patients, yellowish pigmentation isn't necessarily an indication of jaundice. To detect jaundice in these patients, examine the hard palate and the sclerae.

Look for petechiae by examining areas with lighter pigmentation, such as the abdomen, gluteal areas, and the inner aspect of the forearm. To distinguish petechiae and ecchymoses from erythema in dark-skinned patients, apply pressure to the area. Erythematous areas will blanch, but petechiae or ecchymoses won't, because erythema is commonly associated with increased skin warmth.

When you assess edema in dark-skinned patients, remember that the affected area may have decreased color because fluid expands the distance between the pigmented layers and the external epithelium. When you palpate the affected area, it may feel tight.

Cyanosis can be difficult to identify in both white and black patients. Because certain factors, such as cold, affect the lips and nail beds, make sure to assess the conjunctivae, palms, soles, buccal mucosa, and tongue as well.

To detect rashes in black or dark-skinned patients, palpate the area to identify changes in skin texture.

Assessing the eyes, ears, nose, and throat

Initial questions

Eyes

◆ Ask the patient about vision problems, such as myopia, hyperopia, blurred vision, or double vision. Does he wear corrective lenses?
◆ Find out when he had his last eye examination.
◆ Ask whether he has noticed vision disturbances, such as rainbows around lights, blind spots, or flashing lights.
◆ Ask whether he has excessive tearing, dry eyes, itching, burning, pain, inflammation, swelling, color blindness, or photophobia.
◆ Elicit a history of eye infections, eye trauma, glaucoma, cataracts, detached retina, or other eye disorders.
◆ If the patient is older than age 50 or has a family history of glaucoma, ask about the date and results of his last test for glaucoma.

Ears

◆ Find out whether the patient has hearing problems, such as deafness, poor hearing, tinnitus, or vertigo. Is he abnormally sensitive to noise? Has he noticed recent changes in his hearing?
◆ Ask about ear discharge, pain, or tenderness behind the ears.
◆ Ask about frequent or recent ear infections or ear surgery.
◆ Ask the date and result of his last hearing test.
◆ Ask whether he uses a hearing aid.
◆ Determine his ear-care habits, including the use of cotton-tipped applicators to remove ear wax.

◆ Ask about exposure to loud noise, including the use of protective earplugs or headphones.

Nose

◆ Ask about nasal problems, including allergies, sinusitis, discharge, colds, (more than four times a year), rhinitis, trauma, and frequent sneezing.
◆ Determine whether your patient has a nasal obstruction, breathing problems, or an inability to smell. Has he had nosebleeds? Has he had a change in appetite or the sense of smell? Has he used nasal sprays?
◆ Ask whether he has had surgery on his nose or sinuses. If so, ask when, why, and what type.

Mouth and throat

◆ Investigate whether your patient has sores in the mouth or on the tongue. Does he have a history of oral herpes infection?
◆ Find out whether he has toothaches, bleeding gums, loss of taste, voice changes, dry mouth, or frequent sore throats.
◆ If the patient has frequent sore throats, ask when they occur. Are they associated with fever or difficulty swallowing? How have the sore throats been treated medically?
◆ Ask whether the patient has ever had a problem swallowing. If so, does he have trouble swallowing solids or liquids? Is the problem constant or intermittent? What precipitates the difficulty? What makes it go away?
◆ Determine whether he has dental caries or tooth loss. Ask whether he wears dentures or bridges.
◆ Ask about the date and result of his last dental examination.
◆ Ask about his dental hygiene practices, including the use of fluoride toothpaste.

Inspecting the conjunctivae

To inspect the conjunctivae, put on gloves and follow these steps.

Inferior palpebral conjunctiva
◆ Gently evert the patient's lower eyelid with the thumb and index finger, as shown below.

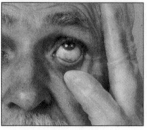

◆ Ask the patient to look up, down, to the left, and to the right as you examine the inferior palpebral conjunctiva. It should be clear and shiny.

Superior palpebral conjunctiva
◆ Check the superior palpebral conjunctiva only if you suspect a foreign body or if the patient has eyelid pain.
◆ Ask the patient to look down while you gently pull the medial eyelashes forward and upward with your thumb and index finger.
◆ While holding the eyelashes, press on the tarsal border with a cotton-tipped applicator to evert the eyelid, as shown below.

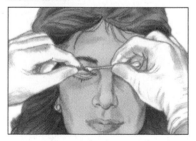

◆ Hold the lashes against the brow and examine the conjunctiva, which should be pink, with no swelling.
◆ To return the eyelid to its normal position, release the eyelashes and ask the patient to look upward. If this doesn't invert the eyelid, grasp the eyelashes and gently pull them forward.

Testing the cardinal positions of gaze

Before testing the cardinal positions of gaze, test the patient's pupillary response to light.
◆ Shine a bright light in the eye, and bring the light in from the side.
◆ Watch the response of the pupil to light in that eye and also in the opposite eye.
◆ Repeat the test on the other eye, and then proceed to assessing the cardinal positions of gaze.

The cardinal positions of gaze evaluate the oculomotor, trigeminal, and abducens nerves as well as the extraocular muscles. To perform the test, follow these steps.
◆ Sit directly in front of the patient, and ask him to remain still.
◆ Hold a small object, such as a pencil, directly in front of his nose at a distance of about 18″ (46 cm).
◆ Ask the patient to follow the object with his eyes without moving his head.
◆ Move the object to each of the six cardinal positions, returning it to the midpoint after each movement. The patient's eyes should remain parallel as they move.
◆ Note abnormal findings, such as nystagmus or the failure of one eye to follow the object.
◆ Test each of the six cardinal positions of gaze: left superior, left lateral, left inferior, right inferior, right lateral, and right superior. The following illus-

trations show testing of the three left positions.

LEFT SUPERIOR

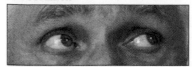

LEFT LATERAL

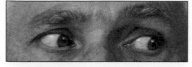

LEFT INFERIOR

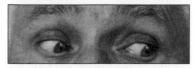

Performing an ophthalmoscopic examination

To use an ophthalmoscope to identify abnormalities of the inner eye, follow these steps.

◆ Before the examination, have the patient remove his eyeglasses or contact lenses if they're tinted, and then darken the room to dilate the patient's pupils.

◆ Sit or stand in front of the patient with your head about 18″ (46 cm) in front of and about 15 degrees to the right of the patient's line of vision in the right eye.

◆ Hold the ophthalmoscope in your right hand with the viewing aperture as close to your right eye as possible.

◆ Place your left thumb on the patient's right eyebrow to keep from hitting him with the ophthalmoscope as you move in close.

◆ Keep your right index finger on the lens selector to adjust the lens as necessary, as shown below.

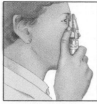

◆ To examine the left eye, perform these steps on the patient's left side. Use your left eye to examine the left eye.

◆ Instruct the patient to look straight ahead at a fixed point on the wall.

◆ Approaching from an oblique angle about 15″ (38 cm) out and with the diopter set at 0, focus a small circle of light on the pupil, as shown below.

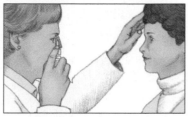

◆ Look for the orange-red glow of the red reflex, which should be sharp and distinct through the pupil. The red reflex indicates that the lens is free from opacity and clouding.

◆ Move closer to the patient, changing the lens selector with your forefinger to keep the retinal structures in focus, as shown below.

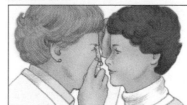

◆ Change the lens selector to a positive diopter to view the vitreous humor, observing for opacity.

◆ View the retina with a strong negative lens setting. Look for a retinal blood vessel, and follow that vessel toward the patient's nose, rotating the lens selector to keep the vessel in focus. Carefully examine all of the retinal structures, including the retinal vessels, optic disk, retinal background, macula, and fovea centralis retinae.

◆ Examine the vessels for color, size ratio of arterioles to veins, arteriole light reflex, and arteriovenous (AV) crossing. The crossing points should be smooth, without nicks or narrowing. The vessels should be free from exudate, bleeding, and narrowing. Retinal vessels normally have an AV ratio of 2:3 or 4:5.

◆ Evaluate the color of the retinal structures. The retina should be light yellow to orange, and the background should be free from hemorrhages, aneurysms, and exudates. The optic disk, located on the nasal side of the retina, should be orange-red with distinct margins. Note the size, shape, clarity, and color of the disk margins. The physiologic cup is normally yellow-white and readily visible.

◆ Examine the macula last, and as briefly as possible, because it's very light-sensitive. The macula, which is darker than the rest of the retinal background, is free from vessels and located temporally to the optic disk. The fovea centralis retinae is a slight depression in the center of the macula.

Using the otoscope

Perform an otoscopic examination to assess the external auditory canal, tympanic membrane, and malleus.

◆ Before you insert the speculum into the patient's ear, check the canal opening for foreign particles or discharge.

◆ Palpate the tragus (the cartilaginous projection anterior to the external opening of the ear) and pull up the auricle. If this area is tender, don't insert the speculum; the patient may have external otitis, and inserting the speculum could be painful.

◆ If the ear canal is clear, straighten the canal by grasping the auricle and pulling it up and back, as shown below. Then gently insert the speculum. For an infant or a toddler, grasp the auricle and pull it down and back.

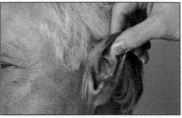

◆ Hold the otoscope as shown below. Avoid hitting the ear canal with the speculum.

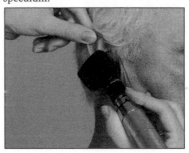

Inspecting the nostrils

◆ Gather a nasal speculum and a small flashlight or penlight.

◆ Have the patient sit in front of you and tilt his head back.

◆ Insert the tip of the closed speculum into one of the nostrils until you reach the point where the blade widens.

◆ Slowly open the speculum as wide as you can without causing discomfort.

◆ Shine the flashlight into the nostril to illuminate the area. The illustration below shows proper placement of the nasal speculum. The inset shows the structures that should be visible during examination of the left nostril.

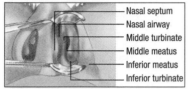

Nasal septum
Nasal airway
Middle turbinate
Middle meatus
Inferior meatus
Inferior turbinate

◆ Note the color and patency of the nostril and the presence of exudate. The mucosa should be moist, pink to red, and free from lesions and polyps. Normally, you wouldn't see drainage, edema, or inflammation of the nasal mucosa, although some tissue enlargement is normal in a pregnant patient.

◆ You should see the choana (posterior air passage), cilia, and the middle and inferior turbinates. Below each turbinate is a groove, or meatus, where the paranasal sinuses drain.

◆ When you've completed your inspection of one nostril, close the speculum and remove it. Then inspect the other nostril.

Inspecting and palpating the frontal and maxillary sinuses

During an inspection, you'll be able to examine the frontal and maxillary sinuses, but not the ethmoidal and sphenoidal sinuses. However, if the frontal and maxillary sinuses are infected, you can assume that the ethmoidal and sphenoidal are infected as well.

◆ Check for swelling around the eyes, especially over the sinus area.

◆ Palpate the frontal and maxillary sinuses for tenderness and warmth.

◆ To palpate the frontal sinuses, place your thumb above the patient's eyes, just under the bony ridges of the upper orbits, and press up. Place your fingertips on his forehead and apply gentle pressure.

◆ To palpate the maxillary sinuses, place your thumbs as shown below. Then apply gentle pressure by pressing your thumbs (or index and middle fingers) up and in on each side of the nose, just below the zygomatic bone (cheekbone).

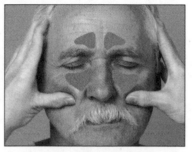

Inspecting and palpating the thyroid gland

◆ To locate the thyroid gland, observe the lower third of the patient's anterior neck.

◆ With the patient's neck extended slightly, look for masses or asymmetry in the gland. Ask him to sip water, with his neck still slightly extended. Watch the thyroid rise and fall with the trachea. You should see slight, symmetrical movement. A fixed thyroid lobe may indicate a mass.

◆ Palpate the thyroid gland while standing in front of the patient. Locate the cricoid cartilage first, and then move one hand to each side to palpate the thyroid lobes. The lobes can be difficult to feel because of their location and the presence of overlying tissues.

◆ Alternatively, stand behind the patient and place the fingers of both hands on the neck, just below the cricoid cartilage. Have the patient swallow, and feel the rise of the thyroid isthmus. Move your fingers down and to the sides to feel the lateral lobes.

◆ To evaluate the size and texture of the thyroid gland, gently displace the thyroid toward the right. Have the patient swallow as you palpate the lateral lobes of the thyroid, as shown below. Displace the thyroid toward the left to examine the left side.

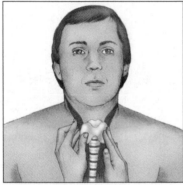

◆ An enlarged thyroid may feel well-defined and finely lobulated.

◆ Thyroid nodules feel like a knot, protuberance, or swelling.

◆ A firm, fixed nodule may indicate a tumor.

◆ Don't confuse thick neck muscles with an enlarged thyroid or goiter.

PART

II

Signs & symptoms

A

Abdominal distention

Abdominal distention refers to increased abdominal girth—the result of increased intra-abdominal pressure forcing the abdominal wall outward. Distention may be mild or severe, depending on the amount of pressure. It may be localized or diffuse and may occur gradually or suddenly. Acute abdominal distention may signal life-threatening peritonitis or acute bowel obstruction.

Abdominal distention may result from fat, flatus, hemorrhage, a fetus (pregnancy or ectopic pregnancy), or fluid. Fluid and gas are normally present in the GI tract but not in the peritoneal cavity. However, if fluid and gas can't pass freely through the GI tract, abdominal distention occurs. In the peritoneal cavity, distention may reflect acute bleeding, accumulation of ascitic fluid, or air from perforation of an abdominal organ.

Abdominal distention doesn't always signal pathology. For example, in anxious patients or those with digestive distress, localized distention in the left upper quadrant can result from aerophagia—the unconscious swallowing of air. Generalized distention can result from ingestion of fruits or vegetables with large quantities of unabsorbable carbohydrates, such as legumes, or from abnormal food fermentation by microbes.

Assessment

If the patient displays abdominal distention, quickly check for signs of hypovolemia, such as pallor, diaphoresis, hypotension, a rapid thready pulse, rapid shallow breathing, decreased urine output, and altered mentation. Ask the patient whether he's experiencing severe abdominal pain or difficulty breathing. Find out about recent accidents, and observe him for signs of trauma and peritoneal bleeding, such as Cullen's sign or Turner's sign. Then auscultate all abdominal quadrants, noting rapid and high-pitched, diminished, or absent bowel sounds. (If you don't hear bowel sounds immediately, listen for at least 5 minutes in each of the four abdominal quadrants.) Gently palpate the abdomen for rigidity. Remember that deep or extensive palpation may increase pain. If you detect abdominal distention and rigidity along with abnormal bowel sounds and if the patient complains of pain, begin emergency interventions. (See *Responding to abdominal distention and rigidity*.)

If the patient's abdominal distention isn't acute, ask about its onset and duration and associated symptoms. A pa-

EMERGENCY INTERVENTIONS

Responding to
abdominal distention and rigidity

If your patient has abdominal distention and rigidity, quickly check his bowel sounds. If you detect abnormal bowel sounds and the patient complains of pain:
◆ Place him in the supine position.
◆ Administer oxygen.

◆ Insert an I.V. catheter for fluid replacement as prescribed.
◆ Prepare to insert a nasogastric tube.
◆ Reassure the patient.
◆ Prepare him for surgery.

tient with localized distention may report a sensation of pressure, fullness, or tenderness in the affected area. A patient with generalized distention may report a bloated feeling, a pounding heart, and difficulty breathing deeply or when lying flat.

The patient may also feel unable to bend at his waist. Make sure to ask about abdominal pain, fever, nausea, vomiting, anorexia, altered bowel habits, and weight gain or loss.

Obtain a medical history, noting GI or biliary disorders that may cause peritonitis or ascites, such as cirrhosis, hepatitis, or inflammatory bowel disease. (See *Detecting ascites,* page 64.) Also note chronic constipation. Has the patient recently had abdominal surgery, which can lead to abdominal distention? Ask about recent accidents, even minor ones, such as falling off a stepladder.

Perform a complete assessment. Don't restrict the assessment to the abdomen because you could miss important clues to the cause of abdominal distention. Next, stand at the foot of the bed and observe the recumbent patient for abdominal asymmetry to determine whether distention is localized or generalized. Then assess abdominal contour by stooping at his side. Inspect for tense, taut skin and bulging flanks,

which may indicate ascites. Observe the umbilicus. An everted umbilicus may indicate ascites or umbilical hernia. An inverted umbilicus may indicate distention from gas; it's also common in obesity. Inspect the abdomen for signs of inguinal or femoral hernia and for incisions that may point to adhesions. Both may lead to intestinal obstruction. Then auscultate for bowel sounds, abdominal friction rubs (indicating peritoneal inflammation), and bruits (indicating an aneurysm).

Next, percuss and palpate the abdomen to determine whether distention results from air, fluid, or both. A tympanic note in the left lower quadrant suggests an air-filled descending or sigmoid colon. A tympanic note throughout a generally distended abdomen suggests an air-filled peritoneal cavity. Dull percussion noted throughout a generally distended abdomen suggests a fluid-filled peritoneal cavity. Shifting of dullness laterally with the patient in the decubitus position also indicates a fluid-filled abdominal cavity. A pelvic or intra-abdominal mass causes local dullness on percussion and should be palpable. Obesity causes a large abdomen without shifting dullness, prominent tympany, or palpable bowel or other masses, with generalized rather then localized dullness.

Detecting ascites

To differentiate ascites from other causes of abdominal distention, check for shifting dullness and fluid wave, as described here.

Shifting dullness

Step 1. With the patient in a supine position, percuss from the umbilicus outward to the flank, as shown. Draw a line on the patient's skin to mark the change from tympany to dullness.

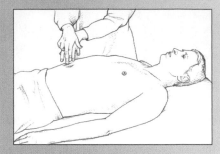

Step 2. Turn the patient onto his side. (Note that this positioning causes ascitic fluid to shift.) Percuss again, and mark the change from tympany to dullness. A difference between these lines can indicate ascites.

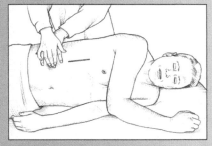

Fluid wave

Have another person press deeply into the patient's midline to prevent vibration from traveling along the abdominal wall. Place one of your palms on one of the patient's flanks. Strike the opposite flank with your other hand. If you feel the blow in the opposite palm, ascitic fluid is present.

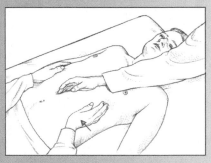

Palpate the abdomen for tenderness, noting whether it's localized or generalized. Watch for peritoneal signs and symptoms, such as rebound tenderness, guarding, rigidity, McBurney's sign, obturator sign, and psoas sign.

Finally, measure the patient's abdominal girth for a baseline value. Mark the flanks with a felt-tipped pen as a reference for subsequent measurements.

Causes

◆ *Abdominal cancer.* Generalized abdominal distention may occur when the cancer—most commonly ovarian, hepatic, or pancreatic—produces ascites (usually in a patient with a known tumor). It's an indication of advanced disease. Shifting dullness and a fluid wave accompany distention. Associated signs and symptoms may include severe abdominal pain, an abdominal mass, anorexia, jaundice, GI hemorrhage, dyspepsia, and weight loss that progresses to muscle weakness and atrophy.

▧ *Abdominal trauma.* When brisk internal bleeding accompanies trauma, abdominal distention may be acute and dramatic. Associated signs and symptoms of this life-threatening disorder include abdominal rigidity with guarding, decreased or absent bowel sounds, vomiting, tenderness, and abdominal bruising. Pain may occur over the trauma site or over the scapula if abdominal bleeding irritates the phrenic nerve. Signs of hypovolemic shock (such as hypotension and rapid, thready pulse) appear with significant blood loss.

▧ *Cirrhosis.* In cirrhosis, ascites causes generalized distention and is confirmed by a fluid wave and shifting dullness. Umbilical eversion and caput medusae (dilated veins around the umbilicus) are common. The patient may report a feeling of fullness or weight gain. Associated findings include vague abdominal pain, fever, anorexia, nausea, vomiting, constipation or diarrhea, bleeding tendencies, severe pruritus, palmar erythema, spider angiomas, leg edema and, possibly, splenomegaly. Hematemesis, encephalopathy, gynecomastia, or testicular atrophy may also be seen. Jaundice is usually a late sign. Hepatomegaly occurs initially, but the liver may not be palpable if the patient has advanced disease.

▧ *Heart failure.* Generalized abdominal distention due to ascites typically accompanies severe cardiovascular impairment and is confirmed by shifting dullness and a fluid wave. Signs and symptoms of heart failure are numerous and depend on the disease stage and degree of cardiovascular impairment. Hallmarks include peripheral edema, jugular vein distention, dyspnea, and tachycardia. Common associated signs and symptoms include hepatomegaly (which may cause right upper quadrant pain), nausea, vomiting, a productive cough, crackles, weight gain, cool extremities, cyanotic nail beds, nocturia, exercise intolerance, nocturnal wheezing, diastolic hypertension, and cardiomegaly.

◆ *Irritable bowel syndrome.* Irritable bowel syndrome may produce intermittent, localized distention—the result of periodic intestinal spasms. Lower abdominal pain or cramping typically accompanies these spasms. The pain is usually relieved by defecation or by passage of intestinal gas and is aggravated by stress. Other possible signs and symptoms include diarrhea that may alternate with constipation or normal bowel function, nausea, dyspepsia, straining and urgency at defecation, a feeling of incomplete evacuation, and small, mucus-streaked stools.

▧ *Large-bowel obstruction.* Dramatic abdominal distention is characteristic in this life-threatening disorder; in fact, loops of the large bowel may become visible on the abdomen. Constipation precedes distention and may be the only symptom for days. Associated findings include tympany, high-pitched bowel sounds, and the sudden onset of colicky lower abdominal pain that becomes persistent. Nausea, fecal vomiting, and diminished peristaltic waves and bowel sounds are late signs.

▧ *Mesenteric artery occlusion (acute).* In this life-threatening disorder, abdominal distention usually occurs several hours after the sudden onset of severe, colicky periumbilical pain that's accompanied by rapid (even forceful) bowel evacuation. The pain later becomes constant and diffuse. Related signs and symptoms include severe abdominal tenderness with guarding and rigidity, absent bowel sounds and, occasionally, a bruit in the right iliac fossa. The patient may also experience vomiting, anorexia, diarrhea, or constipation. Late signs include fever, tachycardia, tachypnea, hypotension, and cool, clammy skin. Abdominal distention or GI bleeding may be the only clue if pain is absent.

◆ *Paralytic ileus.* Paralytic ileus, which produces generalized distention with a tympanic percussion note, is accompanied by absent or hypoactive bowel sounds and, occasionally, mild abdominal pain and vomiting. The patient may be severely constipated or may pass flatus and small, liquid stools.

◼ *Peritonitis.* Peritonitis is a life-threatening disorder in which abdominal distention may be localized or generalized, depending on the extent of the inflammation. Fluid accumulates within the peritoneal cavity and then within the bowel lumen, causing a fluid wave and shifting dullness. Typically, distention is accompanied by sudden and severe abdominal pain that worsens with movement, rebound tenderness, and abdominal rigidity. The skin over the patient's abdomen may appear taut. Associated signs and symptoms usually include hypoactive or absent bowel sounds, fever, chills, hyperalgesia (extreme sensitivity to pain), nausea, and vomiting. Signs of shock, such as tachycardia and hypotension, appear with significant fluid loss into the abdomen.

◼ *Small-bowel obstruction.* Abdominal distention is characteristic in small-bowel obstruction, a life-threatening disorder, and is most pronounced during late obstruction, especially in the distal small bowel. Auscultation reveals hypoactive or hyperactive bowel sounds, whereas percussion produces a tympanic note. Accompanying signs and symptoms include colicky periumbilical pain, constipation, nausea, and vomiting; the higher the obstruction, the earlier and more severe the vomiting. Rebound tenderness reflects intestinal strangulation with ischemia. Associated signs and symptoms include drowsiness, malaise, and signs of dehydration. Signs of hypovolemic shock appear with progressive dehydration and plasma loss.

◼ *Toxic megacolon (acute).* Toxic megacolon is a life-threatening complication of infectious or ulcerative colitis. It produces dramatic abdominal distention that usually develops gradually and is accompanied by a tympanic percussion note, diminished or absent bowel sounds, and mild rebound tenderness. The patient also presents with abdominal pain and tenderness, fever, tachycardia, and dehydration.

Abdominal mass

Commonly detected on routine assessment, an abdominal mass is a localized swelling in one abdominal quadrant. Typically, this sign develops insidiously and may represent an enlarged organ, a neoplasm, an abscess, a vascular defect, or a fecal mass.

Distinguishing an abdominal mass from a normal structure requires skillful palpation. At times, palpation must be repeated with the patient in a different position or performed by a second examiner to verify initial findings. A palpable abdominal mass is an important clinical sign and usually represents a serious—and perhaps life-threatening—disorder.

EMERGENCY INTERVENTIONS

Suspected abdominal aortic aneurysm

If you suspect that your patient has an aortic aneurysm:
◆ Quickly take his vital signs.
◆ Withhold food or fluids until he's examined.
◆ Prepare to administer oxygen.
◆ Prepare to start an I.V. infusion for fluid and blood replacement.
◆ Obtain routine preoperative tests.

◆ Prepare the patient for angiography as prescribed.
◆ Frequently monitor blood pressure, pulse, respirations, and urine output.
◆ Be alert for signs of shock, such as tachycardia, hypotension, and cool, clammy skin, which may indicate significant blood loss.

Assessment

If the patient has a pulsating midabdominal mass and severe abdominal or back pain, suspect an aortic aneurysm and act quickly. (See *Suspected abdominal aortic aneurysm*.)

If the patient's abdominal mass doesn't suggest an aortic aneurysm, continue with a detailed history. Ask the patient whether the mass is painful. If so, ask whether the pain is constant or occurs only on palpation. Is it localized or generalized? Determine whether the patient was already aware of the mass. If he was, find out if he noticed a change in the size or location of the mass.

Next, review the patient's medical history, paying special attention to GI disorders. Ask the patient about GI symptoms, such as constipation, diarrhea, rectal bleeding, abnormally colored stools, and vomiting. Has the patient noticed a change in his appetite? If the patient is female, ask whether her menstrual cycles are regular and when the first day of her last menses was.

A complete assessment should be performed. Begin by inspecting the abdomen. Next, auscultate for bowel sounds in each quadrant. Listen for bruits or friction rubs, and check for enlarged veins. Lightly palpate and then deeply palpate the abdomen, assessing a painful or suspicious areas last. Note the patient's position when you locate the mass. Some masses can be detected only with the patient in a supine position; others require a side-lying position.

Estimate the size of the mass in centimeters. Determine its shape. Is it round or sausage shaped? Describe its contour as smooth, rough, sharply defined, nodular, or irregular. Determine the consistency of the mass. Is it soft, solid, or hard? Also, percuss the mass. A dull sound indicates a fluid-filled mass; a tympanic sound, an air-filled mass.

Next, determine whether the mass moves with your hand or in response to respiration. Is the mass free-floating or attached to intra-abdominal structures? To determine whether the mass is located in the abdominal wall or the abdominal cavity, ask the patient to lift his head and shoulders off the examination table, thereby contracting his abdominal muscles. While these muscles are contracted, try to palpate the mass. If you can, the mass is in the abdominal wall; if you can't, the mass is within the abdominal cavity. (See *Abdominal masses: Locations and common causes.*)

After the abdominal examination is complete, perform pelvic, genital, and rectal examinations.

Causes

◩ *Abdominal aortic aneurysm.* Abdominal aortic aneurysm may persist for years, producing only a pulsating periumbilical mass with a systolic bruit over the aorta. However, it may become life-threatening if the aneurysm expands and its walls weaken. In such cases, the patient initially reports constant upper abdominal pain or, less commonly, low back or dull abdominal pain. If the aneurysm ruptures, he'll report severe abdominal and back pain. After rupture, the aneurysm no longer pulsates.

Associated signs and symptoms of rupture include mottled skin below the waist, absent femoral and pedal pulses, lower blood pressure in the legs than in the arms, mild to moderate tenderness with guarding, and abdominal rigidity. Signs of shock—such as tachycardia, hypotension, and cool, clammy skin—appear with significant blood loss.

◆ *Cholecystitis.* Deep palpation below the liver border may reveal a smooth, firm, sausage-shaped mass. However, with acute inflammation, the gallbladder is usually too tender to be palpated. Cholecystitis can cause severe right upper quadrant pain that may radiate to the right shoulder, chest, or back; abdominal rigidity and tenderness; fever; pallor; diaphoresis; anorexia; nausea; and vomiting. Recurrent attacks usually occur 1 to 6 hours after meals. Murphy's sign (inspiratory arrest elicited when the examiner palpates the right upper quadrant as the patient takes a deep breath) is common.

◆ *Colon cancer.* A right lower quadrant mass may occur with cancer of the right colon, which may also cause occult bleeding with anemia and abdominal aching, pressure, or dull cramps. Associated findings include weakness, fatigue, exertional dyspnea, vertigo, and signs and symptoms of intestinal obstruction, such as obstipation (severe constipation) and vomiting.

Occasionally, cancer of the left colon also causes a palpable mass. It usually produces rectal bleeding, intermittent abdominal fullness or cramping, and rectal pressure. The patient may also report fremitus and pelvic discomfort. Later, he develops obstipation, diarrhea, or pencil-shaped, grossly bloody, or mucus-streaked stools. Typically, defecation relieves pain.

◆ *Crohn's disease.* With Crohn's disease, tender, sausage-shaped masses are usually palpable in the right lower quadrant and, at times, in the left lower quadrant. Attacks of colicky right lower quadrant pain and diarrhea are common. Associated signs and symptoms include fever, anorexia, weight loss, hyperactive bowel sounds, nausea, abdominal tenderness with guarding, and perirectal, skin, or vaginal fistulas.

◆ *Diverticulitis.* Most common in the sigmoid colon, diverticulitis may produce a left lower quadrant mass that's usually tender, firm, and fixed. It also produces intermittent abdominal pain that's relieved by defecation or passage of flatus. Other findings may include alternating constipation and diarrhea, nausea, a low-grade fever, and a distended and tympanic abdomen.

◆ *Gastric cancer.* Advanced gastric cancer may produce an epigastric mass. Early findings include chronic dyspepsia and epigastric discomfort, whereas late findings include weight

Abdominal masses: Locations and common causes

The location of an abdominal mass provides an important clue to the causative disorder. Here are the disorders most commonly responsible for abdominal masses in each of the four abdominal quadrants.

Right upper quadrant
- Aortic aneurysm (epigastric area)
- Cholecystitis or cholelithiasis
- Gallbladder, gastric, or hepatic carcinoma
- Hepatomegaly
- Hydronephrosis
- Pancreatic abscess or pseudocysts
- Renal cell carcinoma

Left upper quadrant
- Aortic aneurysm (epigastric area)
- Gastric carcinoma (epigastric area)
- Hydronephrosis
- Pancreatic abscess (epigastric area)
- Pancreatic pseudocysts (epigastric area)
- Renal cell carcinoma
- Splenomegaly

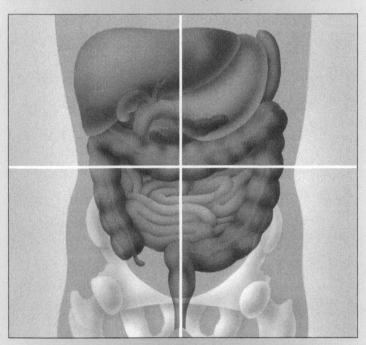

Right lower quadrant
- Bladder distention (suprapubic area)
- Colon cancer
- Crohn's disease
- Ovarian cyst (suprapubic area)
- Uterine leiomyomas (suprapubic area)

Left lower quadrant
- Bladder distention (suprapubic area)
- Colon cancer
- Diverticulitis
- Ovarian cyst (suprapubic area)
- Uterine leiomyomas (suprapubic area)
- Volvulus

loss, a feeling of fullness after eating, fatigue and, occasionally, coffee-ground vomitus or melena.

◆ *Hepatomegaly.* Hepatomegaly produces a firm, blunt, irregular mass in the epigastric region or below the right costal margin. Associated signs and symptoms vary with the causative disorder but commonly include ascites, right upper quadrant pain and tenderness, anorexia, nausea, vomiting, leg edema, jaundice, palmar erythema, spider angiomas, gynecomastia, testicular atrophy and, possibly, splenomegaly.

◆ *Hernia.* The soft and typically tender bulge is usually an effect of prolonged, increased intra-abdominal pressure on weakened areas of the abdominal wall. An umbilical hernia is typically located around the umbilicus; an inguinal hernia, in either the right or left groin. An incisional hernia can occur anywhere along a previous incision. Hernia may be the only sign until strangulation occurs.

◆ *Hydronephrosis.* Enlarging one or both kidneys, hydronephrosis produces a smooth, boggy mass in one or both flanks. Other findings vary with the degree of hydronephrosis. The patient may have severe colicky renal pain or dull flank pain that radiates to the groin, vulva, or testes. Hematuria, pyuria, dysuria, alternating oliguria and polyuria, nocturia, accelerated hypertension, nausea, and vomiting may also occur.

◆ *Ovarian cyst.* A large ovarian cyst may produce a smooth, rounded, fluctuant mass, resembling a distended bladder, in the suprapubic region. Large or multiple cysts may also cause mild pelvic discomfort, lower back pain, menstrual irregularities, and hirsutism. A twisted or ruptured cyst may cause abdominal tenderness, distention, and rigidity.

◆ *Splenomegaly.* Lymphomas, leukemias, hemolytic anemias, and inflammatory diseases are among the many disorders that may cause splenomegaly. Typically, the smooth edge of the enlarged spleen is palpable in the left upper quadrant. Associated signs and symptoms vary with the causative disorder but usually include a feeling of abdominal fullness, left upper quadrant abdominal pain and tenderness, splenic friction rub, splenic bruits, and a low-grade fever.

◆ *Uterine leiomyomas (fibroids).* If large enough, these common, benign uterine tumors produce a round, multinodular mass in the suprapubic region. The patient's chief complaint is usually menorrhagia; she may also experience a feeling of heaviness in the abdomen, and pressure on surrounding organs may cause back pain, constipation, and urinary frequency or urgency. Edema and varicosities of the lower extremities may develop. Rapid fibroid growth in perimenopausal or postmenopausal women needs further evaluation.

Abdominal pain

Abdominal pain usually results from a GI disorder, but it can be caused by a reproductive, genitourinary (GU), musculoskeletal, or vascular disorder; drug use; or ingestion of toxins. At times, such pain signals life-threatening complications.

Abdominal pain arises from the abdominopelvic viscera, the parietal peritoneum, or the capsules of the liver, kidney, or spleen. It may be acute or chronic, diffuse or localized. Visceral pain develops slowly into a deep, dull, aching pain that's poorly localized in the epigastric, periumbilical, or lower midabdominal (hypogastric) region. In contrast, somatic (parietal, peritoneal) pain produces a sharp, more intense, well-localized discomfort that rapidly follows the insult. Movement or coughing aggravates this pain. (See *Abdominal pain: Types and locations.*)

Abdominal pain: Types and locations

AFFECTED ORGAN	VISCERAL PAIN	PARIETAL PAIN	REFERRED PAIN
Appendix	Periumbilical area	Right lower quadrant	Right lower quadrant
Distal colon	Hypogastrium and left flank for descending colon	Over affected area	Left lower quadrant and back (rare)
Gallbladder	Middle epigastrium	Right upper quadrant	Right subscapular area
Ovaries, fallopian tubes, and uterus	Hypogastrium and groin	Over affected area	Inner thighs
Pancreas	Middle epigastrium and left upper quadrant	Middle epigastrium and left upper quadrant	Back and left shoulder
Proximal colon	Periumbilical area and right flank for ascending colon	Over affected site	Right lower quadrant and back (rare)
Small intestine	Periumbilical area	Over affected site	Midback (rare)
Stomach	Middle epigastrium	Middle epigastrium and left upper quadrant	Shoulders
Ureters	Costovertebral angle	Over affected site	Groin: scrotum in men, labia in women (rare)

Pain may also be referred to the abdomen from another site with the same or similar nerve supply. This sharp, well-localized, referred pain is felt in skin or deeper tissues and may coexist with skin hyperesthesia and muscle hyperalgesia.

Mechanisms that produce abdominal pain include stretching or tension of the gut wall, traction on the peritoneum or mesentery, vigorous intestinal contraction, inflammation, ischemia, and sensory nerve irritation.

Assessment

Ask the patient to rate his pain using a pain scale. If the patient is experiencing sudden and severe abdominal pain, you must react quickly. (See *Responding to sudden and severe abdominal pain,* page 72.)

If the patient has no life-threatening signs or symptoms, take his history. Ask him whether he has had this type of pain before. Have him describe the pain in his own words—for example, dull, sharp, stabbing, or burning. Ask whether anything relieves the pain or makes it worse. Ask the patient whether the pain is constant or intermittent

EMERGENCY INTERVENTIONS

Responding to sudden and severe abdominal pain

If your patient develops sudden and severe abdominal pain, you must react quickly:
◆ Take his vital signs.
◆ Palpate pulses below the waist.
◆ Be alert for signs of hypovolemic shock, such as tachycardia and hypotension.

◆ Obtain I.V. access as prescribed.
◆ Determine whether the patient also has mottled skin below the waist and a pulsating epigastric mass or rebound tenderness and rigidity. If so, prepare him for surgery.

and when the pain began. Constant, steady abdominal pain suggests organ perforation, ischemia, or inflammation or blood in the peritoneal cavity. Intermittent, cramping abdominal pain suggests that the patient may have obstruction of a hollow organ.

If pain is intermittent, find out the duration of a typical episode. In addition, ask the patient where the pain is located and if it radiates to other areas.

Find out whether movement, coughing, exertion, vomiting, eating, elimination, or walking worsens or relieves the pain. The patient may report abdominal pain as indigestion or gas pain, so have him describe it in detail.

Ask the patient about substance abuse and a history of vascular, GI, GU, or reproductive disorders. Ask the female patient about the date of her last menses, changes in her menstrual pattern, or dyspareunia.

Ask the patient about appetite changes. Ask about the onset and frequency of nausea or vomiting. Find out about increased flatulence, constipation, diarrhea, and changes in stool consistency. When was the last bowel movement? Ask about urinary frequency, urgency, or pain. Is the urine cloudy or pink?

Perform a physical examination. Take the patient's vital signs, and assess skin turgor and mucous mem-

branes. Inspect his abdomen for distention or visible peristaltic waves and, if indicated, measure his abdominal girth.

Auscultate for bowel sounds, and characterize their motility. Percuss all quadrants, noting the percussion sounds. Palpate the entire abdomen for masses, rigidity, and tenderness. Check for costovertebral angle (CVA) tenderness, abdominal tenderness with guarding, and rebound tenderness.

Causes

◣ *Abdominal aortic aneurysm (dissecting).* Initially, this life-threatening disorder may produce dull lower abdominal, lower back, or severe chest pain. Usually, abdominal aortic aneurysm produces constant upper abdominal pain, which may worsen when the patient lies down and may abate when he leans forward or sits up. Palpation may reveal an epigastric mass that pulsates before rupture but not after it.

Other findings may include mottled skin below the waist, absent femoral and pedal pulses, lower blood pressure in the legs than in the arms, mild to moderate abdominal tenderness with guarding, and abdominal rigidity. Signs of shock, such as hypotension, tachycardia and tachypnea, may appear.

◆ *Abdominal cancer.* Abdominal pain usually occurs late in abdominal cancer. It may be accompanied by anorexia, weight loss, weakness, depression, and abdominal mass and distention.

◼ *Abdominal trauma.* Generalized or localized abdominal pain occurs with ecchymoses of the abdomen, abdominal tenderness, vomiting and, with hemorrhage into the peritoneal cavity, abdominal rigidity. Bowel sounds are decreased or absent. The patient may have signs of hypovolemic shock, such as hypotension and a rapid, thready pulse.

◼ *Acute pancreatitis.* Life-threatening acute pancreatitis produces fulminating, continuous upper abdominal pain that may radiate to both flanks and to the back. To relieve this pain, the patient may bend forward, draw his knees to his chest, or move restlessly about. Early findings include abdominal tenderness, nausea, vomiting, fever, pallor, tachycardia and, in some patients, abdominal rigidity, rebound tenderness, and hypoactive bowel sounds. Turner's sign (ecchymosis of the abdomen or flank) or Cullen's sign (a bluish tinge around the umbilicus) signals hemorrhagic pancreatitis. Jaundice may occur as inflammation subsides.

◼ *Adrenal crisis.* Severe abdominal pain appears early, along with nausea, vomiting, dehydration, profound weakness, anorexia, and fever. Later signs are progressive loss of consciousness; hypotension; tachycardia; oliguria; cool, clammy skin; and increased motor activity, which may progress to delirium or seizures.

◆ *Anthrax (GI).* An acute infectious disease, GI anthrax is caused by the gram-positive, spore-forming bacterium *Bacillus anthracis.* Although the disease most commonly occurs in wild and domestic grazing animals, such as cattle, sheep, and goats, the spores can live in the soil for many years. The disease can occur in humans exposed to infected animals, tissue from infected animals (as can occur by eating meat from an infected animal), or biological warfare. Most natural cases occur in agricultural regions worldwide. Initial signs and symptoms include loss of appetite, nausea, vomiting, and fever. Late signs and symptoms include abdominal pain, severe bloody diarrhea, and hematemesis.

◆ *Appendicitis.* With appendicitis, pain initially occurs in the epigastric or umbilical region. Anorexia, nausea, or vomiting may occur after the onset of pain. Pain localizes at McBurney's point in the right lower quadrant and is accompanied by abdominal rigidity, increasing tenderness (especially over McBurney's point), rebound tenderness, and retractive respirations. Later signs and symptoms include malaise, constipation (or diarrhea), low-grade fever, and tachycardia.

◆ *Cholecystitis.* Severe pain in the right upper quadrant may arise suddenly or increase gradually over several hours, usually after meals. It may radiate to the right shoulder, chest, or back. Accompanying the pain are anorexia, nausea, vomiting, fever, abdominal rigidity, tenderness, pallor, and diaphoresis. Murphy's sign (inspiratory arrest elicited when the examiner palpates the right upper quadrant as the patient takes a deep breath) is common.

◆ *Cholelithiasis.* Patients may suffer sudden, severe, and paroxysmal pain in the right upper quadrant lasting several minutes to several hours. The pain may radiate to the epigastrium, back, or shoulder blades. The pain is accompanied by anorexia, nausea, vomiting (sometimes bilious), diaphoresis, restlessness, and abdominal tenderness with guarding over the gallbladder or biliary duct. The patient may also experience fatty food intolerance and frequent indigestion.

◆ *Chronic pancreatitis.* A nonthreatening disease, chronic pancreatitis produces severe left upper quadrant or epigastric pain that radiates to the back. Abdominal tenderness, a midepigastric mass, jaundice, fever, and splenomegaly may occur. Steatorrhea, weight loss, maldigestion, and diabetes mellitus are common.

◼ *Cirrhosis.* Dull abdominal aching occurs early and is usually accompanied by anorexia, indigestion, nausea, vomiting, constipation, or diarrhea. Subsequent right upper quadrant pain worsens when the patient sits up or leans forward. Associated signs include fever, ascites, leg edema, weight gain, hepatomegaly, jaundice, severe pruritus, bleeding tendencies, palmar erythema, and spider angiomas. Gynecomastia and testicular atrophy may also be present.

◆ *Crohn's disease.* An acute attack in Crohn's disease causes severe cramping pain in the lower abdomen, typically preceded by weeks or months of milder cramping pain. Crohn's disease may also cause diarrhea, hyperactive bowel sounds, dehydration, weight loss, fever, abdominal tenderness with guarding, and possibly a palpable mass in a lower quadrant. Abdominal pain is commonly relieved by defecation. Milder chronic signs and symptoms include right lower quadrant pain with diarrhea, steatorrhea, and weight loss. Complications include perirectal or vaginal fistulas.

◆ *Diverticulitis.* Mild cases of diverticulitis usually produce intermittent, diffuse left lower quadrant pain, which is sometimes relieved by defecation or passage of flatus and worsened by eating. Other signs and symptoms include nausea, constipation or diarrhea, a low-grade fever and, in many cases, a palpable abdominal mass that's usually tender, firm, and fixed. Rupture causes severe left lower quadrant pain, abdominal rigidity and, possibly, signs

and symptoms of sepsis and shock (high fever, chills, and hypotension).

◆ *Drugs.* Salicylates and nonsteroidal anti-inflammatory drugs commonly cause burning, gnawing pain in the left upper quadrant or epigastric area, along with nausea and vomiting.

◆ *Duodenal ulcer.* Localized abdominal pain—described as steady, gnawing, burning, aching, or hungerlike—may occur high in the midepigastrium, slightly off center, usually on the right. The pain usually doesn't radiate unless pancreatic penetration occurs. It typically begins 2 to 4 hours after a meal and may cause nocturnal awakening. Ingestion of food or antacids brings relief until the cycle starts again, but it may also produce weight gain. Other symptoms include changes in bowel habits and heartburn or retrosternal burning.

◼ *Ectopic pregnancy.* Lower abdominal pain may be sharp, dull, or cramping and constant or intermittent in ectopic pregnancy, a potentially life-threatening disorder. Vaginal bleeding, nausea, and vomiting may occur, along with urinary frequency, a tender adnexal mass, and a 1- to 2-month history of amenorrhea. Rupture of the fallopian tube produces sharp lower abdominal pain, which may radiate to the shoulders and neck and become extreme with cervical or adnexal palpation. Signs of shock (such as pallor, tachycardia, and hypotension) may also appear.

◆ *Endometriosis.* Constant, severe pain in the lower abdomen usually begins 5 to 7 days before the start of menses and may be aggravated by defecation. Depending on the location of the ectopic tissue, the pain may be accompanied by constipation, abdominal tenderness, dysmenorrhea, dyspareunia, and deep sacral pain.

◆ *Escherichia coli O157:H7.* E. coli O157:H7 is an aerobic, gram-negative bacillus that causes food-borne illness. Most strains of *E. coli* are harmless and are part of normal intestinal flora of healthy humans and animals. However, *E. coli* O157:H7, one of hundreds of strains of the bacterium, is capable of producing a powerful toxin and can cause severe illness. Eating undercooked beef or other foods contaminated with the bacteria causes the disease. Signs and symptoms include watery or bloody diarrhea, nausea, vomiting, fever, and abdominal cramps. In children younger than age 5 and in elderly patients, hemolytic uremic syndrome may develop, which may ultimately lead to acute renal failure.

◆ *Gastric ulcer.* Diffuse, gnawing, burning pain in the left upper quadrant or epigastric area commonly occurs 1 to 2 hours after meals and may be relieved by ingestion of food or antacids. Vague bloating and nausea after eating are common. Indigestion, weight change, anorexia, and episodes of GI bleeding also occur.

◆ *Gastritis.* With acute gastritis, the patient experiences a rapid onset of abdominal pain that can range from mild epigastric discomfort to burning pain in the left upper quadrant. Other typical features include belching, fever, malaise, anorexia, nausea, bloody or coffee-ground vomitus, and melena. However, significant bleeding is unusual, unless the patient has hemorrhagic gastritis.

◆ *Gastroenteritis.* Cramping or colicky abdominal pain, which can be diffuse, originates in the left upper quadrant and radiates or migrates to the other quadrants, usually in a peristaltic manner. It's accompanied by diarrhea, hyperactive bowel sounds, headache, myalgia, nausea, and vomiting.

◆ *Heart failure.* Right upper quadrant pain commonly accompanies heart failure's hallmarks: jugular vein distention, dyspnea, tachycardia, and peripheral edema. Other findings include nausea, vomiting, ascites, productive cough, crackles, weight gain, cool extremities, and cyanotic nail beds. Clinical signs are numerous and vary according to the stage of the disease and amount of cardiovascular impairment.

◆ *Hepatitis.* Liver enlargement from any type of hepatitis causes discomfort or dull pain and tenderness in the right upper quadrant. Associated signs and symptoms may include dark urine, clay-colored stools, nausea, vomiting, anorexia, jaundice, malaise, and pruritus.

◼ *Intestinal obstruction.* Short episodes of intense, colicky, cramping pain alternate with pain-free intervals in an intestinal obstruction, a life-threatening disorder. Accompanying signs and symptoms may include abdominal distention, tenderness, and guarding; visible peristaltic waves; high-pitched, tinkling, or hyperactive sounds proximal to the obstruction and hypoactive or absent sounds distally; obstipation; and pain-induced agitation. In jejunal and duodenal obstruction, nausea and bilious vomiting occur early. In distal small- or large-bowel obstruction, nausea and vomiting are commonly feculent. Complete obstruction produces absent bowel sounds. Late-stage obstruction produces signs of hypovolemic shock, such as hypotension and tachycardia.

◆ *Irritable bowel syndrome.* Lower abdominal cramping or pain is aggravated by ingestion of coarse or raw foods and may be alleviated by defecation or passage of flatus. Related findings include abdominal tenderness, diurnal diarrhea alternating with constipation or normal bowel function, and small stools with visible mucus. Dyspepsia, nausea, and abdominal distention with a feeling of incomplete evacuation may also occur. Stress, anxiety, and emotional lability intensify the symptoms.

◆ *Listeriosis.* A serious infection, listeriosis is caused by eating food contaminated with the bacterium *Listeria monocytogenes*. This food-borne illness primarily affects pregnant women, neonates, and those with weakened immune systems. Signs and symptoms include fever, myalgia, abdominal pain, nausea, vomiting, and diarrhea. If the infection spreads to the nervous system, meningitis may develop; signs and symptoms include fever, headache, nuchal rigidity, and change in the level of consciousness. *Listeriosis* infection during pregnancy may lead to premature delivery, infection of the neonate, or stillbirth.

◗ *Mesenteric artery ischemia.* Always suspect mesenteric artery ischemia in patients older than age 50 with chronic heart failure, cardiac arrhythmia, cardiovascular infarct, or hypotension who develop sudden, severe abdominal pain after 2 to 3 days of colicky periumbilical pain and diarrhea. Initially, the abdomen is soft and tender with decreased bowel sounds. Associated findings include vomiting, anorexia, alternating periods of diarrhea and constipation and, in late stages, extreme abdominal tenderness with rigidity, tachycardia, tachypnea, absent bowel sounds, and cool, clammy skin.

◆ *Ovarian cyst.* Torsion or hemorrhage causes pain and tenderness in the right or left lower quadrant. Sharp and severe if the patient suddenly stands or stoops, the pain becomes brief and intermittent if the torsion self-corrects or dull and diffuse after several hours if it doesn't. Pain is accompanied by slight fever, mild nausea and vomiting, abdominal tenderness, a palpable abdominal mass and, possibly, amenorrhea. Abdominal distention may occur if the patient has a large cyst. Peritoneal irritation, or rupture and ensuing peritonitis, causes high fever and severe nausea and vomiting.

◆ *Pelvic inflammatory disease.* In this disease, pain in the right or left lower quadrant ranges from vague discomfort worsened by movement to deep, severe, and progressive pain. Sometimes, metrorrhagia precedes or accompanies the onset of pain. Extreme pain accompanies cervical or adnexal palpation. Associated findings include abdominal tenderness, a palpable abdominal or pelvic mass, fever, occasional chills, nausea, vomiting, urinary discomfort, and abnormal vaginal bleeding or purulent vaginal discharge.

◗ *Perforated ulcer.* With perforated ulcer, sudden, severe, and prostrating epigastric pain may radiate through the abdomen to the back or right shoulder. Other signs and symptoms include boardlike abdominal rigidity, tenderness with guarding, generalized rebound tenderness, absent bowel sounds, grunting and shallow respirations and, in many cases, fever, tachycardia, hypotension, and syncope.

◗ *Peritonitis.* With peritonitis, sudden and severe pain can be diffuse or localized in the area of the underlying disorder; movement worsens the pain. The degree of abdominal tenderness usually varies according to the extent of disease. Typical findings include fever; chills; nausea; vomiting; hypoactive or absent bowel sounds; abdominal tenderness, distention, and rigidity; rebound tenderness and guarding; hyperalgesia; tachycardia; hypotension; tachypnea; and positive psoas and obturator signs.

◆ *Prostatitis.* Vague abdominal pain or discomfort in the lower abdomen, groin, perineum, or rectum may develop with prostatitis. Other findings include dysuria, urinary frequency and urgency, fever, chills, lower back pain, myalgia, arthralgia, and nocturia. Scrotal pain, penile pain, and pain on ejaculation may occur in chronic cases.

◆ *Pyelonephritis (acute).* Progressive lower quadrant pain in one or both sides, flank pain, and CVA tenderness characterize this disorder. Pain may radiate to the lower midabdomen or to the groin. Additional signs and symptoms include abdominal and back tenderness, high fever, shaking chills, nausea, vomiting, and urinary frequency and urgency.

◆ *Renal calculi.* Depending on the location of calculi, severe abdominal or back pain may occur. However, the classic symptom is severe, colicky pain that travels from the CVA to the flank, suprapubic region, and external genitalia. The pain may be excruciating or dull and constant. Pain-induced agitation, nausea, vomiting, abdominal distention, fever, chills, hypertension, and urinary urgency with hematuria and dysuria may occur.

◆ *Sickle cell crisis.* Sudden, severe abdominal pain may accompany chest, back, hand, or foot pain. Associated signs and symptoms include weakness, aching joints, dyspnea, and scleral jaundice.

◼ *Smallpox (variola major).* This virus is considered a potential agent for biological warfare. Initial signs and symptoms include high fever, malaise, prostration, severe headache, backache, and abdominal pain. A maculopapular rash develops on the mucosa of the mouth, pharynx, face, and forearms and then spreads to the trunk and legs. Within 2 days, the rash becomes vesicular and later pustular. The lesions develop at the same time, appear identical, and are more prominent on the face and extremities. The pustules are round, firm, and embedded in the skin. After 8 to 9 days, the pustules form a crust, and later the scab separates from the skin, leaving a pitted scar. In fatal cases, death results from encephalitis, extensive bleeding, or secondary infection.

◆ *Splenic infarction.* Fulminating pain in the left upper quadrant occurs along with chest pain that may worsen on inspiration. Pain usually radiates to the left shoulder with splinting of the left diaphragm, abdominal guarding and, occasionally, a splenic friction rub.

◆ *Ulcerative colitis.* Ulcerative colitis may begin with vague abdominal discomfort that leads to cramping lower abdominal pain. As the disorder progresses, pain may become steady and diffuse, increasing with movement and coughing. The most common symptom—recurrent and possibly severe diarrhea with blood, pus, and mucus—may relieve the pain. The abdomen may feel soft and extremely tender. High-pitched, infrequent bowel sounds may accompany nausea, vomiting, anorexia, weight loss, and mild, intermittent fever.

Abdominal rigidity

Detected by palpation, abdominal rigidity refers to abnormal muscle tension or inflexibility of the abdomen. Rigidity may be voluntary or involuntary. Voluntary rigidity reflects the patient's fear or nervousness on palpation; involuntary rigidity reflects potentially life-threatening peritoneal irritation or inflammation. (See *Recognizing voluntary rigidity,* page 78.)

Involuntary rigidity most commonly results from GI disorders but may also result from pulmonary and vascular disorders and from the effects of insect toxins. Usually, it's accompanied by fever, nausea, vomiting, and abdominal tenderness, distention, and pain.

Assessment

After palpating abdominal rigidity, quickly take the patient's vital signs. Even though the patient may not appear gravely ill or have markedly abnormal vital signs, abdominal rigidity calls for emergency interventions. (See *Responding to abdominal rigidity,* page 79.)

If the patient's condition allows further assessment, take a brief history. Find out when the abdominal rigidity began. Is it associated with abdominal pain? If so, did the pain begin at the same time? Determine whether the abdominal rigidity is localized or generalized. Is it always present? Has its site changed or remained constant? Next, ask about aggravating or alleviating factors, such as position changes, coughing, vomiting, elimination, and walking.

Explore other signs and symptoms. Inspect the abdomen for peristaltic waves, which may be visible in very thin patients. Also check for a visibly distended bowel loop. Next, auscultate bowel sounds. Avoid palpation because it may exacerbate abdominal pain and rupture an inflamed organ. Finally, check for poor skin turgor and dry mucous membranes, which indicate dehydration.

Causes

◆ *Abdominal aortic aneurysm (dissecting).* Mild to moderate abdominal rigidity occurs with abdominal aortic aneurysm, a life-threatening disorder. Typically, it's accompanied by constant upper abdominal pain that may radiate to the lower back. The pain may worsen when the patient lies down and may be relieved when he leans forward or sits up. Before rupture, the aneurysm may produce a pulsating mass in the epigastrium, accompanied by a systolic bruit over the aorta. However, the mass stops pulsating after rupture. Associated signs and symptoms include mottled skin below the waist, absent femoral and pedal pulses, lower blood pressure in the legs than in the arms, and mild to moderate tenderness with guarding. Significant blood loss causes signs of shock, such as hypotension, tachycardia, tachypnea, and cool, clammy skin.

◆ *Insect toxins.* Insect stings and bites, especially black widow spider bites, release toxins that can produce generalized, cramping abdominal pain, usually accompanied by rigidity. These toxins may also cause a low-grade fever, nausea, vomiting, tremors, and burning sensations in the hands and feet. Some patients develop increased salivation, hypertension, paresis, and hyperactive reflexes. Children commonly are restless, have an expiratory grunt, and keep their legs flexed.

◆ *Mesenteric artery ischemia.* A life-threatening disorder, mesenteric artery ischemia is characterized by 2 to 3 days of persistent, low-grade abdominal pain and diarrhea leading to sudden, severe abdominal pain and rigidity. Rigidity occurs in the central or periumbilical region and is accompanied by severe abdominal tenderness,

EMERGENCY INTERVENTIONS

Responding to abdominal rigidity

If you detect abdominal rigidity in your patient:
◆ Take his vital signs.
◆ Prepare to administer oxygen.
◆ Prepare to insert an I.V. line for fluid and blood replacement.
◆ Administer drugs to support blood pressure as prescribed.

◆ Prepare to insert an indwelling urinary catheter.
◆ Monitor intake and output closely.
◆ Obtain blood specimens for testing as prescribed.
◆ Prepare the patient for X-rays.
◆ Prepare the patient for emergency surgery, if indicated.

---

fever, and signs of shock, such as tachycardia and hypotension. Other findings may include vomiting, anorexia, and diarrhea or constipation. Always suspect this disorder in patients older than age 50 who have a history of heart failure, arrhythmia, cardiovascular infarct, or hypotension.

◪ *Peritonitis.* Depending on the cause of peritonitis, abdominal rigidity may be localized or generalized. For example, if an inflamed appendix causes local peritonitis, rigidity may be localized in the right lower quadrant. If a perforated ulcer causes widespread peritonitis, rigidity may be generalized and, in severe cases, boardlike.

Peritonitis also causes sudden and severe abdominal pain that can be localized or generalized. In addition, it can produce abdominal tenderness and distention, rebound tenderness, guarding, hyperalgesia, hypoactive or absent bowel sounds, nausea, and vomiting. Usually, the patient displays fever, chills, tachycardia, tachypnea, and hypotension.

Accessory muscle use

When breathing requires extra effort, the accessory muscles—the sternocleidomastoid, scalene, pectoralis major,

trapezius, internal intercostals, and abdominal muscles—stabilize the thorax during respiration. Some accessory muscle use normally takes place during such activities as singing, talking, coughing, defecating, and exercising. (See *Accessory muscles: Locations and functions,* page 80.) However, more pronounced use of these muscles may signal acute respiratory distress, diaphragmatic weakness, or fatigue. It may also result from chronic respiratory disease. Typically, the extent of accessory muscle use reflects the severity of the underlying cause.

Assessment

If the patient displays increased accessory muscle use, immediately look for signs of acute respiratory distress. These include a decreased level of consciousness, shortness of breath when speaking, tachypnea, intercostal and sternal retractions, cyanosis, adventitious breath sounds (such as wheezing or stridor), diaphoresis, nasal flaring, and extreme apprehension or agitation. Quickly auscultate for abnormal, diminished, or absent breath sounds. Check for airway obstruction and, if detected, attempt to restore airway patency and then begin emergency inter-

Accessory muscles: Locations and functions

Physical exertion and pulmonary disease usually increase the work of breathing, taxing the diaphragm and external intercostal muscles. When this happens, accessory muscles provide the extra effort needed to maintain respirations. The upper accessory muscles assist with inspiration, whereas the upper chest, sternum, internal intercostal, and abdominal muscles assist with expiration.

With inspiration, the scalene muscles elevate, fix, and expand the upper chest. The sternocleidomastoid muscles raise the sternum, expanding the chest's anteroposterior and longitudinal dimensions. The pectoralis major elevates the chest, increasing its anteroposterior size, and the trapezius raises the thoracic cage.

With expiration, the internal intercostals depress the ribs, decreasing the chest size. The abdominal muscles pull the lower chest down, depress the lower ribs, and compress the abdominal contents, which exerts pressure on the chest.

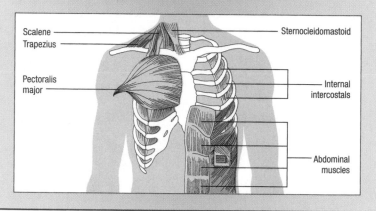

ventions. (See *Responding to increased accessory muscle use.*)

If the patient's condition allows, examine him more closely. Ask him about the onset, duration, and severity of associated signs and symptoms, such as dyspnea, chest pain, cough, or fever.

Explore his medical history, focusing on respiratory disorders, such as infection or chronic obstructive pulmonary disease (COPD). Ask about cardiac disorders, such as heart failure, which may lead to pulmonary edema; also inquire about neuromuscular disorders, such as amyotrophic lateral sclerosis, which may affect respiratory

muscle function. Note a history of allergies or asthma. Because collagen vascular diseases can cause diffuse infiltrative lung disease, ask about such conditions as rheumatoid arthritis and lupus erythematosus.

Ask about recent trauma, especially to the spine or chest. Find out whether the patient has recently undergone pulmonary function tests or received respiratory therapy. Ask about smoking and occupational exposure to chemical fumes or mineral dusts such as asbestos. Explore the family history for such disorders as cystic fibrosis and neurofibromatosis, which can cause diffuse infiltrative lung disease.

EMERGENCY INTERVENTIONS

Responding to increased accessory muscle use

If you notice a patient's accessory muscle use has increased:
◆ Open the patient's airway.
◆ Insert an oral airway and prepare for endotracheal intubation, if necessary.
◆ Assess the patient's oxygen saturation using a pulse oximeter.
◆ Administer oxygen as prescribed.
◆ Insert an I.V. catheter as prescribed.

If the patient has chronic obstructive pulmonary disease (COPD), use a low flow rate of oxygen for mild exacerbations. However, you may need to use a high flow rate initially. In such cases, be attentive to the patient's respiratory drive; giving a patient with COPD too much oxygen may decrease respiratory drive.

Perform a detailed chest examination, noting an abnormal respiratory rate, pattern, or depth. Assess the color, temperature, and turgor of the patient's skin, and check for clubbing.

Causes

◆ *Acute respiratory distress syndrome (ARDS)*. In ARDS, a life-threatening disorder, accessory muscle use increases in response to hypoxia. It's accompanied by intercostal, supracostal, and sternal retractions on inspiration and by grunting on expiration. Other characteristics include tachypnea, dyspnea, diaphoresis, diffuse crackles, and a cough with pink, frothy sputum. Worsening hypoxia produces anxiety, tachycardia, and mental sluggishness.

◆ *Airway obstruction.* Acute upper airway obstruction can be life-threatening—fortunately, most obstructions are subacute or chronic. Typically, this disorder increases accessory muscle use. Its most telling sign, however, is inspiratory stridor. Associated signs and symptoms include dyspnea, tachypnea, gasping, wheezing, coughing, drooling, intercostal retractions, cyanosis, and tachycardia.

◆ *Amyotrophic lateral sclerosis.* Typically, this progressive motor neuron disorder affects the diaphragm more than the accessory muscles. As a result, increased accessory muscle use is characteristic. Other signs and symptoms include fasciculations, muscle atrophy and weakness, spasticity, bilateral Babinski's reflex, and hyperactive deep tendon reflexes. Incoordination makes carrying out routine activities difficult for the patient. Associated signs and symptoms include impaired speech, difficulty chewing or swallowing and breathing, urinary frequency and urgency and, occasionally, choking and excessive drooling. (*Note:* Other neuromuscular disorders may produce similar signs and symptoms.) Although the patient's mental status remains intact, his poor prognosis may cause periodic depression.

◆ *Asthma.* During acute asthma attacks, the patient usually displays increased accessory muscle use. Accompanying it are severe dyspnea, tachypnea, wheezing, a productive cough, nasal flaring, and cyanosis. Auscultation reveals faint or possibly absent breath sounds, musical crackles, and rhonchi. Other signs and symptoms include tachycardia, diaphoresis, and apprehension caused by air hunger. Chronic asthma may also cause barrel chest.

◆ *Chronic bronchitis.* With chronic bronchitis, a form of COPD, increased accessory muscle use may be chronic and is preceded by a productive cough and exertional dyspnea. Chronic bronchitis is accompanied by wheezing, basal crackles, tachypnea, jugular vein distention, prolonged expiration, barrel chest, and clubbing. Cyanosis and weight gain from edema account for the characteristic label of "blue bloater." A low-grade fever may occur with secondary infection.

◆ *Emphysema.* Increased accessory muscle use occurs with progressive exertional dyspnea and a minimally productive cough in this form of COPD. Sometimes called a "pink puffer," the patient will display pursed-lip breathing and tachypnea. Associated signs and symptoms include peripheral cyanosis, anorexia, weight loss, malaise, barrel chest, and clubbing. Auscultation reveals distant heart sounds; percussion detects hyperresonance.

◆ *Pneumonia.* Bacterial pneumonia usually produces increased accessory muscle use. Initially, this infection causes a sudden high fever with chills. Its associated signs and symptoms include chest pain, a productive cough, dyspnea, tachypnea, tachycardia, expiratory grunting, cyanosis, diaphoresis, and fine crackles.

◆ *Pulmonary edema.* With acute pulmonary edema, increased accessory muscle use is accompanied by dyspnea, tachypnea, orthopnea, crepitant crackles, wheezing, and a cough with pink, frothy sputum. Other findings include restlessness, tachycardia, ventricular gallop, and cool, clammy, cyanotic skin.

◆ *Pulmonary embolism.* Although signs and symptoms vary with the size, number, and location of the emboli, pulmonary embolism is a life-threatening disorder that may cause increased accessory muscle use. Typically, it produces dyspnea and tachypnea that may be accompanied by pleuritic or substernal chest pain. Other signs and symptoms include restlessness, anxiety, tachycardia, a productive cough, a low-grade fever and, with a large embolus, hemoptysis, cyanosis, syncope, jugular vein distention, scattered crackles, and focal wheezing.

◆ *Spinal cord injury.* Increased accessory muscle use may occur, depending on the location and severity of the injury. An injury below L1 typically doesn't affect the diaphragm or accessory muscles, whereas an injury between C3 and C5 affects the upper respiratory muscles and diaphragm, causing increased accessory muscle use.

Associated signs and symptoms of spinal cord injury include unilateral or bilateral Babinski's reflex, hyperactive deep tendon reflexes, spasticity, and variable or total loss of pain and temperature sensation, proprioception, and motor function. Horner's syndrome (unilateral ptosis, pupillary constriction, facial anhidrosis) may occur with lower cervical cord injury.

◆ *Thoracic injury.* Increased accessory muscle use may occur, depending on the type and extent of injury. Associated signs and symptoms of this potentially life-threatening injury include an obvious chest wound or bruising, chest pain, dyspnea, cyanosis, and agitation. Signs of shock, such as tachycardia and hypotension, occur with significant blood loss.

Agitation

Agitation refers to a state of hyperarousal, increased tension, and irritability that can lead to confusion, hyperactivity, and overt hostility. Agitation can result from a toxic (poisons), metabolic, or infectious cause; brain injury;

or a psychiatric disorder. It can also result from hypoxia, pain, fever, anxiety, drug use and withdrawal, hypersensitivity reactions, and various disorders. It can arise gradually or suddenly and last for minutes or months. Whether it's mild or severe, agitation worsens with increased hypoxia, fever, pain, stress, or external stimuli.

Agitation alone merely signals a change in the patient's condition. However, it's a useful indicator of a developing disorder. Obtaining a good history is critical to determining the underlying cause of agitation.

Assessment

Determine the severity of the patient's agitation by examining the number and quality of agitation-induced behaviors, such as emotional lability, confusion, memory loss, hyperactivity, and hostility. Obtain a history from the patient or a family member, including diet, known allergies, and use of herbal medicine.

Ask whether the patient is being treated for an illness. Has he had recent infections, trauma, stress, or changes in sleep patterns? Ask the patient about prescribed or over-the-counter drug use, including supplements and herbal medicines. Check for signs of drug abuse, such as needle tracks and dilated pupils. Ask about alcohol intake. Obtain the patient's baseline vital signs and neurologic status for future comparison.

Causes

◆ *Alcohol withdrawal syndrome.* Mild to severe agitation occurs in alcohol withdrawal syndrome, along with hyperactivity, tremors, and anxiety. With delirium, the potentially life-threatening stage of alcohol withdrawal, severe agitation accompanies hallucinations, insomnia, diaphoresis, and a depressed mood. The patient's pulse rate and temperature rise as withdrawal progresses; status epilepticus, cardiac exhaustion, and shock can occur.

◆ *Anxiety.* Anxiety produces varying degrees of agitation. The patient may be unaware of his anxiety or may complain of it without knowing its cause. Other findings include nausea, vomiting, diarrhea, cool and clammy skin, frontal headache, back pain, insomnia, and tremors.

◆ *Dementia.* Mild to severe agitation can result from many common syndromes, such as Alzheimer's and Huntington's diseases. The patient may display a decrease in memory, attention span, problem-solving ability, and alertness. Hypoactivity, wandering behavior, hallucinations, aphasia, and insomnia may also occur.

◆ *Drugs.* Mild to moderate agitation, which is commonly dose related, develops as an adverse reaction to central nervous system stimulants—especially appetite suppressants, such as amphetamines and amphetamine-like drugs; sympathomimetics, such as ephedrine; caffeine; and theophylline.

◆ *Drug withdrawal syndrome.* Mild to severe agitation occurs in drug withdrawal syndrome. Related findings vary with the drug but include anxiety, abdominal cramps, diaphoresis, and anorexia. With opioid or barbiturate withdrawal, a decreased level of consciousness (LOC), seizures, and elevated blood pressure, heart rate, and respiratory rate can also occur.

◆ *Hepatic encephalopathy.* Agitation occurs only with fulminating encephalopathy. Other findings include drowsiness, stupor, fetor hepaticus, asterixis, and hyperreflexia.

◼ *Hypersensitivity reaction.* Moderate to severe agitation appears, possibly as the first sign of a hypersensitivity reaction. Depending on the severity of the reaction, agitation may be accompanied by urticaria, pruritus, and facial and dependent edema.

With anaphylactic shock, a potentially life-threatening reaction, agitation occurs rapidly along with apprehension, urticaria or diffuse erythema, warm and moist skin, paresthesia, pruritus, edema, dyspnea, wheezing, stridor, hypotension, and tachycardia. Abdominal cramps, vomiting, and diarrhea can also occur.

◖ *Hypoxemia.* Beginning as restlessness, agitation rapidly worsens. The patient may be confused and have impaired judgment and motor coordination. He may also have tachycardia, tachypnea, dyspnea, and cyanosis.

◖ *Increased intracranial pressure (ICP).* Agitation usually precedes other early signs and symptoms of increased ICP, such as headache, nausea, and vomiting. Increased ICP also produces respiratory changes, such as Cheyne-Stokes, cluster, ataxic, or apneustic breathing; sluggish, nonreactive, or unequal pupils; widening pulse pressure; tachycardia; decreased LOC; seizures; and such motor changes as decerebrate or decorticate posture.

◆ *Post–head trauma syndrome.* Shortly after, or even years after, a head injury, mild to severe agitation develops, characterized by disorientation, loss of concentration, angry outbursts, and emotional lability. Other findings include fatigue, wandering behavior, and poor judgment.

◆ *Radiographic contrast media.* Reaction to the contrast medium injected during various diagnostic tests produces moderate to severe agitation along with other signs of hypersensitivity.

◆ *Vitamin B_6 deficiency.* Agitation can range from mild to severe. Other effects include seizures, peripheral paresthesia, and dermatitis. Oculogyric crisis (rotation of the eyeballs) may also occur.

Amenorrhea

Amenorrhea, the absence of menstrual flow, can be classified as primary or secondary. With primary amenorrhea, menstruation fails to begin before age 16. With secondary amenorrhea, it begins at an appropriate age but later ceases for 3 or more months in the absence of normal physiologic causes, such as pregnancy, lactation, or menopause.

Pathologic amenorrhea results from anovulation or physical obstruction to menstrual outflow, such as from an imperforate hymen, cervical stenosis, or intrauterine adhesions. Anovulation itself may result from hormonal imbalance, debilitating disease, stress or emotional disturbances, strenuous exercise, malnutrition, obesity, or anatomic abnormalities, such as a congenital absence of the ovaries or uterus. Amenorrhea may also result from drug or hormonal treatments.

Assessment

Begin by determining whether the amenorrhea is primary or secondary. If it's primary, ask the patient at what age her mother first menstruated because age of menarche is fairly consistent in families. Form an overall impression of the patient's physical, mental, and emotional development because these factors as well as heredity and climate may delay menarche until after age 16.

If menstruation began at an appropriate age but has since ceased, determine the frequency and duration of the patient's previous menses. Ask her about the onset and nature of changes in her normal menstrual pattern, and determine the date of her last menses. Find out if she has noticed related signs, such as breast swelling or weight changes.

Determine when the patient last had a physical examination. Review her health history, noting especially long-term illnesses, such as anemia, or use of hormonal contraceptives. Ask about exercise habits, especially running, and whether she experiences stress on the job or at home. Probe the patient's eating habits, including the number and size of daily meals and snacks, and ask whether she has gained weight recently.

Observe her appearance for secondary sex characteristics or signs of virilization. If you're responsible for performing a pelvic examination, check for anatomic aberrations of the outflow tract, such as cervical adhesions, fibroids, or an imperforate hymen.

Causes

◆ *Adrenal tumor.* Amenorrhea may be accompanied by acne, thinning scalp hair, hirsutism, increased blood pressure, truncal obesity, and psychotic changes. Asymmetrical ovarian enlargement in conjunction with the rapid onset of virilizing signs is usually indicative of an adrenal tumor.

◆ *Adrenocortical hyperplasia.* Amenorrhea precedes characteristic cushingoid signs, such as truncal obesity, moon face, buffalo hump, bruises, purple striae, hypertension, renal calculi, psychiatric disturbances, and widened pulse pressure. Acne, thinning scalp hair, and hirsutism typically appear.

◆ *Adrenocortical hypofunction.* In addition to amenorrhea, adrenocortical hypofunction may cause fatigue, irritability, weight loss, increased pigmentation (including bluish black discoloration of the areolas and mucous membranes of the lips, mouth, rectum, and vagina), nausea, vomiting, and orthostatic hypotension.

◆ *Amenorrhea-lactation disorders.* Amenorrhea-lactation disorders, such as Forbes-Albright syndrome (rare endocrine disorder caused by a hormone-secreting tumor of the hypothalamus or pituitary gland that produces excessive amounts of prolactin) and Chiari-Frommel syndrome (rare endocrine disorder that affects women who have recently given birth, in which prolactin secretion is continued and gonadotropin production is decreased), produce secondary amenorrhea accompanied by lactation in the absence of breast-feeding. Associated features include hot flashes, dyspareunia, vaginal atrophy, and large, engorged breasts.

◆ *Anorexia nervosa.* Anorexia nervosa is a psychological disorder that can cause either primary or secondary amenorrhea. Related findings include significant weight loss, a thin or emaciated appearance, compulsive behavior patterns, a blotchy or sallow complexion, constipation, reduced libido, decreased pleasure in once-enjoyable activities, dry skin, loss of scalp hair, lanugo on the face and arms, skeletal muscle atrophy, and sleep disturbances.

◆ *Congenital absence of the ovaries.* This condition results in primary amenorrhea and the absence of secondary sex characteristics.

◆ *Congenital absence of the uterus.* Primary amenorrhea occurs with congenital absence of the uterus; however, the patient may develop breasts.

◆ *Corpus luteum cysts.* Corpus luteum cysts may cause sudden amenorrhea as well as acute abdominal pain and breast swelling. Examination may reveal a tender adnexal mass and vaginal and cervical hyperemia.

◆ *Drugs.* Busulfan, chlorambucil, injectable or implanted contraceptives, cyclophosphamide, and phenothiazines may cause amenorrhea. Hormonal contraceptives may cause anovulation and amenorrhea after they're discontinued.

◆ *Hypothalamic tumor.* In addition to amenorrhea, a hypothalamic tumor can cause endocrine and visual field defects, gonadal underdevelopment or dysfunction, and short stature.

◆ *Hypothyroidism.* Deficient thyroid hormone levels can cause primary or secondary amenorrhea. Typically vague, early findings include fatigue, forgetfulness, cold intolerance, unexplained weight gain, and constipation. Subsequent signs include bradycardia; decreased mental acuity; dry, flaky, inelastic skin; puffy face, hands, and feet; hoarseness; periorbital edema; ptosis; dry, sparse hair; and thick, brittle nails. Other common findings include anorexia, abdominal distention, decreased libido, ataxia, intention tremor, nystagmus, and delayed reflex relaxation time, especially in the Achilles tendon.

◆ *Mosaicism.* Mosaicism, a condition in which an individual has two or more cell lines that differ genetically, results in primary amenorrhea and the absence of secondary sex characteristics.

◆ *Ovarian insensitivity to gonadotropins.* A hormonal disturbance, ovarian insensitivity to gonadotropins leads to amenorrhea and an absence of secondary sex characteristics.

◆ *Pituitary tumor.* Amenorrhea may be the first sign of a pituitary tumor. Associated findings include headache; vision disturbances such as bitemporal hemianopsia; and acromegaly. Cushingoid signs include moon face, buffalo hump, hirsutism, hypertension, truncal obesity, bruises, purple striae, widened pulse pressure, and psychiatric disturbances.

◆ *Polycystic ovary syndrome.* Typically, menarche occurs at a normal age, followed by irregular menstrual cycles, oligomenorrhea, and secondary amenorrhea. Or, periods of profuse bleeding may alternate with periods of amenorrhea. Obesity, hirsutism, slight deepening of the voice, and enlarged, "oyster-like" ovaries may also accompany this disorder.

◆ *Pseudoamenorrhea.* An anatomic anomaly, such as imperforate hymen, obstructs menstrual flow, causing primary amenorrhea and, possibly, cyclic episodes of abdominal pain. Examination may reveal a pink or blue bulging hymen.

◆ *Pseudocyesis.* With pseudocyesis, amenorrhea may be accompanied by lordosis, abdominal distention, nausea, and breast enlargement.

◆ *Radiation therapy.* Irradiation of the abdomen may destroy the endometrium or ovaries, causing amenorrhea.

◆ *Surgery.* Surgical removal of both ovaries or the uterus produces amenorrhea.

◆ *Testicular feminization.* Primary amenorrhea may signal this form of male pseudohermaphroditism. The patient, outwardly female but genetically male, shows breast and external genital development but scant or absent pubic hair.

◆ *Thyrotoxicosis.* Thyroid hormone overproduction may result in amenorrhea. Classic signs and symptoms include an enlarged thyroid (goiter), nervousness, heat intolerance, diaphoresis, tremors, palpitations, tachycardia, dyspnea, weakness, and weight loss despite increased appetite.

◆ *Turner's syndrome.* Primary amenorrhea and failure to develop secondary sex characteristics may signal this syndrome of genetic ovarian dysgenesis. Typical features include short stature, webbing of the neck, low nuchal hairline, a broad chest with widely spaced nipples and poor breast development, underdeveloped genitalia, and edema of the legs and feet.

◆ *Uterine hypoplasia.* Primary amenorrhea results from underdevelopment of the uterus, which is detectable on physical examination.

Amnesia

Amnesia—a disturbance in, or loss of, memory—may be classified as partial or complete and as anterograde or retrograde. Anterograde amnesia denotes memory loss of events that occurred after the onset of the causative trauma or disease; retrograde amnesia, memory loss of events that occurred before the onset. Depending on the cause, amnesia may arise suddenly or slowly and may be temporary or permanent.

Organic (or true) amnesia results from temporal lobe dysfunction, and it characteristically spares patches of memory. A common symptom in patients with seizures or head trauma, organic amnesia can also be an early indicator of Alzheimer's disease. Hysterical amnesia has a psychogenic origin and characteristically causes complete memory loss. Treatment-induced amnesia is usually transient.

Assessment

Because the patient typically isn't aware of his amnesia, you'll usually need help in gathering information from his family or friends. Throughout your assessment, notice the patient's general appearance, behavior, mood, and train of thought. Ask when the amnesia first appeared and what the patient is unable to remember. Can he learn new information? How long does he remember it? Does the amnesia encompass a recent or remote period?

Test the patient's recent memory by asking him to identify and repeat three items. Retest after 3 minutes. Test his intermediate memory by asking, "Who was the president before this one?" and "What was the last type of car you bought?" Test remote memory with such questions as "How old are you?" and "Where were you born?"

Take the patient's vital signs and assess his level of consciousness (LOC). Check his pupils; they should be equal in size and should constrict quickly when exposed to direct light. Also assess his extraocular movements. Test motor function by having the patient move his arms and legs through their range of motion. Evaluate sensory function with pinpricks on the patient's skin.

Causes

◆ *Alzheimer's disease.* Alzheimer's disease usually begins with retrograde amnesia, which progresses slowly over many months or years to include anterograde amnesia, producing severe and permanent memory loss. Associated findings include agitation, inability to concentrate, disregard for personal hygiene, confusion, irritability, and emotional lability. Later signs include aphasia, dementia, incontinence, and muscle rigidity.

◪ *Cerebral hypoxia.* After recovery from hypoxia (brought on by such conditions as carbon monoxide poisoning or acute respiratory failure), the patient may experience total amnesia for the event, along with sensory disturbances, such as numbness and tingling.

◆ *Drugs.* Anterograde amnesia can be precipitated by general anesthetics, especially fentanyl, halothane, and isoflurane; barbiturates, most commonly pentobarbital and thiopental; and certain benzodiazepines, especially triazolam.

◆ *Electroconvulsive therapy.* The sudden onset of retrograde or anterograde amnesia occurs with electroconvulsive therapy. Typically, the amnesia lasts for several minutes to several hours, but severe, prolonged amnesia occurs with treatments given frequently over a prolonged period.

◪ *Head trauma.* Depending on the trauma's severity, amnesia may last for minutes, hours, or longer. Usually, the patient experiences brief retrograde and longer anterograde amnesia as well as persistent amnesia about the traumatic event. 'Severe head trauma can cause permanent amnesia or difficulty retaining recent memories. Related findings may include altered respirations and LOC; headache; dizziness; confusion; visual disturbances, such as blurred or double vision; and motor and sensory disturbances, such as hemiparesis and paresthesia, on the side of the body opposite the injury.

◆ *Herpes simplex encephalitis.* Recovery from herpes simplex encephalitis commonly leaves the patient with severe and possibly permanent amnesia. Associated findings include signs and symptoms of meningeal irritation, such as headache, fever, and altered LOC, along with seizures and various motor and sensory disturbances (such as paresis, numbness, and tingling).

◆ *Hysteria.* Hysterical amnesia, a complete and long-lasting memory loss, begins and ends abruptly and is typically accompanied by confusion.

◆ *Seizures.* In temporal lobe seizures, amnesia occurs suddenly and lasts for several seconds to minutes. The patient may recall an aura or nothing at all. An irritable focus on the left side of the brain primarily causes amnesia for verbal memories, whereas an irritable focus on the right side of the brain causes graphic and nonverbal amnesia. Associated signs and symptoms may include decreased LOC during the seizure, confusion, abnormal mouth movements, and visual, olfactory, and auditory hallucinations.

◆ *Temporal lobe surgery.* Usually performed on only one lobe, this surgery causes brief, slight amnesia. However, removal of both lobes results in permanent amnesia.

◆ *Wernicke-Korsakoff syndrome.* Retrograde and anterograde amnesia can become permanent without treatment in this syndrome. Accompanying signs and symptoms include apathy, an inability to concentrate or to put events into sequence, and confabulation to fill memory gaps. The syndrome may also cause diplopia, decreased LOC, headache, ataxia, and symptoms of peripheral neuropathy, such as numbness and tingling.

Analgesia

Analgesia, the absence of sensitivity to pain, is a sign of central nervous system disease, commonly indicating a specific type and location of spinal cord lesion. It always occurs with loss of temperature sensation (thermanesthesia) because these sensory nerve impulses travel together in the spinal cord. It can also occur with other sensory deficits—such as paresthesia, loss of proprioception and vibratory sense, and tactile anesthesia—in various disorders involving the peripheral nerves, spinal cord, and brain. However, when accompanied only by thermanesthesia, analgesia points to an incomplete lesion of the spinal cord. (See *Suspected spinal cord injury.*)

Analgesia can be classified as partial or total below the level of the lesion and as unilateral or bilateral, depending on the cause and level of the lesion. Its onset may be slow and progressive with a tumor or abrupt with trauma. Transient in many cases, analgesia may resolve spontaneously.

Assessment

After you're satisfied that the patient's spine and respiratory status are stabilized—or if the analgesia isn't severe and isn't accompanied by signs of spinal cord injury—perform a physical assessment and baseline neurologic evaluation. First, take the patient's vital signs and assess his level of con-

EMERGENCY INTERVENTIONS

Suspected spinal cord injury

If you suspect a spinal cord injury, you must take emergency measures to protect your patient. Follow these steps:
◆ Immobilize his spine in proper alignment using a cervical collar and a long backboard, if possible.
◆ If a cervical collar isn't available, assist the patient into a supine position on a flat surface and place sandbags around his head, neck, and torso.
◆ Use correct technique and extreme caution when moving the patient to prevent exacerbating spinal injury.

◆ Continuously monitor respiratory rate and rhythm.
◆ Observe the patient for accessory muscle use because a complete lesion above the T6 level may cause diaphragmatic and intercostal muscle paralysis.
◆ Have an artificial airway and a handheld resuscitation bag immediately available.
◆ Be prepared to initiate emergency resuscitation measures in case of respiratory failure.

sciousness. Then test pupillary, corneal, cough, and gag reflexes to rule out brain stem and cranial nerve involvement. If the patient is conscious, evaluate his speech and ability to swallow.

If possible, observe the patient's gait and posture and assess his balance and coordination. Evaluate muscle tone and strength in all extremities. Test for other sensory deficits over all dermatomes (individual skin segments innervated by a specific spinal nerve) by applying light tactile stimulation with a tongue depressor or cotton swab. Perform a more thorough check of pain sensitivity, if necessary, using a pin. Tell the patient to relax, and explain that you're going to lightly touch areas of his skin with a small pin. Have him close his eyes. Apply the pin firmly enough to produce pain without breaking the skin. (See *Testing for analgesia*, page 90.) Also, test temperature sensation over all dermatomes, using two test tubes—one filled with hot water, the other with cold water. In each arm and leg, test vibration sense (using a tuning fork), proprioception, and su-

perficial and deep tendon reflexes (DTRs). Check for increased muscle tone by extending and flexing the patient's elbows and knees as he tries to relax.

Focus your history taking on the onset of analgesia (sudden or gradual) and on a recent trauma—a fall, sports injury, or automobile accident. Obtain a complete medical history, noting especially an incidence of cancer in the patient or his family.

Causes

◆ *Anterior cord syndrome.* With anterior cord syndrome, analgesia and thermanesthesia occur bilaterally below the level of the lesion, along with flaccid paralysis and hypoactive DTRs.
◪ *Central cord syndrome.* Typically, analgesia and thermanesthesia occur bilaterally in several dermatomes, in many cases extending in a capelike fashion over the arms, back, and shoulders. Early weakness in the hands progresses to weakness and muscle spasms in the arms and shoulder girdle. Hyperactive DTRs and spastic

Testing for analgesia

By carefully and systematically testing the patient's sensitivity to pain, you can determine whether his nerve damage has a segmental or peripheral distribution and help locate the causative lesion.

Starting with the patient's head and face, move down his body, pricking his skin on al-ternating sides. Have the patient report when he feels pain. Use the blunt end of the pin occasionally, and vary your test pattern to gauge the accuracy of his response.

Document your findings thoroughly, clearly marking areas of lost pain sensation on a dermatome chart (shown below).

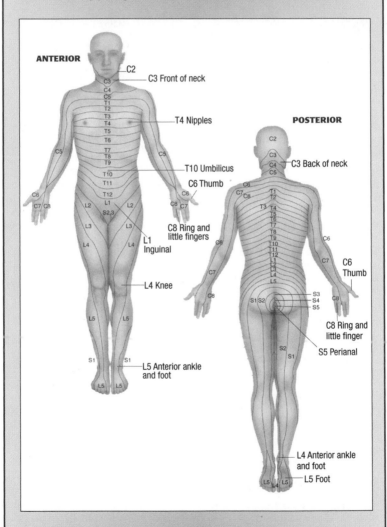

weakness of the legs may develop. However, if the lesion affects the lumbar spine, hypoactive DTRs and flaccid weakness may persist in the legs.

With brain stem involvement, additional findings include facial analgesia and thermanesthesia, vertigo, nystagmus, atrophy of the tongue, and dysarthria. The patient may also have dysphagia, urine retention, anhidrosis, decreased intestinal motility, and hyperkeratosis.

◆ *Drugs.* Analgesia may occur with use of a topical or local anesthetic, although numbness and tingling are more common.

◆ *Spinal cord hemisection.* Contralateral analgesia and thermanesthesia occur below the level of the lesion. In addition, loss of proprioception, spastic paralysis, and hyperactive DTRs develop ipsilaterally. The patient may also experience urine retention with overflow incontinence.

Anhidrosis

Anhidrosis, an abnormal deficiency of sweat, can be classified as generalized (complete) or localized (partial). Generalized anhidrosis can lead to life-threatening impairment of thermoregulation. Localized anhidrosis rarely interferes with thermoregulation because it affects only a small percentage of the body's eccrine (sweat) glands.

Anhidrosis results from neurologic and skin disorders; congenital, atrophic, or traumatic changes to sweat glands; and the use of certain drugs. Neurologic disorders disturb central or peripheral nervous pathways that normally activate sweating, causing retention of excess body heat and perspiration. The absence, obstruction, atrophy, or degeneration of sweat glands can produce anhidrosis at the skin surface, even if neurologic stimulation is normal. (See *Eccrine dysfunction in anhidrosis,* pages 92 and 93.)

Anhidrosis may go unrecognized until significant heat or exertion fails to raise sweat. However, localized anhidrosis commonly provokes compensatory hyperhidrosis in the remaining functional sweat glands—which, in many cases, is the patient's chief complaint.

Assessment

If you detect anhidrosis in a patient whose skin feels hot and flushed, ask him whether he's also experiencing nausea, dizziness, palpitations, and substernal tightness. If he is, quickly take his rectal temperature and other vital signs and assess his level of consciousness. If a rectal temperature higher than 102.2° F (39° C) is accompanied by tachycardia, tachypnea, and altered blood pressure and LOC, suspect life-threatening anhidrotic asthenia (heatstroke). If you suspect anhidrotic asthenia, you must intervene quickly. (See *Suspected anhidrotic asthenia,* page 94.)

If anhidrosis is localized or if the patient reports local hyperhidrosis or unexplained fever, take a brief history. Ask the patient to characterize his sweating during heat spells or strenuous activity. Does he usually sweat slightly or profusely? Ask about recent prolonged or extreme exposure to heat and about the onset of anhidrosis or hyperhidrosis. Obtain a complete medical history, focusing on neurologic disorders; skin disorders such as psoriasis; autoimmune disorders such as scleroderma; systemic diseases that can cause peripheral neuropathies, such as diabetes mellitus; and drug use.

Inspect skin color, texture, and turgor. If you detect skin lesions, document their location, size, color, texture, and pattern.

Eccrine dysfunction in anhidrosis

Eccrine glands, located over most of the skin, help regulate body temperature by secreting sweat. A change or dysfunction in these glands can result in anhidrosis of varying severity. These illustrations show a normal eccrine gland and some common abnormalities.

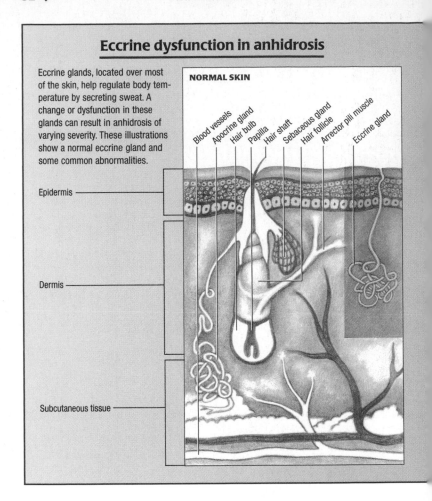

Causes

◆ *Anhidrotic asthenia (heatstroke).* A life-threatening disorder, anhidrotic asthenia causes acute, generalized anhidrosis. In early stages, sweating may still occur and the patient may be rational, but his rectal temperature may already exceed 102.2° F (39° C). Associated signs and symptoms include severe headache and muscle cramps, which later disappear; fatigue; nausea and vomiting; dizziness; palpitations; substernal tightness; and elevated blood pressure followed by hypotension. Within minutes, anhidrosis and hot, flushed skin develop, accompanied by tachycardia, tachypnea, and confusion progressing to seizure or loss of consciousness.

◆ *Burns.* Depending on their severity, burns may cause permanent anhidrosis in affected areas as well as blistering, edema, and increased pain or loss of sensation.

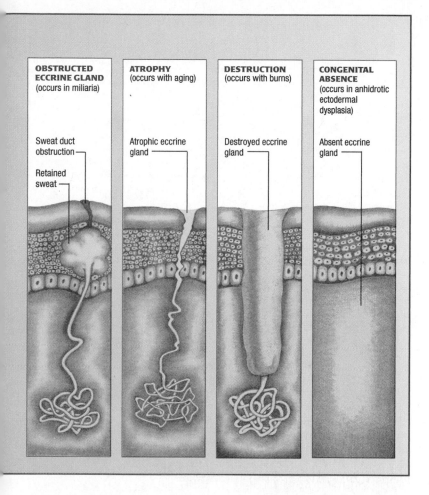

OBSTRUCTED ECCRINE GLAND (occurs in miliaria)

Sweat duct obstruction

Retained sweat

ATROPHY (occurs with aging)

Atrophic eccrine gland

DESTRUCTION (occurs with burns)

Destroyed eccrine gland

CONGENITAL ABSENCE (occurs in anhidrotic ectodermal dysplasia)

Absent eccrine gland

◆ *Drugs.* Anticholinergics, such as atropine and scopolamine, can cause generalized anhidrosis.

◆ *Miliaria crystallina.* This usually innocuous form of miliaria causes anhidrosis and tiny, clear, fragile blisters, usually under the arms and breasts.

◆ *Miliaria profunda.* If severe and extensive, miliaria profunda can progress to life-threatening anhidrotic asthenia. Typically, it produces localized anhidrosis with compensatory facial hyperhidrosis. Whitish papules appear most-ly on the trunk but also on the extremities. Associated signs and symptoms include inguinal and axillary lymphadenopathy, weakness, shortness of breath, palpitations, and fever.

◆ *Miliaria rubra (prickly heat).* Miliaria rubra typically produces localized anhidrosis and can also progress to life-threatening anhidrotic asthenia if it becomes severe and extensive; however, this is a rare occurrence. Small, erythematous papules with centrally placed blisters appear on the trunk and

EMERGENCY INTERVENTIONS

Suspected anhidrotic asthenia

If you suspect that a patient has anhidrotic asthenia, quickly perform these interventions:

◆ Start rapid cooling measures such as immersing him in ice or very cold water.

◆ Administer I.V. fluid replacements.
◆ Check the patient's vital signs and neurologic status frequently until his temperature drops below 102° F (38.9° C).

---

neck and rarely on the face, palms, or soles. Pustules may also appear in extensive and chronic miliaria. Related symptoms include paroxysmal itching and paresthesia.

◆ *Peripheral neuropathy.* Anhidrosis over the legs usually appears with compensatory hyperhidrosis over the head and neck. Associated findings mainly involve extremities and include glossy red skin; paresthesia, hyperesthesia, or anesthesia in the hands and feet; diminished or absent deep tendon reflexes; flaccid paralysis and muscle wasting; footdrop; and burning pain.

◆ *Shy-Drager syndrome.* A degenerative neurologic syndrome, Shy-Drager syndrome causes ascending anhidrosis in the legs. Other signs and symptoms include severe orthostatic hypotension, loss of leg hair, impotence, constipation, urine retention or urgency, decreased salivation and tearing, mydriasis, and impaired visual accommodation. Eventually, focal neurologic signs—such as leg tremors, incoordination, and muscle wasting and fasciculation—may appear.

◆ *Spinal cord lesions.* Anhidrosis may occur symmetrically below the level of the lesion, with compensatory hyperhidrosis in adjacent areas. Other findings depend on the site and extent of the lesion but may include partial or total loss of motor and sensory function below the lesion as well as impaired cardiovascular and respiratory function.

Anorexia

Anorexia, a lack of appetite in the presence of a physiologic need for food, is a common symptom of GI and endocrine disorders and is characteristic of certain severe psychological disturbances such as anorexia nervosa. It can also result from such factors as anxiety, chronic pain, poor oral hygiene, increased body temperature due to hot weather or fever, and changes in taste or smell that normally accompany aging. Anorexia also can result from drug therapy or abuse. Short-term anorexia rarely jeopardizes health, but chronic anorexia can lead to life-threatening malnutrition.

Assessment

Take the patient's vital signs and weight. Find out previous minimum and maximum weights. Ask about involuntary weight loss greater than 10 lb (4.5 kg) in the past month. Explore dietary habits, such as when and what the patient eats. Ask what foods he likes and dislikes and why. The patient may identify tastes and smells that nauseate him and cause loss of appetite. Ask about dental problems that interfere with chewing, including poor-fitting dentures. Ask whether he has difficulty or pain when swallowing or if he vomits or has diarrhea after

Is your patient malnourished?

When assessing a patient with anorexia, make sure to check for these common signs of malnutrition.

Hair. Dull, dry, thin, fine, straight, and easily plucked; areas of lighter or darker spots and hair loss

Face. Generalized swelling, dark areas on cheeks and under eyes, lumpy or flaky skin around the nose and mouth, enlarged parotid glands

Eyes. Dull appearance; dry and either pale or red membranes; triangular, shiny gray spots on conjunctivae; red and fissured eyelid corners; bloodshot ring around cornea

Lips. Red and swollen, especially at corners

Tongue. Swollen, purple, and raw-looking, with sores or abnormal papillae

Teeth. Missing, or emerging abnormally; visible cavities or dark spots; spongy, bleeding gums

Neck. Swollen thyroid gland

Skin. Dry, flaky, swollen, and dark, with lighter or darker spots, some resembling bruises; tight and drawn, with poor skin turgor

Nails. Spoon-shaped, brittle, and ridged

Musculoskeletal system. Muscle wasting, knock-knee or bowlegs, bumps on ribs, swollen joints, musculoskeletal hemorrhages

Cardiovascular system. Heart rate above 100 beats/minute, arrhythmias, elevated blood pressure

Abdomen. Enlarged liver and spleen

Reproductive system. Decreased libido, amenorrhea

Nervous system. Irritability, confusion, paresthesia in hands and feet, loss of proprioception, decreased ankle and knee reflexes

meals. Ask the patient how frequently and intensely he exercises.

Check for a history of stomach or bowel disorders, which can interfere with the ability to digest, absorb, or metabolize nutrients. Find out about changes in bowel habits. Ask about alcohol use and drug use and dosage.

If the medical history doesn't reveal an organic basis for anorexia, consider psychological factors. Ask the patient whether he knows what's causing his decreased appetite. Situational factors—such as a death in the family or problems at school or at work—can lead to depression and a subsequent loss of appetite. Be alert for signs of malnutrition, consistent refusal of food, and a 7% to 10% loss of body weight in the preceding month. (See *Is your patient malnourished?*)

Causes

◆ *Acquired immunodeficiency syndrome.* An infection or Kaposi's sarcoma affecting the GI or respiratory tract may lead to anorexia. Other findings include fatigue, afternoon fevers, night sweats, diarrhea, cough, lymphadenopathy, bleeding, oral thrush, gingivitis, and skin disorders, including persistent herpes zoster and recurrent herpes simplex, herpes labialis, or herpes genitalis.

◆ *Adrenocortical hypofunction.* With adrenocortical hypofunction, anorexia may begin slowly and subtly, causing gradual weight loss. Other common signs and symptoms include nausea and vomiting, abdominal pain, diarrhea, weakness, fatigue, malaise, vitiligo, bronze-colored skin, and purple striae on the breasts, abdomen, shoulders, and hips.

◆ *Alcoholism.* Chronic anorexia commonly accompanies alcoholism, eventually leading to malnutrition. Other findings include signs of liver damage (jaundice, spider angiomas, ascites, edema), paresthesia, tremors, increased blood pressure, bruising, GI bleeding, and abdominal pain.

◆ *Anorexia nervosa.* Chronic anorexia begins insidiously and eventually leads to life-threatening malnutrition, as evidenced by skeletal muscle atrophy, loss of fatty tissue, constipation, amenorrhea, dry and blotchy or sallow skin, alopecia, sleep disturbances, distorted self-image, anhedonia, and decreased libido. Paradoxically, the patient typically exhibits extreme restlessness and vigor and may exercise avidly. He also may have complicated food preparation and eating rituals.

◆ *Appendicitis.* Anorexia closely follows the abrupt onset of generalized or localized epigastric pain, nausea, and vomiting. It can continue as pain localizes in the right lower quadrant (McBurney's point), and other signs and symptoms appear: abdominal rigidity, rebound tenderness, constipation (or diarrhea), a slight fever, and tachycardia.

◆ *Cancer.* Chronic anorexia occurs along with possible weight loss, weakness, apathy, and cachexia.

◆ *Chronic renal failure.* Chronic anorexia is common and insidious. It's accompanied by changes in all body systems, such as nausea, vomiting, mouth ulcers, ammonia breath odor, metallic taste in the mouth, GI bleeding, constipation or diarrhea, drowsiness, confusion, tremors, pallor, dry and scaly skin, pruritus, alopecia, purpuric lesions, and edema.

◼ *Cirrhosis.* Anorexia occurs early in cirrhosis and may be accompanied by weakness, nausea, vomiting, constipation or diarrhea, and dull abdominal pain. It continues after these early signs and symptoms subside and is accompanied by lethargy, slurred speech, bleeding tendencies, ascites, severe pruritus, dry skin, poor skin turgor, hepatomegaly, fetor hepaticus, jaundice, leg edema, gynecomastia, and right upper quadrant pain.

◆ *Crohn's disease.* Chronic anorexia causes marked weight loss. Associated signs vary according to the site and extent of the lesion but may include diarrhea, abdominal pain, fever, an abdominal mass, weakness, perianal or vaginal fistulas and, rarely, clubbing of the fingers. Acute inflammatory signs and symptoms—right lower quadrant pain, cramping, tenderness, flatulence, fever, nausea, diarrhea (including nocturnal), and bloody stools—mimic those of appendicitis.

◆ *Drugs.* Anorexia results from the use of amphetamines; chemotherapeutic agents; sympathomimetics such as ephedrine; and some antibiotics. It also signals digoxin toxicity.

◆ *Gastritis.* With acute gastritis, the onset of anorexia may be sudden. The patient may experience postprandial epigastric distress after a meal, accompanied by nausea, vomiting (commonly with hematemesis), fever, belching, hiccups, and malaise.

◆ *Hepatitis.* With viral hepatitis (hepatitis A, B, C, D, E, or G), anorexia begins in the preicteric phase, accompanied by fatigue, malaise, headache, arthralgia, myalgia, photophobia, nausea and vomiting, a mild fever, hepatomegaly, and lymphadenopathy. It may continue throughout the icteric phase, along with mild weight loss, dark urine, clay-colored stools, jaundice, right upper quadrant pain and, possibly, irritability and severe pruritus.

Signs and symptoms of nonviral hepatitis usually resemble those of viral hepatitis but may vary, depending on the cause and extent of liver damage.

◆ *Hypothyroidism.* Anorexia is common and usually insidious in patients with a thyroid hormone deficiency. Typically, vague early findings include fatigue, forgetfulness, cold intolerance, unexplained weight gain, and constipation. Subsequent findings include decreased mental stability; dry, flaky, and inelastic skin; edema of the face, hands, and feet; ptosis; hoarseness; thick, brittle nails; coarse, broken hair; and signs of decreased cardiac output such as bradycardia. Other common findings include abdominal distention, menstrual irregularities, decreased libido, ataxia, intention tremor, nystagmus, a dull facial expression, and slow reflex relaxation time.

◼ *Ketoacidosis.* Anorexia usually arises gradually and is accompanied by dry, flushed skin; a fruity breath odor; polydipsia; polyuria and nocturia; hypotension; a weak, rapid pulse; a dry mouth; abdominal pain; and vomiting.

◆ *Pernicious anemia.* With pernicious anemia, insidious anorexia may cause considerable weight loss. Related findings include the classic triad of a burning tongue, general weakness, and numbness and tingling in the extremities; alternating constipation and diarrhea; abdominal pain; nausea and vomiting; bleeding gums; ataxia; positive Babinski's and Romberg's signs; diplopia and blurred vision; irritability; headache; malaise; and fatigue.

◆ *Radiation therapy.* Radiation treatments can cause anorexia, possibly as a result of metabolic disturbances.

◆ *Total parenteral nutrition.* Maintenance of blood glucose levels by I.V. therapy may cause anorexia.

Anuria

Clinically defined as urine output of less than 100 ml in 24 hours, anuria indicates either urinary tract obstruction or acute renal failure due to various mechanisms. (See *Major causes of*

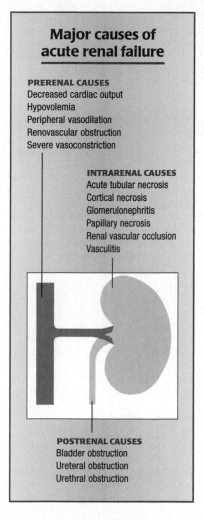

Major causes of acute renal failure

PRERENAL CAUSES
Decreased cardiac output
Hypovolemia
Peripheral vasodilation
Renovascular obstruction
Severe vasoconstriction

INTRARENAL CAUSES
Acute tubular necrosis
Cortical necrosis
Glomerulonephritis
Papillary necrosis
Renal vascular occlusion
Vasculitis

POSTRENAL CAUSES
Bladder obstruction
Ureteral obstruction
Urethral obstruction

acute renal failure.) Fortunately, anuria is rare.

Because urine output is easily measured, anuria rarely goes undetected. However, without immediate treatment, it can rapidly cause uremia and other complications of urine retention.

Assessment

Take the patient's vital signs and obtain a complete history. First, ask about changes in his voiding pattern. Determine the amount of fluid he normally ingests each day, the amount of fluid he ingested in the last 24 to 48 hours, and the time and amount of his last urination. Review his medical history, noting previous kidney disease, urinary tract obstruction or infection, prostate enlargement, renal calculi, neurogenic bladder, or congenital abnormalities. Ask about drug use and about abdominal, renal, or urinary tract surgery.

Inspect and palpate the abdomen for asymmetry, distention, or bulging. Inspect the flank area for edema or erythema, and percuss and palpate the bladder. Palpate the kidneys anteriorly and posteriorly, and percuss them at the costovertebral angle. Auscultate over the renal arteries, listening for bruits.

Causes

◆ *Acute tubular necrosis.* Oliguria (occasionally anuria) is a common finding with acute tubular necrosis. It precedes the onset of diuresis, which is heralded by polyuria. Associated findings reflect the underlying cause and may include signs and symptoms of hyperkalemia (muscle weakness, cardiac arrhythmias), uremia (anorexia, nausea, vomiting, confusion, lethargy, twitching, seizures, pruritus, uremic frost, and Kussmaul's respirations), and heart failure (edema, jugular vein distention, crackles, and dyspnea).
◆ *Cortical necrosis (bilateral).* Cortical necrosis is characterized by a sudden change from oliguria to anuria, along with gross hematuria, flank pain, and fever.
◆ *Diagnostic tests.* Contrast media used in radiographic studies can cause nephrotoxicity, producing oliguria and, rarely, anuria.
◆ *Drugs.* Many classes of drugs can cause anuria or, more commonly, oliguria through their nephrotoxic effects.

Antibiotics, especially the aminoglycosides, are the most commonly seen nephrotoxins. Anesthetics, heavy metals, ethyl alcohol, and organic solvents can also be nephrotoxic. Adrenergics and anticholinergics can cause anuria by affecting the nerves and muscles of micturition to produce urine retention.
◆ *Glomerulonephritis (acute).* Acute glomerulonephritis produces anuria or oliguria. Related effects include a mild fever, malaise, flank pain, gross hematuria, facial and generalized edema, elevated blood pressure, headache, nausea, vomiting, abdominal pain, and signs and symptoms of pulmonary congestion (crackles, dyspnea).
◆ *Hemolytic-uremic syndrome.* Anuria commonly occurs in the initial stages of hemolytic-uremic syndrome and may last from 1 to 10 days. The patient may experience vomiting, diarrhea, abdominal pain, hematemesis, melena, purpura, fever, elevated blood pressure, hepatomegaly, ecchymoses, edema, hematuria, and pallor. He may also show signs of upper respiratory tract infection.
◆ *Renal artery occlusion (bilateral).* Bilateral renal artery occlusion produces anuria or severe oliguria, commonly accompanied by severe, continuous upper abdominal and flank pain; nausea and vomiting; decreased bowel sounds; a fever up to 102° F (38.9° C); and diastolic hypertension.
◆ *Renal vein occlusion (bilateral).* Bilateral renal vein occlusion occasionally causes anuria; more typical signs and symptoms include acute lower back pain, fever, flank tenderness, and hematuria. Development of pulmonary emboli—a common complication—produces sudden dyspnea, pleuritic pain, tachypnea, tachycardia, crackles, pleural friction rub and, possibly, hemoptysis.
◆ *Urinary tract obstruction.* Severe urinary tract obstruction can produce acute and sometimes total anuria, al-

ternating with or preceded by burning and pain on urination, overflow incontinence or dribbling, increased urinary frequency and nocturia, voiding of small amounts, or an altered urine stream. Associated findings include bladder distention, pain and a sensation of fullness in the lower abdomen and groin, upper abdominal and flank pain, nausea and vomiting, and signs of secondary infection, such as fever, chills, malaise, and cloudy, foul-smelling urine.

◆ *Vasculitis.* Vasculitis occasionally produces anuria. More typical findings include malaise, myalgia, polyarthralgia, fever, elevated blood pressure, hematuria, proteinuria, arrhythmia, pallor and, possibly, skin lesions, urticaria, and purpura.

Anxiety

Anxiety is the most common psychiatric symptom and can result in significant impairment. A subjective reaction to a real or imagined threat, anxiety is a nonspecific feeling of uneasiness or dread. It may be mild, moderate, or severe. Mild anxiety may cause slight physical or psychological discomfort. Severe anxiety may be incapacitating or even life-threatening.

Everyone experiences anxiety from time to time—it's a normal response to actual danger, prompting the body (through stimulation of the sympathetic and parasympathetic nervous systems) to purposeful action. It's also a normal response to physical and emotional stress, which can be produced by virtually any illness. In addition, anxiety can be precipitated or exacerbated by many nonpathologic factors, including lack of sleep, poor diet, and excessive intake of caffeine or other stimulants. However, excessive, unwarranted anxiety may indicate an underlying psychological problem.

Assessment

If the patient displays acute, severe anxiety, quickly take his vital signs and determine his chief complaint; these findings will serve as a guide for how to proceed. For example, if the patient's anxiety occurs with chest pain and shortness of breath, you might suspect myocardial infarction and act accordingly. While examining the patient, try to keep him calm. Suggest relaxation techniques, and talk to him in a reassuring, soothing voice. Uncontrolled anxiety can alter vital signs and exacerbate the causative disorder.

If the patient displays mild or moderate anxiety, ask about its duration. Is the anxiety constant or sporadic? Did he notice precipitating factors? Find out if the anxiety is exacerbated by stress, lack of sleep, or caffeine intake and alleviated by rest, tranquilizers, or exercise.

Obtain a complete medical history, especially noting drug use. Then perform a physical examination, focusing on complaints that may trigger or be aggravated by anxiety.

If the patient's anxiety isn't accompanied by significant physical signs, suspect a psychological basis. Determine the patient's level of consciousness (LOC), and observe his behavior. If appropriate, refer the patient for psychiatric evaluation.

Causes

◆ *Acute respiratory distress syndrome.* Acute anxiety occurs along with tachycardia, mental sluggishness and, in severe cases, hypotension. Other respiratory signs and symptoms include dyspnea, tachypnea, intercostal and suprasternal retractions, crackles, and rhonchi.

◆ *Anaphylactic shock.* Acute anxiety usually signals the onset of anaphylactic shock. It's accompanied by urticaria, angioedema, pruritus, and shortness of breath. Soon, other signs and symptoms develop: light-headedness, hypotension, tachycardia, nasal congestion, sneezing, wheezing, dyspnea, a barking cough, abdominal cramps, vomiting, diarrhea, and urinary urgency and incontinence.

◆ *Angina pectoris.* Acute anxiety may either precede or follow an attack of angina pectoris. An attack produces sharp and crushing substernal or anterior chest pain that may radiate to the back, neck, arms, or jaw. The pain may be relieved by nitroglycerin or rest, which eases anxiety.

◆ *Asthma.* With allergic asthma attacks, acute anxiety occurs with dyspnea, wheezing, a productive cough, accessory muscle use, hyperresonant lung fields, diminished breath sounds, coarse crackles, cyanosis, tachycardia, and diaphoresis.

◆ *Autonomic hyperreflexia.* The earliest signs of autonomic hyperreflexia may be acute anxiety accompanied by severe headache and dramatic hypertension. Pallor and motor and sensory deficits occur below the level of the lesion; flushing occurs above it.

◢ *Cardiogenic shock.* Acute anxiety is accompanied by cool, pale, clammy skin; tachycardia; a weak, thready pulse; tachypnea; ventricular gallop; crackles; jugular vein distention; decreased urine output; hypotension; narrowing pulse pressure; and peripheral edema.

◆ *Chronic obstructive pulmonary disease (COPD).* Acute anxiety, exertional dyspnea, cough, wheezing, crackles, hyperresonant lung fields, tachypnea, and accessory muscle use characterize COPD.

◆ *Drugs.* Many drugs cause anxiety, especially sympathomimetics and central nervous system stimulants. In addition, many antidepressants may cause paradoxical anxiety.

◆ *Heart failure.* With heart failure, acute anxiety is commonly the first symptom of inadequate oxygenation. Associated findings include restlessness, shortness of breath, tachypnea, decreased LOC, edema, crackles, ventricular gallop, hypotension, weight gain, diaphoresis, and cyanosis.

◆ *Hyperthyroidism.* Acute anxiety may be an early sign of hyperthyroidism. Classic signs and symptoms include heat intolerance, weight loss despite increased appetite, nervousness, tremor, palpitations, sweating, an enlarged thyroid, and diarrhea. Exophthalmos may occur.

◆ *Mitral valve prolapse.* Panic may occur in patients with mitral valve prolapse, referred to as the click-murmur syndrome. The disorder may also cause paroxysmal palpitations accompanied by sharp, stabbing, or aching precordial pain. Its hallmark is a midsystolic click, followed by an apical systolic murmur.

◆ *Mood disorder.* Anxiety may be the patient's chief complaint in the depressive or manic form of mood disorder. With the depressive form, chronic anxiety occurs with varying severity. Associated findings include dysphoria; anger; insomnia or hypersomnia; decreased libido, interest, energy, and concentration; appetite disturbance; multiple somatic complaints; and suicidal thoughts. With the manic form, the patient's chief complaint may be a reduced need for sleep, hyperactivity, increased energy, rapid or pressured speech and, in severe cases, paranoid ideas and other psychotic symptoms.

◢ *Myocardial infarction (MI).* With MI, a life-threatening disorder, acute anxiety commonly occurs with persistent, crushing substernal pain that may radiate to the left arm, jaw, neck, or shoulder blades. It can be accompanied by shortness of breath, nausea, vomiting, diaphoresis, and cool, pale skin.

◆ *Obsessive-compulsive disorder.* Chronic anxiety occurs with obsessive-compulsive disorder, along with recurrent, unshakable thoughts or impulses to perform ritualistic acts. The patient recognizes these acts as irrational but is unable to control them. Anxiety builds if he can't perform these acts and diminishes after he does.

◆ *Pheochromocytoma.* Acute, severe anxiety accompanies pheochromocytoma's cardinal sign: persistent or paroxysmal hypertension. Common associated signs and symptoms include tachycardia, diaphoresis, orthostatic hypotension, tachypnea, flushing, a severe headache, palpitations, nausea, vomiting, epigastric pain, and paresthesia.

◆ *Phobias.* With phobias, chronic anxiety occurs along with a persistent fear of an object, activity, or situation that results in a compelling desire to avoid it. The patient recognizes the fear as irrational but can't suppress it.

◆ *Pneumonia.* Acute anxiety may occur with pneumonia because of hypoxemia. Other findings include a productive cough, pleuritic chest pain, fever, chills, crackles, diminished breath sounds, and hyperresonant lung fields.

◤ *Pneumothorax.* Acute anxiety occurs in moderate to severe pneumothorax associated with profound respiratory distress. It's accompanied by sharp pleuritic pain, coughing, shortness of breath, cyanosis, asymmetrical chest expansion, pallor, jugular vein distention, and a weak, rapid pulse.

◆ *Postconcussion syndrome.* Postconcussion syndrome may produce chronic anxiety or periodic attacks of acute anxiety. Associated signs and symptoms include irritability, insomnia, dizziness, and a mild headache. The anxiety is usually most pronounced in situations demanding attention, judgment, or comprehension.

◆ *Posttraumatic stress disorder.* Posttraumatic stress disorder occurs in the patient who has experienced an extreme traumatic event. It produces chronic anxiety of varying severity and is accompanied by intrusive, vivid memories and thoughts of the traumatic event. The patient also relives the event in dreams and nightmares. Insomnia, depression, and feelings of numbness and detachment are common.

◤ *Pulmonary edema.* With pulmonary edema, acute anxiety occurs with dyspnea, orthopnea, cough with frothy sputum, tachycardia, tachypnea, crackles, ventricular gallop, hypotension, and a thready pulse. The patient's skin may be cool, clammy, and cyanotic.

◤ *Pulmonary embolism.* With pulmonary embolism, acute anxiety is usually accompanied by dyspnea, tachypnea, chest pain, tachycardia, blood-tinged sputum, and a low-grade fever.

◆ *Rabies.* Anxiety signals the beginning of the acute phase of rabies, a rare disorder, which is commonly accompanied by painful laryngeal spasms associated with difficulty swallowing and, as a result, hydrophobia.

◆ *Somatoform disorder.* Somatoform disorder, which usually begins in young adulthood, is characterized by anxiety and multiple somatic complaints that can't be explained physiologically. The symptoms aren't produced intentionally but are severe enough to significantly impair functioning. Pain disorder, conversion disorder, and hypochondriasis are examples of somatoform disorder.

Aphasia

Aphasia—impaired expression or comprehension of written or spoken language—reflects disease or injury of the brain's language centers. Depending on its severity, aphasia may slightly impede communication or may make it impossible. It can be classified as Bro-

Identifying types of aphasia

TYPE	LOCATION OF LESION	SIGNS AND SYMPTOMS
Anomic aphasia	Temporal-parietal area; may extend to angular gyrus but is sometimes poorly localized	The patient's understanding of written and spoken language is relatively unimpaired. His speech, although fluent, lacks meaningful content. Word-finding difficulty and circumlocution are characteristic. Rarely, the patient also displays paraphasias.
Broca's aphasia (expressive aphasia)	Broca's area; usually in third frontal convolution of the left hemisphere	The patient's understanding of written and spoken language is relatively spared, but speech is nonfluent, evidencing word-finding difficulty, jargon, paraphasias, limited vocabulary, and simple sentence construction. He can't repeat words and phrases. If Wernicke's area is intact, he recognizes speech errors and shows frustration. He's commonly hemiparetic.
Global aphasia	Broca's and Wernicke's areas	The patient has profoundly impaired receptive and expressive ability. He can't repeat words or phrases and can't follow directions. His occasional speech is marked by paraphasias or jargon.
Wernicke's aphasia (receptive aphasia)	Wernicke's area; usually in posterior or superior temporal lobe	The patient has difficulty understanding written and spoken language. He can't repeat words or phrases and can't follow directions. His speech is fluent but may be rapid and rambling, with paraphasias. He has difficulty naming objects (anomia) and is unaware of speech errors.

ca's, Wernicke's, anomic, or global aphasia. Anomic aphasia eventually resolves in more than 50% of patients, but global aphasia is usually irreversible. (See *Identifying types of aphasia.*)

Assessment

If the patient doesn't display signs of increased intracranial pressure (ICP) or if his aphasia has developed gradually, perform a thorough neurologic examination, starting with the patient history. You'll probably need to obtain this history from the patient's family or companion because of the patient's im-

pairment. Ask whether the patient has a history of headaches, hypertension, seizure disorders, or drug use. Also ask about the patient's ability to communicate and to perform routine activities before aphasia began.

Check for obvious signs of neurologic deficit, such as ptosis or fluid leakage from the nose and ears. Take the patient's vital signs and assess his level of consciousness (LOC). Be aware, however, that assessing LOC is usually difficult because the patient's verbal responses may be unreliable. Also, recognize that dysarthria (impaired articulation due to weakness or paralysis of the muscles necessary for speech) or speech apraxia (inability to voluntarily control the muscles of speech) may accompany aphasia; therefore, speak slowly and distinctly, and allow the patient ample time to respond. Assess the patient's pupillary response, eye movements, and motor function, especially his mouth and tongue movement, swallowing ability, and spontaneous movements and gestures. To best assess motor function, first demonstrate the motions and then have the patient imitate them.

Causes

◆ *Alzheimer's disease.* With this degenerative disease, anomic aphasia may begin insidiously and then progress to severe global aphasia. Associated signs and symptoms include behavioral changes, loss of memory, poor judgment, restlessness, myoclonus, and muscle rigidity. Incontinence is usually a late sign.

◼ *Brain abscess.* Any type of aphasia may occur with brain abscess. Usually, aphasia develops insidiously and may be accompanied by hemiparesis, ataxia, facial weakness, and signs of increased ICP.

◆ *Brain tumor.* A brain tumor may cause any type of aphasia. As the tumor enlarges, other aphasias may occur along with behavioral changes, memory loss, motor weakness, seizures, auditory hallucinations, visual field deficits, and increased ICP.

◆ *Creutzfeldt-Jakob disease.* A rapidly progressive dementia, Creutzfeldt-Jakob disease is accompanied by neurologic signs and symptoms, such as myoclonic jerking, ataxia, aphasia, vision disturbances, and paralysis. It generally affects adults ages 40 to 65.

◼ *Encephalitis.* Encephalitis usually produces transient aphasia. Its early signs and symptoms include fever, headache, and vomiting. Seizures, con-

fusion, stupor or coma, hemiparesis, asymmetrical deep tendon reflexes, positive Babinski's reflex, ataxia, myoclonus, nystagmus, ocular palsies, and facial weakness may accompany aphasia.

◼ *Head trauma.* Any type of aphasia may accompany severe head trauma; typically, it occurs suddenly and may be transient or permanent, depending on the extent of brain damage. Associated signs and symptoms include blurred or double vision, headache, pallor, diaphoresis, numbness and paresis, cerebrospinal otorrhea or rhinorrhea, altered respirations, tachycardia, disorientation, behavioral changes, and signs of increased ICP.

◆ *Seizures.* Seizures and the postictal state may cause transient aphasia if the seizures involve the language centers.

◼ *Stroke.* The most common cause of aphasia, stroke may produce Wernicke's, Broca's, or global aphasia. Associated findings include decreased LOC, right-sided hemiparesis, homonymous hemianopsia, paresthesia, and loss of sensation. (These signs and symptoms may appear on the left side if the right hemisphere contains the language centers.)

◆ *Transient ischemic attack.* Transient ischemic attacks can produce any type of aphasia, which occurs suddenly and resolves within 24 hours of the attack. Associated signs and symptoms include transient hemiparesis, hemianopsia, and paresthesia (all usually right-sided), dizziness, and confusion.

Apnea

Apnea, the cessation of spontaneous respiration, is occasionally temporary and self-limiting, as occurs during Cheyne-Stokes and Biot's respirations. More commonly, however, it's a life-threatening emergency that requires

Causes of apnea

Apnea results from several pathophysiologic mechanisms. The list below details the numerous causes of this life-threatening disorder.

Airway obstruction
◆ Asthma
◆ Bronchospasm
◆ Chronic bronchitis
◆ Chronic obstructive pulmonary disease
◆ Foreign body aspiration
◆ Hemothorax or pneumothorax
◆ Mucus plug
◆ Obstruction by tongue or tumor
◆ Obstructive sleep apnea
◆ Secretion retention
◆ Tracheal or bronchial rupture

Brain stem dysfunction
◆ Brain abscess
◆ Brain stem injury
◆ Brain tumor
◆ Central nervous system depressants
◆ Central sleep apnea
◆ Cerebral hemorrhage
◆ Cerebral infarction
◆ Encephalitis
◆ Head trauma
◆ Increased intracranial pressure
◆ Medullary or pontine hemorrhage or infarction
◆ Meningitis
◆ Transtentorial herniation

Neuromuscular failure
◆ Amyotrophic lateral sclerosis
◆ Botulism
◆ Diphtheria
◆ Guillain-Barré syndrome
◆ Myasthenia gravis
◆ Phrenic nerve paralysis
◆ Rupture of the diaphragm
◆ Spinal cord injury

Parenchymatous disease
◆ Acute respiratory distress syndrome
◆ Diffuse pneumonia
◆ Emphysema
◆ Near drowning
◆ Pulmonary edema
◆ Pulmonary fibrosis
◆ Secretion retention

Pleural pressure gradient disruption
◆ Flail chest
◆ Open chest wounds

Pulmonary capillary perfusion decrease
◆ Arrhythmias
◆ Cardiac arrest
◆ Myocardial infarction
◆ Pulmonary embolism
◆ Pulmonary hypertension
◆ Shock

immediate intervention to prevent death.

Apnea usually results from one or more of six pathophysiologic mechanisms, each of which has numerous causes. Common causes include trauma, cardiac arrest, neurologic disease, aspiration of foreign objects, bronchospasm, and drug overdose. (See *Causes of apnea*.)

Assessment

If you detect apnea, you must intervene quickly. (See *Responding to apnea*.) When the patient's respiratory and cardiac status is stable, investigate the underlying cause of apnea. Ask him (or, if he's unable to answer, anyone who witnessed the episode) about the onset of apnea and events immedi-

EMERGENCY INTERVENTIONS

Responding to apnea

Perform these interventions if your patient develops apnea:
◆ Place the patient in a supine position, and open his airway using the head-tilt, chin-lift technique; if the patient has an obvious or suspected head or neck injury, use the jaw-thrust technique.
◆ Quickly look, listen, and feel for spontaneous respiration.

◆ If spontaneous respirations are absent, begin artificial ventilation until spontaneous respirations occur or until mechanical ventilation can be initiated.
◆ Assess the patient's carotid pulse immediately after you've established a patent airway. If the patient is an infant or small child, assess the brachial pulse instead.
◆ If the patient's pulse is absent, begin cardiac compressions.

ately preceding it. The cause may become readily apparent, as in trauma.

Take a patient history, noting especially reports of headache, chest pain, muscle weakness, sore throat, or dyspnea. Ask about a history of respiratory, cardiac, or neurologic disease and about allergies and drug use.

Inspect the head, face, neck, and trunk for soft-tissue injury, hemorrhage, or skeletal deformity. Don't overlook obvious clues, such as oral and nasal secretions reflecting fluid-filled airways and alveoli or facial soot and singed nasal hair suggesting thermal injury to the tracheobronchial tree.

Auscultate over all lung lobes for adventitious breath sounds, particularly crackles and rhonchi, and percuss the lung fields for increased dullness or hyperresonance. Move on to the heart, auscultating for murmurs, pericardial friction rub, and arrhythmias. Check for cyanosis, pallor, jugular vein distention, and edema. If appropriate, perform a neurologic assessment. Evaluate the patient's level of consciousness (LOC), orientation, and mental status; test cranial nerve function and motor function, sensation, and reflexes in all extremities.

Causes

◙ *Airway obstruction.* Occlusion or compression of the trachea, central airways, or smaller airways can cause sudden apnea by blocking the patient's airflow and producing acute respiratory failure.

◙ *Brain stem dysfunction.* Primary or secondary brain stem dysfunction can cause apnea by destroying the brain stem's ability to initiate respirations. Apnea may arise suddenly (as in trauma, hemorrhage, or infarction) or gradually (as in degenerative disease or tumor). Apnea may be preceded by a decreased LOC and by various motor and sensory deficits.

◆ *Drugs.* Central nervous system (CNS) depressants may cause hypoventilation and apnea. Benzodiazepines may cause respiratory depression and apnea when given I.V. along with other CNS depressants to elderly or acutely ill patients. Neuromuscular blockers—such as curariform drugs and anticholinesterases—may produce sudden apnea because of respiratory muscle paralysis.

◙ *Neuromuscular failure.* Trauma or disease can disrupt the mechanics of respiration, causing sudden or gradual apnea. Associated findings include di-

aphragmatic or intercostal muscle paralysis from injury or respiratory weakness or paralysis from acute or degenerative disease.

◪ *Parenchymatous lung disease.* An
accumulation of fluid within the alveoli
produces apnea by interfering with pulmonary gas exchange and producing
acute respiratory failure. Apnea may
arise suddenly, as in near drowning
and acute pulmonary edema, or gradually, as in emphysema. Apnea may also
be preceded by crackles and labored
respirations with accessory muscle use.

◪ *Pleural pressure gradient disruption.*
Conversion of normal negative pleural
air pressure to positive pressure by
chest wall injuries (such as flail chest)
causes lung collapse, producing respiratory distress and, if untreated, apnea.
Associated signs include an asymmetrical chest wall and asymmetrical or
paradoxical respirations.

◆ *Pulmonary capillary perfusion decrease.* Apnea can stem from obstructed pulmonary circulation, most commonly due to heart failure or lack of
circulatory patency. It occurs suddenly
in cardiac arrest, massive pulmonary
embolism, and most cases of severe
shock. In contrast, it occurs progressively in septic shock and pulmonary
hypertension. Related findings include
hypotension, tachycardia, and edema.

◆ *Sleep-related apneas.* These repetitive apneas occur during sleep as a result of airflow obstruction or brain
stem dysfunction.

Apneustic respirations

Apneustic respirations are characterized by prolonged, gasping inspiration,
with a pause at full inspiration. This irregular breathing pattern is an important localizing sign of severe brain
stem damage.

Involuntary breathing is primarily
regulated by groups of neurons located
in respiratory centers in the medulla
oblongata and pons. In the medulla,
neurons react to impulses from the
pons and other areas to regulate respiratory rate and depth. In the pons, two
respiratory centers regulate respiratory
rhythm by interacting with the medullary respiratory center to smooth the
transition from inspiration to expiration
and back. The apneustic center in the
pons stimulates inspiratory neurons in
the medulla to precipitate inspiration.
These inspiratory neurons, in turn,
stimulate the pneumotaxic center in
the pons to precipitate expiration. Destruction of neural pathways by pontine lesions disrupts normal regulation
of respiratory rhythm, causing apneustic respirations.

Assessment

If you suspect that your patient is experiencing apneustic respirations, provide adequate ventilation. The patient
may require an artificial airway, oxygen, and mechanical ventilation. Make
sure you differentiate apneustic respirations from bradypnea and hyperpnea
(disturbances in rate and depth but not
in rhythm), Cheyne-Stokes respirations
(rhythmic alterations in rate and depth
followed by periods of apnea), and
Biot's respirations (irregularly alternating periods of hyperpnea and apnea).
Next, thoroughly evaluate the patient's
neurologic status using a standardized
tool such as the Glasgow Coma Scale.
Finally, obtain a brief patient history
from a family member, if possible.

Causes

◪ *Pontine lesions.* Apneustic respirations usually result from extensive
damage to the upper or lower pons due
to infarction, hemorrhage, herniation,

severe infection, tumor, or trauma. Typically, these respirations are accompanied by profound stupor or coma; pinpoint midline pupils; ocular bobbing (a spontaneous downward jerk, followed by a slow drift up to midline); quadriplegia or, less commonly, hemiplegia with the eyes pointing toward the weak side; a positive Babinski's reflex; negative oculocephalic and oculovestibular reflexes; and, possibly, decorticate posture.

Arm pain

Arm pain usually results from musculoskeletal disorders, but it can also stem from neurovascular or cardiovascular disorders. (See *Causes of local pain*, page 108.) In some cases, it may be referred pain from another area, such as the chest, neck, or abdomen. Its location, onset, and character provide clues to its cause. The pain may affect the entire arm or only the upper arm or forearm. It may arise suddenly or gradually and may be constant or intermittent. Arm pain can be described as sharp or dull, burning or numbing, and shooting or penetrating. Diffuse arm pain, however, may be difficult to describe, especially if it isn't associated with injury.

Assessment

If the patient reports arm pain after an injury, take a brief history of the injury from the patient. Then quickly assess him for severe injuries requiring immediate treatment. If you've ruled out severe injuries, check pulses, capillary refill time, sensation, and movement distal to the affected area because circulatory impairment or nerve injury may require immediate surgery. Inspect the arm for deformities, assess the level of pain, and immobilize the arm to prevent further injury.

If the patient reports continuous or intermittent arm pain, ask him to describe it and to relate when it began. Is the pain associated with repetitive or specific movements or positions? Ask him to point out other painful areas because arm pain may be referred. For example, left arm pain commonly accompanies the characteristic chest pain of myocardial infarction, and right shoulder pain may be referred from the right upper quadrant abdominal pain of cholecystitis. Ask the patient whether the pain worsens in the morning or in the evening, prevents him from performing his job, or restricts movement. Also ask whether heat, rest, or drugs relieve it. Finally, ask about preexisting illnesses, a family history of gout or arthritis, and current drug therapy.

Next, perform a focused examination. Observe the way the patient walks, sits, and holds his arm. Inspect the entire arm, comparing it with the opposite arm for symmetry, movement, and muscle atrophy. (You'll need to determine whether the patient is right- or left-handed.) Palpate the entire arm for swelling, nodules, and tender areas. In both arms, compare active range of motion, muscle strength, and reflexes.

If the patient reports numbness or tingling, check his sensation to vibration, temperature, and pinprick. Compare bilateral hand grasps and shoulder strength to detect weakness.

If a patient has a cast, splint, or restrictive dressing, check for circulation, sensation, and mobility distal to the dressing. Ask the patient about edema and whether the pain has worsened within the last 24 hours.

Examine the neck for pain on motion, point tenderness, muscle spasms, or arm pain when the neck is extended with the head toward the involved side.

Causes of local pain

Various disorders cause hand, wrist, elbow, or shoulder pain. In some disorders, pain may radiate from the injury site to other areas.

Hand pain

◆ Arthritis
◆ Buerger's disease
◆ Carpal tunnel syndrome
◆ Dupuytren's contracture
◆ Elbow tunnel syndrome
◆ Fracture
◆ Ganglion
◆ Infection
◆ Occlusive vascular disease
◆ Radiculopathy
◆ Raynaud's disease
◆ Shoulder-hand syndrome (reflex sympathetic dystrophy)
◆ Sprain or strain
◆ Thoracic outlet syndrome
◆ Trigger finger

Wrist pain

◆ Arthritis
◆ Carpal tunnel syndrome
◆ Fracture
◆ Ganglion
◆ Sprain or strain
◆ Tenosynovitis (de Quervain's disease)

Elbow pain

◆ Arthritis
◆ Bursitis

◆ Dislocation
◆ Fracture
◆ Lateral epicondylitis (tennis elbow)
◆ Tendinitis
◆ Ulnar neuritis

Shoulder pain

◆ Acromioclavicular separation
◆ Acute pancreatitis
◆ Adhesive capsulitis (frozen shoulder)
◆ Angina pectoris
◆ Arthritis
◆ Bursitis
◆ Cholecystitis or cholelithiasis
◆ Clavicle fracture
◆ Diaphragmatic pleurisy
◆ Dislocation
◆ Dissecting aortic aneurysm
◆ Gastritis
◆ Humeral neck fracture
◆ Infection
◆ Pancoast's syndrome
◆ Perforated ulcer
◆ Pneumothorax
◆ Ruptured spleen (left shoulder)
◆ Shoulder-hand syndrome
◆ Subphrenic abscess
◆ Tendinitis

Causes

◆ *Angina.* Angina may cause inner arm pain as well as chest and jaw pain. Typically, the pain follows exertion and persists for a few minutes. Accompanied by dyspnea, diaphoresis, and apprehension, the pain is relieved by rest or by vasodilators such as nitroglycerin.

◆ *Biceps rupture.* Rupture of the biceps after excessive weight lifting or osteoarthritic degeneration of bicipital tendon insertion at the shoulder can cause pain in the upper arm. Forearm flexion and supination aggravate the pain. Other signs and symptoms include muscle weakness, deformity, and edema.

◆ *Cellulitis.* Typically, cellulitis affects the legs, but it can also affect the arms. It produces pain as well as redness, tenderness, edema and, at times, fever, chills, tachycardia, headache, and hypotension. Cellulitis usually follows an injury or insect bite.

◆ *Cervical nerve root compression.* Compression of the cervical nerves supplying the upper arm produces chronic arm and neck pain, which may worsen with movement or prolonged sitting. The patient may also experience muscle weakness, paresthesia, and decreased reflex response.

◆ *Compartment syndrome.* Severe pain with passive muscle stretching is the cardinal symptom of compartment syndrome. It may also impair distal circulation and cause muscle weakness, decreased reflex response, paresthesia, and edema. Ominous signs include paralysis and an absent pulse.

◆ *Fractures.* In fractures of the cervical vertebrae, humerus, scapula, clavicle, radius, or ulna, pain can occur at the injury site and radiate throughout the entire arm. Pain at a fresh fracture site is intense and worsens with movement. Associated signs and symptoms include crepitus, felt and heard from bone ends rubbing together (don't attempt to elicit this sign); deformity, if bones are misaligned; local ecchymosis and edema; impaired distal circulation; paresthesia; and decreased sensation distal to the injury site. Fractures of the small wrist bones can manifest with pain and swelling several days after the trauma.

◆ *Muscle contusion.* Muscle contusion may cause generalized pain in the area of injury. It may also cause local swelling and ecchymosis.

◆ *Muscle strain.* Acute or chronic muscle strain causes mild to severe pain with movement. The resultant reduction in arm movement may cause muscle weakness and atrophy.

🔋 *Myocardial infarction (MI).* An MI is a life-threatening disorder in which the patient may complain of left arm pain as well as the characteristic deep and crushing chest pain. He may display weakness, pallor, nausea, vomiting, diaphoresis, altered blood pressure, tachycardia, dyspnea, and feelings of apprehension or impending doom.

◆ *Neoplasms of the arm.* Neoplasms of the arm produce continuous, deep, and penetrating arm pain that worsens at night. Occasionally, redness and swelling accompany arm pain; later, skin breakdown, impaired circulation, and paresthesia may occur.

◆ *Osteomyelitis.* Osteomyelitis typically begins with vague and evanescent localized arm pain and fever and is accompanied by local tenderness, painful and restricted movement and, later, swelling. Associated findings include malaise and tachycardia.

Asterixis

A bilateral, coarse movement, asterixis is characterized by the sudden relaxation of muscle groups holding a sustained posture. This elicited sign is most commonly observed in the wrists and fingers but may also appear during any sustained voluntary action. Typically, it signals hepatic, renal, or pulmonary disease.

To elicit asterixis, have the patient extend his arms, dorsiflex his wrists, and spread his fingers (or do this for him, if necessary). Briefly observe him for asterixis. Alternatively, if the patient has a decreased level of consciousness (LOC) but can follow verbal commands, ask him to squeeze two of your fingers. Consider rapid clutching and unclutching indications of asterixis. Alternatively, elevate the patient's leg off the bed and dorsiflex the foot. Briefly check for asterixis in the ankle. If the patient can tightly close his eyes and mouth, watch for irregular tremulous movements of the eyelids and corners of the mouth. If he can stick out his tongue, observe the patient for continuous quivering. (See *Recognizing asterixis,* page 110.)

Recognizing asterixis

With asterixis, the patient's wrists and fingers are observed to "flap" because there's a brief, rapid relaxation of dorsiflexion of the wrist.

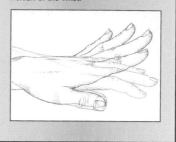

Assessment

Because asterixis may signal serious metabolic deterioration, quickly evaluate the patient's neurologic status and vital signs. Compare these data with baseline measurements, and watch carefully for acute changes. Continue to closely monitor his neurologic status, vital signs, and urine output.

Watch for signs of respiratory insufficiency, and be prepared to provide endotracheal intubation and ventilatory support. Also, be alert for complications of end-stage hepatic, renal, or pulmonary disease.

If the patient has hepatic disease, assess him for early indications of hemorrhage, including restlessness, tachypnea, and cool, moist, pale skin. (If the patient is jaundiced, check for pallor in the conjunctiva and mucous membranes of the mouth.)

If the patient has renal disease, briefly review the therapy he has received. If he's on dialysis, ask about the frequency of treatments to help gauge the severity of disease. Question

a family member if the patient's LOC is significantly decreased.

Then assess the patient for hyperkalemia and metabolic acidosis. Look for tachycardia, nausea, diarrhea, abdominal cramps, muscle weakness, hyperreflexia, and Kussmaul's respirations. If the patient has pulmonary disease, check for labored respirations, tachypnea, accessory muscle use, and cyanosis, which are critical signs.

Causes

◆ *Drugs.* Certain drugs, such as the anticonvulsant phenytoin, may cause asterixis.

◪ *Hepatic encephalopathy.* A life-threatening disorder, hepatic encephalopathy initially causes mild personality changes and a slight tremor. The tremor progresses into asterixis—a hallmark of hepatic encephalopathy—and is accompanied by lethargy, aberrant behavior, and apraxia. Eventually, the patient becomes stuporous and displays hyperventilation. When he slips into a coma, hyperactive reflexes, a positive Babinski's sign, and fetor hepaticus are characteristic signs. The patient may also experience bradycardia, decreased respirations, and seizures.

◪ *Severe respiratory insufficiency.* Characterized by life-threatening respiratory acidosis, severe respiratory insufficiency initially produces headache, restlessness, confusion, apprehension, and decreased reflexes. Eventually, the patient becomes somnolent and may demonstrate asterixis before slipping into a coma. Associated signs and symptoms of respiratory insufficiency include difficulty breathing and rapid, shallow respirations. The patient may be hypertensive in early disease but hypotensive later.

◪ *Uremic syndrome.* A life-threatening disorder, uremic syndrome initially causes lethargy, somnolence, confusion, disorientation, behavior changes, and irritability. Eventually, signs and symptoms appear in diverse body systems. Asterixis is accompanied by stupor, paresthesia, muscle twitching, fasciculations, and footdrop. Other signs and symptoms include polyuria and nocturia followed by oliguria and, then, anuria; elevated blood pressure; signs of heart failure and pericarditis; deep, gasping respirations (Kussmaul's respirations); anorexia; nausea; vomiting; diarrhea; GI bleeding; weight loss; ammonia breath odor; and metallic taste (dysgeusia).

Ataxia

Classified as cerebellar or sensory, ataxia refers to incoordination and irregularity of voluntary, purposeful movements. Cerebellar ataxia results from disease of the cerebellum and its pathways to and from the cerebral cortex, brain stem, and spinal cord. It causes gait, trunk, limb, and possibly speech disorders. Sensory ataxia, which causes gait disorders, results from impaired position sense (proprioception) due to the interruption of afferent nerve fibers in the peripheral nerves, posterior roots, posterior columns of the spinal cord, or medial lemnisci. Occasionally, sensory ataxia is caused by a lesion in both parietal lobes. (See *Identifying ataxia*, page 112.)

Ataxia occurs in acute and chronic forms. Acute ataxia may result from stroke, hemorrhage, or a large tumor in the posterior fossa. With this life-threatening condition, the cerebellum may herniate downward through the foramen magnum behind the cervical spinal cord or upward through the tentorium on the cerebral hemispheres. Herniation may also compress the brain stem. Acute ataxia may also re-

sult from drug toxicity or poisoning. Chronic ataxia can be progressive and, at times, can result from acute disease. It can also occur in metabolic and chronic degenerative neurologic disease.

Assessment

If ataxic movements suddenly develop, examine the patient for signs of increased intracranial pressure and impending herniation. Determine his level of consciousness (LOC), and be alert for pupillary changes, motor weakness or paralysis, neck stiffness or pain, and vomiting. Check his vital signs, especially respirations; abnormal respiratory patterns may quickly lead to respiratory arrest.

If the patient isn't in distress, review his history. Ask about multiple sclerosis, diabetes, central nervous system infection, neoplastic disease, previous stroke, and a family history of ataxia. Also ask about chronic alcohol abuse or prolonged exposure to industrial toxins such as mercury. Find out whether the patient's ataxia developed suddenly or gradually.

If necessary, perform Romberg's test to help distinguish between cerebellar and sensory ataxia. Instruct the patient to stand with his feet together and his arms at his side. Note his posture and balance, first with his eyes open and then closed. Test results may indicate normal posture and balance (minimal swaying), cerebellar ataxia (swaying and inability to maintain balance with eyes open or closed), or sensory ataxia (increased swaying and inability to maintain balance with eyes closed). Stand close to the patient during this test to prevent his falling.

If you test for gait and limb ataxia, be aware that motor weakness may mimic ataxic movements, so check motor strength as well. Gait ataxia may be

Identifying ataxia

Ataxia may be observed in the patient's speech, in the movements of his trunk and limbs, or in his gait.

Cerebellar ataxia

With cerebellar ataxia, the patient may stagger or lurch in zigzag fashion, turn with extreme difficulty, and lose his balance when his feet are together.

Gait ataxia

With gait ataxia, the patient's gait is wide based, unsteady, and irregular.

Limb ataxia

With limb ataxia, the patient loses the ability to gauge distance, speed, and power of movement, resulting in poorly controlled, variable, and inaccurate voluntary movements. He may move too quickly or too slowly, or his movements may break down into component parts, giving him the appearance of a puppet or a robot. Other effects include a coarse, irregular tremor in purposeful movement (but not at rest) and reduced muscle tone.

Sensory ataxia

With sensory ataxia, the patient moves abruptly and stomps or taps his feet. This occurs because he throws his feet forward and outward and then brings them down first on the heels and then on the toes. The patient also fixes his eyes on the ground, watching his steps. However, if he can't watch them, staggering worsens. When he stands with his feet together, he sways or loses his balance.

Speech ataxia

Speech ataxia is a form of dysarthria in which the patient typically speaks slowly and stresses usually unstressed words and syllables. Speech content is unaffected.

Truncal ataxia

Truncal ataxia is a disturbance in equilibrium in which the patient can't sit or stand without falling. Also, his head and trunk may bob and sway (titubation). If he can walk, his gait is reeling.

severe, even when limb ataxia is minimal. With gait ataxia, ask the patient whether he tends to fall to one side, or if falling occurs more frequently at night. With truncal ataxia, remember that the patient's inability to walk or stand, combined with the absence of other signs while he's lying down, may give the impression of hysteria or drug or alcohol intoxication.

Causes

◼ *Cerebellar abscess.* Cerebellar abscess commonly causes limb ataxia on the same side as the lesion as well as gait and truncal ataxia. Typically, the initial symptom is a headache localized behind the ear or in the occipital region, followed by oculomotor palsy, fever, vomiting, an altered LOC, and coma.

◼ *Cerebellar hemorrhage.* With cerebellar hemorrhage, a life-threatening disorder, ataxia is usually acute but transient. Unilateral or bilateral ataxia affects the trunk, gait, or limbs. The patient initially experiences repeated vomiting, occipital headache, vertigo, oculomotor palsy, dysphagia, and dysarthria. Later signs, such as a decreased LOC or coma, signal impending herniation.

🔰 *Creutzfeldt-Jakob disease.* Creutzfeldt-Jakob disease is a rapidly progressive dementia that's accompanied by neurologic signs and symptoms, such as myoclonic jerking, ataxia, aphasia, vision disturbances, and paralysis. It generally affects adults ages 40 to 65.

◆ *Diabetic neuropathy.* Peripheral nerve damage due to diabetes mellitus may cause sensory ataxia, extremity pain, slight leg weakness, skin changes, and bowel and bladder dysfunction.

🔰 *Diphtheria.* Within 4 to 8 weeks of the onset of symptoms, a life-threatening neuropathy can produce sensory ataxia. Diphtheria can be accompanied by fever, paresthesia, and paralysis of the limbs and, sometimes, the respiratory muscles.

◆ *Drugs.* Toxic levels of anticonvulsants, especially phenytoin, may result in gait ataxia. Toxic levels of anticholinergics and tricyclic antidepressants may also result in ataxia. Aminoglutethimide causes ataxia in about 10% of patients; however, this effect usually disappears 4 to 6 weeks after drug therapy is discontinued.

🔰 *Encephalomyelitis.* Encephalomyelitis is a complication of measles, smallpox, chickenpox, or rubella or of rabies or smallpox vaccination that may damage cerebrospinal white matter. Rarely, it's accompanied by cerebellar ataxia. Other signs and symptoms include headache, fever, vomiting, an altered LOC, paralysis, seizures, oculomotor palsy, and pupillary changes.

◆ *Friedreich's ataxia.* A progressive familial disorder, Friedreich's ataxia affects the spinal cord and cerebellum. It causes gait ataxia, followed by truncal, limb, and speech ataxia. Other signs and symptoms include pes cavus (abnormally high arch in the foot), kyphoscoliosis, cranial nerve palsy, and motor and sensory deficits. A positive Babinski's reflex may appear.

◆ *Guillain-Barré syndrome.* Peripheral nerve involvement usually follows a mild viral infection, rarely leading to sensory ataxia. Guillain-Barré syndrome also causes ascending paralysis and, possibly, respiratory distress.

◆ *Hepatocerebral degeneration.* Patients who survive hepatic coma are occasionally left with residual neurologic defects, including mild cerebellar ataxia with a wide-based, unsteady gait. Ataxia may be accompanied by an altered LOC, dysarthria, rhythmic arm tremors, and choreoathetosis of the face, neck, and shoulders.

◆ *Multiple sclerosis (MS).* Nystagmus and cerebellar ataxia commonly occur in MS, but they aren't always accompanied by limb weakness and spasticity. Speech ataxia (especially scanning) may occur as well as sensory ataxia from spinal cord involvement. During remissions, ataxia may subside or even disappear. During exacerbations, it may reappear, worsen, or even become permanent. MS also causes optic neuritis, optic atrophy, numbness and weakness, diplopia, dizziness, and bladder dysfunction.

◆ *Olivopontocerebellar atrophy.* This condition produces gait ataxia and, later, limb and speech ataxia. Rarely, it produces an intention tremor. It's accompanied by choreiform movements, dysphagia, and loss of sphincter tone.

◆ *Poisoning.* Chronic arsenic poisoning may cause sensory ataxia, along with headache, seizures, an altered LOC, motor deficits, and muscle aching. Chronic mercury poisoning causes gait and limb ataxia, principally of the arms. It also causes tremors of the extremities, tongue, and lips; mental confusion; mood changes; and dysarthria.

◆ *Polyneuropathy.* Carcinomatous and myelomatous polyneuropathy may occur before detection of the primary tumor in cancer, multiple myeloma, or Hodgkin's disease. Signs and symptoms include ataxia, severe motor weakness, muscle atrophy, and sensory loss in the limbs. Pain and skin changes may also occur.

◆ *Porphyria.* Porphyria affects the sensory and, more frequently, the motor nerves, possibly leading to ataxia. It also causes abdominal pain, mental disturbances, vomiting, headache, focal neurologic defects, an altered LOC, generalized seizures, and skin lesions.

◆ *Posterior fossa tumor.* Gait, truncal, or limb ataxia is an early sign and may worsen as the tumor enlarges. It's accompanied by vomiting, headache, papilledema, vertigo, oculomotor palsy, a decreased LOC, and motor and sensory impairments on the same side as the lesion.

◆ *Spinocerebellar ataxia.* With spinocerebellar ataxia, the patient may initially experience fatigue, followed by stiff-legged gait ataxia. Eventually, limb ataxia, dysarthria, static tremor, nystagmus, cramps, paresthesia, and sensory deficits occur.

◼ *Stroke.* In stroke, occlusions in the vertebrobasilar arteries halt blood flow to cause infarction in the medulla, pons, or cerebellum that may lead to ataxia. Ataxia may occur at the onset of stroke and remain as a residual deficit. Worsening ataxia during the acute phase may indicate extension of the stroke or severe swelling. Ataxia may be accompanied by unilateral or bilateral motor weakness, a possible altered LOC, sensory loss, vertigo, nausea, vomiting, oculomotor palsy, and dysphagia.

◆ *Wernicke's disease.* The result of thiamine deficiency, Wernicke's disease produces gait ataxia and, rarely, intention tremor or speech ataxia. With severe ataxia, the patient may be unable to stand or walk. Ataxia decreases with thiamine therapy. Associated signs and symptoms include nystagmus, diplopia, ocular palsies, confusion, tachycardia,

exertional dyspnea, and orthostatic hypotension.

Aura

An aura is a sensory or motor phenomenon, idea, or emotion that marks the initial stage of a seizure or the approach of a classic migraine headache. Auras may be classified as cognitive, affective, psychosensory, or psychomotor. (See *Recognizing types of auras.*)

When associated with a seizure, an aura stems from an irritable focus in the brain that spreads throughout the cortex. Although an aura was once considered a sign of impending seizure, it's now considered the first stage of a seizure. Typically, it occurs seconds to minutes before the ictal phase. Its intensity, duration, and type depend on the origin of the irritable focus. For example, an aura of bitter taste commonly accompanies a frontal lobe lesion. Unfortunately, an aura is difficult to describe because the postictal phase of a seizure temporarily alters the patient's level of consciousness, impairing his memory of the event.

The aura associated with a classic migraine headache results from cranial vasoconstriction. Diagnostically important, it helps distinguish a classic migraine from other types of headaches.

Typically, an aura develops over 10 to 30 minutes and varies in intensity and duration. If the patient recognizes the aura as a warning sign, he may be able to prevent the headache by taking appropriate drugs.

Assessment

When an aura rapidly progresses to the ictal phase of a seizure, quickly evaluate the seizure and be alert for life-threatening complications such as apnea. When an aura heralds a classic

Recognizing types of auras

Determining whether an aura marks the patient's thought processes, emotions, or sensory or motor function requires keen observation. An aura typically is difficult to describe and is only dimly remembered when associated with seizure activity. Below you'll find the types of auras the patient may experience.

Affective auras
◆ Fear
◆ Paranoia
◆ Other emotions

Cognitive auras
◆ Déjà vu (familiarity with unfamiliar events or environments)
◆ Flashback of past events
◆ Jamais vu (unfamiliarity with a known event)
◆ Time standing still

Psychomotor auras
◆ Automatisms (inappropriate, repetitive movements): lip smacking, chewing, swallowing, grimacing, picking at clothes, climbing stairs

Psychosensory auras
◆ Auditory: buzzing or ringing in the ears
◆ Gustatory: acidic, metallic, or bitter tastes
◆ Olfactory: foul odors
◆ Tactile: numbness or tingling
◆ Vertigo
◆ Visual: flashes of light (scintillations)

migraine, make the patient as comfortable as possible. Obtain a thorough history of the patient's headaches or seizure history, asking him to describe any sensory or motor phenomena that precede each headache or seizure. Find out how long each headache or seizure typically lasts. Does anything make it worse, such as bright lights, noise, or caffeine? Does anything make it better? Ask the patient about drugs he takes for pain relief.

Causes

◆ *Classic migraine headache.* A migraine is preceded by a vague premonition and then, usually, a visual aura involving flashes of light. The aura lasts 10 to 30 minutes and may intensify until it completely obscures the patient's vision. A classic migraine may cause numbness or tingling of the lips, face, or hands; slight confusion; and dizziness before the characteristic unilateral, throbbing headache appears. It slowly intensifies; when it peaks, it may cause photophobia, nausea, and vomiting.
◆ *Seizure (generalized tonic-clonic).* A generalized tonic-clonic seizure may begin with or without an aura. The patient loses consciousness and falls to the ground. His body stiffens (tonic phase), and then he experiences rapid, synchronous muscle jerking and hyperventilation (clonic phase). The seizure usually lasts 2 to 5 minutes.

B

Babinski's reflex

Babinski's reflex—dorsiflexion of the great toe with extension and fanning of the other toes—is an abnormal reflex elicited by firmly stroking the lateral aspect of the sole of the foot with a moderately sharp object. (See *How to elicit Babinski's reflex*.) An indicator of corticospinal damage, Babinski's reflex may occur unilaterally or bilaterally and may be temporary or permanent. A temporary Babinski's reflex commonly occurs during the postictal phase of a seizure, whereas a permanent Babinski's reflex occurs with corticospinal damage. A positive Babinski's reflex is normal in neonates and in infants younger than age 2.

Assessment

After eliciting a positive Babinski's reflex, evaluate the patient for other neurologic signs. Evaluate muscle strength in each extremity by having the patient push or pull against your resistance. Passively flex and extend the extremity to assess muscle tone. Intermittent resistance to flexion and extension indicates spasticity, and a lack of resistance indicates flaccidity.

Next, check for evidence of incoordination by asking the patient to perform a repetitive activity. Test deep tendon reflexes (DTRs) in the patient's elbow, antecubital area, wrist, knee, and ankle by striking the tendon with a reflex hammer. An exaggerated muscle response indicates hyperactive DTRs; little or no muscle response indicates hypoactivity.

Then evaluate pain sensation and proprioception in the feet. As you move the patient's toes up and down, ask him to identify the direction in which the toes have been moved without looking at his feet.

Causes

◆ *Amyotrophic lateral sclerosis (ALS).* In ALS, a progressive motor neuron disorder, bilateral Babinski's reflex may occur with hyperactive DTRs and spasticity. Typically, ALS produces fasciculations accompanied by muscle atrophy and weakness. Incoordination makes carrying out activities of daily living difficult for the patient. Associated signs and symptoms include impaired speech; difficulty chewing, swallowing, and breathing; urinary frequency and urgency; and, occasionally, choking and excessive drooling. Although his mental status remains intact, the patient's poor prognosis may cause periodic depression. Progressive bulbar palsy involves the brain stem

◆

How to elicit Babinski's reflex

To elicit Babinski's reflex, stroke the lateral aspect of the sole of the patient's foot with your thumbnail or another moderately sharp object. Normally, this elicits flexion of all toes (a negative Babinski's reflex), as shown below in the left illustration. With a positive Babinski's reflex, the great toe dorsiflexes and the other toes fan out, as shown in the right illustration.

NORMAL TOE FLEXION

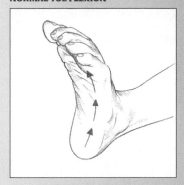

POSITIVE BABINSKI'S REFLEX

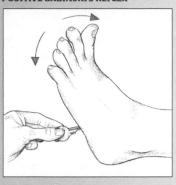

and may cause episodes of crying or inappropriate laughter.

◆ *Brain tumor.* A brain tumor that involves the corticospinal tract may produce Babinski's reflex. The reflex may be accompanied by hyperactive DTRs (unilateral or bilateral), spasticity, seizures, cranial nerve dysfunction, hemiparesis or hemiplegia, decreased pain sensation, an unsteady gait, incoordination, headache, emotional lability, and a decreased level of consciousness (LOC).

◆ *Head trauma.* Unilateral or bilateral Babinski's reflex may occur as the result of primary corticospinal damage or secondary injury associated with increased intracranial pressure and is commonly accompanied by hyperactive DTRs and spasticity. The patient may also have weakness and incoordination. Other signs and symptoms vary with the type of head trauma and include headache, vomiting, behavior changes, altered vital signs, and a decreased LOC with abnormal pupil size and response to light.

◆ *Hepatic encephalopathy.* Babinski's reflex occurs late in hepatic encephalopathy when the patient slips into a coma. It's accompanied by hyperactive DTRs and fetor hepaticus (abnormal breath odor).

◆ *Meningitis.* With meningitis, bilateral Babinski's reflex commonly follows fever, chills, and malaise and is accompanied by nausea and vomiting. As meningitis progresses, it causes a decreased LOC, nuchal rigidity, positive Brudzinski's and Kernig's signs, hyperactive DTRs, and opisthotonos. Associated signs and symptoms include irritability, photophobia, diplopia, delirium, and a deep stupor that may progress to a coma.

◆ *Rabies.* Bilateral Babinski's reflex—possibly elicited by nonspecific noxious stimuli alone—appears in the excitation phase of rabies. This phase occurs 2 to 10 days after the onset of prodromal signs and symptoms, such as fever, malaise, and irritability (which occur 30 to 40 days after a bite from an infected animal). Rabies is characterized by marked restlessness and extremely painful pharyngeal muscle spasms. Difficulty swallowing causes excessive drooling and hydrophobia in about 50% of affected patients. Seizures and hyperactive DTRs may also occur.

◆ *Spinal cord injury.* With acute spinal cord injury, spinal shock temporarily erases all reflexes. As shock resolves, Babinski's reflex occurs—unilaterally when an injury affects only one side of the spinal cord (Brown-Séquard syndrome), bilaterally when an injury affects both sides. Rather than signaling the return of neurologic function, this reflex confirms corticospinal damage. It's accompanied by hyperactive DTRs, spasticity, and variable or total loss of pain and temperature sensation, proprioception, and motor function. Horner syndrome, marked by unilateral ptosis, pupillary constriction, and facial anhidrosis, may occur with lower cervical cord injury.

◆ *Spinal cord tumor.* With spinal cord tumor, bilateral Babinski's reflex occurs with variable loss of pain and temperature sensation, proprioception, and motor function. Spasticity, hyperactive DTRs, absent abdominal reflexes, and incontinence are also characteristic. Diffuse pain may occur at the level of the tumor.

◆ *Spinal paralytic poliomyelitis.* Unilateral or bilateral Babinski's reflex occurs 5 to 7 days after the onset of fever. It's accompanied by progressive weakness, paresthesia, muscle tenderness, spasticity, irritability and, later, atrophy. Resistance to neck flexion is characteristic, as are Hoyne's, Kernig's, and Brudzinski's signs.

◆ *Spinal tuberculosis (TB).* Spinal TB may produce bilateral Babinski's reflex accompanied by variable loss of pain and temperature sensation, proprioception, and motor function. It also causes spasticity, hyperactive DTRs, bladder incontinence, and absent abdominal reflexes.

◆ *Stroke.* Babinski's reflex varies with the site of the stroke. If it involves the cerebrum, it produces unilateral Babinski's reflex accompanied by hemiplegia or hemiparesis, unilateral hyperactive DTRs, hemianopsia, and aphasia. If it involves the brain stem, it produces bilateral Babinski's reflex accompanied by bilateral weakness or paralysis, bilateral hyperactive DTRs, cranial nerve dysfunction, incoordination, and an unsteady gait. Generalized signs and symptoms of stroke include headache, vomiting, fever, disorientation, nuchal rigidity, seizures, and coma.

◆ *Syringomyelia.* With syringomyelia (chronic, progressive disease of the spinal cord), bilateral Babinski's reflex occurs with muscle atrophy and weakness that may progress to paralysis. It's accompanied by spasticity, ataxia and, occasionally, deep pain. DTRs may be hypoactive or hyperactive. Cranial nerve dysfunction, such as dysphagia and dysarthria, commonly appears late in the disorder.

Back pain

Back pain affects an estimated 80% of the population; in fact, it's the second leading reason—after the common cold—for time lost from work. Although this symptom may herald a spondylogenic disorder, it may also result from a genitourinary, GI, cardiovascular, or neoplastic disorder or the postural imbalance associated with pregnancy.

The onset, location, intensity, and distribution of pain and its response to activity and rest provide important clues about the cause. It may remain localized in the back or radiate along the spine or down one or both legs.

Intrinsic back pain results from muscle spasm, nerve root irritation, fracture, or a combination of these disorders. It usually occurs in the lumbosacral area, but may also be referred from the abdomen or flank.

Assessment

If the patient reports acute, severe back pain, quickly take his vital signs, and then perform a rapid evaluation to rule out life-threatening causes. Typically, visceral-referred back pain is unaffected by activity and rest. In contrast, spondylogenic-referred back pain worsens with activity and improves with rest. Pain of neoplastic origin is usually relieved by walking and worsens at night. If the patient describes deep lumbar pain unaffected by activity, palpate for a pulsating epigastric mass, which may indicate a dissecting abdominal aortic aneurysm. If the patient describes severe epigastric pain that radiates through the abdomen to the back, assess him for absent bowel sounds and abdominal rigidity and tenderness, which may indicate a perforated ulcer or acute pancreatitis.

If the patient's pain isn't acute and severe, obtain a medical history, including past injuries, surgeries, and illnesses, and a family history. Ask about diet and alcohol intake. Also take a drug history, including past and present prescriptions and over-the-counter drugs. Ask the patient to describe the location of the pain and to rate it according to a pain scale.

Next, perform a thorough assessment. Be aware of the patient's expressions of pain as you do so. Observe skin color and palpate skin temperature. Palpate femoral, popliteal, posterior tibial, and pedal pulses. Ask about unusual sensations in the legs, such as numbness and tingling. Observe the patient's posture if pain doesn't prohibit standing. Observe the level of the shoulders and pelvis and the curvature of the back. Ask the patient to bend forward, backward, and from side to side while you palpate for paravertebral muscle spasms. Palpate the dorsolumbar spine for point tenderness. Then ask the patient to walk—first on his heels and then on his toes; protect him from falling as he does so. Weakness may reflect a muscular disorder or spinal nerve root irritation. Have the patient sit to evaluate and compare patellar tendon (knee), Achilles tendon, and Babinski's reflexes. To reproduce leg and back pain, position the patient in a supine position on the examining table. Grasp his heel and slowly lift his leg. If he feels pain, note its exact location and the angle between the table and his leg when it occurs. Repeat this maneuver with the opposite leg. Pain along the sciatic nerve may indicate disk herniation or sciatica. Also note the range of motion of the hip and knee. Palpate the flanks and percuss with the fingertips or perform fist percussion to elicit costovertebral angle (CVA) tenderness.

Causes

◢ *Abdominal aortic aneurysm (dissecting).* Life-threatening dissection of this aneurysm may initially cause lower back pain or dull abdominal pain. It commonly produces constant upper abdominal pain. A pulsating abdominal mass may be palpated in the epigastrium; however, after rupture it no longer pulses. Aneurysmal dissection can also cause mottled skin below the waist, absent femoral and pedal pulses, lower blood pressure in the legs than in the arms, mild to moderate tenderness with guarding, and abdominal rigidity. Observe for signs of shock.

◆ *Ankylosing spondylitis.* Ankylosing spondylitis is a chronic, progressive disorder that causes sacroiliac pain, which radiates up the spine and is aggravated by lateral pressure on the pelvis. The pain is usually most severe in the morning or after a period of inactivity and isn't relieved by rest. Abnormal rigidity of the lumbar spine with forward flexion is also characteristic. This disorder can cause local tenderness, fatigue, fever, anorexia, weight loss, and occasional iritis.

◳ *Appendicitis.* Appendicitis is a life-threatening disorder in which a vague and dull discomfort in the epigastric or umbilical region migrates to McBurney point in the right lower quadrant. With retrocecal appendicitis, pain may also radiate to the back. The shift in pain is preceded by anorexia and nausea and is accompanied by fever, occasional vomiting, abdominal tenderness (especially over McBurney point), and rebound tenderness. Some patients also have painful, urgent urination.

◆ *Cholecystitis.* Cholecystitis produces severe pain in the right upper quadrant of the abdomen that may radiate to the right shoulder, chest, or back. The pain may arise suddenly or may increase gradually over several hours. Accompanying signs and symptoms include anorexia, fever, nausea, vomiting, right upper quadrant tenderness, abdominal rigidity, pallor, and sweating.

◆ *Chordoma.* A chordoma is a slow-developing malignant tumor that usually occurs in the sacrum, coccyx, or at the base of the skull but can also occur other places in the spine. As the tumor expands, constipation and bowel or bladder incontinence may accompany persistent pain in the lower back, sacrum, and coccyx.

◆ *Endometriosis.* Endometriosis causes deep sacral pain and severe, cramping pain in the lower abdomen. The pain worsens just before or during menstruation and may be aggravated by defecation. It's accompanied by constipation, abdominal tenderness, and dyspareunia.

◆ *Intervertebral disk rupture.* Intervertebral disk rupture produces lower back pain with or without leg pain (sciatica). It rarely produces leg pain alone. The pain usually begins in the back and radiates to the buttocks and legs. The pain is exacerbated by activity, coughing, and sneezing and is eased by rest. It's accompanied by paresthesia (most commonly, numbness or tingling in the lower leg and foot), paravertebral muscle spasm, and decreased reflexes on the affected side. This disorder also affects posture and gait. The patient's spine is slightly flexed and he leans toward the painful side. He walks slowly and rises from a sitting to a standing position with extreme difficulty.

◆ *Lumbosacral sprain.* Lumbosacral sprain causes aching, localized pain and tenderness associated with muscle spasm on lateral motion. A recumbent patient typically flexes his knees and hips to help ease the pain. Flexion of the spine and movement intensify the pain, whereas rest helps relieve it.

◆ *Metastatic tumors.* Metastatic tumors commonly spread to the spine, causing lower back pain. Typically, the pain begins abruptly, is accompanied by cramping muscular pain (usually worse at night), and isn't relieved by rest.

◆ *Myeloma.* Back pain caused by myeloma, a primary malignant tumor, usually begins abruptly and worsens with exercise. It may be accompanied by arthritic signs and symptoms, such as achiness, joint swelling, and tenderness. Other signs and symptoms include fever, malaise, peripheral paresthesia, and weight loss.

◳ *Pancreatitis (acute).* Pancreatitis is a life-threatening disorder that usually produces fulminating, continuous upper abdominal pain that may radiate to both flanks and to the back. To relieve this pain, the patient may bend forward, draw his knees to his chest, or move restlessly. Early associated signs and symptoms include abdominal tenderness, nausea, vomiting, fever, pallor, tachycardia and, in some cases, abdominal guarding, rigidity, rebound tenderness, and hypoactive bowel sounds. A late sign may be jaundice. Occurring as inflammation subsides, Turner's sign (ecchymosis of the abdomen or flank) or Cullen's sign (bluish discoloration of skin around the umbilicus and on both flanks) signals hemorrhagic pancreatitis.

◪ *Perforated ulcer.* In some patients, perforation of a duodenal or gastric ulcer causes sudden, prostrating epigastric pain that may radiate throughout the abdomen and to the back. This life-threatening disorder also causes board-like abdominal rigidity, tenderness with guarding, generalized rebound tenderness, absent bowel sounds, and grunting, shallow respirations. Associated signs include fever, tachycardia, and hypotension.

◆ *Prostate cancer.* Chronic aching back pain may be the only symptom of prostate cancer. It may also produce hematuria and decrease the urine stream.

◆ *Pyelonephritis (acute).* Pyelonephritis produces progressive flank and lower abdominal pain accompanied by back pain or tenderness (especially over the CVA). Other signs and symptoms include high fever and chills, nausea and vomiting, flank and abdominal tenderness, and urinary frequency and urgency.

◆ *Renal calculi.* The colicky pain of renal calculi usually travels from the CVA to the flank, suprapubic region, and external genitalia. Its intensity varies but may become excruciating if calculi travel down a ureter. If calculi are in the renal pelvis and calyces, dull

and constant flank pain may occur. Renal calculi also cause nausea, vomiting, urinary urgency (if a calculus lodges near the bladder), and hematuria. The pain resolves or significantly decreases after calculi move to the bladder.

◆ *Sacroiliac strain.* Sacroiliac strain causes sacroiliac pain that may radiate to the buttock, hip, and lateral aspect of the thigh. The pain is aggravated by weight bearing on the affected extremity and by abduction with resistance of the leg. An associated symptom may be tenderness of the symphysis pubis.

◆ *Spinal neoplasm (benign).* Spinal neoplasm typically causes severe, localized back pain and scoliosis.

◆ *Spinal stenosis.* Resembling a ruptured intervertebral disk, spinal stenosis produces back pain that commonly affects both legs. The pain may radiate to the toes and may progress to numbness or weakness unless the patient rests.

◆ *Spondylolisthesis.* Spondylolisthesis (displacement of a lumbar vertebra) may cause lower back pain, with or without nerve root involvement. Symptoms associated with nerve root involvement include paresthesia, buttock pain, and pain that radiates down the leg. Palpation of the lumbar spine may reveal a "step-off" of the spinous process. Flexion of the spine may be limited.

◆ *Transverse process fracture.* Transverse process fracture causes severe localized back pain with muscle spasm.

◆ *Vertebral compression fracture.* Initially, vertebral compression fracture may be painless. Several weeks later, it causes back pain aggravated by weight bearing and local tenderness. Fracture of a thoracic vertebra may cause referred pain in the lumbar area.

◆ *Vertebral osteomyelitis.* Initially, vertebral osteomyelitis causes insidious back pain. As it progresses, the pain

may become constant, more pronounced at night, and aggravated by spinal movement. Accompanying signs and symptoms include vertebral and hamstring spasms, tenderness of the spinous processes, fever, and malaise.
◆ *Vertebral osteoporosis.* Vertebral osteoporosis causes chronic, aching back pain that's aggravated by activity and somewhat relieved by rest. Tenderness may also occur.

Battle's sign

Battle's sign—ecchymosis over the mastoid process of the temporal bone—is commonly the only outward sign of a basilar skull fracture. In fact, this type of fracture may go undetected even by skull X-rays. If left untreated, it can be fatal because of associated injury to the nearby cranial nerves and brain stem as well as to blood vessels and the meninges.

Appearing behind one or both ears, Battle's sign is easily overlooked or hidden by the patient's hair. During emergency care of a trauma victim, it may be overshadowed by imminently life-threatening or more apparent injuries.

A force that's strong enough to fracture the base of the skull causes Battle's sign by damaging supporting tissues of the mastoid area and causing seepage of blood from the fracture site to the mastoid. Battle's sign usually develops 24 to 36 hours after a fracture and may persist for several days to weeks.

Assessment

Perform a complete neurologic assessment. Begin with the history. Ask the patient about recent trauma to the head. Did he sustain a severe blow to the head? Was he involved in a motor vehicle accident? Note the patient's level of consciousness as he responds. Does he respond quickly or slowly? Are his answers appropriate, or does he appear confused?

Check the patient's vital signs; stay alert for hypertension, widening pulse pressure, and bradycardia, signs of increased intracranial pressure. Assess cranial nerve function in nerves II, III, IV, VI, VII, and VIII. Evaluate pupil size and response to light as well as motor and verbal responses. Relate these data to the Glasgow Coma Scale. Also note cerebrospinal fluid (CSF) leakage from the nose or ears. Ask about postnasal drip, which may reflect CSF drainage down the throat. Look for the halo sign—a blood stain encircled by a yellowish ring—on bed linens or dressings. To confirm that drainage is CSF, test it with a Dextrostix; CSF is positive for glucose, whereas mucus isn't. Follow up the neurologic assessment with a complete physical assessment to detect other injuries associated with basilar skull fracture.

Causes

◪ *Basilar skull fracture.* Battle's sign may be the only outward sign of basilar skull fracture, or it may be accompanied by periorbital ecchymosis (raccoon eyes), conjunctival hemorrhage, nystagmus, ocular deviation, epistaxis, anosmia, a bulging tympanic membrane (from CSF or blood accumulation), visible fracture lines on the external auditory canal, tinnitus, difficulty hearing, facial paralysis, or vertigo.

Biot's respirations

A late and ominous sign of neurologic deterioration, Biot's respirations are characterized by an irregular and unpredictable rate, rhythm, and depth.

Identifying Biot's respirations

Biot's respirations, also known as *ataxic respirations,* have a completely irregular pattern. Shallow and deep breaths occur randomly, with haphazard, irregular pauses. The respiratory rate tends to be slow and may progressively decelerate to apnea.

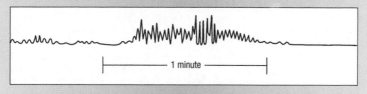

|————— 1 minute —————|

EMERGENCY INTERVENTIONS

Responding to Biot's respirations

If you detect Biot's respirations in a patient, perform these interventions:
◆ Assess the patient's respiratory status.
◆ Prepare to intubate the patient and provide mechanical ventilation.
◆ Take the patient's vital signs, especially noting increased systolic blood pressure.

This rare breathing pattern may appear abruptly and may reflect increased pressure on the medulla coinciding with brain stem compression.

Assessment

Observe the patient's breathing pattern for several minutes to avoid confusing Biot's respirations with other respiratory patterns. (See *Identifying Biot's respirations.*) Perform emergency interventions as needed. (See *Responding to Biot's respirations.*)

Causes

 Brain stem compression. Biot's respirations are characteristic in brain stem compression, a neurologic emergency. Rapidly enlarging lesions may cause ataxic respirations and lead to complete respiratory arrest.

Bladder distention

Bladder distention—abnormal enlargement of the bladder—results from an inability to excrete urine, which results in its accumulation. Distention can be caused by a mechanical or anatomic obstruction, neuromuscular disorder, or the use of certain drugs. Relatively common in all ages and both sexes, it's most common in older men with prostate disorders that cause urine retention.

Distention usually develops gradually, but it occasionally has a sudden onset. Gradual distention usually produces no symptoms until stretching of the bladder produces discomfort. Acute distention produces suprapubic fullness, pressure, and pain. If severe distention isn't corrected promptly by catheterization or massage, the bladder rises within the abdomen, its walls become thin, and the bladder may rupture.

Assessment

If distention is severe, insert an indwelling urinary catheter to prevent bladder rupture. If distention isn't severe, begin by reviewing the patient's voiding patterns. Find out the time and amount of the patient's last voiding and the amount of fluid consumed since then. Ask if he has difficulty urinating. Does he urinate with urgency or without warning? Is urination painful or irritating? Ask about the force and continuity of his urine stream and whether he feels that his bladder is empty after voiding.

Explore the patient's history of urinary tract obstruction or infections; venereal disease; neurologic, intestinal, or pelvic surgery; lower abdominal or urinary tract trauma; and systemic or neurologic disorders. Note his drug history, including his use of over-the-counter drugs.

Take the patient's vital signs, and percuss and palpate the bladder. (Remember that if the bladder is empty, it can't be palpated through the abdominal wall.) Inspect the urethral meatus, and measure its diameter. Describe the appearance and amount of any discharge. Finally, test for perineal sensation and anal sphincter tone.

Causes

◆ *Benign prostatic hyperplasia (BPH).* With BPH, bladder distention typically develops gradually as the prostate enlarges. Occasionally, its onset is acute.

Initially, the patient experiences urinary hesitancy, straining, and frequency; reduced force of and the inability to stop the urine stream; nocturia; and postvoiding dribbling. As the disorder progresses, it produces sensations of suprapubic fullness and incomplete bladder emptying, perineal pain, constipation, and hematuria.

◆ *Bladder cancer.* By blocking the urethral orifice, neoplasms can cause bladder distention. Associated signs and symptoms include hematuria (most common sign); urinary frequency and urgency; nocturia; dysuria; pyuria; pain in the bladder, rectum, pelvis, flank, back, or legs; vomiting; diarrhea; and sleeplessness. A mass may be palpable on bimanual examination.

◆ *Drugs.* Parasympatholytics, anticholinergics, ganglionic blockers, sedatives, anesthetics, and opiates can produce urine retention and bladder distention.

◆ *Multiple sclerosis (MS).* With MS, a neuromuscular disorder, urine retention and bladder distention result from the interruption of upper motor neuron control of the bladder. Associated signs and symptoms include optic neuritis, paresthesia, impaired position and vibratory senses, diplopia, nystagmus, dizziness, abnormal reflexes, dysarthria, muscle weakness, emotional lability, Lhermitte's sign (transient, electric-like shocks that spread down the body when the head is flexed), Babinski's sign, and ataxia.

◆ *Prostate cancer.* Prostate cancer eventually causes bladder distention in about 25% of patients. Usual signs and symptoms include dysuria, urinary frequency and urgency, nocturia, weight loss, fatigue, perineal pain, and constipation. For some patients, urine retention and bladder distention are the only signs.

◆ *Prostatitis.* Bladder distention is rare with chronic prostatitis. With acute prostatitis, bladder distention occurs rapidly along with perineal discomfort and suprapubic fullness. Other signs and symptoms include perineal pain; a tense, boggy, tender, and warm enlarged prostate; decreased libido; impotence; decreased force of the urine stream; dysuria; hematuria; and urinary frequency and urgency. Additional signs and symptoms include fatigue, malaise, myalgia, fever, chills, nausea, and vomiting.

◆ *Spinal neoplasms.* Disrupting upper neuron control of the bladder, spinal neoplasms cause neurogenic bladder and resultant distention. Associated signs and symptoms include a sense of pelvic fullness, continuous overflow dribbling, back pain that typically mimics sciatic pain, constipation, tender vertebral processes, sensory deficits, and muscle weakness, flaccidity, and atrophy. Signs and symptoms of urinary tract infection may also occur.

◆ *Urethral calculi.* With urethral calculi, urethral obstruction leads to bladder distention. The obstruction causes pain radiating to the penis or vulva and referred to the perineum or rectum. It may also produce a urethral discharge.

◆ *Urethral stricture.* Urethral stricture results in urine retention and bladder distention with chronic urethral discharge (most common sign), urinary frequency (also common), dysuria, urgency, decreased force and diameter of the urine stream, and pyuria. Urinoma (urine that's encapsulated by fibrous tissue) and urosepsis may also develop.

Blood pressure decrease

Low blood pressure refers to inadequate intravascular pressure to maintain the oxygen requirements of the body's tissues. Although commonly linked to shock, this sign may also result from a cardiovascular, respiratory, neurologic, or metabolic disorder. Hypoperfusion states especially affect the kidneys, brain, and heart, and may lead to renal failure, a change in the patient's level of consciousness (LOC), or myocardial ischemia. Low blood pressure may be drug-induced or may accompany diagnostic tests—most commonly those using contrast media. It may stem from stress or change of position—specifically, rising abruptly from a supine or sitting position to a standing position (orthostatic hypotension).

Normal blood pressure varies considerably; what qualifies as low blood pressure for one person may be normal for another. Therefore, every blood pressure reading must be compared against the patient's baseline. Typically, a reading below 90/60 mm Hg is considered low blood pressure.

Low blood pressure can reflect an expanded intravascular space (as in severe infections, allergic reactions, or adrenal insufficiency), reduced intravascular volume (as in dehydration and hemorrhage), or decreased cardiac output (as in impaired cardiac muscle contractility). Because the body's pressure-regulating mechanisms are complex and interrelated, a combination of these factors usually contributes to low blood pressure.

◆ **ALERT** Low blood pressure is dangerous when it occurs abruptly or is accompanied by such symptoms as dizziness or syncope.

Assessment

If the patient's systolic pressure is less than 80 mm Hg, or 30 mm Hg below his baseline, suspect shock. Quickly evaluate the patient for a decreased

EMERGENCY INTERVENTIONS

Responding to severe hypotension

If your patient develops severe hypotension, take these steps:
◆ Elevate the patient's legs above the level of his heart, or place him in Trendelenburg's position if the bed can be adjusted.
◆ Insert an I.V. catheter using a large-bore needle to replace fluids and blood or to administer drugs.
◆ Prepare to administer oxygen with mechanical ventilation, if necessary.
◆ Monitor the patient's intake and output,
and insert an indwelling urinary catheter to accurately measure urine output.
◆ Assist with a central venous catheter or a pulmonary artery catheter insertion to facilitate monitoring his fluid status, if necessary.
◆ Prepare for cardiac monitoring to evaluate cardiac rhythm.
◆ Be ready to insert a nasogastric tube, if prescribed, to prevent aspiration in the comatose patient.

LOC. Check his apical pulse for tachycardia and his respirations for tachypnea. Also, inspect the patient for cool, clammy skin. Then take appropriate action. (See *Responding to severe hypotension.*)

If the patient is conscious, ask him about associated symptoms. For example, does he feel unusually weak or fatigued? Has he had nausea, vomiting, or dark or bloody stools? Is his vision blurred? Is his gait unsteady? Does he have palpitations? Does he have chest or abdominal pain or difficulty breathing? Has he had episodes of dizziness or fainting? Do these episodes occur when he stands up suddenly? If so, take the patient's blood pressure while he's lying down, sitting, and then standing; compare readings. (See *Ensuring accurate blood pressure measurement.*) A drop in systolic or diastolic pressure of 20 mm Hg or more and an increase in heart rate of more than 15 beats/minute between position changes suggest orthostatic hypotension.

Next, continue with a physical assessment. Inspect the skin for pallor, sweat, and clamminess. Palpate periph-
eral pulses. Note paradoxical pulse (an accentuated fall in systolic pressure during inspiration), which suggests pericardial tamponade. Then auscultate for abnormal heart sounds (gallops, murmurs), rate (bradycardia, tachycardia), or rhythm. Auscultate the lungs for abnormal breath sounds (diminished sounds, crackles, wheezing), rate (bradypnea, tachypnea), or rhythm (agonal or Cheyne-Stokes respirations). Look for signs of hemorrhage, including visible bleeding and palpable masses, bruising, and tenderness. Assess the patient for abdominal rigidity and rebound tenderness; auscultate for abnormal bowel sounds. Also, carefully assess the patient for possible sources of infection such as open wounds.

Causes

◆ *Acute adrenal insufficiency.* Orthostatic hypotension is characteristic with acute adrenal insufficiency, accompanied by fatigue, weakness, nausea, vomiting, abdominal discomfort, weight loss, fever, and tachycardia. The patient may also have hyperpigmentation of the fingers, nails, nipples, scars,

Ensuring accurate blood pressure measurement

When taking the patient's blood pressure, begin by applying the cuff properly, as shown here.

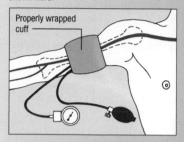

Properly wrapped cuff

Stay alert for these common pitfalls to avoid recording an inaccurate blood pressure measurement:

◆ *Wrong-sized cuff.* Select the appropriate-sized cuff for the patient. Doing so makes sure that adequate pressure is applied to compress the brachial artery during cuff inflation. If the cuff bladder is too narrow, a false-high reading will be obtained; too wide, a false-low reading. The cuff bladder width should be about 40% of the circumference of the midpoint of the limb; bladder length should be twice the width. If the arm circumference is less than 13″ (33 cm), select a regular-sized cuff; if it's 13″ to 16″ (33 to 40.5 cm), a large-sized cuff; if it's more than 16″, a thigh cuff. Pediatric cuffs are also available.

◆ *Slow cuff deflation, causing venous congestion in the extremity.* Don't deflate the cuff more slowly than 2 mm Hg/heartbeat because you'll get a false-high reading.

◆ *Cuff wrapped too loosely, reducing its effective width.* Tighten the cuff to avoid a false-high reading.

◆ *Mercury column not read at eye level.* Read the mercury column at eye level. If the column is below eye level, you may record a false-low reading; if it's above eye level, a false-high reading.

◆ *Tilted mercury column.* Keep the mercury column vertical to avoid a false-high reading.

◆ *Poorly timed measurement.* Don't take the patient's blood pressure if he appears anxious or if he has just eaten or ambulated; you'll get a false-high reading.

◆ *Incorrect position of the arm.* Keep the patient's arm level with his heart to avoid a false-low reading.

◆ *Cuff overinflation, causing venospasm or pain.* Don't overinflate the cuff because you'll get a false-high reading.

◆ *Failure to notice an auscultatory gap* (sound fades out for 10 to 15 mm Hg and then returns). To avoid missing the top Korotkoff's sound, estimate systolic pressure by palpation first. Then inflate the cuff rapidly—at a rate of 2 to 3 mm Hg/second—to about 30 mm Hg above the palpable systolic pressure.

◆ *Inaudibility of feeble sounds.* Before reinflating the cuff, have the patient raise his arm to reduce venous pressure and amplify low-volume sounds. After inflating the cuff, lower the patient's arm, and then deflate the cuff and listen. Alternatively, with the patient's arm positioned at heart level, inflate the cuff and have the patient make a fist. Have him rapidly open and close his hand 10 times before you begin to deflate the cuff, and then listen. Be sure to document that the blood pressure reading was augmented.

and body folds; pale, cool, clammy skin; restlessness; decreased urine output; tachypnea; and coma.

◼ *Anaphylactic shock.* Following exposure to an allergen, such as penicillin or insect venom, a dramatic fall in blood pressure and narrowed pulse pressure signal an anaphylactic reaction. Initially, anaphylactic shock causes anxiety, restlessness, a feeling of doom, intense itching (especially of the hands and feet), and a pounding headache. Later, it may also produce weakness, sweating, nasal congestion, coughing, difficulty breathing, nausea, abdominal cramps, involuntary defecation, seizures, flushing, change or loss of voice due to laryngeal edema, urinary incontinence, and tachycardia.

◨ *Anthrax (inhalation)*. Anthrax is an acute infectious disease that's caused by the spore-forming bacterium *Bacillus anthracis*. The disease can occur in humans who are exposed to infected animals (wild and domestic grazing animals), tissue from infected animals, or biological warfare. Most natural cases occur in agricultural regions worldwide because the spores can live in the soil for many years. Anthrax may occur in the cutaneous, inhalation, or GI form.

Inhalation anthrax is caused by inhaling aerosolized spores. Initial signs and symptoms are flulike and include fever, chills, weakness, cough, and chest pain. The disease generally occurs in two stages with a period of recovery after the initial signs and symptoms. The second stage develops abruptly with rapid deterioration marked by fever, dyspnea, stridor, and hypotension, generally leading to death within 24 hours.

◨ *Cardiac arrhythmias*. With an arrhythmia, blood pressure may fluctuate between normal and low readings. Dizziness, chest pain, difficulty breathing, light-headedness, weakness, fatigue, and palpitations may also occur.

◆ *Cardiac contusion*. With cardiac contusion, low blood pressure occurs along with tachycardia and, at times, anginal pain and dyspnea.

◨ *Cardiac tamponade*. An accentuated fall in systolic pressure (more than 10 mm Hg) during inspiration, known as *paradoxical pulse,* is characteristic in patients with cardiac tamponade. This disorder also causes narrowed pulse

pressure, restlessness, cyanosis, tachycardia, jugular vein distention, muffled heart sounds, dyspnea, and Kussmaul's sign (increased venous distention with inspiration).

◨ *Cardiogenic shock*. A fall in systolic pressure to less than 80 mm Hg or to 30 mm Hg less than the patient's baseline because of decreased cardiac contractility is characteristic in cardiogenic shock. Accompanying low blood pressure are tachycardia, narrowed pulse pressure, diminished Korotkoff sounds, peripheral cyanosis, and pale, cool, clammy skin. Associated signs and symptoms include angina, dyspnea, jugular vein distention, oliguria, ventricular gallop, tachypnea, and restlessness and anxiety, which may progress to disorientation and confusion.

◨ *Diabetic ketoacidosis*. Low blood pressure associated with diabetic ketoacidosis results from hypovolemia, caused by osmotic diuresis occurring with hyperglycemia. It typically occurs in patients with type 1 diabetes mellitus. Other symptoms include polydipsia, polyuria, polyphagia, dehydration, weight loss, abdominal pain, nausea, vomiting, fruity breath odor, Kussmaul's respirations, tachycardia, confusion, and stupor that may progress to a coma.

◆ *Drugs*. Calcium channel blockers, diuretics, vasodilators, alpha- and beta-adrenergic blockers, general anesthetics, opioid analgesics, monoamine oxidase inhibitors, anxiolytics (such as benzodiazepines), tranquilizers, and most I.V. antiarrhythmics can cause low blood pressure.

◆ *Heart failure*. With heart failure, blood pressure may fluctuate between normal and low readings. However, a precipitous drop in blood pressure may signal cardiogenic shock. Other signs and symptoms of heart failure include exertional dyspnea, dyspnea of abrupt or gradual onset, paroxysmal nocturnal dyspnea or difficulty breathing in the supine position (orthopnea), fatigue, weight gain, pallor or cyanosis, sweating, and anxiety. Auscultation reveals ventricular gallop, tachycardia, bilateral crackles, and tachypnea. Dependent edema, jugular vein distention, increased capillary refill time, and hepatomegaly may also occur.

◆ *Hyperosmolar hyperglycemic nonketotic syndrome (HHNS).* HHNS, which occurs in patients with type 2 diabetes mellitus, decreases blood pressure—at times dramatically—because of significant fluid loss from diuresis caused by severe hyperglycemia and hyperosmolarity. It also produces dry mouth, poor skin turgor, tachycardia, confusion progressing to coma and, occasionally, generalized tonic-clonic seizure.

◼ *Hypovolemic shock.* A fall in systolic pressure to less than 80 mm Hg or 30 mm Hg less than the patient's baseline, secondary to acute blood loss or dehydration, is characteristic in hypovolemic shock. It's accompanied by diminished Korotkoff sounds, narrowed pulse pressure, and a rapid, weak, and irregular pulse. Other signs and symptoms include oliguria, confusion, disorientation, restlessness, anxiety, and peripheral vasoconstriction (which causes cyanosis of the extremities and pale, cool, clammy skin).

◼ *Hypoxemia.* Initially, blood pressure may be normal or slightly elevated; however, as hypoxemia becomes more pronounced, blood pressure drops. The patient may also display tachycardia, tachypnea, dyspnea, restlessness, and confusion and may progress from stupor to a coma.

◼ *Myocardial infarction (MI).* With MI, a life-threatening disorder, blood pressure may be low or high. However, a precipitous drop in blood pressure may signal cardiogenic shock. Associated signs and symptoms may include chest pain that may radiate to the jaw,

shoulder, arm, or epigastrium; dyspnea; anxiety; nausea or vomiting; sweating; and cool, pale, or cyanotic skin. Auscultation may reveal an atrial gallop, a murmur and, occasionally, an irregular pulse.

◼ *Neurogenic shock.* The result of sympathetic denervation due to cervical injury or anesthesia, neurogenic shock produces low blood pressure and bradycardia. However, the patient's skin remains warm and dry because of cutaneous vasodilation and sweat gland denervation. Depending on the cause of shock, there may be motor weakness of the limbs or diaphragm.

◼ *Pulmonary embolism.* Pulmonary embolism causes sudden, sharp chest pain and dyspnea accompanied by a cough and, occasionally, a low-grade fever. Low blood pressure occurs with narrowed pulse pressure and diminished Korotkoff sounds. Associated signs include tachycardia, tachypnea, restlessness, paradoxical pulse, jugular vein distention, and hemoptysis.

◼ *Septic shock.* Initially, septic shock produces fever and chills. Low blood pressure, tachycardia, and tachypnea may also develop early, but the patient's skin remains warm. Later, low blood pressure becomes increasingly severe—less than 80 mm Hg or 30 mm Hg less than the patient's baseline—and is accompanied by narrowed pulse pressure. Other late signs and symptoms include pale skin, cyanotic extremities, apprehension, restlessness, thirst, oliguria, and coma.

◆ *Vasovagal syncope.* Vasovagal syncope is the transient loss or near-loss of consciousness that's characterized by low blood pressure, pallor, cold sweats, nausea, palpitations or slowed heart rate, and weakness following stressful, painful, or claustrophobic experiences.

Blood pressure increase

Elevated blood pressure—an intermittent or sustained increase in blood pressure exceeding 119/79 mm Hg—may develop suddenly or gradually. A sudden, severe rise in pressure—exceeding 180/110 mm Hg—may indicate life-threatening hypertensive crisis. However, even a less dramatic rise may be equally significant. An elevation of the diastolic of 15 degrees or more, or a rise in the systolic of 30 degrees or more is typically cause for concern.

Usually associated with essential hypertension, elevated blood pressure may also result from a renal or endocrine disorder; a treatment that affects fluid status, such as dialysis; or a drug's adverse effect. Ingestion of large amounts of certain foods, such as black licorice and cheddar cheese, may temporarily elevate blood pressure. (See *Pathophysiology of elevated blood pressure*.)

Sometimes, elevated blood pressure may simply reflect inaccurate blood pressure measurement. (See *Ensuring accurate blood pressure measurement*, page 127.) However, careful measurement alone doesn't ensure a clinically useful reading. To be useful, each blood pressure reading must be compared with the patient's baseline. Serial readings may be necessary to establish elevated blood pressure. Also, remember that normally, blood pressure in children is lower than in adults. (See *Normal pediatric blood pressure*, page 132.)

Assessment

If you detect sharply elevated blood pressure, quickly rule out possible life-threatening causes, and then complete a more leisurely assessment. Determine if the patient has a history of cardiovascular or cerebrovascular disease, diabetes, or renal disease. Ask about a family history of high blood pressure—a likely finding with essential hypertension, pheochromocytoma, or polycystic kidney disease. Then ask about its onset. Did high blood pressure appear abruptly? Ask the patient's age. The sudden onset of high blood pressure in middle-aged or elderly patients suggests renovascular stenosis. Although essential hypertension may begin in childhood, it typically isn't diagnosed until near age 35. Pheochromocytoma and primary aldosteronism usually occur between ages 40 and 60. If you suspect either, check for orthostatic hypotension. Take the patient's blood pressure with him lying down, sitting, and then standing. Normally, systolic pressure falls and diastolic pressure rises on standing. With orthostatic hypotension, both pressures fall.

Note headache, palpitations, blurred vision, and sweating. Ask about wine-colored urine and decreased urine output; these signs suggest glomerulonephritis, which can cause elevated blood pressure.

Obtain a drug history, including past and present prescriptions, herbal preparations, and over-the-counter (OTC) drugs (especially decongestants). If the patient is already taking an antihypertensive, determine how well he complies with the regimen. Ask about his perception of elevated blood pressure. How serious does he believe it is? Does he expect drug therapy to help? Explore psychosocial or environmental factors that may impact blood pressure control.

Follow up the history with a thorough physical assessment. Using a funduscope, check for intraocular hemorrhage, exudate, and papilledema, which characterize severe hypertension. Check for carotid bruits and jugu-

Pathophysiology of elevated blood pressure

Blood pressure—the force blood exerts on vessels as it flows through them—depends on cardiac output, peripheral resistance, and blood volume. A brief review of its regulating mechanisms—nervous system control, capillary fluid shifts, kidney excretion, and hormonal changes—will help you understand how elevated blood pressure develops.

◆ *Nervous system control* involves the sympathetic system, chiefly baroreceptors and chemoreceptors, which promotes moderate vasoconstriction to maintain normal blood pressure. When this system responds inappropriately, increased vasoconstriction enhances peripheral resistance, resulting in elevated blood pressure.

◆ *Capillary fluid shifts* regulate blood volume by responding to arterial pressure. Increased pressure forces fluid into the interstitial space; decreased pressure allows it to be drawn back into the arteries by osmosis. However, this fluid shift may take several hours to adjust blood pressure.

◆ *Kidney excretion* also helps regulate blood volume by increasing or decreasing urine formation. Normally, a mean arterial pressure of about 60 mm Hg maintains urine output. When pressure drops below this reading, urine formation ceases, thereby increasing blood volume. Conversely, when arterial pressure exceeds this reading, urine formation increases, thereby reducing blood volume. Like capillary fluid shifts, this mechanism may take several hours to adjust blood pressure.

◆ *Hormonal changes* reflect stimulation of the kidney's renin-angiotensin-aldosterone system in response to low arterial pressure. This system affects vasoconstriction, which increases arterial pressure, and stimulates aldosterone release, which regulates sodium retention—a key determinant of blood volume.

Elevated blood pressure signals the breakdown or inappropriate response of these pressure-regulating mechanisms. Its associated signs and symptoms concentrate in the target organs and tissues illustrated below.

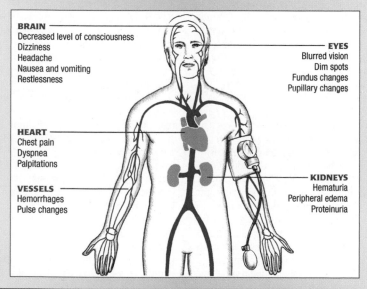

BRAIN
Decreased level of consciousness
Dizziness
Headache
Nausea and vomiting
Restlessness

EYES
Blurred vision
Dim spots
Fundus changes
Pupillary changes

HEART
Chest pain
Dyspnea
Palpitations

VESSELS
Hemorrhages
Pulse changes

KIDNEYS
Hematuria
Peripheral edema
Proteinuria

Normal pediatric blood pressure

This chart shows normal blood pressures in children, which are lower than normal rates in adults. Normal blood pressure varies depending on the child's age.

AGE	NORMAL SYSTOLIC PRESSURE	NORMAL DIASTOLIC PRESSURE
Birth to 3 months	40 to 80 mm Hg	Not detectable
3 months to 1 year	80 to 100 mm Hg	Not detectable
1 to 4 years	100 to 108 mm Hg	60 mm Hg
4 to 12 years	108 to 120 mm Hg	60 to 70 mm Hg

lar vein distention. Assess skin color, temperature, and turgor. Palpate peripheral pulses. Auscultate for abnormal heart and breath sounds as well as abnormal rates or rhythms.

Palpate the abdomen for tenderness, masses, or liver enlargement. Auscultate for abdominal bruits. Renal artery stenosis produces bruits over the upper abdomen or in the costovertebral angles. Easily palpable, enlarged kidneys and a large, tender liver suggest polycystic kidney disease. Obtain a urine sample to check for microscopic hematuria. (See *Responding to elevated blood pressure.*)

Causes

◆ *Anemia.* Accompanying elevated systolic pressure in anemia are pulsations in the capillary beds, bounding pulse, tachycardia, systolic ejection murmur, pale mucous membranes and, in patients with sickle cell anemia, ventricular gallop and crackles.

◆ *Aortic aneurysm (dissecting).* Initially, this life-threatening disorder causes a sudden rise in systolic pressure (which may be the precipitating event), but no change in diastolic pressure.

However, this increase is brief. The body's ability to compensate fails, resulting in hypotension.

◆ *Atherosclerosis.* With atherosclerosis, systolic pressure rises while diastolic pressure commonly remains normal or slightly elevated. The patient may show no other signs, or he may have a weak pulse, flushed skin, tachycardia, angina, and claudication.

◆ *Cushing's syndrome.* Cushing's syndrome causes elevated blood pressure and widened pulse pressure as well as truncal obesity, moon face, and other cushingoid signs. It's usually caused by corticosteroid use.

◆ *Drugs.* Central nervous system stimulants (such as amphetamines), sympathomimetics, corticosteroids, nonsteroidal anti-inflammatory drugs, hormonal contraceptives, monoamine oxidase inhibitors, and OTC cold remedies can increase blood pressure, as can cocaine abuse.

◆ *Hypertension.* Essential hypertension is characterized by a gradual increase in blood pressure from decade to decade. Except for this high blood pressure, the patient may be asymptomatic or (rarely) may complain of sub-

EMERGENCY INTERVENTIONS

Responding to elevated blood pressure

Elevated blood pressure can signal various life-threatening disorders. However, if pressure exceeds 180/110 mm Hg, the patient may be experiencing hypertensive crisis and may require prompt treatment. Maintain a patent airway in case the patient vomits, and institute seizure precautions. Prepare to administer an I.V. antihypertensive and diuretic. You'll also need to insert an indwelling urinary catheter to accurately monitor urine output.

If blood pressure is less severely elevated, continue to rule out other life-threatening causes. If the patient is pregnant, suspect preeclampsia or eclampsia. Place her on bed rest, and insert an I.V. catheter. If ordered, administer magnesium sulfate (to decrease neuromuscular irritability) and an antihypertensive. Monitor her vital signs closely for the next 24 hours. If diastolic blood pressure continues to exceed 100 mm Hg despite drug therapy, you may need to prepare the patient for induced labor and delivery or for cesarean birth. Offer emotional support if she must face delivery of a premature neonate.

If the patient isn't pregnant, quickly observe for equally obvious clues. Assess the patient for exophthalmos and an enlarged thyroid gland. If these signs are present, ask about a history of hyperthyroidism. Then look for other associated signs and symptoms,

including tachycardia, widened pulse pressure, palpitations, severe weakness, diarrhea, fever exceeding 100° F (37.8° C), and nervousness. Prepare to administer an antithyroid drug orally or by nasogastric tube, if ordered. Also, evaluate fluid status; look for signs of dehydration such as poor skin turgor. Prepare the patient for I.V. fluid replacement and temperature control using a cooling blanket, if necessary.

If the patient shows signs of increased intracranial pressure (such as a decreased level of consciousness, bradycardia, and widened pulse pressure), ask him or a family member if he has recently experienced head trauma. Then check for an increased respiratory rate. You'll need to maintain a patent airway in case the patient vomits. In addition, institute seizure precautions, and prepare to give an I.V. diuretic. Insert an indwelling urinary catheter, if ordered, and monitor intake and output. Check his vital signs every 5 to 15 minutes (depending on the patient's condition) until he's stable.

If the patient has absent or weak peripheral pulses, ask about chest pressure or pain, which suggests a dissecting aortic aneurysm. Enforce bed rest until a diagnosis has been established. If ordered, give the patient an I.V. antihypertensive or prepare him for surgery.

---

occipital headache, light-headedness, tinnitus, and fatigue.

With malignant hypertension, diastolic pressure abruptly rises above 110 mm Hg, and systolic pressure may exceed 180 mm Hg. Typically, the patient has pulmonary edema marked by jugular vein distention, dyspnea, tachypnea, tachycardia, and coughing of pink, frothy sputum. Other characteristic signs and symptoms include severe headache, confusion, blurred vision, tinnitus, epistaxis, muscle twitching, chest pain, nausea, and vomiting.

◪ *Increased intracranial pressure (ICP).* Increased ICP initially causes tachypnea, followed by increased systolic pressure and widened pulse pressure. It affects the heart rate last, causing bradycardia. Associated signs and symptoms include headache, projectile vomiting, a decreased level of consciousness, and fixed or dilated pupils.

◼ *Myocardial infarction (MI)*. MI is a life-threatening disorder that may cause high or low blood pressure. Common findings include crushing chest pain that may radiate to the jaw, shoulder, arm, or epigastrium. Other findings include dyspnea, anxiety, nausea, vomiting, weakness, diaphoresis, atrial gallop, and murmurs.

◆ *Pheochromocytoma*. Pheochromocytoma is characterized by paroxysmal or sustained elevated blood pressure and may be accompanied by orthostatic hypotension. Associated signs and symptoms include anxiety, diaphoresis, palpitations, tremors, pallor, nausea, weight loss, and headache.

◆ *Polycystic kidney disease*. Elevated blood pressure with polycystic kidney disease is typically preceded by flank pain. Other signs and symptoms include enlarged kidneys; an enlarged, tender liver; and intermittent gross hematuria.

◼ *Preeclampsia and eclampsia*. Potentially life-threatening to the mother and fetus, preeclampsia and eclampsia characteristically increase blood pressure. They're defined as a reading of 140/90 mm Hg, an increase of 30 mm Hg above the patient's baseline systolic pressure, or an increase of 15 mm Hg above the patient's baseline diastolic pressure when measured on two occasions, 6 hours apart. Accompanying elevated blood pressure are generalized edema, sudden weight gain of 3 lb (1.4 kg) or more per week during the second trimester or of more than 1 lb (0.5 kg) per week during the third trimester, severe frontal headache, blurred or double vision, decreased urine output, proteinuria, midabdominal pain, neuromuscular irritability, nausea and, possibly, seizures (eclampsia).

◆ *Renovascular stenosis*. Renovascular stenosis produces abruptly elevated systolic and diastolic pressures. Other signs and symptoms include bruits over the upper abdomen or in the costovertebral angles, hematuria, and acute flank pain.

◼ *Thyrotoxicosis*. Accompanying the elevated systolic pressure associated with thyrotoxicosis, a potentially life-threatening disorder, are widened pulse pressure, tachycardia, bounding pulse, pulsations in the capillary nail beds, palpitations, weight loss, exophthalmos, an enlarged thyroid gland, weakness, diarrhea, a fever over 100° F (37.8° C), and warm, moist skin. The patient may appear nervous and emotionally unstable, displaying occasional outbursts or even psychotic behavior. Heat intolerance, exertional dyspnea and, in females, decreased or absent menses may also occur.

Bowel sounds, absent

Absent bowel sounds refers to an inability to hear bowel sounds with a stethoscope in any quadrant after listening for at least 5 minutes in each quadrant. Bowel sounds cease when mechanical or vascular obstruction or neurogenic inhibition halts peristalsis. When peristalsis stops, gas from bowel contents and fluid secreted from the intestinal walls accumulate and distend the lumen, leading to life-threatening complications, such as perforation, peritonitis, and sepsis, or hypovolemic shock.

Simple mechanical obstruction, resulting from adhesions, hernia, or tumor, causes loss of fluids and electrolytes and induces dehydration. Vascular obstruction cuts off circulation to the intestinal walls, leading to ischemia, necrosis, and shock. Neurogenic

Are bowel sounds really absent?

Before concluding that the patient has absent bowel sounds, ask yourself these three questions:
1. *Did you use the diaphragm of your stethoscope to auscultate for the bowel sounds?*
The diaphragm detects high-frequency sounds, such as bowel sounds, whereas the bell detects low-frequency sounds, such as a vascular bruit or venous hum.
2. *Did you listen for bowel sounds in the same spot for at least 5 minutes?*
Normally, bowel sounds occur every 5 to 15 seconds, but the duration of a single sound may be less than 1 second.
3. *Did you listen for bowel sounds in all quadrants?*
Bowel sounds may be absent in one quadrant but present in another.

inhibition, affecting innervation of the intestinal wall, may result from infection, bowel distention, or trauma. It may also follow metabolic imbalances such as hypokalemia.

Abrupt cessation of bowel sounds, when accompanied by abdominal pain, rigidity, and distention, signals a life-threatening crisis requiring immediate intervention. Absent bowel sounds following a period of hyperactive sounds may be equally ominous. (See *Are bowel sounds really absent?*)

Assessment

If you fail to detect bowel sounds and the patient reports sudden, severe abdominal pain and cramping or exhibits severe abdominal distention, you must intervene quickly. (See *Responding to absent bowel sounds.*)

If the patient's pain isn't severe or accompanied by other life-threatening signs or symptoms, obtain a detailed medical and surgical history and perform a complete physical assessment.

EMERGENCY INTERVENTIONS

Responding to absent bowel sounds

Take these steps if your patient has absent bowel sounds accompanied by sudden, severe abdominal pain and cramping or severe abdominal distention:
◆ Prepare to insert a nasogastric or intestinal tube to suction lumen contents and decompress the bowel.
◆ Prepare to administer I.V. fluids and electrolytes, as prescribed, to offset dehydration and imbalances caused by the dysfunctioning bowel.
◆ Withhold oral intake in case the patient requires surgery.
◆ Take the patient's vital signs; stay alert for signs of shock.
◆ Measure abdominal girth as a baseline for gauging subsequent changes.
◆ Check emesis (if present) for occult blood.
◆ Notify the practitioner immediately.

Start with abdominal pain. When did it begin? Has it gotten worse? Where does he feel it? Ask about a sensation of bloating and about flatulence. Find out if the patient has had diarrhea or has passed pencil-thin stools—possible signs of a developing luminal obstruction. The patient may have had no bowel movements at all—a possible sign of complete obstruction or paralytic ileus.

Ask about conditions that commonly lead to mechanical obstruction, such as abdominal tumors, hernias, and adhesions from past surgery. Determine if the patient was involved in an accident—even a seemingly minor one—which may have caused vascular clots. Check for a history of acute pancreatitis, diverticulitis, or gynecologic infection, which may have led to intra-abdominal infection and bowel dysfunction. Be sure to ask about previous toxic conditions, such as uremia, and about spinal cord injury, which can lead to paralytic ileus.

Start your physical assessment by inspecting the abdominal contour. Stoop at the recumbent patient's side and then at the foot of his bed to detect localized or generalized distention. Auscultate in all quadrants, listening for 5 minutes each. Percuss and palpate the abdomen gently. Listen for dullness over fluid-filled areas and tympany over pockets of gas. Palpate for abdominal rigidity and guarding, which suggest peritoneal irritation that can lead to paralytic ileus.

Causes

◪ *Complete mechanical intestinal obstruction.* With complete mechanical intestinal obstruction, absent bowel sounds follow a period of hyperactive bowel sounds—a potentially life-threatening disorder. This silence accompanies acute, colicky abdominal pain that arises in the quadrant of obstruction and may radiate to the flank or lumbar regions. Associated signs and symptoms include abdominal distention and bloating, constipation, and nausea and vomiting (the higher the blockage, the earlier and more severe the vomiting). In late stages, signs of shock may occur with fever, rebound tenderness, and abdominal rigidity.

◆ *Mesenteric artery occlusion.* With mesenteric artery occlusion, bowel sounds disappear after a brief period of hyperactive sounds. Sudden, severe midepigastric or periumbilical pain occurs next, followed by abdominal distention, bruits, vomiting, constipation, fever, and signs of shock. Abdominal rigidity may appear later.

◆ *Paralytic (adynamic) ileus.* The cardinal sign of paralytic ileus is absent bowel sounds. Associated signs and symptoms include abdominal distention, generalized discomfort, and constipation or the passage of small, liquid stools. If paralytic ileus follows acute abdominal infection, the patient may also experience fever and abdominal pain.

Bowel sounds, hyperactive

Sometimes audible without a stethoscope, hyperactive bowel sounds reflect increased intestinal motility (peristalsis). They're commonly characterized as rapid, rushing, gurgling waves of sounds. (See *Characteristics of bowel sounds*.) They may stem from life-threatening bowel obstruction or GI hemorrhage or from GI infection, inflammatory bowel disease (which usually follows a chronic course), food allergies, or stress.

Assessment

After detecting hyperactive bowel sounds, quickly check the patient's vital signs and ask him about associated symptoms, such as abdominal pain, vomiting, and diarrhea. If he reports cramping abdominal pain or vomiting, continue to auscultate for bowel sounds. If bowel sounds stop abruptly, suspect complete bowel obstruction.

If you've ruled out life-threatening conditions, obtain a detailed medical and surgical history. Ask the patient if he has had a hernia or abdominal surgery because these may cause mechanical intestinal obstruction. Does he have a history of inflammatory bowel disease? Also, ask about recent eruptions of gastroenteritis among family members, friends, or coworkers. If the patient has traveled recently, even within the United States, was he aware of any endemic illnesses?

In addition, determine whether stress may have contributed to the patient's problem. Ask about food allergies and recent ingestion of unusual foods or fluids. Check for fever, which suggests infection. Having already auscultated, now gently inspect, percuss, and palpate the abdomen.

Causes

◆ *Crohn's disease.* Hyperactive bowel sounds usually arise insidiously with Crohn's disease. Associated signs and symptoms include diarrhea, cramping abdominal pain that may be relieved by defecation, anorexia, a low-grade fever, abdominal distention and tenderness and, in many cases, a fixed mass in the right lower quadrant. Perianal and vaginal lesions are common. Muscle wasting, weight loss, and signs of dehydration may occur as Crohn's disease progresses.

Characteristics of bowel sounds

The sounds of swallowed air and fluid moving through the GI tract are known as *bowel sounds.* These sounds usually occur every 5 to 15 seconds, but their frequency may be irregular. For example, bowel sounds are normally more active just before and after a meal. Bowel sounds may last less than 1 second or up to several seconds.

Key descriptive terms
◆ *Normal bowel sounds* can be characterized as murmuring, gurgling, or tinkling.
◆ *Hyperactive bowel sounds* can be characterized as loud, gurgling, splashing, and rushing; they're higher pitched and occur more frequently than normal sounds.
◆ *Hypoactive bowel sounds* can be characterized as softer or lower in tone and less frequent than normal sounds.

◆ *Food hypersensitivity.* Malabsorption—typically lactose intolerance—may cause hyperactive bowel sounds. Associated signs and symptoms include diarrhea and, possibly, nausea and vomiting, angioedema, and urticaria.
◆ *Gastroenteritis.* Gastroenteritis typically causes hyperactive bowel sounds that follow sudden nausea and vomiting and accompany "explosive" diarrhea. Abdominal cramping or pain is common, usually after a peristaltic wave. Fever may occur, depending on the causative organism.
◆ *GI hemorrhage.* Hyperactive bowel sounds provide the most immediate indication of persistent upper GI bleeding. Other findings include hematemesis, coffee-ground vomitus, abdominal distention, bloody diarrhea, rectal pas-

sage of bright red clots and jellylike material or melena, and pain during bleeding. Decreased urine output, tachycardia, and hypotension accompany blood loss.

◩ *Mechanical intestinal obstruction.* Hyperactive bowel sounds occur simultaneously with cramping abdominal pain every few minutes in patients with mechanical intestinal obstruction, a potentially life-threatening disorder; bowel sounds may later become hypoactive and then disappear. With small-bowel obstruction, nausea and vomiting occur earlier and with greater severity than in large-bowel obstruction. With complete bowel obstruction, abdominal distention and constipation also accompany hyperactive sounds, although the part of the bowel distal to the obstruction may continue to empty for up to 3 days.

◆ *Ulcerative colitis (acute).* Hyperactive bowel sounds arise abruptly in patients with ulcerative colitis and are accompanied by bloody diarrhea, anorexia, abdominal pain, nausea and vomiting, fever, and tenesmus (a painful anal sphincter spasm accompanied by an urgent desire to evacuate the bowel, involuntary straining, and the passage of a small amount of fecal matter). Weight loss, arthralgia, and arthritis may occur.

Bowel sounds, hypoactive

Hypoactive bowel sounds, detected by auscultation, are diminished in regularity, tone, and loudness from normal bowel sounds. In themselves, hypoactive bowel sounds don't herald an emergency; in fact, they're considered normal during sleep. However, they may lead to absent bowel sounds, which can indicate a life-threatening disorder.

Hypoactive bowel sounds result from decreased peristalsis, which, in turn, can result from a developing bowel obstruction. The obstruction may be mechanical (as from a hernia, tumor, or twisting), vascular (as from an embolism or thrombosis), or neurogenic (as from mechanical, ischemic, or toxic impairment of bowel innervation). Hypoactive bowel sounds can also result from the use of certain drugs, abdominal surgery, and radiation therapy.

Assessment

After detecting hypoactive bowel sounds, look for related symptoms. Ask the patient about the location, onset, duration, frequency, and severity of any pain. Cramping or colicky abdominal pain usually indicates a mechanical bowel obstruction, whereas diffuse abdominal pain usually indicates intestinal distention related to paralytic ileus.

Ask the patient about recent vomiting. When did it begin? How often does it occur? Does the vomitus look bloody? Also ask about changes in bowel habits. Does he have a history of constipation? When was the last time he had a bowel movement or expelled gas?

Obtain a detailed medical and surgical history of conditions that may cause mechanical bowel obstruction, such as an abdominal tumor or hernia. Does the patient have a history of severe pain; trauma; conditions that can cause paralytic ileus, such as pancreatitis; bowel inflammation or gynecologic infection, which may produce peritonitis; or toxic conditions such as uremia? Has he recently had radiation therapy or abdominal surgery or ingested a drug, such as an opiate, which can decrease peristalsis and cause hypoactive bowel sounds?

After the history is complete, perform a careful physical assessment. Inspect the abdomen for distention, noting surgical incisions and obvious masses. Gently percuss and palpate the abdomen for masses, gas, fluid, tenderness, and rigidity. Measure abdominal girth to detect a subsequent increase in distention. Also check for poor skin turgor, hypotension, narrowed pulse pressure, tachycardia, and other signs of dehydration and electrolyte imbalance, which may result from paralytic ileus.

Causes

◆ *Drugs.* Certain classes of drugs reduce intestinal motility and thus produce hypoactive bowel sounds. These include opiates, such as codeine; anticholinergics, such as propantheline bromide (Pro-Banthine); phenothiazines, such as chlorpromazine (Thorazine); and vinca alkaloids, such as vincristine (Oncovin). General or spinal anesthetics produce transient hypoactive sounds.

◆ *Mechanical intestinal obstruction.* With mechanical intestinal obstruction, bowel sounds may become hypoactive after a period of hyperactivity. The patient may also have acute colicky abdominal pain in the quadrant of obstruction, possibly radiating to the flank or lumbar region; nausea and vomiting (the higher the obstruction, the earlier and more severe the vomiting); constipation; and abdominal distention and bloating. If the obstruction becomes complete, signs of shock may occur.

◣ *Mesenteric artery occlusion.* With mesenteric artery occlusion, bowel sounds become hypoactive after a brief period of hyperactivity and then quickly disappear, signifying a life-threaten-

ing crisis. Associated signs and symptoms include fever; a history of colicky abdominal pain leading to sudden and severe midepigastric or periumbilical pain, followed by abdominal distention and possible bruits; vomiting; constipation; and signs of shock. Abdominal rigidity may appear late.

◆ *Paralytic (adynamic) ileus.* Bowel sounds are hypoactive and may become absent with paralytic ileus. Associated signs and symptoms include abdominal distention, generalized discomfort, and constipation or passage of small, liquid stools and flatus. If the disorder follows acute abdominal infection, fever and abdominal pain may occur.

◆ *Radiation therapy.* Hypoactive bowel sounds and abdominal tenderness may occur after irradiation of the abdomen.

◆ *Surgery.* Hypoactive bowel sounds may occur after surgical manipulation of the bowel. Motility and bowel sounds in the small intestine usually resume within 24 hours; colonic bowel sounds, in 3 to 5 days.

Bradycardia

Bradycardia refers to a heart rate of less than 60 beats/minute. It occurs normally in young adults, trained athletes, and elderly people as well as during sleep. It's also a normal response to vagal stimulation caused by coughing, vomiting, or straining during defecation. When bradycardia results from these causes, the heart rate rarely drops below 40 beats/minute. However, when it results from pathologic causes (such as cardiovascular disorders), the heart rate may be slower.

By itself, bradycardia is a nonspecific sign. However, in conjunction with such symptoms as chest pain, hypotension, dizziness, syncope, and shortness

EMERGENCY INTERVENTIONS

Managing severe bradycardia

Bradycardia can signal a life-threatening disorder when accompanied by pain, shortness of breath, dizziness, syncope, prolonged exposure to cold, or head or neck trauma. In such a patient, perform these interventions:
◆ Quickly take his vital signs.
◆ Connect him to a cardiac monitor, and insert an I.V. catheter. Depending on the cause of bradycardia, you'll need to administer fluids, atropine, or thyroid medication, as prescribed.
◆ If ordered, insert an indwelling urinary catheter.
◆ Anticipate orders for intubation, mechanical ventilation, or placement of a pacemaker if the patient's respiratory rate falls.
◆ If appropriate, perform a focused evaluation to help locate the cause of bradycardia. For example, ask about pain. Viselike pressure or crushing or burning chest pain that

radiates to the arms, back, or jaw may indicate an acute myocardial infarction (MI); a severe headache, increased intracranial pressure. Also, ask about nausea, vomiting, or shortness of breath—signs and symptoms associated with an acute MI and cardiomyopathy. Observe the patient for peripheral cyanosis, edema, or jugular vein distention, which may indicate cardiomyopathy. Look for a thyroidectomy scar because severe bradycardia may result from hypothyroidism caused by failure to take thyroid hormone replacement therapy.
◆ If the cause of bradycardia is evident, provide supportive care. For example, keep the hypothermic patient warm by applying blankets, and monitor his core temperature until it reaches 99° F (37.2° C); stabilize the head and neck of a trauma patient until cervical spinal injury is ruled out.

of breath, it can signal a life-threatening disorder.

Assessment

After detecting bradycardia, check for related signs of life-threatening disorders. (See *Managing severe bradycardia*.) If the patient's bradycardia isn't accompanied by untoward signs, ask the patient if he or a family member has a history of a slow pulse rate. Also, find out if he has an underlying metabolic disorder such as hypothyroidism, which can precipitate bradycardia. Ask which medications he's taking and if he's complying with the prescribed schedule and dosage. Monitor his vital signs, temperature, pulse,

respirations, blood pressure, and oxygen saturation.

Causes

◪ *Cardiac arrhythmia.* Depending on the type of cardiac arrhythmia and the patient's tolerance of it, bradycardia may be transient or sustained, benign or life-threatening. Related findings include hypotension, palpitations, dizziness, weakness, syncope, and fatigue.
◪ *Cardiomyopathy.* Cardiomyopathy is a potentially life-threatening disorder that may cause transient or sustained bradycardia. Other findings include dizziness, syncope, edema, fatigue, jugular vein distention, orthopnea, dyspnea, and peripheral cyanosis.

◆ *Drugs.* Beta-adrenergic blockers and some calcium channel blockers, cardiac glycosides, topical miotics (such as pilocarpine [Pilopine HS]), protamine, quinidine (Quinalan) and other antiarrhythmics, and sympatholytics may cause transient bradycardia. Failure to take thyroid replacement therapy as directed may cause bradycardia.

◆ *Hypothermia.* Bradycardia usually appears with hypothermia when the core temperature drops below 89.6° F (32° C). It's accompanied by shivering, peripheral cyanosis, muscle rigidity, bradypnea, and confusion leading to stupor.

◆ *Hypothyroidism.* Hypothyroidism causes severe bradycardia in addition to fatigue, constipation, unexplained weight gain, and sensitivity to cold. Related signs include cool, dry, thick skin; sparse, dry hair; facial swelling; periorbital edema; thick, brittle nails; and confusion leading to stupor.

◆ *Invasive treatments.* Suctioning can induce hypoxia and vagal stimulation, causing bradycardia. Cardiac surgery can cause edema or damage to conduction tissues, causing bradycardia.

◆ *Myocardial infarction (MI).* Sinus bradycardia is the most common arrhythmia associated with an acute MI. Accompanying signs and symptoms may include an aching, burning, or viselike pressure in the chest that may radiate to the jaw, shoulder, arm, back, or epigastric area; nausea and vomiting; cool, clammy, and pale or cyanotic skin; anxiety; and dyspnea. Blood pressure may be increased or decreased. Auscultation may reveal abnormal heart sounds.

Bradypnea

Commonly preceding life-threatening apnea or respiratory arrest, bradypnea is a pattern of regular respirations with a rate of less than 10 breaths/minute. This sign results from neurologic and metabolic disorders and drug overdose, which depress the brain's respiratory control centers. (See *Understanding how the nervous system controls breathing,* page 142.)

Assessment

Depending on the degree of central nervous system (CNS) depression, the patient with severe bradypnea may require constant stimulation to breathe. Take the patient's vital signs and assess his neurologic status by checking pupil size and reactions. Also evaluate his level of consciousness (LOC) and his ability to move his extremities. Place the patient on an apnea monitor and pulse oximeter, and keep emergency airway equipment readily available.

Obtain a brief medical history from the patient, if possible. Alternatively, obtain this information from whoever accompanied him to your facility. Ask if he's experiencing a drug overdose and, if so, try to determine what drugs he took, how much, when, and by what route. Check his arms for needle marks, indicating possible drug abuse. The practitioner may need to order I.V. naloxone (Narcan), an opioid antagonist.

If you rule out a drug overdose, ask about chronic illnesses, such as diabetes and renal failure. Check for a medical identification bracelet or an identification card that names an underlying condition. Also ask whether the patient has a history of head trauma, brain tumor, neurologic infection, or stroke.

Because respiratory rates are higher in children than in adults, bradypnea in children is defined according to age. (See *Respiratory rates in children,* page 143.)

Understanding how the nervous system controls breathing

Stimulation from external sources and from higher brain centers acts on respiratory centers in the pons and medulla. These centers, in turn, send impulses to the various parts of the respiratory system to alter respiration patterns.

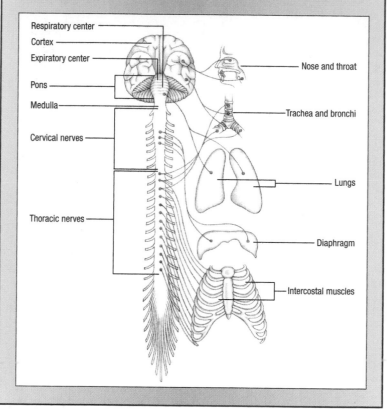

Causes

◆ *Diabetic ketoacidosis.* Bradypnea occurs late in patients with severe, uncontrolled diabetes. Patients with severe ketoacidosis may experience Kussmaul's respirations. Associated signs and symptoms include hypotension, decreased LOC, tachycardia, fatigue, weakness, fruity breath odor, and oliguria.

◆ *Drugs.* Overdose with an opioid analgesic or, less commonly, a sedative, barbiturate, phenothiazine, or other CNS depressant can cause bradypnea. The use of any of these drugs with alcohol can also cause bradypnea.

◆ *Hepatic failure.* Occurring with end-stage hepatic failure, bradypnea may be accompanied by coma, hyperactive reflexes, asterixis, a positive Babinski's sign, and fetor hepaticus (abnormal breath odor).

◈ *Increased intracranial pressure (ICP).* A late sign of increased ICP, a life-threatening condition, bradypnea is preceded by a decreased LOC, deteriorating motor function, and fixed, dilated pupils. The triad of bradypnea, bradycardia, and hypertension is a classic sign of late medullary strangulation.

◆ *Renal failure.* Occurring with end-stage renal failure, bradypnea may be accompanied by convulsions, a decreased LOC, GI bleeding, hypotension or hypertension, and uremic frost.

◈ *Respiratory failure.* Bradypnea occurs with end-stage respiratory failure along with cyanosis, diminished breath sounds, tachycardia, mildly increased blood pressure, and a decreased LOC.

Breast dimpling

Breast dimpling—the puckering or retraction of skin on the breast—results from abnormal attachment of the skin to underlying tissue. It suggests an inflammatory or malignant mass beneath the skin surface and usually represents a late sign of breast cancer. Dimpling usually affects women older than age 40, but occasionally affects men.

Because breast dimpling occurs over a mass or induration, the patient usually discovers other signs before becoming aware of the dimpling. However, a thorough breast examination may reveal dimpling and alert the patient and nurse to a problem.

Assessment

Obtain a medical, reproductive, and family history, noting factors that place the patient at high risk for breast cancer. Ask about pregnancy history because a woman who hasn't had a full-term pregnancy before age 30 is at higher risk for developing breast cancer. Ask if her mother or a sister had breast cancer. Has she herself had a previous malignancy, especially cancer in the other breast? Ask about the patient's dietary habits because a high-fat diet predisposes women to breast cancer.

Ask the patient if she has noticed changes in the shape of her breast. Is

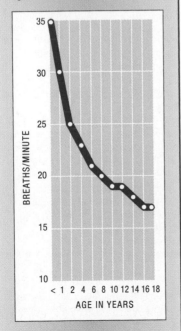

Respiratory rates in children

This graph shows normal respiratory rates in children, which are higher than normal rates in adults. Accordingly, bradypnea in children is defined by the age of the child.

BREATHS/MINUTE

35
30
25
20
15
10

< 1 2 4 6 8 10 12 14 16 18

AGE IN YEARS

any area painful or tender, and is the pain cyclic? If she's breast-feeding, has she recently experienced high fever, chills, malaise, muscle aches, fatigue, or other flulike signs or symptoms? Can she remember sustaining trauma to the breast?

Carefully inspect the dimpled area. Is it swollen, red, or warm to the touch? Do you see bruises or contusions? Ask the patient to tense her pectoral muscles by pressing her hips with both hands or by raising her hands over her head. Does the puckering increase? Gently pull the skin up toward the clavicle. Is the dimpling exaggerated?

Observe the breast for nipple retraction. Do both nipples point in the same direction? Are the nipples flattened or inverted? Does the patient report nipple discharge? If so, ask her to describe the color and character of the discharge. Observe the contour of both breasts. Are they symmetrical?

Examine both breasts with the patient lying down, sitting, and then leaning forward. Does the skin move freely over both breasts? If you can palpate a lump, describe its size, location, consistency, mobility, and delineation. What relation does the lump have to the breast dimpling? Gently mold the breast skin around the lump. Is the dimpling exaggerated? Also examine breast and axillary lymph nodes, noting any enlargement.

Causes

◆ *Breast abscess.* Breast dimpling sometimes accompanies a chronic breast abscess. Associated findings include a firm, irregular, nontender lump and signs of nipple retraction, such as deviation, inversion, or flattening. Axillary lymph nodes may be enlarged.
◆ *Breast cancer.* Breast dimpling is an important, but somewhat late sign of breast cancer. A neoplasm that causes dimpling is usually close to the skin and at least 1 cm in diameter. It feels irregularly shaped and fixed to underlying tissue, and it's usually painless. Other signs of breast cancer include peau d'orange, changes in breast symmetry or size, nipple retraction, and a unilateral, spontaneous, nonmilky nipple discharge that's serous or bloody. Axillary lymph nodes may be enlarged. Pain may be present, but isn't a reliable symptom of breast cancer. A breast ulcer may appear as a late sign.
◆ *Fat necrosis.* Breast dimpling from fat necrosis follows inflammation and trauma to the fatty tissue of the breast. Tenderness, erythema, bruising, and contusions may occur. Other findings include a hard, indurated, poorly delineated lump, which is fibrotic and fixed to underlying tissue or overlying skin as well as signs of nipple retraction. Fat necrosis is difficult to differentiate from breast cancer.
◆ *Mastitis.* Breast dimpling may signal bacterial mastitis, which usually results from duct obstruction and milk stasis during lactation. Heat, erythema, swelling, induration, pain, and tenderness usually accompany mastitis. Dimpling is more likely to occur with diffuse induration than with a single hard mass. The skin on the breast may feel fixed to underlying tissue. Other possible findings include nipple retraction, nipple cracks, a purulent discharge, and enlarged axillary lymph nodes. Flulike signs and symptoms, such as fever, malaise, fatigue, and aching, commonly occur.

Breast nodule

A commonly reported gynecologic sign, a breast nodule has two chief causes: benign breast disease and cancer. Benign breast disease, the leading cause of nodules, can stem from cyst formation in obstructed and dilated lactiferous ducts, hypertrophy or tumor formation in the ductal system, inflammation, or infection.

Although fewer than 20% of breast nodules are malignant, the signs and symptoms of breast cancer aren't easily distinguished from those of benign breast disease. Breast cancer is a leading cause of death among women, but can occur occasionally in men, with signs and symptoms mimicking those found in women. Thus, breast nodules in both sexes should always be evaluated.

A woman who's familiar with the feel of her breasts and performs monthly breast self-examinations can detect a nodule 6.4 mm or less in size, considerably smaller than the 1-cm nodule that's readily detectable by an experienced examiner. However, a woman may fail to report a nodule because of the fear of breast cancer.

Assessment

If the patient reports a lump, ask her how and when she discovered it. Does the size and tenderness of the lump vary with her menstrual cycle? Has the lump changed since she first noticed it? Has she noticed other breast signs, such as a change in breast shape, size, or contour; discharge; or nipple changes?

Is she breast-feeding? Does she have fever, chills, fatigue, or other flulike signs or symptoms? Ask her to describe any pain or tenderness associated with the lump. Is the pain in one breast only? Has she sustained recent trauma to the breast?

Explore the patient's medical and family history for factors that increase her risk of breast cancer. These include a high-fat diet, having a mother or sister with breast cancer, or having a history of cancer, especially cancer in the other breast. Other risk factors include nulliparity and a first pregnancy after age 30.

Next, perform a thorough breast examination. Pay special attention to the upper outer quadrant of each breast, where one-half of the ductal tissue is located. This is the most common site of malignant breast tumors.

Carefully palpate a suspected breast nodule, noting its location, shape, size, consistency, mobility, and delineation. Does the nodule feel soft, rubbery, and elastic or hard? Is it mobile, slipping away from your fingers as you palpate it, or firmly fixed to adjacent tissue? Does the nodule seem to limit the mobility of the entire breast? Note the nodule's delineation. Are the borders clearly defined or indefinite? Does the area feel more like hardness or diffuse induration than a nodule with definite borders?

Do you feel one nodule or several small ones? Is the shape round, oval, lobular, or irregular? Inspect and palpate the skin over the nodule for warmth, redness, and edema. Palpate the lymph nodes of the breast and axilla for enlargement.

Observe the contour of the breasts, looking for asymmetry and irregularities. Be alert for signs of retraction, such as skin dimpling and nipple deviation, retraction, or flattening. (To exaggerate dimpling, have your patient raise her arms over her head or press her hands against her hips.) Gently pull the breast skin toward the clavicle. Is dimpling evident? Mold the breast skin and again observe the area for dimpling.

Stay alert for a nipple discharge that's spontaneous, unilateral, and nonmilky (serous, bloody, or purulent). Be careful not to confuse it with the grayish discharge that can be elicited from the nipples of a woman who has been pregnant.

Causes

◆ *Adenofibroma.* The extremely mobile or "slippery" feel of an adenofibroma, a benign neoplasm, helps distinguish it from other breast nodules. The nodule usually occurs singly and characteristically feels firm, elastic, and round or lobular, with well-defined margins. It doesn't cause pain or tenderness, can vary from pinhead size to very large, commonly grows rapidly, and usually lies around the nipple or on the lateral side of the upper outer quadrant.

◆ *Areolar gland abscess.* Areolar gland abscess is a tender, palpable mass on the periphery of the areola following an inflammation of Montgomery's glands. Fever may also be present.

◆ *Breast abscess.* A localized, hot, tender, fluctuant mass with erythema and peau d'orange typifies an acute breast abscess. Associated signs and symptoms include fever, chills, malaise, and general discomfort. With a chronic abscess, the nodule is nontender, irregular, and firm and may feel like a thick wall of fibrous tissue. It's commonly accompanied by skin dimpling, peau d'orange, nipple retraction and, sometimes, axillary lymphadenopathy.

◆ *Breast cancer.* A hard, poorly delineated nodule that's fixed to the skin or underlying tissue suggests breast cancer. Malignant nodules typically cause breast dimpling, nipple deviation or retraction, or flattening of the nipple or breast contour. Between 40% and 50% of malignant nodules occur in the upper outer quadrant.

Nodules usually occur singly, although satellite nodules may surround the main one. They're usually nontender. Nipple discharge may be serous or bloody. (A bloody nipple discharge in the presence of a nodule is a classic sign of breast cancer.) Additional findings include edema (peau d'orange) of the skin overlying the mass, erythema, tenderness, and axillary lymphadenopathy. A breast ulcer may occur as a late sign. Breast pain, an unreliable symptom, may be present.

◆ *Fibrocystic breast disease.* The most common cause of breast nodules, fibrocystic breast disease produces smooth, round, slightly elastic nodules, which increase in size and tenderness just before menstruation. The nodules may occur in fine, granular clusters in both breasts or as widespread, well-defined lumps of varying sizes. A thickening of adjacent tissue may be palpable. Cystic nodules are mobile, which helps differentiate them from malignant ones. Because cystic nodules aren't fixed to underlying breast tissue, they don't produce retraction signs, such as nipple deviation or dimpling. Signs and symptoms of premenstrual syndrome—including headache, irritability, bloating, nausea, vomiting, and abdominal cramping—may also be present.

◆ *Mammary duct ectasia.* The rubbery breast nodule in mammary duct ectasia, a menopausal or postmenopausal disorder, usually lies under the areola. It's commonly accompanied by transient pain, itching, tenderness, and erythema of the areola; thick, sticky, multicolored nipple discharge from multiple ducts; and nipple retraction. The skin overlying the mass may be bluish green or exhibit peau d'orange. Axillary lymphadenopathy is possible.

◆ *Mastitis.* With mastitis, breast nodules are firm and indurated or tender, flocculent (fluffy), and distinct. Gentle palpation defines the area of maximum purulent accumulation. Skin dimpling and nipple deviation, retraction, or flattening may be present, and the nipple may show a crack or abrasion. Accompanying signs and symptoms include breast warmth, erythema, tenderness, and peau d'orange as well as a high fever, chills, malaise, and fatigue.

◆ *Paget's disease.* Paget's disease is a slow-growing intraductal carcinoma that begins as a scaling, eczematoid unilateral nipple lesion. The nipple later becomes reddened and excoriated and may eventually be completely destroyed. The disease process extends along the skin as well as in the ducts, usually progressing to a deep-seated mass.

Breast pain

An unreliable indicator of cancer, breast pain commonly results from benign breast disease. It may occur during rest or movement and may be aggravated by manipulation or palpation. Breast pain may be unilateral or bilateral; cyclic, intermittent, or constant; and dull or sharp. It may result from surface cuts, furuncles, contusions, or similar lesions (superficial pain); nipple fissures or inflammation in the papillary ducts or areolae (severe localized pain); stromal distention in the breast parenchyma; a tumor that affects nerve endings (severe, constant pain); or inflammatory lesions that distend the stroma (the framework of connective tissue) and irritate sensory nerve endings (severe, constant pain). Breast pain may radiate to the back, arms and, sometimes, the neck.

Breast *tenderness* refers to pain elicited by physical contact. Breast tenderness in women may occur before menstruation and during pregnancy. Before menstruation, breast pain or tenderness stems from increased mammary blood flow due to hormonal changes. During pregnancy, breast tenderness and throbbing, tingling, or pricking sensations may occur, also due to hormonal changes.

In men, breast pain may stem from gynecomastia (especially during puberty and old age), reproductive tract anomalies, or organic disease of the liver or pituitary, adrenal cortex, or thyroid glands.

Assessment

Begin by asking the patient if breast pain is constant or intermittent. For either type, ask about onset and character. If it's intermittent, determine the relationship of pain to the phase of the menstrual cycle. Is the patient breast-feeding? If not, ask about nipple discharge and have her describe it. Is she pregnant? Has she reached menopause? Has she recently experienced flulike symptoms or sustained injury to the breast? Has she noticed a change in breast shape or contour? Ask the patient to describe the pain. Determine if the pain affects one breast or both, and ask the patient to point to the painful area.

Start your examination with the patient's arms at her sides. Inspect the breasts. Note their size, symmetry, and contour and the appearance of the skin. Remember that breast shape and size vary and that breasts normally change during menses, pregnancy, and lactation and with aging. Are the breasts red or edematous? Are the veins prominent? Note the size, shape, and symmetry of the nipples and areolae. Do you detect ecchymosis, a rash, ulceration, or discharge? Do the nipples point in the same direction? Do you see signs of retraction, such as skin dimpling or nipple inversion or flattening? Repeat your inspection with the patient's arms raised above her head and then with her hands pressed against her hips.

Palpate the breasts, first with the patient seated and then with her lying down and a pillow placed under her shoulder on the side being examined. Use the pads of your fingers to compress breast tissue against the chest wall. Proceed systematically from the sternum to the midline and from the axilla to the midline, noting warmth, tenderness, nodules, masses, or irregularities. Palpate the nipple, noting tenderness and nodules, and check for discharge. Palpate axillary lymph nodes, noting enlargement.

Causes

◆ *Areolar gland abscess.* Areolar gland abscess is a tender, palpable mass on the periphery of the areola following an inflammation of Montgomery's glands. Fever may also occur.

◆ *Breast abscess (acute).* An acute breast abscess causes local pain, tenderness, erythema, peau d'orange, and warmth. Malaise, fever, and chills may also occur.

◆ *Breast cyst.* A breast cyst that enlarges rapidly may cause acute, localized, and usually unilateral pain.

◆ *Fat necrosis.* Local pain and tenderness may develop in fat necrosis, a benign disorder. A history of trauma is usually present. Associated findings include ecchymosis; erythema of the overriding skin; a firm, irregular, fixed mass; and skin retraction signs, such as skin dimpling and nipple retraction. Fat necrosis may be hard to differentiate from cancer.

◆ *Fibrocystic breast disease.* Fibrocystic breast disease is a common cause of breast pain that's associated with the development of cysts that may cause pain before menstruation and produce no symptoms afterward. Later in the course of the disorder, pain and tenderness may persist throughout the cycle. The cysts feel firm, mobile, and well defined. Many are bilateral and found in the upper outer quadrant of the breast; others are unilateral and generalized. Signs and symptoms of premenstrual syndrome—including headache, irritability, bloating, nausea, vomiting,

and abdominal cramping—may also be present.

◆ *Mammary duct ectasia.* Although ectasia (duct dilation) commonly produces no symptoms at first, burning pain and itching around the areola may occur. The history may include one or more episodes of inflammation with pain, tenderness, erythema, and acute fever, or with pain and tenderness alone, which develop and then subside spontaneously within 7 to 10 days. Other findings include a rubbery, subareolar breast nodule; swelling and erythema around the nipple; nipple retraction; a bluish green discoloration or peau d'orange of the skin overlying the nodule; a thick, sticky, multicolored nipple discharge from multiple ducts; and axillary lymphadenopathy. A breast ulcer may occur in late stages.

◆ *Mastitis.* Unilateral pain may be severe, particularly when the inflammation occurs near the skin surface. Breast skin is typically red and warm at the inflammation site; peau d'orange may be present. Palpation reveals a firm area of induration. Skin retraction signs—such as breast dimpling and nipple deviation, inversion, or flattening—may be present. Systemic signs and symptoms—such as high fever, chills, malaise, and fatigue—may also occur.

◆ *Sebaceous cyst (infected).* Breast pain may be reported with sebaceous cyst, a cutaneous cyst. Associated signs and symptoms include a small, well-delineated nodule, localized erythema, and induration.

Breast ulcer

Appearing on the nipple, areola, or the breast itself, an ulcer indicates destruction of the skin and subcutaneous tissue. A breast ulcer is usually a late sign of cancer, appearing well after the confirming diagnosis. Breast ulcers can also result from trauma, infection, or radiation.

Assessment

Begin the history by asking when the patient first noticed the ulcer and if it was preceded by other breast changes, such as nodules, edema, or nipple discharge, deviation, or retraction. Does the ulcer seem to be getting better or worse? Does it cause pain or produce drainage? Has she noticed a change in breast shape? Has she had a skin rash? If she has been treating the ulcer at home, find out how.

Review the patient's personal and family history for factors that increase the risk of breast cancer. Ask about previous cancer, especially of the breast, and mastectomy. Determine whether the patient's mother or a sister has had breast cancer. Ask the patient's age at menarche and menopause because more than 30 years of menstrual activity increases the risk of breast cancer. Also ask about pregnancy because nulliparity or birth of a first child after age 30 increases the risk of breast cancer.

If the patient recently gave birth, ask if she breast-feeds her infant or has recently weaned him. Ask if she's currently taking an oral antibiotic and if she's diabetic. All these factors predispose the patient to *Candida* infections.

Inspect the patient's breast, noting asymmetry or flattening. Look for a rash, scaling, cracking, or red excoriation on the nipples, areola, and inframammary fold. Check especially for skin changes, such as warmth, erythema, or peau d'orange. Palpate the breast for masses, noting induration beneath the ulcer. Then carefully palpate for tenderness or nodules around the areola and the axillary lymph nodes.

Causes

◆ *Aging.* Breast ulcers can result from normal skin changes that occur as a person ages, such as thinning, decreased vascularity, and loss of elasticity. They may also result from poor skin hygiene, tight brassieres, falls, or abuse.

◆ *Breast cancer.* A breast ulcer that doesn't heal within a month usually indicates cancer. Ulceration along a mastectomy scar may indicate metastatic cancer; a nodule beneath the ulcer may be a late sign of a fulminating tumor. Other signs include skin dimpling, nipple retraction, bloody or serous nipple discharge, erythema, peau d'orange, and enlarged axillary lymph nodes. A breast ulcer may be the presenting sign of breast cancer in men, who are more apt to miss or dismiss earlier breast changes.

◆ *Breast trauma.* Tissue destruction with inadequate healing may produce breast ulcers. Associated signs depend on the type of trauma, but may include ecchymosis, lacerations, abrasions, swelling, and hematoma.

◆ Candida albicans *infection.* Severe *Candida* infection can cause maceration of breast tissue followed by ulceration. Well-defined, bright-red papular patches—usually with scaly borders—characterize the infection, which can develop in the breast folds. Cracked nipples predispose breast-feeding women to infection. Women describe the pain, felt when the infant sucks, as a burning pain that penetrates into the chest wall.

◆ *Paget's disease.* With Paget's disease, bright-red nipple excoriation can extend to the areola and ulcerate. Serous or bloody nipple discharge and extreme nipple itching may accompany ulceration. Symptoms are usually unilateral.

◆ *Radiation therapy.* After radiation therapy, the breasts appear "sunburned." Subsequently, the skin ulcerates and the surrounding area becomes red and tender.

Breath with ammonia odor

The odor of ammonia on the breath—described as urinous or "fishy" breath—typically occurs in end-stage chronic renal failure. This sign improves slightly after hemodialysis and persists throughout the course of the disorder.

Ammonia breath odor reflects the long-term metabolic disturbances and biochemical abnormalities associated with uremia. It's produced by metabolic end products being blown off by the lungs and the breakdown of urea (to ammonia) in the saliva; however, a specific uremic toxin hasn't been identified. In animals, breath odor analysis has revealed toxic metabolites, such as dimethylamine and trimethylamine, which contribute to the "fishy" odor. The source of these amines, although still unclear, may be intestinal bacteria acting on dietary chlorine.

Assessment

When you detect ammonia breath odor, the diagnosis of chronic renal failure will probably be well established. Look for associated GI symptoms so that palliative care and support can be individualized.

Inspect the patient's oral cavity for bleeding, swollen gums or tongue, and ulceration with drainage. Ask the patient if he has experienced a metallic taste, loss of smell, increased thirst, heartburn, difficulty swallowing, loss of appetite at the sight of food, or early morning vomiting. Because GI bleeding is common in patients with chronic renal failure, ask about bowel habits, noting especially melenic stools or constipation.

Take the patient's vital signs. Watch for indications of hypertension (the patient with end-stage chronic renal failure is usually somewhat hypertensive) or hypotension. Stay alert for other signs of shock and altered mental status. Significant changes can indicate complications, such as massive GI bleeding or pericarditis with tamponade.

Causes

◆ *End-stage chronic renal failure.* Ammonia breath odor is a late finding of this disorder. Accompanying signs and symptoms include anuria, skin pigmentation changes and excoriation, brown arcs under the nail margins, tissue wasting, Kussmaul's respirations, neuropathy, lethargy, somnolence, confusion, disorientation, behavior changes with irritability, and mood lability. Later neurologic signs that signal impending uremic coma include muscle twitching and fasciculation, asterixis, paresthesia, and footdrop. Cardiovascular findings include hypertension and signs of myocardial infarction, heart failure, pericarditis, and stroke. GI findings include anorexia, nausea, heartburn, vomiting, constipation, and hiccups. Oral signs and symptoms include stomatitis, gum ulceration and bleeding, a coated tongue, and a metallic taste in the mouth. The patient has an increased risk of peptic ulceration and acute pancreatitis. Weight loss is common; uremic frost, pruritus, and signs of hormonal changes, such as impotence or amenorrhea, also appear.

Breath with fecal odor

Fecal breath odor typically accompanies fecal vomiting associated with a long-standing intestinal obstruction or gastrojejunocolic fistula. It represents an important late diagnostic clue to a potentially life-threatening GI disorder because complete obstruction of any part of the bowel, if untreated, can cause death within hours from vascular collapse and shock.

When the obstructed or adynamic intestine attempts self-decompression by regurgitating its contents, vigorous peristaltic waves propel bowel contents backward into the stomach. When the stomach fills with intestinal fluid, further reverse peristalsis results in vomiting. The odor of feculent vomitus lingers in the mouth.

Fecal breath odor may also occur in patients with a nasogastric (NG) or intestinal tube. The odor is detected only while the underlying disorder persists and abates soon after its resolution.

Assessment

Because fecal breath odor signals a potentially life-threatening intestinal obstruction, you'll need to quickly evaluate the patient's condition. Monitor his vital signs, and stay alert for signs of shock, such as hypotension, tachycardia, narrowed pulse pressure, and cool, clammy skin. Ask the patient if he's experiencing nausea or has vomited. Find out the frequency of vomiting as well as the color, odor, amount, and consistency of the vomitus. Have an emesis basin nearby to collect and accurately measure the vomitus. Anticipate possible surgery to relieve an obstruction or repair a fistula.

If the patient's condition permits, ask about previous abdominal surgery because adhesions can cause an obstruction. Also ask about loss of appetite. Is the patient experiencing abdominal pain? If so, have him describe its onset, duration, intensity, and location. Ask if the pain is intense, persistent, or spasmodic. Have the patient describe his normal bowel habits, especially noting constipation, diarrhea, or leakage of stool. Ask when the patient's last bowel movement occurred, and have him describe the stool's color and consistency.

Auscultate for bowel sounds—hyperactive, high-pitched sounds may indicate *impending* bowel obstruction, whereas hypoactive or absent sounds occur *late* in obstruction and paralytic ileus. Inspect the abdomen, noting its contour and any surgical scars. Measure abdominal girth to provide baseline data for subsequent assessment of distention. Palpate for tenderness, distention, and rigidity. Percuss for tympany, indicating a gas-filled bowel, and dullness, indicating fluid.

Rectal and pelvic examinations should be performed. All patients with a suspected bowel obstruction should have a flat and upright abdominal X-ray; some will also need a chest X-ray, sigmoidoscopy, and barium enema.

Causes

◆ *Distal small-bowel obstruction.* With late obstruction, nausea is present although vomiting may be delayed. Vomitus initially consists of gastric contents, then changes to bilious contents, followed by fecal contents with resultant fecal breath odor. Accompanying symptoms include achiness, malaise, drowsiness, and polydipsia. Bowel changes (ranging from diarrhea to constipation) are accompanied by abdominal distention, persistent epigastric or periumbilical colicky pain, and hyperactive bowel sounds and borborygmi.

As the obstruction becomes complete, bowel sounds become hypoactive or absent. Fever, hypotension, tachycardia, and rebound tenderness may indicate strangulation or perforation.

◆ *Gastrojejunocolic fistula.* With gastrojejunocolic fistula, symptoms may be variable and intermittent because of temporary plugging of the fistula. Fecal vomiting with resultant fecal breath odor may occur, but the most common chief complaint is diarrhea, accompanied by abdominal pain. Related GI findings include anorexia, weight loss, abdominal distention and, possibly, marked malabsorption.

◆ *Large-bowel obstruction.* Vomiting is usually absent initially, but fecal vomiting with resultant fecal breath odor occurs as a late sign. Typically, symptoms develop more slowly than in small-bowel obstruction. Colicky abdominal pain appears suddenly, followed by continuous hypogastric pain. Marked abdominal distention and tenderness occur, and loops of large bowel may be visible through the abdominal wall. Although constipation develops, defecation may continue for up to 3 days after complete obstruction because of stool remaining in the bowel below the obstruction. Leakage of stool is common with partial obstruction.

Breath with fruity odor

Fruity breath odor results from respiratory elimination of excess acetone. This sign characteristically occurs with ketoacidosis—a potentially life-threatening condition that requires immediate treatment to prevent severe dehydration, irreversible coma, and death.

Ketoacidosis results from the excessive catabolism of fats for cellular energy in the absence of usable carbohydrates. This process begins when insulin levels are insufficient to transport glucose into the cells, as in diabetes mellitus, or when glucose is unavailable and hepatic glycogen stores are depleted, as in low-carbohydrate diets and malnutrition. Lacking glucose, the cells burn fat faster than enzymes can handle the ketones, the acidic end products. As a result, ketones accumulate in blood and urine. To compensate for increased acidity, Kussmaul's respirations expel carbon dioxide with enough acetone to scent the breath. Eventually, this compensatory mechanism fails, producing ketoacidosis.

Assessment

When you detect fruity breath odor, check for Kussmaul's respirations and examine the patient's level of consciousness (LOC). Take his vital signs and check skin turgor. Stay alert for fruity breath odor that accompanies rapid, deep respirations, stupor, and poor skin turgor. Try to obtain a brief history, noting especially diabetes mellitus, nutritional problems such as anorexia nervosa, and fad diets with little or no carbohydrates. If the patient is in distress, intervene immediately. (See *Responding to a patient in distress.*)

If the patient isn't in severe distress, obtain a thorough history. Ask about the onset and duration of fruity breath odor. Find out about changes in breathing pattern. Ask about increased thirst, frequent urination, weight loss, fatigue, and abdominal pain. Obtain a complete medication history, including over-the-counter medications. Ask the female patient if she has had candidal vaginitis or vaginal secretions with itching. If the patient has a history of diabetes mellitus, ask about stress, infections, and noncompliance with therapy—the most common causes of ketoacidosis in known diabetics. If the patient is suspected of having anorexia

EMERGENCY INTERVENTIONS

Responding to a patient in distress

If your patient has a decreased level of consciousness, fruity breath odor, and Kussmaul's respirations you must intervene quickly:

◆ Obtain initial venous and arterial blood samples for glucose, complete blood count, and electrolyte, acetone, and arterial blood gas (ABG) levels.

◆ Obtain a urine specimen to test for glucose and acetone.

◆ Prepare to administer I.V. fluids and electrolytes to maintain hydration and electrolyte balance.

◆ Give regular insulin, as ordered, to reduce blood glucose levels in the patient with diabetic ketoacidosis.

◆ If the patient is obtunded, prepare for endotracheal intubation.

◆ Prepare for central venous catheter and arterial line insertions.

◆ Insert a nasogastric tube and an indwelling urinary catheter, as prescribed.

◆ Attach the patient to a continuous cardiac monitor.

◆ Monitor the patient's vital signs and neurologic status frequently.

◆ Draw blood as prescribed to continue monitoring glucose, electrolyte, acetone, and ABG levels.

---

nervosa, obtain a dietary and weight history.

Causes

◆ *Anorexia nervosa.* Severe weight loss associated with anorexia nervosa may produce fruity breath, usually with nausea, constipation, and cold intolerance as well as dental enamel erosion and scars or calluses in the dorsum of the hand (both related to induced vomiting).

◆ *Drugs.* Drugs known to cause metabolic acidosis, such as nitroprusside and salicylates, can result in fruity breath odor.

◆ *Ketoacidosis.* Fruity breath odor accompanies alcoholic ketoacidosis, which is usually seen in poorly nourished alcoholics with vomiting, abdominal pain, and only minimal food intake over several days. Kussmaul's respirations begin abruptly and accompany dehydration, abdominal pain and distention, and absent bowel sounds.

Blood glucose levels are normal or slightly decreased.

With diabetic ketoacidosis, fruity breath odor commonly occurs as ketoacidosis develops over 1 to 2 days. Other findings include polydipsia, polyuria, nocturia, a weak and rapid pulse, hunger, weight loss, weakness, fatigue, nausea, vomiting, and abdominal pain. Eventually, Kussmaul's respirations, orthostatic hypotension, dehydration, tachycardia, confusion, and stupor occur. Signs and symptoms may lead to coma.

Starvation ketoacidosis is a potentially life-threatening disorder that has a gradual onset. Besides fruity breath odor, typical findings include signs of cachexia and dehydration, a decreased LOC, bradycardia, and a history of severely limited food intake.

◆ *Low-carbohydrate diets.* Diets low in carbohydrates, which encourage little or no carbohydrate intake, may cause ketoacidosis and the resulting fruity breath odor.

Brudzinski's sign

A positive Brudzinski's sign (flexion of the hips and knees in response to passive flexion of the neck) signals meningeal irritation. Passive flexion of the neck stretches the nerve roots, causing pain and involuntary flexion of the knees and hips. It's a common and important early indicator of life-threatening meningitis and subarachnoid hemorrhage. It can be elicited in children as well as adults, although more reliable indicators of meningeal irritation exist for infants.

Testing for Brudzinski's sign

Here's how to test for Brudzinski's sign when you suspect meningeal irritation:
With the patient in a supine position, place your hands behind her neck and lift her head toward her chest.

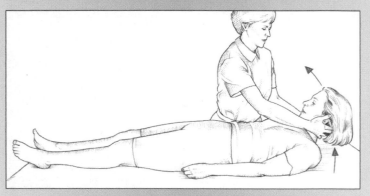

If your patient has meningeal irritation, she'll flex her hips and knees in response to the passive neck flexion.

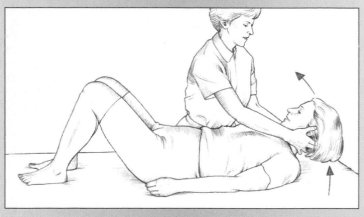

Testing for Brudzinski's sign isn't part of the routine assessment unless meningeal irritation is suspected. (See *Testing for Brudzinski's sign.*)

Assessment

If the patient is alert, ask him about headache, neck pain, nausea, and vision disturbances—all possible indications of increased intracranial pressure (ICP). Also observe the patient for signs and symptoms of increased ICP, such as an altered level of consciousness (LOC), pupillary changes, bradycardia, widened pulse pressure, irregular respiratory patterns, vomiting, and moderate fever.

Continue your neurologic assessment by evaluating the patient's cranial nerve function, noting motor or sensory deficits. Be sure to look for Kernig's sign (resistance to knee extension after flexion of the hip), which is a further indication of meningeal irritation. Also look for signs of central nervous system infection such as nuchal rigidity.

Ask the patient or his family, if necessary, about a history of hypertension, spinal arthritis, a sudden onset of headaches, or recent head trauma. Also ask about dental work and abscessed teeth, endocarditis, and I.V. drug abuse.

Causes

◆ *Arthritis.* With severe spinal arthritis, a positive Brudzinski's sign can occasionally be elicited. The patient may also report back pain (especially after weight bearing) and limited mobility.
◤ *Meningitis.* A positive Brudzinski's sign can usually be elicited 24 hours after the onset of meningitis, a life-threatening disorder. Additional findings may include headache, nuchal rigidity, irritability or restlessness, deep stupor, vertigo, fever, chills, muscular hypotonia, opisthotonos, papilledema, ocular and facial palsies, nausea and vomiting, photophobia, diplopia, and unequal, sluggish pupils. As ICP rises, arterial hypertension, bradycardia, widened pulse pressure, Cheyne-Stokes or Kussmaul's respirations, and coma may develop.
◤ *Subarachnoid hemorrhage.* Brudzinski's sign may be elicited within minutes after initial bleeding in subarachnoid hemorrhage, a life-threatening disorder. Accompanying signs and symptoms include the sudden onset of severe headache, nuchal rigidity, an altered LOC, dizziness, cranial nerve palsies, nausea and vomiting, and fever. Focal signs—such as hemiparesis, vision disturbances, or aphasia—may also occur. As ICP rises, arterial hypertension, bradycardia, widened pulse pressure, Cheyne-Stokes or Kussmaul's respirations, and coma may develop.

Bruits

Commonly an indicator of life- or limb-threatening vascular disease, bruits are swishing sounds caused by turbulent blood flow. They're characterized by location, duration, intensity, pitch, and the time of onset in the cardiac cycle. Loud bruits produce intense vibration and a palpable thrill.

Bruits are most significant when heard over the abdominal aorta; the renal, carotid, femoral, popliteal, or subclavian artery; or the thyroid gland. (See *Preventing false bruits,* page 156.) They're also significant when heard consistently despite changes in patient position and when heard during diastole.

Preventing false bruits

Auscultating bruits accurately requires practice and skill. These sounds typically stem from arterial luminal narrowing or arterial dilation, but they can also result from excessive pressure applied to the stethoscope's bell during auscultation. This pressure compresses the artery, creating turbulent blood flow and a false bruit.

To prevent false bruits, place the bell lightly on the patient's skin. If you're auscultating for a popliteal bruit, help the patient to a supine position, place your hand behind his ankle, and lift his leg slightly before placing the bell behind the knee.

NORMAL BLOOD FLOW, NO BRUIT

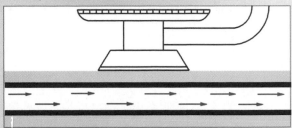

TURBULENT BLOOD FLOW AND TRUE BRUIT CAUSED BY ANEURYSM

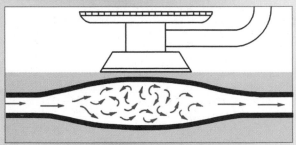

TURBULENT BLOOD FLOW AND FALSE BRUIT CAUSED BY COMPRESSION OF ARTERY

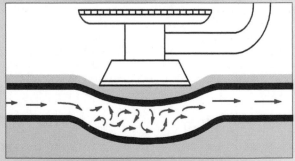

Assessment

If you detect bruits over the abdominal aorta, check for a pulsating mass or a bluish discoloration around the umbilicus (Cullen's sign). Either of these signs may signal life-threatening dissection of an aortic aneurysm. Also, check peripheral pulses, comparing intensity in the upper versus lower extremities. If you suspect dissection, monitor the patient's vital signs constantly, and withhold food and oral fluids until a definitive diagnosis is made. Watch for signs and symptoms of hypovolemic shock.

If you detect bruits over the thyroid gland, ask the patient if he has a history or signs and symptoms of hyperthyroidism. Watch for signs and symptoms of life-threatening thyroid storm, such as tremor, restlessness, diarrhea, abdominal pain, and hepatomegaly.

If you detect carotid artery bruits, stay alert for signs and symptoms of a transient ischemic attack (TIA), which may indicate an impending stroke. Evaluate the patient frequently for changes in neurologic and muscle function.

If you detect bruits over the femoral, popliteal, or subclavian artery, assess the patient for signs and symptoms of decreased or absent peripheral circulation. Ask if he has a history of intermittent claudication. Watch for the sudden absence of a pulse, pallor, or coolness, which may indicate a threat to the affected limb.

Causes

◪ *Abdominal aortic aneurysm.* A pulsating periumbilical mass accompanied by a systolic bruit over the aorta characterizes an abdominal aortic aneurysm. Associated signs and symptoms include mottled skin, diminished peripheral pulses, and a rigid, tender abdomen. Sharp, tearing pain in the ab-

domen, flank, or lower back signals imminent dissection.

◆ *Abdominal aortic atherosclerosis.* Loud systolic bruits in the epigastric and midabdominal areas are common in this disorder. They may be accompanied by leg weakness, numbness, paresthesia, or paralysis; leg pain; or decreased or absent femoral, popliteal, or pedal pulses. Abdominal pain is rarely present.

◆ *Anemia.* In patients with severe anemia, short systolic bruits may be heard over both carotid arteries and may be accompanied by headache, fatigue, dizziness, pallor, palpitations, mild tachycardia, dyspnea, nausea, and anorexia.

◆ *Carotid artery stenosis.* Systolic bruits can be heard over one or both carotid arteries. Dizziness, vertigo, headache, syncope, aphasia, dysarthria, sudden vision loss, hemiparesis, or hemiparalysis signals a TIA and may herald a stroke.

◆ *Carotid cavernous fistula.* Continuous bruits heard over the eyeballs and temples are characteristic of carotid cavernous fistula, as are vision disturbances and protruding, pulsating eyeballs.

◆ *Peripheral arteriovenous fistula.* A rough, continuous bruit with systolic accentuation may be heard over a peripheral arteriovenous fistula; a palpable thrill is also common.

◆ *Peripheral vascular disease.* Peripheral vascular disease characteristically produces bruits over the femoral artery and other arteries in the legs. It can also cause diminished or absent femoral, popliteal, or pedal pulses; intermittent claudication; numbness, weakness, pain, and cramping in the legs, feet, and hips; and cool, shiny skin and hair loss on the affected extremity. It also predisposes the patient to lower-extremity ulcers that heal with difficulty.

◆ *Renal artery stenosis.* Systolic bruits are commonly heard over the abdominal midline and flank on the side affected with renal artery stenosis. Hypertension, headache, palpitations, tachycardia, anxiety, dizziness, retinopathy, hematuria, and mental sluggishness may also appear.

◆ *Subclavian steal syndrome.* With subclavian steal syndrome, systolic bruits may be heard over one or both subclavian arteries as a result of arterial lumen narrowing. They may be accompanied by decreased blood pressure and claudication in the affected arm, hemiparesis, vision disturbances, vertigo, and dysarthria.

◆ *Thyrotoxicosis.* With thyrotoxicosis, a systolic bruit is commonly heard over the thyroid gland. The most common accompanying signs and symptoms include thyroid enlargement, fatigue, nervousness, tachycardia, heat intolerance, sweating, tremor, diarrhea, and weight loss despite increased appetite. Exophthalmos may also be present.

Butterfly rash

The presence of a butterfly rash is typically a sign of systemic lupus erythematosus (SLE), but it can also signal dermatologic disorders. Typically, a butterfly rash appears across the nose and cheeks. (See *Recognizing butterfly rash.*) Similar rashes may appear on the neck, scalp, and other areas. Butterfly rash is sometimes mistaken for sunburn because it can be provoked or aggravated by ultraviolet rays; however, it has more substance, is more sharply demarcated, and has a thicker feel in relation to surrounding skin.

Assessment

Ask the patient when he first noticed the butterfly rash and if he has recently been exposed to the sun. Has he noticed a rash elsewhere on his body? Also, ask about recent weight or hair loss. Does he have a family history of lupus? Is he taking hydralazine or procainamide (Pronestyl), which are common causes of drug-induced lupus erythematosus (LE)?

Inspect the rash, noting macules, papules, pustules, or scaling. Is the rash edematous? Are areas of hypopigmentation or hyperpigmentation present? Look for blisters or ulcers in the mouth, and note inflamed lesions. Check for rashes elsewhere on the body.

Causes

◆ *Discoid lupus erythematosus.* With discoid lupus erythematosus, a localized form of LE, the patient may have a unilateral or butterfly rash that consists of erythematous, raised, sharply demarcated plaques with follicular plugging and central atrophy. The rash may also involve the scalp, ears, chest, or any part of the body exposed to the sun. Other accompanying signs include conjunctival redness, dilated capillaries of the nail fold, bilateral parotid gland enlargement, oral lesions, and mottled, reddish blue skin on the legs.

◆ *Erysipelas.* Erysipelas, an acute cellulitis, causes rosy or crimson swollen lesions, mainly on the neck and head and commonly along the nasolabial fold. It may cause hemorrhagic pus-filled blisters. Other signs and symptoms include fever, chills, cervical lymphadenopathy, and malaise.

◆ *Polymorphous light eruption.* Polymorphous light eruption is provoked by ultraviolet rays. A butterfly rash appears as erythema, vesicles, plaques, and multiple small papules that may later become eczematized, lichenified, and excoriated. The rash appears on the cheeks and bridge of the nose, the hands and arms, and other areas, beginning a few hours to several days after exposure. It may be accompanied by pruritus.

◆ *Rosacea.* Initially with rosacea, a butterfly rash may appear as a prominent, nonscaling, intermittent erythema limited to the lower one-half of the nose or including the chin, cheeks, and central forehead. As it develops, the duration of the rash increases. With advanced rosacea, the skin is oily, with papules, pustules, nodules, and telangiectasis restricted to the central oval of the face. Men with severe rosacea may also have rhinophyma—a thickened, lobulated overgrowth of sebaceous glands and epithelial connective tissue on the lower one-half of the nose and, possibly, the adjacent cheeks.

◆ *Seborrheic dermatitis.* With seborrheic dermatitis, a rash appears as greasy and scaling with slightly yellow macules and papules of varying size on the cheeks and the bridge of the nose, in a "butterfly" pattern. The scalp, beard, eyebrows, portions of the forehead above the bridge of the nose, nasolabial fold, or trunk may also be involved. Associated signs and symptoms include crusts and fissures (particularly when the external ear and scalp are involved), pruritus, redness, blepharitis, styes, and severe acne. Severe seborrheic dermatitis of the face occurs in acquired immunodeficiency syndrome.

◆ *Systemic lupus erythematosus.* Occurring in about 40% of patients with SLE, butterfly rash appears as a red, usually scaly, sharply demarcated macular eruption. The rash may be transient in patients with acute SLE or may progress slowly to include the forehead, chin, area around the ears, and other exposed areas. Common associated skin findings include scaling, patchy alopecia, mucous membrane lesions, mottled erythema of the palms and fin-

Recognizing butterfly rash

With classic butterfly rash, lesions appear on the cheeks and the bridge of the nose, creating a characteristic butterfly pattern. The rash may vary in severity from malar erythema to discoid lesions (plaques).

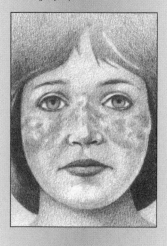

gers, periungual erythema with edema, reddish purple macular lesions on the volar surfaces of the fingers, telangiectasia of the base of the nails or eyelids, purpura, petechiae, and ecchymoses.

Joint pain, stiffness, and deformities may accompany the butterfly rash. Related findings include periorbital and facial edema, dyspnea, a low-grade fever, malaise, weakness, fatigue, weight loss, anorexia, nausea, vomiting, lymphadenopathy, photosensitivity, and hepatosplenomegaly.

C

Capillary refill time, increased

Capillary refill time is the duration required for color to return to the nail bed of a finger or toe after application of slight pressure, which causes blanching. This duration reflects the quality of peripheral vasomotor function. Normal capillary refill time is less than 3 seconds.

Increased refill time isn't diagnostic of a disorder, but must be evaluated along with other signs and symptoms. However, this sign usually signals obstructive peripheral arterial disease or decreased cardiac output.

Capillary refill time is typically tested during a routine cardiovascular assessment. It isn't tested with suspected life-threatening disorders because other, more characteristic signs and symptoms appear earlier.

Assessment

If you detect increased capillary refill time, take the patient's vital signs and check pulses in the affected limb. Does the limb feel cold or look cyanotic? Does the patient report pain or unusual or decreased sensations in his fingers or toes, especially after exposure to cold?

Take a brief medical history, especially noting previous peripheral vascular disease. Obtain a complete medication history, including over-the-counter drugs.

Causes

◤ *Aortic aneurysm (dissecting).* Capillary refill time is increased in the fingers and toes with a dissecting aneurysm in the thoracic aorta and is prolonged in just the toes with a dissecting aneurysm in the abdominal aorta. Common accompanying signs and symptoms include a pulsating abdominal mass, a systolic bruit, and substernal back or abdominal pain.

◆ *Aortic arch syndrome.* Increased capillary refill time in the fingers occurs early in a patient with aortic arch syndrome. Other signs and symptoms include fever, night sweats, arthralgia, weight loss, anorexia, nausea, malaise, a skin rash, splenomegaly, and pallor. Later, the patient displays absent carotid pulses and, possibly, unequal radial pulses.

◆ *Arterial occlusion (acute).* Increased capillary refill time occurs early with arterial occlusion. Arterial pulses are usually absent distal to the obstruction; the affected limb appears cool and pale or cyanotic. Intermittent claudication, moderate to severe pain,

◆

numbness, and paresthesia or paralysis of the affected limb may occur.

◆ *Buerger's disease.* With Buerger's disease, capillary refill time is increased in the toes. Exposure to low temperatures turns the feet cold, cyanotic, and numb; later, they redden, become hot, and tingle. Other findings include intermittent claudication of the instep and weak peripheral pulses. If the disease affects the hands, increased capillary refill time may accompany painful fingertip ulcerations.

🔰 *Cardiac tamponade.* Increased capillary refill time represents a late sign of cardiac tamponade. Associated signs include paradoxical pulse, tachycardia, cyanosis, dyspnea, jugular vein distention, hypotension, and narrowed pulse pressure.

◆ *Drugs.* Drugs that cause vasoconstriction (particularly alpha-adrenergic blockers) increase capillary refill time.

🔰 *Hypothermia.* Increased capillary refill time may appear early as a compensatory response with hypothermia. Associated signs and symptoms depend on the degree of hypothermia and may include shivering, fatigue, weakness, a decreased level of consciousness, slurred speech, ataxia, muscle stiffness or rigidity, tachycardia or bradycardia, hyporeflexia or areflexia, diuresis, oliguria, bradypnea, decreased blood pressure, and cold, pale skin.

◆ *Peripheral arterial trauma.* Trauma to a peripheral artery that reduces distal blood flow also increases capillary refill time in the affected extremity. Related findings in that extremity include bruising or pulsating bleeding, a weakened pulse, cyanosis, paresthesia, sensory loss, and cool, pale skin.

◆ *Peripheral vascular disease.* Increased capillary refill time in the affected extremities is a late sign of peripheral vascular disease. Peripheral pulses gradually weaken and then disappear. Intermittent claudication, coolness, pallor, and decreased hair growth are associated signs.

◆ *Raynaud's disease.* With Raynaud's disease, capillary refill time is prolonged in the fingers, the usual site of this disease's characteristic episodic arterial vasospasm. Exposure to cold or stress produces blanching in the fingers, then cyanosis, and then erythema before the fingers return to normal temperature. Warmth relieves the symptoms, which may include paresthesia. Chronic disease may produce trophic changes, such as sclerodactyly (stiff, tight skin on the fingers with atrophy of the soft tissues), ulcerations, or chronic paronychia (nailbed fold inflammation).

◆ *Volkmann's contracture.* Increased capillary refill time results from vasospasm that occurs with Volkmann's contracture. Associated signs include the loss of mobility and loss of strength in the affected extremity.

Carpopedal spasm

Carpopedal spasm is the violent, painful contraction of the muscles in the hands and feet. (See *Recognizing carpopedal spasm,* page 162.) It's an important sign of tetany, a potentially life-threatening condition characterized by increased neuromuscular excitation and sustained muscle contraction. It's commonly associated with hypocalcemia.

Carpopedal spasm requires prompt evaluation and intervention. If the primary event isn't treated promptly, the patient can also develop laryngospasm, seizures, cardiac arrhythmias, and cardiac and respiratory arrest.

Recognizing carpopedal spasm

Carpopedal spasm of the hand nvolves adduction of the thumb over the palm, followed by flexion of the metacarpophalangeal joints, extension of the interphalangeal joints (fingers together), adduction of the hyperextended fingers, and flexion of the wrist and elbow joints. Similar effects occur in the joints of the feet.

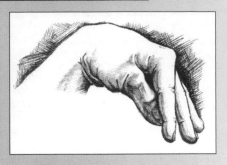

Assessment

If you detect carpopedal spasm, quickly examine the patient for signs of respiratory distress, which may indicate hypocalcemia. Connect the patient to a cardiac monitor to assess for arrhythmias. Obtain blood specimens for electrolyte analysis (especially calcium), and obtain an electrocardiogram as ordered.

If the patient isn't in distress, obtain a detailed history. Ask about the onset and duration of the spasms and ask for a description of the pain they produce. Also ask about related signs and symptoms of hypocalcemia, such as numbness and tingling of the fingertips and feet, other muscle cramps or spasms, and nausea, vomiting, and abdominal pain. Check for previous neck surgery, calcium or magnesium deficiency, tetanus exposure, and hypoparathyroidism.

During the history, form a general impression of the patient's mental status and behavior. If possible, ask family members or friends if they've noticed changes in the patient's behavior. Mental confusion or even personality changes may occur with hypocalcemia.

Inspect the patient's skin and fingernails, noting dryness or scaling and ridged, brittle nails.

Causes

◆ *Hypocalcemia.* Carpopedal spasm is an early sign of hypocalcemia. It's usually accompanied by paresthesia of the fingers, toes, and perioral area; muscle weakness, twitching, and cramping; hyperreflexia; chorea; fatigue; and palpitations. Positive Chvostek's and Trousseau's signs can be elicited. Laryngospasm, stridor, and seizures may appear in severe hypocalcemia.

Chronic hypocalcemia may be accompanied by mental status changes; cramps; dry, scaly skin; brittle nails; and thin, patchy hair and eyebrows.

◼ *Tetanus.* Tetanus develops when *Clostridium tetani* enters a wound in a nonimmunized individual. The patient develops muscle spasms and painful seizures. Difficulty swallowing and a low-grade fever are also present. If the patient isn't treated or treatment is delayed, the mortality rate is very high.

◆ *Treatments.* Multiple blood transfusions and parathyroidectomy may cause hypocalcemia, resulting in carpopedal spasm. Surgical procedures that impair calcium absorption, such as ileostomy formation and gastric resection with gastrojejunostomy, may also cause hypocalcemia.

Chest expansion, asymmetrical

Asymmetrical chest expansion is the uneven extension of portions of the chest wall during inspiration. During normal respiration, the thorax uniformly expands upward and outward, and then contracts downward and inward. When this process is disrupted, breathing becomes uncoordinated, resulting in asymmetrical chest expansion.

Asymmetrical chest expansion may develop suddenly or gradually and may affect one or both sides of the chest wall. It may occur as delayed expiration (chest lag), as abnormal movement during inspiration (for example, intercostal retractions, paradoxical movement, or chest-abdomen asynchrony), or as a unilateral absence of movement. This sign usually results from pleural disorders, such as hemothorax or tension pneumothorax. (See *Recognizing life-threatening causes of asymmetrical chest expansion,* page 164.) However, it can also result from a musculoskeletal or urologic disorder, airway obstruction, or trauma. Regardless of its underlying cause, asymmetrical chest expansion produces rapid and shallow or deep respirations that increase the work of breathing.

Assessment

If you detect asymmetrical chest expansion, first consider traumatic injury to the patient's ribs or sternum, which can cause flail chest, a life-threatening emergency characterized by paradoxical chest movement. Quickly take the patient's vital signs and look for signs of acute respiratory distress—rapid and shallow respirations, tachycardia, and cyanosis.

◆ **ALERT** Because any form of asymmetrical chest expansion can compromise the patient's respiratory status, don't leave the patient unattended and stay alert for signs of respiratory distress.

If the patient isn't experiencing acute respiratory distress, obtain a brief history. Asymmetrical chest expansion commonly results from mechanical airflow obstruction, so find out if the patient is experiencing dyspnea or pain during breathing. If so, does he feel short of breath constantly or intermittently? Does the pain worsen his feeling of breathlessness? Does repositioning, coughing, or other activity relieve or worsen the patient's dyspnea or pain? Is the pain more noticeable during inspiration or expiration? Can he inhale deeply?

Ask if the patient has a history of pulmonary or systemic illness, such as frequent upper respiratory tract infections, asthma, tuberculosis, pneumonia, or cancer. Has he had thoracic surgery? Also ask about blunt or penetrating chest trauma, which may have caused pulmonary injury. Obtain an occupational history to find out if the patient may have inhaled toxic fumes or aspirated a toxic substance.

Next, perform a physical examination. Begin by gently palpating the trachea for midline positioning. (Deviation of the trachea usually indicates an acute problem requiring immediate intervention.) Then examine the posterior chest wall for areas of tenderness or deformity. To evaluate the extent of asymmetrical chest expansion, place your hands—fingers together and thumbs abducted toward the spine—flat on both sections of the lower posterior chest wall. Position your thumbs at the 10th rib, and grasp the lateral rib cage with your hands. As the patient

Recognizing life-threatening causes of asymmetrical chest expansion

Asymmetrical chest expansion can result from several life-threatening disorders. Two common causes—bronchial obstruction and flail chest—produce distinctive chest wall movements that provide important clues about the underlying disorder.

With *bronchial obstruction*, only the unaffected portion of the chest wall expands during inspiration. Intercostal bulging during expiration and hyperresonance on percussion may indicate that air is trapped in the chest.

With *flail chest*—a disruption of the thorax due to multiple rib fractures—the unstable portion of the chest wall collapses inward at inspiration and balloons outward at expiration.

INSPIRATION

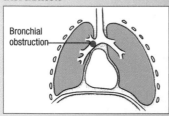

Bronchial obstruction

INSPIRATION

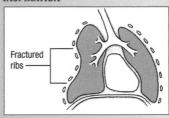

Fractured ribs

EXPIRATION

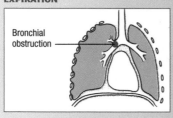

Bronchial obstruction

EXPIRATION

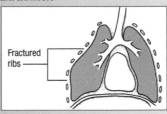

Fractured ribs

inhales, note the uneven separation of your thumbs, and gauge the distance between them. Then repeat this technique on the upper posterior chest wall. Next, use the ulnar surface of your hand to palpate for vocal or tactile fremitus on both sides of the chest. To check for vocal fremitus, ask the patient to repeat "99" as you proceed. Note asymmetrical vibrations and areas of enhanced, diminished, or absent fremitus. Then percuss and auscultate to detect air and fluid in the lungs and

pleural spaces. Finally, auscultate all lung fields for normal and adventitious breath sounds. Examine the patient's anterior chest wall, using the same assessment techniques.

Causes

◆ *Bronchial obstruction.* Bronchial obstruction can produce asymmetrical chest expansion that may occur gradually or suddenly. Typically, a lack of chest movement indicates complete obstruction; chest lag signals partial obstruction. You may also note dyspnea, accessory muscle use, decreased or absent breath sounds, and retractions.

◆ *Flail chest.* With flail chest, the patient may have ecchymoses, severe localized pain, or other signs of traumatic injury to the chest wall. He may also exhibit rapid, shallow respirations, tachycardia, and cyanosis.

❧ *Hemothorax.* Hemothorax causes chest lag during inspiration. Other findings include signs of traumatic chest injury, stabbing pain at the injury site, anxiety, restlessness, dullness on percussion, tachypnea, tachycardia, and hypoxemia. If hypovolemia occurs, you'll note signs of shock, such as hypotension and a rapid, weak pulse.

◆ *Kyphoscoliosis.* Abnormal curvature of the thoracic spine in the anteroposterior direction (kyphosis) and the lateral direction (scoliosis) gradually compresses one lung and distends the other. This produces decreased chest wall movement on the compressed lung side and expands the intercostal muscles during inspiration on the opposite side. It can also produce ineffective coughing, dyspnea, back pain, and fatigue.

◆ *Myasthenia gravis.* With myasthenia gravis, progressive loss of ventilatory muscle function produces asynchrony of the chest and abdomen during inspiration, which can lead to the onset of acute respiratory distress. Typically, the patient's shallow respirations and increased muscle weakness cause severe dyspnea, tachypnea, and possible apnea.

◆ *Pleural effusion.* Chest lag at end-inspiration occurs gradually with pleural effusion. Usually, some combination of dyspnea, tachypnea, and tachycardia precedes chest lag; the patient may also have pleuritic pain that worsens with coughing or deep breathing. The area of the effusion is delineated by dullness on percussion and by egopho-

ny, bronchophony, whispered pectoriloquy, decreased or absent breath sounds, and decreased tactile fremitus.

◆ *Pneumonia.* Depending on whether fluid consolidation in the lungs develops unilaterally or bilaterally with pneumonia, asymmetrical chest expansion occurs as inspiratory chest lag or as chest-abdomen asynchrony. The patient typically has a fever, chills, tachycardia, tachypnea, and dyspnea along with crackles, rhonchi, and chest pain that worsens during deep breathing. He may also be fatigued and anorexic and have a productive cough.

❧ *Pneumothorax.* With pneumothorax, entrapment of air in the pleural space can cause chest lag at end-inspiration. Typical signs and symptoms include sudden, stabbing chest pain that may radiate to the arms, face, back, or abdomen and dyspnea unrelated to the chest pain's severity. Other findings include tachypnea, decreased tactile fremitus, tympany on percussion, decreased or absent breath sounds over the trapped air, tachycardia, restlessness, and anxiety.

With tension pneumothorax, which rapidly compresses the heart and great vessels and causes cyanosis and hypotension, the same signs and symptoms occur as in pneumothorax but they're much more severe. The patient may also develop subcutaneous crepitation of the upper trunk, neck, and face and mediastinal and tracheal deviation away from the affected side. A crunching sound over the precordium with each heartbeat indicates pneumomediastinum.

❧ *Pulmonary embolism.* Pulmonary embolism is an acute, life-threatening disorder that causes chest lag, tachycardia, and sudden, stabbing chest pain. The patient usually has severe dyspnea, blood-tinged sputum, a pleural friction rub, acute anxiety, and restlessness.

Chest pain

Chest pain usually results from disorders that affect thoracic or abdominal organs—the heart, pleurae, lungs, esophagus, rib cage, gallbladder, pancreas, or stomach. An important indicator of several life-threatening disorders, it can also result from a musculoskeletal or hematologic disorder, anxiety, and drug therapy.

Chest pain can arise suddenly or gradually, and its cause may be difficult to ascertain initially. The pain can radiate to the arms, neck, jaw, or back. It can be steady or intermittent, mild or severe. It can range in character from a sharp shooting sensation to a feeling of heaviness, fullness, or even indigestion. It can be provoked or aggravated by stress, anxiety, exertion, deep breathing, or eating certain foods. (See *Managing severe chest pain,* pages 168 and 169.)

Assessment

If the chest pain isn't severe, proceed with the history. Ask if the patient feels diffuse pain or can point to the painful area. Ask whether he has discomfort radiating to his neck, jaw, arms, or back. If he does, ask him to describe it. Is it a dull, aching, pressurelike sensation or a sharp, stabbing pain? Does he feel it on the surface or deep inside? Find out whether it's constant or intermittent and how long it lasts. Ask if movement, exertion, breathing, or eating certain foods worsens or helps to relieve the pain. Does anything in particular seem to bring it on? Review the patient's history for cardiac or pulmonary disease, chest trauma, intestinal disease, or sickle cell anemia. Find out which medications he's taking, including over-the-counter drugs, and ask about recent dosage changes.

Take the patient's vital signs, noting tachypnea, fever, tachycardia, oxygen saturation, paradoxical pulse, and hypertension or hypotension. Also, look for jugular vein distention and peripheral edema. Observe the patient's breathing pattern. Auscultate his lungs for a pleural friction rub, crackles, rhonchi, wheezing, or diminished or absent breath sounds. Next, auscultate for murmurs, clicks, gallops, or a pericardial friction rub. Palpate for thrills, gallops, tactile fremitus, and abdominal masses or tenderness.

Causes

◆ *Angina pectoris.* With angina pectoris, the patient may experience a feeling of tightness or pressure in the chest that he describes as pain or a sensation of indigestion or expansion. The pain usually occurs in the retrosternal region. It may radiate to the neck, jaw and, classically, to the inner aspect of the left arm. Angina tends to begin gradually, builds to its maximum, and then slowly subsides. Provoked by exertion, emotional stress, or a heavy meal, the pain typically lasts 2 to 10 minutes. Associated findings include dyspnea, nausea, vomiting, tachycardia, dizziness, diaphoresis, belching, and palpitations.

With Prinzmetal's angina, caused by vasospasm of coronary vessels, chest pain typically occurs when the patient is at rest; it may even awaken him. Other findings may be shortness of breath, nausea, vomiting, dizziness, and palpitations.
◆ *Anxiety.* Acute anxiety can produce intermittent, sharp, stabbing chest pain, commonly located behind the left breast. The pain typically lasts only a few seconds, but the patient may experience a precordial ache or a sensation of heaviness that lasts for hours or days.

◣ *Aortic aneurysm (dissecting).* The chest pain associated with a dissecting aortic aneurysm usually begins suddenly and is most severe at its onset. The patient describes an excruciating tearing, ripping, stabbing pain in his chest and neck that radiates to his upper back, abdomen, and lower back. He may also have abdominal tenderness, a palpable abdominal mass, tachycardia, syncope, loss of consciousness, a lower blood pressure in the legs than in the arms, and weak or absent femoral or pedal pulses. His skin is pale, cool, diaphoretic, and may be mottled below the waist. Capillary refill time is increased, and palpation reveals decreased pulsation in the carotid arteries.

◆ *Asthma.* In an asthma attack, diffuse and painful chest tightness arises suddenly along with a dry cough and mild wheezing, which progress to a productive cough, audible wheezing, and severe dyspnea. Related respiratory findings include rhonchi, crackles, prolonged expirations, intercostal and supraclavicular retractions on inspiration, accessory muscle use, flaring nostrils, and tachypnea. Other findings include restlessness, anxiety, tachycardia, diaphoresis, flushing, and cyanosis.

◆ *Bronchitis.* In its acute form, bronchitis produces a burning chest pain or a sensation of substernal tightness. It also produces a cough, initially dry but later productive, that worsens the chest pain.

◆ *Interstitial lung disease.* As interstitial lung disease advances, the patient may experience pleuritic chest pain along with progressive dyspnea, cellophane-type crackles, a nonproductive cough, clubbing, and cyanosis.

◆ *Lung abscess.* Pleuritic chest pain develops insidiously in lung abscess along with a cough that raises copious amounts of purulent, foul-smelling, blood-tinged sputum. The patient also displays diaphoresis, anorexia, weight loss, fever, chills, fatigue, weakness, dyspnea, and clubbing.

◆ *Lung cancer.* The chest pain associated with lung cancer is commonly described as intermittent aching, felt deep within the chest. If the tumor metastasizes to the ribs or vertebrae, the pain becomes localized, continuous, and gnawing.

◆ *Mitral valve prolapse.* Most patients with mitral valve prolapse are asymptomatic, but some may experience a sharp, stabbing precordial chest pain or ache. The pain can last for seconds or hours and occasionally mimics the pain of ischemic heart disease. Patients may experience dizziness, weakness, dyspnea, tachycardia, and palpitations.

◣ *Myocardial infarction (MI).* The chest pain felt during an MI may last for hours. Typically a crushing substernal pain unrelieved by rest or nitroglycerin, it may radiate to the patient's left arm, jaw, neck, or shoulder blades. Other findings include pallor, clammy skin, dyspnea, nausea, vomiting, hypotension or hypertension, anxiety, and crackles.

◆ *Pericarditis.* Pericarditis produces precordial or retrosternal pain aggravated by deep breathing, coughing, position changes and, occasionally, swallowing. The pain is commonly sharp or cutting and radiates to the shoulder and neck. Associated signs and symptoms include a pericardial friction rub, fever, tachycardia, and dyspnea.

◆ *Pleurisy.* The chest pain of pleurisy arises abruptly and reaches maximum intensity within a few hours. The pain is sharp, usually unilateral, and located in the lower and lateral aspects of the chest. Deep breathing, coughing, or thoracic movement aggravates it.

◆ *Pneumonia.* Pneumonia produces pleuritic chest pain that increases with deep inspiration and is accompanied
(Text continues on page 170.)

EMERGENCY INTERVENTIONS

Managing severe chest pain

Sudden, severe chest pain may result from several life-threatening disorders. Your evaluation and interventions will vary, depending on the pain's location and character. This flowchart will help you establish priorities for managing this emergency successfully.

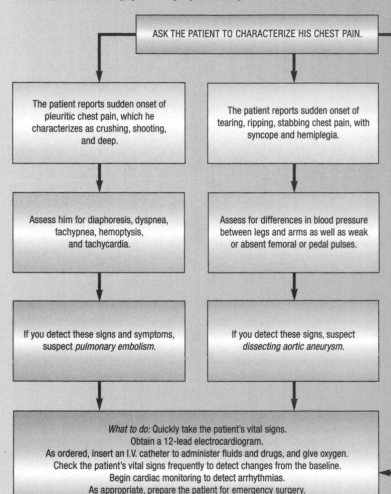

ASK THE PATIENT TO CHARACTERIZE HIS CHEST PAIN.

The patient reports sudden onset of pleuritic chest pain, which he characterizes as crushing, shooting, and deep.

The patient reports sudden onset of tearing, ripping, stabbing chest pain, with syncope and hemiplegia.

Assess him for diaphoresis, dyspnea, tachypnea, hemoptysis, and tachycardia.

Assess for differences in blood pressure between legs and arms as well as weak or absent femoral or pedal pulses.

If you detect these signs and symptoms, suspect *pulmonary embolism.*

If you detect these signs, suspect *dissecting aortic aneurysm.*

What to do: Quickly take the patient's vital signs.
Obtain a 12-lead electrocardiogram.
As ordered, insert an I.V. catheter to administer fluids and drugs, and give oxygen.
Check the patient's vital signs frequently to detect changes from the baseline.
Begin cardiac monitoring to detect arrhythmias.
As appropriate, prepare the patient for emergency surgery.
Prepare the patient with pulmonary embolism or myocardial infarction (MI)
for possible thrombolytic therapy.

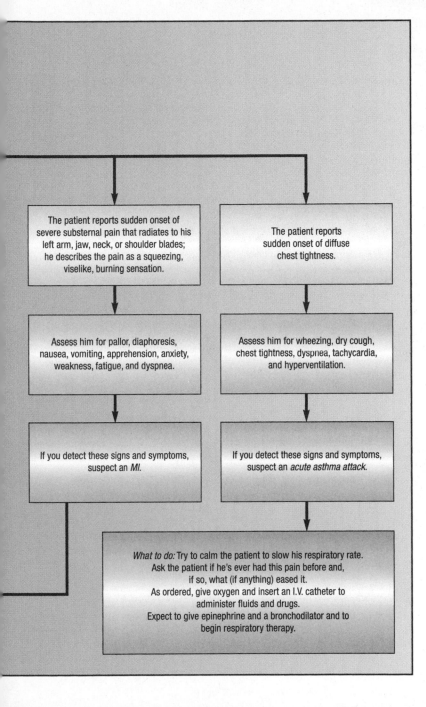

The patient reports sudden onset of severe substernal pain that radiates to his left arm, jaw, neck, or shoulder blades; he describes the pain as a squeezing, viselike, burning sensation.

Assess him for pallor, diaphoresis, nausea, vomiting, apprehension, anxiety, weakness, fatigue, and dyspnea.

If you detect these signs and symptoms, suspect an *MI.*

The patient reports sudden onset of diffuse chest tightness.

Assess him for wheezing, dry cough, chest tightness, dyspnea, tachycardia, and hyperventilation.

If you detect these signs and symptoms, suspect an *acute asthma attack.*

What to do: Try to calm the patient to slow his respiratory rate. Ask the patient if he's ever had this pain before and, if so, what (if anything) eased it. As ordered, give oxygen and insert an I.V. catheter to administer fluids and drugs. Expect to give epinephrine and a bronchodilator and to begin respiratory therapy.

by shaking chills and fever. The patient has a dry cough that later becomes productive. Other signs and symptoms include crackles, rhonchi, tachycardia, tachypnea, dyspnea, cyanosis, decreased breath sounds, and diaphoresis.

◆ *Pneumothorax.* Spontaneous pneumothorax causes sudden sharp chest pain that's severe, typically unilateral, and rarely localized. When the pain is centrally located and radiates to the neck, it may mimic that of an MI. Breath sounds are decreased or absent on the affected side with hyperresonance or tympany, subcutaneous crepitation, and decreased vocal fremitus. Other findings include anxiety, restlessness, tachypnea, tachycardia, and hypoxemia.

◪ *Pulmonary embolism.* Typically, the patient with a pulmonary embolism experiences sudden dyspnea with intense angina-like or pleuritic chest pain aggravated by deep breathing and thoracic movement. Other findings include tachycardia, tachypnea, cough, diaphoresis, crackles, diffuse wheezing, dullness to percussion, signs of circulatory collapse, signs of cerebral ischemia, and restlessness. A patient with a large embolus may have cyanosis and jugular vein distention.

◆ *Sickle cell crisis.* Chest pain associated with sickle cell crisis typically has a bizarre distribution. It may start as a vague pain, commonly located in the back, hands, or feet. As the pain worsens, it becomes generalized or localized to the abdomen or chest, causing severe pleuritic pain. The patient may also have abdominal distention and rigidity, dyspnea, fever, and jaundice.

◆ *Thoracic outlet syndrome.* Thoracic outlet syndrome may be confused with angina, especially when it causes paresthesia along the ulnar distribution of the left arm. The patient usually experiences angina-like pain after lifting his arms above his head, working with his hands above his shoulders, or lifting a weight. The pain disappears as soon as he lowers his arms. Other signs include pale skin and a difference in blood pressure between both arms.

◆ *Tuberculosis (TB).* In a patient with TB, pleuritic chest pain and fine crackles occur after coughing. Associated signs and symptoms include night sweats, anorexia, weight loss, fever, malaise, dyspnea, a mild to severe productive cough, occasional hemoptysis, dullness to percussion, increased tactile fremitus, and amphoric breath sounds (sounds similar to those produced by blowing across the top of a bottle).

◆ *Tularemia.* Tularemia is an infectious disease that's caused by the bacterium *Francisella tularensis*. Signs and symptoms following inhalation of the organism include the abrupt onset of fever, chills, headache, generalized myalgia, a nonproductive cough, dyspnea, pleuritic chest pain, and empyema (pus in a body cavity such as the pleural cavity).

Cheyne-Stokes respirations

Cheyne-Stokes respirations are characterized by a waxing and waning period of hyperpnea that alternates with a shorter period of apnea. Although this pattern can occur normally in patients who live at high altitudes or in those with heart or lung disease, it usually indicates increased intracranial pressure (ICP) from a deep cerebral or brain stem lesion or a metabolic disturbance.

Cheyne-Stokes respirations typically indicate a major change in the patient's condition—usually deterioration. For example, in a patient who has had head trauma or brain surgery, Cheyne-

Stokes respirations may signal increasing ICP.

Assessment

If the patient's condition permits, obtain a brief history. Ask especially about drug use. However, if you detect Cheyne-Stokes respirations in a patient with a history of head trauma, recent brain surgery, or another brain insult, quickly take his vital signs. Keep his head elevated 30 degrees, and perform a rapid neurologic assessment. Reevaluate the patient's neurologic status frequently. If ICP continues to rise, you'll detect changes in the patient's level of consciousness (LOC), pupillary reactions, and ability to move his extremities.

Time the periods of hyperpnea and apnea for 3 to 4 minutes to evaluate respirations and to obtain baseline data. Stay alert for prolonged periods of apnea. Frequently check the patient's vital signs and oxygen saturation, and prepare for endotracheal intubation, if necessary.

Causes

◆ *Drugs.* Large doses of an opioid, hypnotic, or barbiturate can precipitate Cheyne-Stokes respirations.
◆ *Heart failure.* With left-sided heart failure, Cheyne-Stokes respirations may occur with exertional dyspnea and orthopnea. Related findings include fatigue, weakness, tachycardia, tachypnea, and crackles. The patient may also have a cough, generally nonproductive but occasionally producing clear or blood-tinged sputum.
◼ *Hypertensive encephalopathy.* Hypertensive encephalopathy is a life-threatening disorder in which severe hypertension precedes Cheyne-Stokes respirations. The patient's LOC is decreased, and he may experience vomit-

ing, seizures, severe headaches, vision disturbances (including transient blindness), or transient paralysis.
◼ *Increased ICP.* As ICP rises, Cheyne-Stokes respirations are the first irregular respiratory pattern to occur. It's preceded by a decreased LOC and accompanied by hypertension, headache, vomiting, impaired or unequal motor movement, and vision disturbances (blurring, diplopia, photophobia, and pupillary changes).
◆ *Renal failure.* With end-stage chronic renal failure, Cheyne-Stokes respirations may occur in addition to bleeding gums, oral lesions, ammonia breath odor, and marked changes in every body system.

Chills

Chills are extreme, involuntary muscle contractions with characteristic paroxysms of violent shivering and teeth chattering. Commonly accompanied by fever, chills tend to arise suddenly, usually heralding the onset of infection. Certain diseases, such as pneumococcal pneumonia, produce only a single, shaking chill. Other diseases, such as malaria, produce intermittent chills with a recurring high fever. Still others produce continuous chills for up to 1 hour, precipitating a high fever. (See *Why chills accompany fever,* page 172.)

Chills can also result from lymphomas, blood transfusion reactions, and certain drugs. Chills without fever occur as a normal response to exposure to cold. (See *Rare causes of chills,* page 173.)

Assessment

Ask the patient when the chills began and whether they're continuous or intermittent. Because fever commonly ac-

Why chills accompany fever

Fever usually occurs when exogenous pyrogens activate endogenous pyrogens to reset the body's thermostat to a higher level. At this higher set point, the body feels cold and responds through several compensatory mechanisms, including rhythmic muscle contractions or chills. These muscle contractions generate body heat and help produce fever. This flow-chart outlines the events that link chills to fever.

Exogenous pyrogens
(infectious organisms, immune
complexes, toxins) enter the body.

↓

Phagocytic leukocytes release
endogenous pyrogens.

↓

Endogenous pyrogens—
possibly with prostaglandins—
stimulate temperature-sensitive
receptors in the hypothalamus and
raise the thermostatic set point
to a higher level.

↓

Descending efferent pathways
from the hypothalamus
innervate effectors, such as skeletal
muscles, and stimulate them to
rhythmically contract.

↓

Rhythmic muscle contractions, or
chills, generate body heat, which
helps produce fever.

companies or follows chills, take his rectal temperature to obtain a baseline reading. Then check his temperature often to monitor fluctuations and to determine his temperature curve. Typically, a localized infection produces a sudden onset of shaking chills, sweats, and high fever. A systemic infection produces intermittent chills with recurring episodes of high fever or continuous chills that may last up to 1 hour and precipitate a high fever.

Ask about related signs and symptoms, such as headache, dysuria, diarrhea, confusion, abdominal pain, cough, sore throat, or nausea. Does the patient have known allergies, an infection, or a recent history of an infectious disorder? Find out which medications he's taking and whether a drug has improved or worsened his symptoms. Has he received treatment that may predispose him to an infection? Ask about recent exposure to farm animals, guinea pigs, hamsters, dogs, and such birds as pigeons, parrots, and parakeets. Also ask about recent insect or animal bites, travel to foreign countries, and contact with persons who have an active infection.

Causes

◆ *Acquired immunodeficiency syndrome (AIDS).* AIDS is caused by infection with the human immunodeficiency virus. The patient usually develops lymphadenopathy and may also experience fatigue, anorexia and weight loss, diarrhea, diaphoresis, skin disorders, and signs of upper respiratory tract infection.

⚡ *Anthrax (inhalation).* Anthrax is an acute infectious disease that can occur in humans exposed to infected animals (wild and domestic grazing animals), tissue from infected animals, or biological warfare. Most natural cases occur in agricultural regions worldwide because the spores can live in the soil for many years. Anthrax may occur in the cutaneous, inhalation, or GI form.

Inhalation anthrax is caused by inhaling aerosolized spores. Initial signs and symptoms are flulike and include fever, chills, weakness, cough, and chest pain. The disease generally occurs in two stages with a period of recovery after the initial signs and symptoms. The second stage develops abruptly with rapid deterioration marked by fever, dyspnea, stridor, and hypotension, generally leading to death within 24 hours.

◆ *Cholangitis.* Charcot's triad—chills with spiking fever, abdominal pain, and jaundice—characterizes cholangitis, a sudden obstruction of the common bile duct. The patient may have associated pruritus, weakness, and fatigue.

◆ *Gram-negative bacteremia.* Gram-negative bacteremia causes sudden chills and a fever, nausea, vomiting, diarrhea, and prostration.

◆ *Hemolytic anemia.* With acute hemolytic anemia, fulminating chills occur with a fever and abdominal pain. The patient rapidly develops jaundice and hepatomegaly and may develop splenomegaly.

◆ *Hepatic abscess.* Hepatic abscess usually arises abruptly, with chills, fever, nausea, vomiting, diarrhea, anorexia, and severe upper abdominal tenderness and pain that may radiate to the right shoulder.

◆ *Infective endocarditis.* Infective endocarditis produces the abrupt onset of intermittent, shaking chills with fever. Petechiae commonly develop. The patient may also have Janeway lesions (red, flat, painless macules) on his hands and feet and Osler's nodes (small, tender, nodular, cutaneous lesions) on his palms and soles.

◆ *Influenza.* Initially, influenza causes an abrupt onset of chills, a high fever,

Rare causes of chills

Chills can result from disorders that rarely occur in the United States, but may be fairly common worldwide. Remember to ask about recent foreign travel when you obtain a patient's history. Here's a partial list of rare disorders that produce chills.

◆ Brucellosis (undulant fever)
◆ Dengue fever (breakbone fever)
◆ Epidemic typhus (louse-borne typhus)
◆ Leptospirosis
◆ Lymphocytic choriomeningitis
◆ Plague
◆ Pulmonary tularemia
◆ Rat bite fever
◆ Relapsing fever

malaise, headache, myalgia, and a nonproductive cough. Some patients may also suddenly develop rhinitis, rhinorrhea, laryngitis, conjunctivitis, hoarseness, and a sore throat. Chills generally subside after the first few days, but an intermittent fever, weakness, and a cough may persist for up to 1 week.

◧ *Legionnaires' disease.* Within 12 to 48 hours after the onset of Legionnaires' disease, the patient suddenly develops chills and a high fever. Prodromal signs and symptoms characteristically include malaise, headache and, possibly, diarrhea, anorexia, diffuse myalgia, and general weakness. An initially nonproductive cough progresses to a productive cough with mucoid or mucopurulent sputum. The patient usually also develops nausea and vomiting, confusion, mild temporary amnesia, pleuritic chest pain, dyspnea, tachypnea, crackles, tachycardia, and flushed and mildly diaphoretic skin.

◆ *Malaria.* The paroxysmal cycle of malaria begins with a period of chills lasting 1 to 2 hours. This is followed by a high fever lasting 3 to 4 hours and then 2 to 4 hours of profuse diaphoresis. The patient also has a headache, muscle pain and, possibly, hepatosplenomegaly.

◆ *Pelvic inflammatory disease.* Pelvic inflammatory disease causes chills and fever with, typically, lower abdominal pain and tenderness; profuse, purulent vaginal discharge; or abnormal menstrual bleeding. The patient may also develop nausea and vomiting, an abdominal mass, and dysuria.

◆ *Pneumonia.* A single shaking chill usually heralds the sudden onset of pneumococcal pneumonia; other pneumonias characteristically cause intermittent chills. With any type of pneumonia, related findings may include fever, a productive cough with bloody sputum, pleuritic chest pain, dyspnea, tachypnea, and tachycardia. The patient may be cyanotic and diaphoretic, with bronchial breath sounds and crackles, rhonchi, increased tactile fremitus, and grunting respirations. He may also experience achiness, anorexia, fatigue, and headache.

◆ *Puerperal or postabortal sepsis.* Chills and a high fever occur as early as 6 hours or as late as 10 days postpartum or postabortion. The patient may also have a purulent vaginal discharge, an enlarged and tender uterus, abdominal pain, backache and, possibly, nausea, vomiting, and diarrhea.

◆ *Pyelonephritis.* With acute pyelonephritis, the patient develops chills, a high fever and, possibly, nausea and vomiting over several hours to days. He generally also has anorexia, fatigue, myalgia, flank pain, costovertebral angle (CVA) tenderness, hematuria or cloudy urine, and urinary frequency, urgency, and burning.

◆ *Q fever.* Cattle, sheep, and goats are most likely to carry the organism that causes Q fever, a highly infectious rickettsial disease. Human infection results from exposure to contaminated milk, urine, feces, or other fluids from infected animals or from inhalation of contaminated barnyard dust. Signs and symptoms include fever, chills, severe headache, malaise, chest pain, nausea, vomiting, and diarrhea. The fever may last up to 2 weeks.

◆ *Renal abscess.* Renal abscess initially produces sudden chills and fever. Later effects include flank pain, CVA tenderness, abdominal muscle spasm, and transient hematuria.

◆ *Rocky Mountain spotted fever.* Rocky Mountain spotted fever begins with a sudden onset of chills, fever, malaise, an excruciating headache, and muscle, bone, and joint pain. Typically, the patient's tongue is covered with a thick white coating that gradually turns brown. After 2 to 6 days of fever and occasional chills, a macular or maculopapular rash appears on the hands and feet and then becomes generalized; after a few days, the rash becomes petechial.

◆ *Septic arthritis.* Chills and fever accompany the characteristic red, swollen, and painful joints caused by septic arthritis.

◆ *Septic shock.* Initially, septic shock produces chills, fever and, possibly, nausea, vomiting, and diarrhea. The patient's skin is typically flushed, warm, and dry; his blood pressure is normal or slightly low; and he has tachycardia and tachypnea. As septic shock progresses, the patient's arms and legs become cool and cyanotic, and he develops oliguria, thirst, anxiety, restlessness, confusion, and hypotension.

◆ *Sinusitis.* With acute sinusitis, chills occur along with fever, headache, and pain, tenderness, and swelling over the affected sinuses. The primary indicator of sinusitis is nasal discharge, which is commonly bloody for 24 to 48 hours before it gradually becomes purulent.

◼ *Snake bite.* Most snake bites that result in envenomization cause chills, typically with a fever. Other signs and symptoms include sweating, weakness, dizziness, fainting, hypotension, nausea, vomiting, diarrhea, and thirst. The area around the snake bite may be marked by immediate swelling and tenderness, pain, ecchymoses, petechiae, blebs, bloody discharge, and local necrosis. The patient may have difficulty speaking, blurred vision, paralysis, and may also show bleeding tendencies and signs of respiratory distress and shock.

◆ *Transfusion reaction.* A hemolytic reaction may cause chills during the transfusion or immediately afterward. The patient also experiences chest pain, dyspnea, facial flushing, hypotension, flank pain, and oliguria. A nonhemolytic febrile reaction may also cause chills. Other signs and symptoms of this reaction include headache, facial flushing, palpitations, cough, tachycardia, chest tightness, and flank pain.

◆ *Tularemia.* Tularemia is an infectious disease that's found in wild animals, water, and moist soil. It's transmitted to humans through the bite of an infected insect or tick, handling infected animal carcasses, drinking contaminated water, or inhaling the bacteria. Signs and symptoms following inhalation of the organism include the abrupt onset of fever, chills, headache, generalized myalgia, a nonproductive cough, dyspnea, pleuritic chest pain, and empyema (pus in a body cavity such as the pleural cavity).

◆ *Typhus.* Typhus is a rickettsial disease transmitted to humans by fleas, mites, or body lice. Initial signs and symptoms include headache, myalgia,

arthralgia, and malaise followed by an abrupt onset of chills, fever, nausea, and vomiting. A maculopapular rash may be present in some cases.

◆ *Violin spider bite.* The violin spider bite produces chills, fever, malaise, weakness, nausea, vomiting, and joint pain within 24 to 48 hours. The patient may also develop a rash and delirium.

Chvostek's sign

Chvostek's sign is an abnormal spasm of the facial muscles that's elicited by lightly tapping the patient's facial nerve near his lower jaw. (See *Eliciting Chvostek's sign*, page 176.) This sign usually suggests hypocalcemia, but can occur normally in about 25% of cases. Typically, it precedes other signs of hypocalcemia and persists until the onset of tetany. It can't be elicited during tetany because of strong muscle contractions.

Assessment

Obtain a brief history. Find out if the patient has had his parathyroid glands surgically removed or if he has a history of hypoparathyroidism, hypomagnesemia, or a malabsorption disorder. Ask if he has had mental status changes, such as depression or slowed responses, which can accompany chronic hypocalcemia.

Causes

◆ *Hypocalcemia.* The degree of muscle spasm elicited reflects the patient's serum calcium level. Initially, hypocalcemia produces paresthesia in the fingers, toes, and circumoral area that progresses to muscle tension and carpopedal spasms. The patient may also complain of muscle weakness, fatigue,

Eliciting Chvostek's sign

Eliciting Chvostek's sign is usually attempted only in patients with suspected hypocalcemic disorders. However, because the parathyroid gland regulates calcium balance, it may also be tested in patients before neck surgery.

To elicit Chvostek's sign:
◆ Tell the patient to relax his facial muscles.
◆ Stand directly in front of him, and tap the facial nerve either just anterior to the earlobe and below the zygomatic arch or between the zygomatic arch and the corner of his mouth.
◆ A positive response varies from twitching of the lip at the corner of the mouth to spasm of all facial muscles, depending on the severity of hypocalcemia.

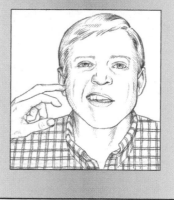

Clubbing

A nonspecific sign of pulmonary and cyanotic cardiovascular disorders, clubbing is the painless, usually bilateral increase in soft tissue around the terminal phalanges of the fingers or toes. It doesn't involve changes in the underlying bone. With early clubbing, the normal 160-degree angle between the nail and the nail base approximates 180 degrees. As clubbing progresses, this angle widens and the base of the nail becomes visibly swollen. With late clubbing, the angle where the nail meets the now-convex nail base extends more than halfway up the nail. (See *Rare causes of clubbing.*)

Assessment

You'll probably detect clubbing while evaluating other signs of known pulmonary or cardiovascular disease. Review the patient's current treatment plan because clubbing may resolve with correction of the underlying disorder. Be sure to evaluate the extent of clubbing in the fingers as well as the toes. (See *Checking for clubbed fingers.*)

Causes

◆ *Bronchiectasis.* Clubbing commonly occurs in the late stage of bronchiectasis. Other classic signs include a cough that produces copious, foul-smelling, and mucopurulent sputum; hemoptysis; and coarse crackles over the affected area, heard during inspiration. The patient may complain of weight loss,

scaly skin; brittle nails; and thin, patchy scalp and eyebrow hair.

and palpitations. Muscle twitching, hyperactive deep tendon reflexes, choreiform movements, and muscle cramps may also occur. The patient with chronic hypocalcemia may have mental status changes; diplopia; difficulty swallowing; abdominal cramps; dry, fatigue, weakness, and exertional dyspnea. He may also have rhonchi, fever, malaise, and halitosis.

◆ *Bronchitis.* With chronic bronchitis, clubbing may occur as a late sign; it's unrelated to the severity of the disease. The patient has a chronic productive cough and may display barrel chest, dyspnea, wheezing, increased accessory muscle use, cyanosis, tachypnea, crackles, scattered rhonchi, and prolonged expiration.

◆ *Emphysema.* Clubbing occurs late in emphysema. The patient may have a barrel chest, anorexia, malaise, dyspnea, tachypnea, diminished breath sounds, peripheral cyanosis, pursed-lip breathing, and a productive cough.

◆ *Endocarditis.* With subacute infective endocarditis, clubbing may be accompanied by fever, anorexia, pallor, weakness, night sweats, fatigue, tachy-

Rare causes of clubbing

Clubbing is typically a sign of pulmonary or cardiovascular disease, but it can result from certain hepatic and GI disorders, such as cirrhosis, Crohn's disease, and ulcerative colitis. Clubbing occurs only rarely in these disorders, however, so first check for their more common signs and symptoms. For example, a patient with cirrhosis usually experiences right upper quadrant pain and hepatomegaly, a patient with Crohn's disease typically has abdominal cramping and tenderness, and a patient with ulcerative colitis may develop diffuse abdominal pain and blood-streaked diarrhea.

Checking for clubbed fingers

Clubbing indicates chronic tissue hypoxia. Normally, the angle between the fingernail and the point where the nail enters the skin is about 160 degrees. Clubbing occurs when that angle increases to 180 degrees or more, as shown below.

NORMAL FINGERS

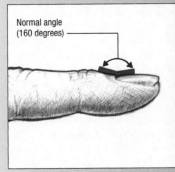

Normal angle (160 degrees)

CLUBBED FINGERS

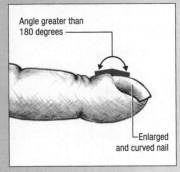

Angle greater than 180 degrees

Enlarged and curved nail

cardia, weight loss, and cardiac murmurs. The patient may also develop arthralgia, petechiae, Osler's nodes (small, tender, nodular, cutaneous lesions), splinter hemorrhages, Janeway lesions (red, flat, painless macules), splenomegaly, and Roth's spots (round, white retinal spots surrounded by hemorrhage).

◆ *Heart failure.* Clubbing occurs as a late sign in heart failure along with wheezing, dyspnea, and fatigue. Other findings include jugular vein distention, hepatomegaly, tachypnea, palpitations, dependent edema, unexplained weight gain, nausea, anorexia, chest tightness, a slowed mental response, hypotension, diaphoresis, narrow pulse pressure, pallor, oliguria, a gallop rhythm (a third heart sound), and crackles on inspiration.

◆ *Interstitial fibrosis.* Clubbing usually occurs in the patient with advanced interstitial fibrosis. Typically, he also develops intermittent chest pain, dyspnea, crackles, fatigue, weight loss and, possibly, cyanosis.

◆ *Lung abscess.* Initially, lung abscess produces clubbing, which may reverse with resolution of the abscess. It can also cause pleuritic chest pain; dyspnea; crackles; a productive cough with a lot of purulent, foul-smelling, usually bloody sputum; and halitosis. The patient may also experience weakness, fatigue, anorexia, headache, malaise, weight loss, and fever with chills. You may hear decreased breath sounds.

◆ *Lung and pleural cancer.* Clubbing occurs commonly in lung and pleural cancers. Associated findings include hemoptysis, dyspnea, wheezing, chest pain, weight loss, anorexia, fatigue, and fever.

Cogwheel rigidity

Cogwheel rigidity is a cardinal sign of Parkinson's disease, marked by muscle rigidity that reacts with superimposed ratchetlike movements when the muscle is passively stretched. This sign can be elicited by stabilizing the patient's forearm and then moving his wrist through the range of motion. (Cogwheel rigidity usually appears in the arms but is sometimes elicited in the ankle.) The patient and examiner can see and feel these characteristic movements, thought to be a combination of rigidity and tremor.

Assessment

After you have elicited cogwheel rigidity, take the patient's history to determine when he first noticed associated signs of Parkinson's disease. For example, has he experienced tremors? Does he have "pill-rolling" hand movements? When did he first notice that his movements were becoming slower? How long has he been experiencing stiffness in his arms and legs? Has his handwriting gotten smaller? While taking the history, observe him for signs of pronounced parkinsonism, such as drooling, masklike facies, dysphagia, monotone speech, and an altered gait.

Find out which medications the patient is taking, and ask if they have helped relieve some of his symptoms. If he's taking levodopa (Dopar) and his symptoms have worsened, find out if he has exceeded the prescribed dosage. If you suspect an overdose, withhold the drug. If the patient has been taking a phenothiazine or another antipsychotic drug and has no history of Parkinson's disease, he may be having an adverse reaction. Withhold the drug, as appropriate.

CONFUSION

♦ 179

Causes

♦ *Drugs.* Phenothiazines and other antipsychotics (such as haloperidol [Haldol], thiothixene [Navane], and loxapine [Loxitane]) can cause cogwheel rigidity. Metoclopramide (Reglan) infrequently causes it.
♦ *Parkinson's disease.* With Parkinson's disease, cogwheel rigidity occurs with an insidious tremor, which usually begins in the fingers (unilateral pillroll tremor), increases during stress or anxiety, and decreases with purposeful movement and sleep. Bradykinesia (slow voluntary movements and speech) also occurs. The patient walks with short, shuffling steps; his gait lacks normal parallel motion and may be retropulsive or propulsive. He has a monotone way of speaking and a masklike facial expression. He may also experience drooling, dysphagia, dysarthria, and the loss of posture control, causing him to walk with his body bent forward. An oculogyric crisis (eyes fixed upward and involuntary tonic movements) or blepharospasm (complete eyelid closure) may also occur.

Confusion

An umbrella term for puzzling or inappropriate behavior or responses, confusion is the inability to think quickly and coherently. Depending on the cause, it may arise suddenly or gradually and may be temporary or irreversible. Aggravated by stress and sensory deprivation, confusion commonly occurs in hospitalized patients—especially elderly patients, in whom it may be mistaken for senility.

When severe confusion arises suddenly and the patient also has hallucinations and psychomotor hyperactivity, his condition is classified as delirium. Long-term, progressive confusion with deterioration of all cognitive functions is classified as dementia.

Confusion can result from fluid and electrolyte imbalances or hypoxemia due to pulmonary disorders. It can also have a metabolic, neurologic, cardiovascular, cerebrovascular, or nutritional origin, or it can result from a severe systemic infection or the effects of toxins, drugs, or alcohol. Confusion may signal the worsening of an underlying and perhaps irreversible disease.

Assessment

When you take his history, ask the patient to describe what's bothering him. He may not report confusion as his chief complaint, but may say he suffers from memory loss, persistent apprehension, or the inability to concentrate. He may be unable to respond logically to direct questions. Check with a family member or friend about its onset and frequency. Find out if the patient has a history of head trauma or a cardiopulmonary, metabolic, cerebrovascular, or neurologic disorder. Obtain a complete medication history, including over-the-counter medications and herbal remedies. Ask about changes in eating or sleeping habits and drug or alcohol use.

Perform an assessment to determine the presence of systemic disorders. Check the patient's vital signs, and assess him for changes in blood pressure, temperature, and pulse. Next, perform a neurologic assessment to establish the patient's level of consciousness.

Causes

♦ *Brain tumor.* In the early stages of a brain tumor, confusion is usually mild and difficult to detect. As the tumor impinges on cerebral structures, however, confusion worsens and the patient may exhibit personality changes, bizarre behavior, sensory and motor deficits, visual field deficits, and aphasia.

◆ *Cerebrovascular disorders.* Cerebrovascular disorders produce confusion due to tissue hypoxia and ischemia. Confusion may be insidious and fleeting, as in a transient ischemic attack, or acute and permanent, as in a stroke.

◆ *Decreased cerebral perfusion.* Mild confusion is an early symptom of decreased cerebral perfusion. Associated findings usually include hypotension, tachycardia or bradycardia, an irregular pulse, edema, and cyanosis.

◆ *Drugs.* Large doses of central nervous system (CNS) depressants produce confusion that can persist for several days after the drug is discontinued. Opioid and barbiturate withdrawal also cause acute confusion, possibly with delirium. Other drugs that commonly cause confusion include lidocaine (LidoPen), indomethacin (Indocin), cycloserine (Seromycin), chloroquine (Aralen), atropine (AtroPen), and cimetidine (Tagamet). Herbal remedies, such as St. John's wort, can cause confusion, especially when taken in conjunction with an antidepressant or other serotonergic drug.

◆ *Fluid and electrolyte imbalance.* The extent of imbalance determines the severity of the patient's confusion. Typically, he'll show signs of dehydration, such as lassitude, poor skin turgor, dry skin and mucous membranes, and oliguria. He may also develop hypotension and a low-grade fever.

◆ *Head trauma.* Concussion, contusion, and brain hemorrhage may produce confusion at the time of injury, shortly afterward, or months or even years afterward. The patient may be delirious, with periodic loss of consciousness. Vomiting, a severe headache, pupillary changes, and sensory and motor deficits are also common.

◆ *Heatstroke.* Heatstroke causes pronounced confusion that gradually worsens as the patient's body temperature rises. Initially, he may be irritable and dizzy; later, he may become delirious, have seizures, and lose consciousness.

◆ *Hypothermia.* Confusion may be an early sign of hypothermia. Typically, the patient displays slurred speech, cold and pale skin, hyperactive deep tendon reflexes, a rapid pulse, and decreased blood pressure and respirations. As his body temperature continues to drop, his confusion progresses to stupor and coma, his muscles become rigid, and his respiratory rate decreases.

◆ *Hypoxemia.* Acute pulmonary disorders that result in hypoxemia produce confusion that can range from mild disorientation to delirium. Chronic pulmonary disorders produce persistent confusion.

◆ *Infection.* Severe generalized infection, such as sepsis, typically produces delirium. CNS infections, such as meningitis, cause varying degrees of confusion along with a headache and nuchal rigidity.

◆ *Metabolic encephalopathy.* Hyperglycemia and hypoglycemia can produce sudden confusion. A patient with hypoglycemia may also experience transient delirium and seizures. Uremic and hepatic encephalopathies produce gradual confusion that may progress to seizures and coma. Usually, the patient also experiences tremors and restlessness.

◆ *Nutritional deficiencies.* Inadequate dietary intake of thiamine, niacin, or vitamin B_{12} produces insidious, progressive confusion and possible mental deterioration.

◆ *Seizure disorders.* Mild to moderate confusion may immediately follow any type of seizure. The confusion usually disappears within several hours.

Constipation

Constipation is defined as small, infrequent, or difficult bowel movements. Because normal bowel movements can vary in frequency and from individual to individual, constipation is relative and must be determined in relation to the patient's normal elimination pattern. Untreated, constipation can affect the patient's health, lifestyle, and well-being.

Because the autonomic nervous system controls bowel movements—by sensing rectal distention from fecal contents and by stimulating the external sphincter—any factor that influences this system may cause bowel dysfunction. Acute constipation usually has a physiological cause, such as an anal or a rectal disorder. Chronic constipation typically has a functional cause and may be related to stress. (See *How habits and stress cause constipation,* page 182.)

Assessment

Ask the patient to describe the frequency of his bowel movements and the size and consistency of his stools. How long has he had constipation? Does the patient have pain related to constipation? If so, when did he first notice the pain, and where is it located? Ask the patient if defecation worsens or helps to relieve the pain. Ask the patient to describe a typical day's diet; estimate his daily fiber and fluid intake. Ask him about changes in eating habits, medication or alcohol use, or physical activity. Has he experienced recent emotional distress or job stress? Find out whether the patient has a history of GI, rectoanal, neurologic, or metabolic disorders; abdominal surgery; or radiation therapy. Then ask about the medications that he's taking, including over-the-counter preparations.

Inspect the abdomen for distention or scars from previous surgery. Then auscultate for bowel sounds, percuss all four quadrants, and gently palpate for abdominal tenderness, a palpable mass, and hepatomegaly. Next, expose the anus and inspect for inflammation, lesions, scars, fissures, and external hemorrhoids. Palpate the anal sphincter for laxity or stricture. Use caution in a patient with a cardiac history. Finally, obtain a stool sample and test it for occult blood.

Causes

◆ *Anal fissure.* A crack or laceration in the lining of the anal wall can cause acute constipation, usually due to the patient's fear of the severe tearing or burning pain associated with bowel movements.
◆ *Anorectal abscess.* In anorectal abscess, constipation occurs together with severe, throbbing, localized pain and tenderness at the abscess site. The patient may also have localized inflammation, swelling, and purulent drainage.
◆ *Cirrhosis.* In the early stages of cirrhosis, the patient experiences constipation along with nausea and vomiting and a dull pain in the right upper quadrant. He may also have indigestion, anorexia, fatigue, malaise, and flatulence.
◆ *Diabetic neuropathy.* Diabetic neuropathy produces episodic constipation or diarrhea. Other signs and symptoms include dysphagia, orthostatic hypotension, syncope, and painless bladder distention with overflow incontinence.

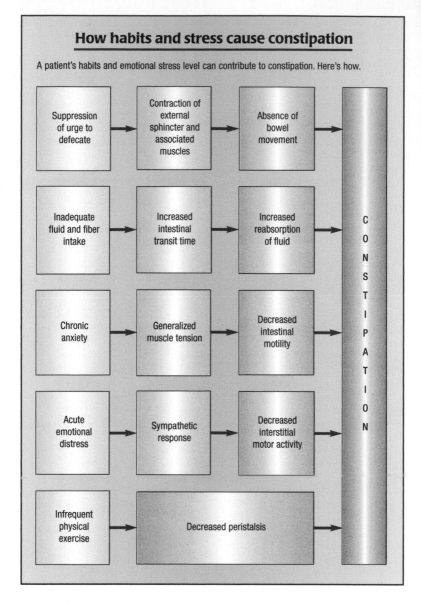

How habits and stress cause constipation

A patient's habits and emotional stress level can contribute to constipation. Here's how.

			C
Suppression of urge to defecate	→ Contraction of external sphincter and associated muscles	→ Absence of bowel movement	→
Inadequate fluid and fiber intake	→ Increased intestinal transit time	→ Increased reabsorption of fluid	→
Chronic anxiety	→ Generalized muscle tension	→ Decreased intestinal motility	→
Acute emotional distress	→ Sympathetic response	→ Decreased interstitial motor activity	→
Infrequent physical exercise	→ Decreased peristalsis		→

C O N S T I P A T I O N

◆ *Diverticulitis.* In diverticulitis, constipation or diarrhea occurs with left lower quadrant pain and tenderness. The patient may develop mild nausea, flatulence, or a low-grade fever.

◆ *Drugs.* Patients commonly experience constipation when taking an opioid analgesic or other drugs, including vinca alkaloids, calcium channel blockers, antacids containing aluminum or calcium, and drugs with anticholinergic effects. Constipation may also be caused by the excessive use of laxatives or enemas.

◆ *Hemorrhoids.* Thrombosed hemorrhoids cause constipation as the patient tries to avoid the pain of defecation.

◆ *Hepatic porphyria.* Abdominal pain precedes constipation in hepatic porphyria. The patient may also have fever, tachycardia, hypertension, diaphoresis, vomiting, photophobia, urine retention and, possibly, visual hallucinations.

◆ *Hypercalcemia.* With hypercalcemia, constipation usually occurs along with anorexia, nausea, vomiting, polyuria, and polydipsia. The patient may also display arrhythmias, bone pain, and personality changes.

◆ *Hypothyroidism.* Constipation occurs early and insidiously in patients with hypothyroidism in addition to fatigue, sensitivity to cold, anorexia with weight gain, menorrhagia in women, decreased memory, and muscle cramps.

◆ *Intestinal obstruction.* Constipation associated with an intestinal obstruction varies in severity and onset, depending on the location and extent of the obstruction. With partial obstruction, constipation may alternate with leakage of liquid stools. With complete obstruction, obstipation may occur.

◆ *Irritable bowel syndrome (IBS).* IBS commonly produces chronic constipation, although some patients have diarrhea and others complain of alternating constipation and diarrhea. Stress may trigger nausea and abdominal distention, which are usually relieved by defecation. Typically, stools are scybalous (a hard, round, thickened mass) and contain visible mucus.

◼ *Mesenteric artery ischemia.* Mesenteric artery ischemia is a life-threatening disorder that produces sudden constipation with failure to expel stool or flatus. Initially, the abdomen is soft and nontender, but soon severe abdominal pain, tenderness, vomiting, and anorexia occur.

◆ *Spinal cord lesion.* Constipation may occur with a spinal cord lesion in addition to urine retention, sexual dysfunction, pain and, possibly, motor weakness, paralysis, or sensory impairment below the level of the lesion.

Corneal reflex, absent

The corneal reflex is tested by drawing a fine-pointed wisp of sterile cotton from a corner of each eye to the cornea. Normally, even though only one eye is tested at a time, the patient blinks bilaterally each time either cornea is touched—this is the corneal reflex. When this reflex is absent, neither eyelid closes when the cornea of one is touched. It usually signifies damage to the trigeminal or facial nerve. (See *Eliciting the corneal reflex,* page 184.)

Assessment

If you can't elicit the corneal reflex, look for other signs of trigeminal nerve dysfunction. To test the three sensory portions of the nerve, touch each side of the patient's face on the brow, cheek, and jaw with a cotton wisp, and ask him to compare the sensations.

If you suspect facial nerve involvement, note if the upper face (brow and eyes) and lower face (cheek, mouth, and chin) are weak bilaterally. An absent corneal reflex may signify a progressive neurologic disorder, so ask the patient about associated symptoms—facial pain, dysphagia, and limb weakness.

Eliciting the corneal reflex

To elicit the corneal reflex, have the patient turn her eyes away from you to avoid involuntary blinking during the procedure. Then approach the patient from the opposite side, out of her line of vision, and brush the cornea lightly with a fine wisp of sterile cotton. Repeat the procedure on the other eye.

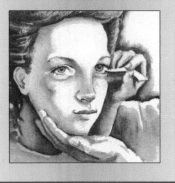

Causes

◆ *Acoustic neuroma.* Acoustic neuroma affects the trigeminal nerve, causing a diminished or absent corneal reflex, tinnitus, and unilateral hearing impairment. Facial palsy and anesthesia, palate weakness, and signs of cerebellar dysfunction may result if the tumor impinges on the adjacent cranial nerves, brain stem, and cerebellum.

◆ *Bell's palsy.* A common cause of diminished or absent corneal reflex, Bell's palsy causes paralysis of the facial nerve. It can also produce complete hemifacial weakness or paralysis and drooling on the affected side, which also sags and appears masklike. The eye on this side can't be shut and tears constantly.

◆ *Brain stem infarction or injury.* An absent corneal reflex can occur on the side opposite a lesion when infarction or injury affects the trigeminal or facial nerve or their connection in the central trigeminal tract. Other findings include a decreased level of consciousness, dysphagia, dysarthria, contralateral limb weakness, headache, and vomiting.

◆ *Guillain-Barré syndrome.* With this polyneuropathic disorder, a diminished or absent corneal reflex accompanies ipsilateral loss of facial muscle control. Muscle weakness occurs, which typically starts in the legs, and then extends to the arms and facial nerves within 72 hours. Other findings include dysarthria, dysphagia, paresthesia, respiratory muscle paralysis, respiratory insufficiency, orthostatic hypotension, incontinence, diaphoresis, and tachycardia.

Costovertebral angle tenderness

Costovertebral angle (CVA) tenderness indicates sudden distention of the renal capsule. It almost always accompanies dull, constant flank pain in the CVA just lateral to the sacrospinalis muscle and below the 12th rib. This associated pain typically travels anteriorly in the subcostal region toward the umbilicus.

Percussing the CVA elicits tenderness, if present. (See *Eliciting CVA tenderness.*) A patient who doesn't have this symptom will perceive a thudding, jarring, or pressurelike sensation when tested, but no pain.

Assessment

After detecting CVA tenderness, determine the possible extent of renal damage. First, find out if the patient has other symptoms of renal or urologic dysfunction. Ask about voiding habits:

Eliciting CVA tenderness

To elicit costovertebral angle (CVA) tenderness, have the patient sit upright facing away from you or have him lie in a prone position. Place the palm of your left hand over the left CVA, and then strike the back of your left hand with the ulnar surface of your right fist (as shown). Repeat this percussion technique over the right CVA. A patient with CVA tenderness will experience intense pain.

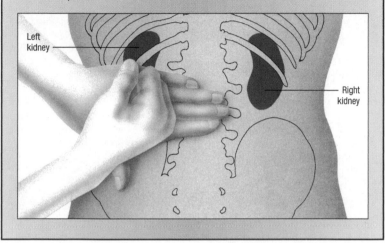

Left kidney

Right kidney

How frequently does he urinate, and in what amounts? Has he noticed a change in urine output? Ask about fluid intake before judging his output as abnormal. Does he have nocturia? Ask about pain or burning during urination or difficulty starting a stream. Does the patient strain to urinate without being able to do so? Ask about urine color; brown or bright red urine may contain blood.

Explore other signs and symptoms. For example, if the patient is experiencing pain in his flank, abdomen, or back, when did he first notice the pain? How severe is it, and where is it located? Find out if the patient has a history of urinary tract infections, congenital anomalies, calculi, or other obstructive nephropathies or uropathies. Also, ask about a history of renovascular disorders such as occlusion of the renal arteries or veins.

Perform a brief physical examination. Begin by taking the patient's vital signs. A fever and chills in a patient with CVA tenderness may indicate acute pyelonephritis. If the patient has hypertension and bradycardia, stay alert for other autonomic effects of renal pain, such as diaphoresis and pallor. Inspect, auscultate, and gently palpate the abdomen for clues to the underlying cause of CVA tenderness. Stay alert for abdominal distention, hypoactive bowel sounds, and palpable masses.

Causes

◆ *Calculi.* Infundibular and ureteropelvic or ureteral calculi produce CVA tenderness and waves of waxing and waning flank pain that may radiate to the groin, testicles, suprapubic area, or labia. The patient may also develop nausea, vomiting, severe abdominal pain, abdominal distention, and decreased bowel sounds.

◆ *Perirenal abscess.* Causing CVA tenderness, perirenal abscess may also produce severe unilateral flank pain, dysuria, a persistent high fever, chills, erythema of the skin and, sometimes, a palpable abdominal mass.

◆ *Pyelonephritis (acute).* Perhaps the most common cause of CVA tenderness, acute pyelonephritis is commonly accompanied by a persistent high fever, chills, flank pain, anorexia, nausea and vomiting, weakness, dysuria, hematuria, nocturia, urinary urgency and frequency, and tenesmus.

◆ *Renal artery occlusion.* With renal artery occlusion, the patient experiences flank pain as well as CVA tenderness. Other findings include nausea, vomiting, decreased bowel sounds, a high fever, and severe, continuous upper abdominal pain.

◆ *Renal vein occlusion.* The patient with renal vein occlusion has CVA tenderness and flank pain. He may also have fever, oliguria, edema, hematuria, and severe, continuous upper abdominal pain.

Cough, barking

Resonant, brassy, and harsh, a barking cough is part of a complex of signs and symptoms that occur with croup syndrome, a group of pediatric disorders marked by some degree of respiratory distress. A barking cough indicates edema of the larynx and surrounding tissue, which can rapidly lead to airway occlusion—a life-threatening emergency.

Assessment

Ask the child's parents when the barking cough began and what other signs and symptoms accompanied it. Has he had previous episodes of croup syndrome? Did his condition improve upon exposure to cold air? Quickly assess the child's respiratory status, and then take his vital signs. Stay alert for tachycardia, signs of hypoxemia, and a decreased level of consciousness. Find out if the child may have aspirated a small object. Observe the child for retractions, nasal flaring, and shallow respirations. Observe the child's body position, activity level, and facial expressions. Is he lethargic and difficult to arouse? If the child shows signs of severe respiratory distress, prepare for possible endotracheal intubation or tracheotomy.

Causes

◾ *Aspiration of foreign body.* Partial obstruction of the upper airway first produces sudden hoarseness and then a barking cough and inspiratory stridor. Other signs include gagging, tachycardia, dyspnea, decreased breath sounds, wheezing and, possibly, cyanosis.

◾ *Epiglottitis.* A medical emergency, epiglottitis occurs nocturnally, heralded by a barking cough and a high fever. The child is hoarse, dysphagic, dyspneic, and restless and appears extremely ill and panicky. The cough may progress to severe respiratory distress with sternal and intercostal retractions, nasal flaring, cyanosis, and tachycardia. The child will struggle to get sufficient air as epiglottic edema increases.

◆ *Laryngotracheobronchitis (acute).* Also known as *viral croup,* laryngotracheobronchitis is most common in children 9 to 18 months and usually occurs in the fall and early winter. It initially produces a fever, runny nose, poor appetite, and infrequent cough. When the infection descends into the laryngotracheal area, a barking cough, hoarseness, and inspiratory stridor occur. Sleeping in a dry room worsens these signs.

◆ *Spasmodic croup.* Acute spasmodic croup usually occurs during sleep with the abrupt onset of a barking cough that awakens the child. Typically, he doesn't have a fever, but may be hoarse, restless, and dyspneic. The signs usually subside within a few hours, but attacks tend to recur.

Cough, nonproductive

A nonproductive cough is a noisy, forceful expulsion of air from the lungs that doesn't yield sputum or blood. Coughing is a necessary protective mechanism that clears airway passages. However, a nonproductive cough is ineffective and can cause damage, such as airway collapse or rupture of alveoli or blebs. A nonproductive cough that later becomes productive is a classic sign of progressive respiratory disease. An acute cough has a sudden onset and may be self-limiting. A cough that persists beyond 1 month is considered chronic.

The cough reflex generally occurs when mechanical, chemical, thermal, inflammatory, or psychogenic stimuli activate cough receptors. (See *Reviewing the cough mechanism,* page 188.) However, external pressure and certain drugs, such as angiotensin-converting enzyme inhibitors, may also cause a nonproductive cough.

Assessment

Ask the patient when his cough began and whether body position, the time of day, or a specific activity affects it.

How does the cough sound? Next, ask about the frequency and intensity of the coughing. If he has pain associated with coughing, breathing, or activity, when did it begin? Where is it located? Ask the patient about recent illness, surgery, or trauma. Also ask about exposure or hypersensitivity to drugs, foods, pets, dust, irritating fumes, chemicals, smoke, or pollen. Find out which medications the patient takes, and ask about recent changes in dosages. As you're taking his history, observe the patient's general appearance and manner.

Next, perform a physical examination. Start by taking the patient's vital signs. Check the depth and rhythm of his respirations, and note if wheezing or "crowing" noises occur with breathing. Check his nose and mouth for congestion, inflammation, drainage, or signs of infection. Inspect his neck for distended jugular veins and tracheal deviation, and palpate for masses or enlarged lymph nodes. Examine his chest, observing its configuration and looking for abnormal chest wall motion. Percuss for dullness, tympany, or flatness. Auscultate for wheezing, crackles, rhonchi, pleural friction rubs, and decreased or absent breath sounds. Finally, examine his abdomen for distention, tenderness, masses, or abnormal bowel sounds.

Causes

◩ *Airway occlusion.* Partial occlusion of the upper airway produces a sudden onset of dry, paroxysmal coughing. The patient is gagging, wheezing, and hoarse, with stridor, tachycardia, and decreased breath sounds.

◩ *Aortic aneurysm (thoracic).* Aortic aneurysm causes a brassy cough with dyspnea, hoarseness, wheezing, and a substernal ache in the shoulders, lower back, or abdomen. The patient may

Reviewing the cough mechanism

Cough receptors are thought to be located in the nose, sinuses, auditory canals, nasopharynx, larynx, trachea, bronchi, pleurae, diaphragm and, possibly, the pericardium and GI tract. When a cough receptor is stimulated, the vagus and glossopharyngeal nerves transmit the impulse to the "cough center" in the medulla. From there, the impulse is transmitted to the larynx and to the inter-costal and abdominal muscles. Deep inspiration (1) is followed by closure of the glottis (2), relaxation of the diaphragm, and contraction of the abdominal and intercostal muscles. The resulting increased pressure in the lungs opens the glottis to release the forceful, noisy expiration known as a cough (3).

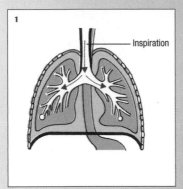

1

Inspiration

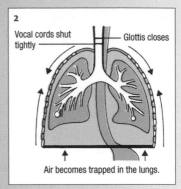

2

Vocal cords shut tightly

Glottis closes

Air becomes trapped in the lungs.

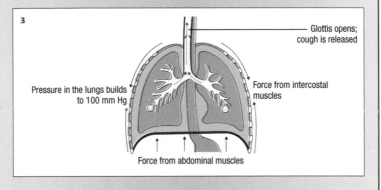

3

Glottis opens; cough is released

Pressure in the lungs builds to 100 mm Hg

Force from intercostal muscles

Force from abdominal muscles

also have facial or neck edema, jugular vein distention, dysphagia, prominent veins over his chest, stridor and, possibly, paresthesia or neuralgia.

◆ *Asthma.* Asthma attacks typically occur at night, starting with a nonpro-ductive cough and mild wheezing, which progresses to severe dyspnea, audible wheezing, chest tightness, and a cough that produces thick mucus.

◆ *Atelectasis.* As lung tissue deflates with atelectasis, it stimulates cough receptors, causing a nonproductive cough. The patient may also have pleuritic chest pain, anxiety, dyspnea, tachypnea, tachycardia, and tracheal deviation.

◆ *Bronchitis (chronic).* Bronchitis starts with a nonproductive, hacking cough that later becomes productive. Other findings include prolonged expiration, wheezing, dyspnea, barrel chest, cyanosis, tachypnea, crackles, and rhonchi.

◆ *Bronchogenic carcinoma.* The earliest indicators of bronchogenic carcinoma may be dyspnea, vague chest pain, and a chronic, nonproductive cough. The patient may also be wheezing.

◆ *Common cold.* The common cold generally starts with a nonproductive, hacking cough and progresses to a mix of sneezing, headaches, malaise, fatigue, rhinorrhea, myalgia, arthralgia, nasal congestion, and sore throat.

◆ *Esophageal achalasia.* In esophageal achalasia, regurgitation and aspiration produce a dry cough. The patient may also have recurrent pulmonary infections and dysphagia.

◆ *Esophageal diverticula.* Esophageal diverticula cause a nocturnal nonproductive cough, dyspepsia, regurgitation and aspiration, and dysphagia. The patient may also exhibit a swollen neck and gurgling sounds, halitosis, and weight loss.

◆ *Esophageal occlusion.* Esophageal occlusion is marked by immediate nonproductive coughing and gagging, with a sensation of something stuck in the throat. Other findings include neck or chest pain and the inability to swallow.

◆ *Hantavirus pulmonary syndrome.* Hantavirus pulmonary syndrome is a disease transmitted by infected rodents through urine, droppings, or saliva. Humans can become infected by inhaling particles infected with the virus. It causes a nonproductive cough as well as noncardiogenic pulmonary edema.

Other findings include headache, myalgia, fever, nausea, and vomiting.

◆ *Hypersensitivity pneumonitis.* With hypersensitivity pneumonitis, an acute nonproductive cough, fever, dyspnea, and malaise usually occur 5 to 6 hours after exposure to an antigen.

◆ *Interstitial lung disease.* A patient with interstitial lung disease has a nonproductive cough and progressive dyspnea. He may also be cyanotic and have clubbing, fine crackles, fatigue, variable chest pain, and weight loss.

◆ *Laryngeal tumor.* A mild, nonproductive cough is an early sign of a laryngeal tumor in addition to minor throat discomfort and hoarseness. Later, dysphagia, dyspnea, cervical lymphadenopathy, stridor, and an earache may occur.

◆ *Laryngitis.* In its acute form, laryngitis causes a nonproductive cough with localized pain as well as fever and malaise. Hoarseness can range from mild to complete loss of voice.

◆ *Lung abscess.* Lung abscess typically begins with a nonproductive cough, weakness, dyspnea, and pleuritic chest pain. The patient may also exhibit diaphoresis, fever, headache, malaise, fatigue, anorexia, and weight loss.

◆ *Pleural effusion.* A nonproductive cough along with dyspnea, pleuritic chest pain, and decreased chest motion are characteristic of pleural effusion.

◆ *Pneumonia.* Bacterial pneumonia usually starts with a nonproductive, hacking, painful cough that rapidly becomes productive. Other findings include chills, fever, dyspnea, chest pain, grunting respirations, and nasal flaring.

With mycoplasma pneumonia, a nonproductive cough arises 2 to 3 days after the onset of malaise, headache, and sore throat. The cough may be paroxysmal, causing substernal chest pain.

Viral pneumonia causes a nonproductive, hacking cough and the onset of malaise, headache, and a low-grade fever.

◪ *Pneumothorax.* Pneumothorax causes a dry cough and signs of respiratory distress, such as dyspnea, tachycardia, tachypnea, restlessness, and cyanosis. The patient experiences sudden, sharp chest pain that worsens with chest movement.

◪ *Pulmonary edema.* Pulmonary edema initially causes a dry cough, exertional and paroxysmal nocturnal dyspnea, orthopnea, tachycardia, tachypnea, dependent crackles, and a ventricular gallop. If pulmonary edema is severe, the coughing produces frothy, bloody sputum.

◪ *Pulmonary embolism.* A pulmonary embolism may produce a dry cough along with dyspnea and chest pain. Typically, however, the cough produces blood-tinged sputum. Tachycardia and a low-grade fever are also common.

◆ *Sarcoidosis.* With sarcoidosis, dyspnea, substernal pain, and malaise accompany a nonproductive cough. The patient may also develop tachypnea, lymphadenopathy, skin lesions, visual impairment, and difficulty swallowing.

◪ *Severe acute respiratory syndrome (SARS).* SARS is an acute infectious disease that generally begins with a fever. Other symptoms include headache; malaise; a dry, nonproductive cough; and dyspnea.

◆ *Tracheobronchitis (acute).* Initially, tracheobronchitis produces a dry cough, which follows the onset of chills, sore throat, fever, muscle and back pain, and substernal tightness.

Cough, productive

Productive coughing is the body's mechanism for clearing airway passages of accumulated secretions that normal mucociliary action doesn't remove. It's a sudden, forceful, noisy expulsion of air from the lungs that contains sputum, blood, or both. The sputum's color, consistency, and odor provide important clues about the patient's condition. A productive cough can occur as a single cough or as paroxysmal coughing, and it can be voluntarily induced, although it's usually a reflexive response to stimulation of the airway mucosa.

Productive coughing commonly results from an acute or chronic infection that causes inflammation, edema, and increased mucus production in the airways. However, it can also result from the inhalation of antigenic or irritating substances or foreign bodies. The most common cause of chronic productive coughing is cigarette smoking.

Assessment

Assess the patient before you take his history because a patient with a productive cough can develop acute respiratory distress from thick or excessive secretions, bronchospasm, or fatigue. Take his vital signs and check the rate, depth, and rhythm of respirations. Stay alert for nasal flaring and cyanosis. (See *Responding to respiratory distress.*)

When the patient's condition permits, ask when the cough began, and find out how much sputum he's coughing up each day. At what time of day does he cough up the most sputum? Ask him if he has noticed an increase in sputum production since his coughing began. Also ask about the color, odor, and consistency of the sputum. Blood-tinged or rust-colored sputum may result from trauma due to coughing or from an underlying condition. Foul-smelling sputum may result from an infection.

How does the cough sound? A hacking cough results from laryngeal involvement, whereas a "brassy" cough indicates major airway involve-

EMERGENCY INTERVENTIONS

Responding to respiratory distress

If your patient with a productive cough develops respiratory distress, you must act quickly:
◆ Keep his airway patent.
◆ Be prepared to administer supplemental oxygen if he becomes restless or confused or if his respirations become shallow, irregular, rapid, or slow.
◆ Elevate the head of the bed at least 30 degrees.
◆ Listen for stridor, wheezing, choking, or gurgling.
◆ Clear excess mucus with tracheal suctioning, if necessary.
◆ Prepare for endotracheal intubation and mechanical ventilation if respiratory distress worsens.

ment. Does the patient feel pain associated with his productive cough? If so, ask about its location and severity and whether it radiates to other areas.

Next, ask the patient about his cigarette, drug, and alcohol use and whether his weight or appetite has changed. Find out if he has a history of asthma, allergies, or respiratory disorders, and ask about recent illnesses, surgery, or trauma. What medications is he taking? Does he work around chemicals or respiratory irritants such as silicone?

Examine the patient's mouth and nose for congestion, drainage, or inflammation. Note his breath odor; halitosis can be a sign of pulmonary infection. Inspect his neck for distended veins, and palpate for tenderness and masses or enlarged lymph nodes. Observe his chest for accessory muscle use, retractions, and uneven chest expansion, and percuss for dullness, tympany, or flatness. Finally, auscultate for a pleural friction rub and abnormal breath sounds—rhonchi, crackles, or wheezes.

Causes

◆ *Actinomycosis.* Actinomycosis, an infectious disease caused by *Actinomyces israelii,* begins with a cough that produces purulent sputum. Fever, weight loss, fatigue, weakness, dyspnea, night sweats, pleuritic chest pain, and hemoptysis may also occur.
◆ *Aspiration pneumonitis.* Aspiration pneumonitis causes coughing that produces pink, frothy and, possibly, purulent sputum. The patient also has marked dyspnea, fever, tachypnea, tachycardia, wheezing, and cyanosis.
◆ *Bronchiectasis.* The chronic cough of bronchiectasis produces copious, mucopurulent sputum that has characteristic layering (top, frothy; middle, clear; bottom, dense with purulent particles). The patient has halitosis and his sputum may smell foul or sickeningly sweet.
◆ *Bronchitis (chronic).* The cough with bronchitis is initially nonproductive. Eventually, it produces mucoid sputum that becomes purulent. Secondary infection can also cause mucopurulent sputum, which may become blood-tinged and foul-smelling. The coughing usually occurs when the

patient is recumbent or rises from sleep.

◆ *Chemical pneumonitis.* Chemical pneumonitis causes a cough with purulent sputum. It can also cause dyspnea, wheezing, orthopnea, fever, malaise, and crackles; mucous membrane irritation of the conjunctivae, throat, and nose; laryngitis; or rhinitis.

◆ *Common cold.* When the common cold causes productive coughing, the sputum is mucoid or mucopurulent. Early indications include sneezing, headache, malaise, fatigue, rhinorrhea, nasal congestion, sore throat, and myalgia.

◆ *Lung abscess (ruptured).* The cardinal sign of a ruptured lung abscess is coughing that produces copious amounts of purulent, foul-smelling, and possibly blood-tinged sputum. It can also cause diaphoresis, anorexia, weakness, fatigue, fever with chills, dyspnea, malaise, pleuritic chest pain, halitosis, and inspiratory crackles.

◆ *Lung cancer.* One of the earliest signs of bronchogenic carcinoma is a chronic cough that produces small amounts of purulent (or mucopurulent), blood-streaked sputum. In a patient with bronchoalveolar cancer, however, coughing produces large amounts of frothy sputum.

◆ *Nocardiosis.* Nocardiosis is an acute or chronic infection of the lungs that may spread to any organ (particularly the brain), causing abscess formation. The infection results in a productive cough with purulent, thick, tenacious sputum and fever that may last several months. Other findings include night sweats, pleuritic pain, anorexia, malaise, fatigue, and weight loss.

◆ *North American blastomycosis.* North American blastomycosis produces coughing that's dry and hacking or produces bloody or purulent sputum. Other findings include pleuritic chest pain, fever, chills, anorexia, weight loss, malaise, fatigue, night sweats, cutaneous lesions (small, painless, nonpruritic macules or papules), and prostration.

◆ *Plague* (Yersinia pestis). Clinical forms of plague include bubonic, septicemic, and pneumonic. Signs and symptoms of the bubonic form include fever, chills, and swollen, inflamed, and tender lymph nodes near the site of a flea bite. Septicemic plague develops as a fulminant illness, generally with the bubonic form. The pneumonic form may be contracted via the respiratory system. Pulmonary signs and symptoms include a productive cough, chest pain, tachypnea, dyspnea, hemoptysis, increasing respiratory distress, and cardiopulmonary insufficiency.

◆ *Pneumonia.* Bacterial pneumonia usually starts with a nonproductive, hacking, painful cough that rapidly becomes productive. Other findings include chills, fever, dyspnea, chest pain, grunting respirations, and nasal flaring. The cough with mycoplasma pneumonia may produce scant blood-flecked sputum but it's usually nonproductive.

◆ *Psittacosis.* As psittacosis progresses, the characteristic hacking cough, nonproductive at first, may later produce a small amount of mucoid, blood-streaked sputum. The infection may begin abruptly, with chills, fever, headache, myalgia, and prostration.

◆ *Pulmonary coccidioidomycosis.* Pulmonary coccidioidomycosis causes a nonproductive or slightly productive cough with fever, pleuritic chest pain, sore throat, headache, backache, malaise, marked weakness, anorexia, hemoptysis, and an itchy macular rash.

◆ *Pulmonary edema.* When severe, pulmonary edema causes a cough that produces frothy, bloody sputum. Early signs and symptoms include an initially dry cough, exertional and paroxysmal nocturnal dyspnea, orthopnea, tachycardia, tachypnea, dependent crackles, and a ventricular gallop.

◗ *Pulmonary embolism.* The cough with pulmonary embolism typically produces blood-tinged sputum. Other common signs and symptoms include dyspnea, chest pain, tachycardia, diaphoresis, restlessness, and a low-grade fever.

◆ *Pulmonary tuberculosis (TB).* Pulmonary TB causes a mild to severe productive cough along with a combination of hemoptysis, malaise, dyspnea, and pleuritic chest pain. Sputum may be scant and mucoid or copious and purulent.

◆ *Silicosis.* A productive cough with mucopurulent sputum is the earliest sign of silicosis. The patient also has exertional dyspnea, tachypnea, weight loss, fatigue, general weakness, and recurrent respiratory infections.

◆ *Tracheobronchitis.* With tracheobronchitis, inflammation initially causes a nonproductive cough. Later, it becomes productive as secretions increase. The sputum is mucoid, mucopurulent, or purulent.

Crackles

A common finding in patients with certain cardiovascular and pulmonary disorders, crackles are nonmusical popping or rattling noises heard during auscultation of breath sounds. They usually occur during inspiration and can be unilateral or bilateral, moist or dry. They're characterized by their pitch, loudness, location, persistence, and occurrence during the respiratory cycle. Crackles indicate abnormal movement of air through fluid-filled airways. They can be irregularly dispersed, as in pneumonia, or localized, as in bronchiectasis. Usually, crackles indicate the degree of an underlying illness. (See *How crackles occur,* page 194.)

Assessment

If the patient has a cough, ask when it began and if it's constant or intermittent. If the cough is productive, determine the sputum's consistency, amount, odor, and color. Ask the patient if he has pain. If so, where and does it radiate to other areas? Also ask what worsens or helps to relieve his pain. Is the patient lying still or moving about restlessly?

Obtain a brief medical history. Does the patient have cancer or a respiratory or cardiovascular problem? Ask about recent surgery, trauma, illness, and exposure to irritants, such as vapors, fumes, or smoke. Is he experiencing hoarseness or difficulty swallowing? Find out which medications he's taking. Also ask about recent weight loss, anorexia, nausea, vomiting, fatigue, weakness, vertigo, and syncope.

Next, perform a physical examination. Examine the patient's nose and mouth for signs of infection, such as inflammation or increased secretions. Note his breath odor; halitosis could indicate pulmonary infection. Check his neck for abnormalities. Inspect the patient's chest for uneven expansion. Percuss for dullness, tympany, or flatness, auscultate his lungs, and listen to his heart. Check his hands and feet for edema or clubbing.

Causes

◗ *Acute respiratory distress syndrome (ARDS).* ARDS causes diffuse, fine to coarse crackles usually heard in the dependent portions of the lungs. It produces cyanosis, nasal flaring, tachypnea, and grunting respirations.

◆ *Bronchiectasis.* With bronchiectasis, persistent, coarse crackles are heard over the affected area of the lung. They're accompanied by a chronic

How crackles occur

Crackles occur when air passes through fluid-filled airways, causing collapsed alveoli to pop open as the airway pressure equalizes. They can also occur when membranes lining the chest cavity and the lungs become inflamed. The illustrations below show a normal alveolus and two pathologic alveolar changes that cause crackles.

NORMAL ALVEOLUS

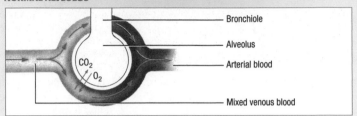

- Bronchiole
- Alveolus
- Arterial blood
- Mixed venous blood

ALVEOLUS IN PULMONARY EDEMA

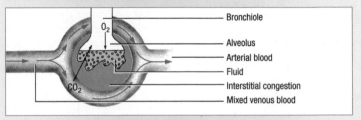

- Bronchiole
- Alveolus
- Arterial blood
- Fluid
- Interstitial congestion
- Mixed venous blood

ALVEOLUS IN INFLAMMATION

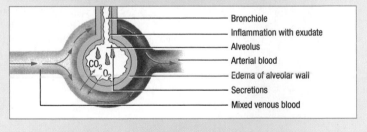

- Bronchiole
- Inflammation with exudate
- Alveolus
- Arterial blood
- Edema of alveolar wall
- Secretions
- Mixed venous blood

cough that produces copious amounts of mucopurulent sputum.

◆ *Bronchitis (chronic)*. Bronchitis causes coarse crackles that are usually heard at the lung bases. Prolonged expirations, wheezing, rhonchi, exertional dyspnea, tachypnea, and a persistent, productive cough also occur.

◈ *Legionnaires' disease*. Legionnaires' disease produces diffuse, moist crackles and a cough that produces scant mucoid, nonpurulent and, possibly, blood-streaked sputum.

◆ *Pneumonia.* Bacterial pneumonia produces diffuse fine crackles, high fever, tachypnea, pleuritic chest pain, cyanosis, grunting respirations, and nasal flaring. Mycoplasma pneumonia produces medium to fine crackles, a nonproductive cough, malaise, sore throat, headache, and fever. The patient may have blood-flecked sputum. Viral pneumonia causes gradually developing, diffuse crackles. The patient may also have a nonproductive cough.

◪ *Pulmonary edema.* Moist, bubbling crackles on inspiration are one of the first signs of pulmonary edema. Other early findings include exertional and paroxysmal nocturnal dyspnea and coughing, which may be initially nonproductive but later produces frothy, bloody sputum.

◪ *Pulmonary embolism.* A pulmonary embolism may cause fine to coarse crackles and a cough that may be dry or that may produce blood-tinged sputum. Usually, the first sign of pulmonary embolism is severe dyspnea, which may be accompanied by angina or pleuritic chest pain.

◆ *Pulmonary tuberculosis (TB).* With pulmonary TB, fine crackles occur after coughing. The patient has a combination of hemoptysis, malaise, dyspnea, and pleuritic chest pain. Sputum may be scant and mucoid or copious and purulent.

◆ *Tracheobronchitis.* In its acute form, tracheobronchitis produces moist or coarse crackles along with a productive cough, chills, sore throat, fever, muscle and back pain, and substernal tightness.

Crepitation, bony

Bony crepitation is a palpable vibration or an audible crunching sound that results when one bone grates against an-

other. This sign commonly results from a fracture, but can happen when bones that have been stripped of their protective articular cartilage grind against each other as they articulate.

Eliciting bony crepitation can help confirm the diagnosis of a fracture, but it can also cause further soft tissue, nerve, or vessel injury. Always evaluate distal pulses and perform neurologic checks distal to the suspected fracture site before manipulating an extremity. After the initial detection of crepitation in a patient with a fracture, avoid subsequent elicitation of this sign.

Assessment

If you detect bony crepitation in a patient with a suspected fracture, ask him if he feels pain and if he can point to the painful area. Find out how and when the injury occurred. Palpate pulses distal to the injury site and check the skin for pallor or coolness. Test motor and sensory function distal to the injury site. To prevent lacerating nerves, blood vessels, or soft tissue, it's very important to immobilize the affected area by applying a splint that includes the joints above and below the affected area. Elevate the affected area, if possible, and apply cold packs. Inspect for abrasions or lacerations. If the patient doesn't have a suspected fracture, ask about a history of osteoarthritis or rheumatoid arthritis. Which medications does he take? Take the patient's vital signs and test his joint range of motion (ROM).

Causes

◆ *Fracture.* In addition to bony crepitation, a fracture causes acute local pain, hematoma, and edema. Other findings may include deformity, point tenderness, discoloration of the limb, and loss of limb function. Neurovascular damage may cause increased capillary refill time, diminished or absent pulses, mottled cyanosis, paresthesia, and decreased sensation (all distal to the fracture site). An open fracture produces an obvious skin wound.

◆ *Osteoarthritis.* In advanced osteoarthritis, joint crepitation may be elicited during ROM testing. Soft fine crepitus on palpation may indicate roughening of the articular cartilage; coarse grating may indicate badly damaged cartilage. The cardinal symptom of osteoarthritis is joint pain, especially during motion and weight bearing.

◆ *Rheumatoid arthritis.* In advanced rheumatoid arthritis, bony crepitation is heard when the affected joint is rotated. However, rheumatoid arthritis usually develops insidiously, producing nonspecific signs and symptoms, such as fatigue, malaise, anorexia, a persistent low-grade fever, weight loss, lymphadenopathy, and vague arthralgia and myalgia. Later, more specific and localized articular signs develop, commonly at the proximal finger joints.

Crepitation, subcutaneous

When bubbles of air or other gases, such as carbon dioxide, are trapped in subcutaneous tissue, palpating or stroking the skin produces a crackling sound called *subcutaneous crepitation* or *subcutaneous emphysema.* The bubbles feel like small, unstable nodules and aren't painful, even though subcutaneous crepitation is commonly associated with painful disorders. Usually, the affected tissue is visibly edematous, which can lead to airway occlusion if edema affects the neck or upper chest.

The air or gas bubbles enter the tissues through open wounds from the action of anaerobic microorganisms or from traumatic or spontaneous rupture or perforation of pulmonary or GI organs.

Assessment

Because subcutaneous crepitation can indicate a life-threatening disorder, you'll need to perform a rapid initial evaluation and intervene if necessary. (See *Responding to subcutaneous crepitation.*)

When the patient's condition permits, palpate the affected skin to evaluate the location and extent of subcutaneous crepitation and to obtain baseline information. Delineate the borders of the area of crepitus with a marker. Palpate the area frequently to determine if the subcutaneous crepitation is increasing. Ask the patient if he's experiencing pain or having difficulty breathing. If he's in pain, find out where the pain is located, how severe it is, and when it began. Ask about recent thoracic surgery, diagnostic tests, and respiratory therapy or a history of trauma or chronic pulmonary disease.

Causes

◆ *Gas gangrene.* Subcutaneous crepitation is the hallmark of gas gangrene, a rare but commonly fatal infection. It's accompanied by local pain, swelling, and discoloration, with the formation of bullae and necrosis. The skin over the wound may rupture, revealing dark red or black necrotic muscle and producing foul-smelling, watery, or frothy discharge. Related findings include tachycardia, tachypnea, a moderate fever, cyanosis, and lassitude.

◆ *Orbital fracture.* An orbital fracture allows air from the nasal sinuses to es-

EMERGENCY INTERVENTIONS

Responding to subcutaneous crepitation

Subcutaneous crepitation occurs when air or gas bubbles escape into tissues. It may signal life-threatening rupture of an air-filled or gas-producing organ or a fulminating anaerobic infection.

Organ rupture

If the patient shows signs of respiratory distress—such as severe dyspnea, tachypnea, accessory muscle use, nasal flaring, air hunger, or tachycardia—quickly test for Hamman's sign to detect trapped air bubbles in the mediastinum.

To test for Hamman's sign, help the patient assume a left-lateral recumbent position. Then place your stethoscope over the precordium. If you hear a loud crunching sound that synchronizes with his heartbeat, the patient has a positive Hamman's sign.

Depending on which organ is ruptured, be prepared for endotracheal intubation, an emergency tracheotomy, or chest tube insertion. Start administering supplemental oxygen immediately. Insert an I.V. catheter to administer fluids and medication, and connect the patient to a cardiac monitor.

Anaerobic infection

If the patient has an open wound with a foul odor and local swelling and discoloration, you must act quickly. Take the patient's vital signs, checking especially for fever, tachycardia, hypotension, and tachypnea. Next, insert an I.V. catheter to administer fluids and medication, and provide supplemental oxygen.

In addition, be prepared for emergency surgery to drain and debride the wound. If the patient's condition is life-threatening, you may need to prepare him for transfer to a facility with a hyperbaric chamber.

---

cape into subcutaneous tissue, causing subcutaneous crepitation of the eyelid and orbit. The most common sign of this fracture is periorbital ecchymosis. Visual acuity is usually normal, although a swollen lid may prevent accurate testing. The patient has facial edema, diplopia, a hyphema and, occasionally, a dilated or unreactive pupil on the affected side.

◼ *Pneumothorax.* Severe pneumothorax produces subcutaneous crepitation in the upper chest and neck. Typically, the patient has unilateral chest pain that's rarely localized initially and increased on inspiration. Dyspnea, cyanosis, tachypnea, tachycardia, restlessness, asymmetrical chest expansion,

and a nonproductive cough can also occur. Breath sounds are absent or decreased and hyperresonance or tympany may be heard on the affected side.

◼ *Rupture of the esophagus.* A ruptured esophagus usually produces subcutaneous crepitation in the neck, chest wall, or supraclavicular fossa, although this sign doesn't always occur. With a rupture of the cervical esophagus, the patient has excruciating pain in the neck or supraclavicular area, his neck is resistant to passive motion, and he has local tenderness, soft-tissue swelling, dysphagia, odynophagia, and orthostatic vertigo.

Life-threatening rupture of the intrathoracic esophagus can produce mediastinal emphysema confirmed by a positive Hamman's sign (crunching, rasping sound that occurs with the heartbeat). The patient has severe retrosternal, epigastric, neck, or scapular pain and edema of the chest wall and neck. He may also display dyspnea, tachypnea, asymmetrical chest expansion, nasal flaring, cyanosis, diaphoresis, tachycardia, hypotension, dysphagia, and fever.

◪ *Rupture of the trachea or major bronchus.* Rupture of the trachea or major bronchus is a life-threatening injury that produces abrupt subcutaneous crepitation of the neck and anterior chest wall. The patient has severe dyspnea with nasal flaring, tachycardia, accessory muscle use, hypotension, cyanosis, extreme anxiety and, possibly, hemoptysis and mediastinal emphysema, with a positive Hamman's sign.

Cry, high-pitched

A high-pitched cry is a brief, sharp, piercing vocal sound produced by a neonate or infant. Whether acute or chronic, this cry is a late sign of increased intracranial pressure (ICP). The acute onset of a high-pitched cry demands emergency treatment to prevent permanent brain damage or death.

A change in the volume of one of the brain's components—brain tissue, cerebrospinal fluid, and blood—may cause increased ICP. In neonates, increased ICP may result from intracranial bleeding associated with birth trauma or from congenital malformations. In infants, increased ICP may result from meningitis, head trauma, or child abuse.

Assessment

Take the infant's vital signs, and then obtain a brief history. Did the infant fall recently or experience even minor head trauma? Be sure to ask the parents about changes in the infant's behavior during the past 24 hours. Has he been vomiting? Has he seemed restless or unlike himself? Has his sucking reflex diminished? Does he cry when he's moved? Suspect child abuse if the infant's history is inconsistent with physical findings.

Next, perform a neurologic examination. Remember that neurologic responses in a neonate or young infant are primarily reflex responses. Determine the infant's level of consciousness (LOC). Is he awake, irritable, or lethargic? Does he reach for an attractive object or turn toward the sound of a rattle? Observe his posture. Is he in the normal flexed position or in extension or opisthotonos? Examine muscle tone and observe the infant for signs of seizure.

Examine the size and shape of the infant's head. Is the anterior fontanel bulging? Measure the infant's head circumference, and check pupillary size and response to light. Unilateral or bilateral dilation and a sluggish response to light may accompany increased ICP. Finally, test the infant's reflexes; expect the Moro reflex to be diminished.

Elevate the infant's head to promote cerebral venous drainage and decrease ICP. Prepare to insert an I.V. catheter, and give a diuretic and corticosteroid as ordered. Make sure that endotracheal intubation equipment is readily available if needed.

Causes

◪ *Increased ICP.* Typically, the infant with a high-pitched cry also displays bulging fontanels, increased head circumference, and widened sutures. Earlier signs and symptoms of increasing ICP include seizures, bradycardia, dilated pupils, decreased LOC, increased systolic blood pressure, widened pulse pressure, an altered respiratory pattern and, possibly, vomiting.

Cyanosis

Cyanosis—a bluish or bluish black discoloration of the skin and mucous membranes—results from excessive concentration of unoxygenated hemoglobin in the blood. It may develop abruptly or gradually and can be classified as central or peripheral, although the two types may coexist.

Central cyanosis reflects inadequate oxygenation of systemic arterial blood. It may occur anywhere on the skin and mucous membranes of the mouth, lips, and conjunctiva.

Peripheral cyanosis reflects sluggish peripheral circulation caused by vasoconstriction, reduced cardiac output, or vascular occlusion. It may be widespread or may occur locally in one extremity. It doesn't affect mucous membranes.

Although cyanosis is an important sign of cardiovascular and pulmonary disorders, it isn't always an accurate gauge of oxygenation. Severe cyanosis is quite obvious, whereas mild cyanosis is more difficult to detect, even in natural, bright light. In dark-skinned patients, cyanosis is most apparent in the mucous membranes and nail beds. Transient, nonpathologic cyanosis may result from environmental factors.

Assessment

Perform a thorough examination if you detect cyanosis in your patient. Begin with a history, focusing on cardiac, pulmonary, and hematologic disorders. Ask the patient when he first noticed the cyanosis. Does it subside and recur? What aggravates or relieves the cyanosis? Next, evaluate the patient's level of consciousness. Ask about headaches, dizziness, or blurred vision. Ask about pain in the arms and legs (especially with walking) and about abnormal sensations, such as numbness, tingling, and coldness. Ask about chest pain and its severity, if present. Does the patient have a cough? If productive, have him describe the sputum. Ask about sleep apnea. Does the patient sleep with his head propped up on pillows? Also, ask about nausea, anorexia, and weight loss.

Begin the physical examination by taking the patient's vital signs. Inspect his skin and mucous membranes to determine the extent of cyanosis. Then test his motor strength. Check the skin for coolness, pallor, redness, pain, and ulceration. Palpate peripheral pulses, and test capillary refill time. Also assess for edema and clubbing. Auscultate heart rate and rhythm, especially noting gallops and murmurs, and auscultate the abdominal aorta and femoral arteries to detect bruits. Evaluate his respiratory rate and rhythm. Check for nasal flaring and asymmetrical chest expansion or barrel chest. Percuss the lungs for dullness or hyperresonance, and auscultate for decreased or adventitious breath sounds. Inspect the abdomen for ascites, and test for shifting dullness or fluid wave. Percuss and palpate for liver enlargement and tenderness.

Causes

◆ *Arteriosclerotic occlusive disease (chronic).* With arteriosclerotic occlusive disease, peripheral cyanosis occurs in the legs whenever they're in a dependent position. Associated signs and symptoms include intermittent claudication and burning pain at rest, paresthesia, muscle atrophy, and weak leg pulses. Late signs are leg ulcers and gangrene.

◆ *Bronchiectasis.* Bronchiectasis produces chronic central cyanosis. Its classic sign, however, is a chronic productive cough with copious, foul-smelling, mucopurulent sputum or hemoptysis.

◆ *Buerger's disease.* With Buerger's disease, exposure to cold initially causes the feet to become cold, cyanotic, and numb; later, they redden, become hot, and tingle. Intermittent claudication of the instep is characteristic. An associated sign is weak peripheral pulses.

◆ *Chronic obstructive pulmonary disease (COPD).* Chronic central cyanosis occurs in advanced stages of COPD and may be aggravated by exertion. Associated signs and symptoms include exertional dyspnea, a productive cough with thick sputum, anorexia, weight loss, pursed-lip breathing, tachypnea, and accessory muscle use.

◆ *Deep vein thrombosis.* With deep vein thrombosis, acute peripheral cyanosis occurs in the affected extremity associated with tenderness, painful movement, edema, and warmth. Homans' sign can also be elicited.

◆ *Heart failure.* Acute or chronic cyanosis may occur in patients as a late sign of heart failure. Central cyanosis occurs with left-sided heart failure, and peripheral cyanosis occurs with right-sided heart failure.

◆ *Lung cancer.* Lung cancer causes chronic central cyanosis accompanied by fever, weakness, weight loss, anorexia, dyspnea, chest pain, hemoptysis, and wheezing.

◆ *Peripheral arterial occlusion (acute).* Peripheral arterial occlusion produces acute cyanosis of one arm or leg or, occasionally, both legs. The cyanosis is accompanied by sharp or aching pain that worsens when the patient moves.

◼ *Pneumonia.* With pneumonia, acute central cyanosis is usually preceded by fever, shaking chills, a cough with purulent sputum, crackles, rhonchi, and pleuritic chest pain that's exacerbated by deep inspiration.

◆ *Pneumothorax.* A cardinal sign of pneumothorax, acute central cyanosis is accompanied by sharp chest pain that's exacerbated by movement, deep breathing, and coughing.

◆ *Polycythemia vera.* A ruddy complexion that can appear cyanotic is characteristic in polycythemia vera, which is a chronic myeloproliferative disorder. Other findings include aquagenic pruritus and coagulation defects.

◼ *Pulmonary edema.* With pulmonary edema, acute central cyanosis occurs with dyspnea, orthopnea, tachycardia, dependent crackles, hypotension, restlessness, and frothy, blood-tinged sputum.

◼ *Pulmonary embolism.* Usually, the first sign of pulmonary embolism is severe dyspnea, which may be accompanied by angina or pleuritic chest pain. Acute central cyanosis occurs when a large embolus causes significant obstruction of the pulmonary circulation. Syncope and jugular vein distention may also occur.

◆ *Raynaud's disease.* With Raynaud's disease, exposure to cold or stress causes the fingers or hands first to blanch and turn cold, become cyanotic, and finally to redden with a return to a normal temperature. The same findings are present with Raynaud's phenomenon when associated with other disorders, such as rheumatoid arthritis, scleroderma, or lupus erythematosus.

◤ *Shock.* With shock, acute peripheral cyanosis develops in the hands and feet, which may also be cold, clammy, and pale. Other signs and symptoms include hypotension, confusion, an increased capillary refill time, and a rapid, weak pulse.

◆ *Sleep apnea.* When chronic and severe, sleep apnea causes pulmonary hypertension and cor pulmonale (right-sided heart failure), which can produce chronic cyanosis.

D

Decerebrate posture

Decerebrate posture is characterized by internal rotation and extension of the arms with the wrists pronated and the fingers flexed. The legs are stiffly extended with forced plantar flexion of the feet. In severe cases, the back is acutely arched (opisthotonos). This sign indicates upper brain stem damage.

Decerebrate posture may be elicited by noxious stimuli or may occur spontaneously. It may be unilateral or bilateral and may affect only the arms with the legs remaining flaccid. Alternatively, decerebrate posture may affect one side of the body and decorticate posture the other. The two postures may also alternate as the patient's neurologic status fluctuates. (See *Comparing decerebrate and decorticate postures.*)

Assessment

After taking the patient's vital signs, determine his level of consciousness, using the Glasgow Coma Scale as a reference. Then evaluate the pupils for size, equality, and response to light. Test deep tendon reflexes (DTRs) and cranial nerve reflexes and check for doll's eye sign.

Next, explore the history of the patient's coma. If you can't obtain this information, look for clues to the causative disorder. Obtain information from the patient's family if available.

Causes

◪ *Brain stem infarction.* Brain stem infarction that produces a coma may elicit decerebrate posture. Other findings vary with the severity of the infarction. With deep coma, all normal reflexes are usually lost.

◪ *Cerebral lesion.* A cerebral lesion that increases intracranial pressure (ICP) may, in later stages, produce decerebrate posture. Associated findings vary with the lesion's site and extent, but commonly include coma, abnormal pupil size and response to light, bradycardia, increasing systolic blood pressure, and widening pulse pressure.

◪ *Diagnostic tests.* Relief from high ICP that results from removing spinal fluid during a lumbar puncture may precipitate cerebral compression of the brain stem and cause decerebrate posture and coma.

◪ *Hypoglycemic encephalopathy.* Hypoglycemic encephalopathy, characterized by extremely low blood glucose levels, may produce decerebrate posture and coma. It also causes dilated pupils, slow respirations, and bradycar-

Comparing decerebrate and decorticate postures

Decerebrate posture results from damage to the upper brain stem. In this posture, the arms are adducted and extended with the wrists pronated and the fingers flexed. The legs are stiffly extended with plantar flexion of the feet.

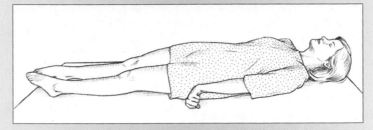

Decorticate posture results from damage to one or both corticospinal tracts. In this posture, the arms are adducted and flexed with the wrists and fingers flexed on the chest. The legs are stiffly extended and internally rotated with plantar flexion of the feet.

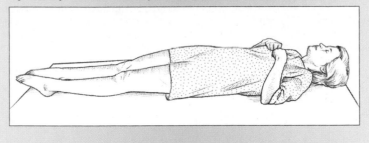

dia. Muscle spasms, twitching, and seizures eventually progress to flaccidity.

◼ *Hypoxic encephalopathy.* Severe hypoxia may produce decerebrate posture—the result of brain stem compression associated with anaerobic metabolism and increased ICP. Other findings include coma, a positive Babinski's reflex, an absent doll's eye sign, hypoactive DTRs and, possibly, fixed pupils and respiratory arrest.

◼ *Pontine hemorrhage.* Typically, pontine hemorrhage rapidly leads to decer-

ebrate posture and coma. Other signs include total paralysis, an absent doll's eye sign, a positive Babinski's reflex, and small, reactive pupils.

◼ *Posterior fossa hemorrhage.* The early signs and symptoms of posterior fossa hemorrhage include vomiting, headache, vertigo, ataxia, stiff neck, drowsiness, papilledema, and cranial nerve palsies. In later stages, as ICP increases, decerebrate posturing occurs.

Decorticate posture

A sign of corticospinal damage, decorticate posture is characterized by adduction of the arms and flexion of the elbows, with wrists and fingers flexed on the chest. The legs are extended and internally rotated, with plantar flexion of the feet. This posture may occur unilaterally or bilaterally.

Although a serious sign, decorticate posture carries a more favorable prognosis than decerebrate posture. However, if the causative disorder extends lower in the brain stem, decorticate posture may progress to decerebrate posture. (See *Comparing decerebrate and decorticate postures*, page 203.)

Assessment

Test the patient's motor and sensory functions. Evaluate pupil size, equality, and response to light. Then test cranial nerve function and deep tendon reflexes. Ask about headache, dizziness, nausea, vision changes, numbness, and tingling. Also ask about the patient's recent and previous medical history.

Causes

◆ *Brain abscess.* Decorticate posture may occur with brain abscess. Accompanying findings vary depending on the size and location of the abscess, but may include aphasia, hemiparesis, headache, dizziness, seizures, and nausea.
◆ *Brain tumor.* A brain tumor may produce decorticate posture that's usually bilateral. Related findings include headache, memory loss, vision changes, seizures, ataxia, aphasia, paresis, sensory loss, and paresthesia.
◆ *Head injury.* Decorticate posture may be among the variable findings of a head injury, depending on the site and severity of the injury. Other findings include headache, nausea and vomiting, dizziness, irritability, aphasia, hemiparesis, unilateral numbness, seizures, and pupillary dilation.

◼ *Stroke.* Typically, a stroke involving the cerebral cortex produces unilateral decorticate posture, also called *spastic hemiplegia*. Other findings include dysarthria, dysphagia, unilateral sensory loss, apraxia, aphasia, and memory loss.

Deep tendon reflexes, hyperactive

A hyperactive deep tendon reflex (DTR) is an abnormally brisk muscle contraction that occurs in response to a sudden stretch induced by sharply tapping the muscle's tendon of insertion.

The corticospinal tract and other descending tracts govern the reflex arc— the relay cycle that produces a reflex response. A corticospinal lesion above the level of the reflex arc or abnormal neuromuscular transmission at the end of the reflex arc may result in hyperactive DTRs. For example, a calcium or magnesium deficiency may cause hyperactive DTRs because they regulate neuromuscular excitability. (See *Tracing the reflex arc,* pages 206 and 207.)

Hyperactive DTRs typically accompany other neurologic findings but usually lack specific diagnostic value.

Assessment

After eliciting hyperactive DTRs, take the patient's history. Ask about pregnancy, injury, or other trauma and about prolonged exposure to cold, wind, or water. Ask about the onset and progression of other signs and symptoms. Next, perform a neurologic examination. Evaluate the patient's level of consciousness, and test motor and sensory function in the limbs. Check for ataxia or tremors and for speech and visual deficits. Test for Chvostek's and Trousseau's signs and for carpedal spasm. Be sure to check the patient's vital signs.

Causes

◆ *Amyotrophic lateral sclerosis (ALS).* ALS produces generalized hyperactive DTRs accompanied by hand or forearm weakness and leg spasticity.

◆ *Brain tumor.* A cerebral tumor causes hyperactive DTRs. Associated signs and symptoms develop slowly and may include unilateral paresis or paralysis, anesthesia, visual field deficits, spasticity, and a positive Babinski's reflex.

◆ *Hypocalcemia.* Hypocalcemia may produce a sudden or gradual onset of generalized hyperactive DTRs with paresthesia, muscle twitching and cramping, positive Chvostek's and Trousseau's signs, carpopedal spasm, and tetany.

◆ *Hypomagnesemia.* Hypomagnesemia results in the gradual onset of generalized hyperactive DTRs accompanied by muscle cramps, hypotension, tachycardia, paresthesia, ataxia, tetany and, possibly, seizures.

◆ *Hypothermia.* Mild hypothermia produces generalized hyperactive DTRs. Other findings include shivering, fatigue, weakness, lethargy, slurred speech, ataxia, muscle stiffness, tachycardia, diuresis, bradypnea, and hypotension.

◆ *Preeclampsia.* Preeclampsia may cause a gradual onset of generalized hyperactive DTRs. Other findings include increased blood pressure, abnormal weight gain, oliguria, severe headache, blurred or double vision,

epigastric pain, nausea and vomiting, shortness of breath, and edema of the face, fingers, and abdomen after bed rest.

◆ *Spinal cord lesion.* Incomplete spinal cord lesions cause hyperactive DTRs below the level of the lesion. Other findings include paralysis and sensory loss below the level of the lesion, urine retention and overflow incontinence, and alternating constipation and diarrhea. A lesion above T6 may also produce autonomic hyperreflexia with diaphoresis and flushing above the level of the lesion, headache, nasal congestion, and increased blood pressure.

◆ *Stroke.* A stroke that affects the origin of the corticospinal tracts causes the sudden onset of hyperactive DTRs. The patient may also have unilateral paresis or paralysis, visual field deficits, spasticity, and a positive Babinski's reflex.

◆ *Tetanus.* With tetanus, the sudden onset of generalized hyperactive DTRs accompanies tachycardia, diaphoresis, a low-grade fever, painful and involuntary muscle contractions, and trismus (lockjaw).

Deep tendon reflexes, hypoactive

A hypoactive deep tendon reflex (DTR) is an abnormally diminished muscle contraction that occurs in response to a sudden stretch induced by sharply tapping the muscle's tendon of insertion. It may be graded as minimal or absent. Symmetrically diminished reflexes may be normal. Hypoactive DTRs may result from damage to the reflex arc involving the specific muscle, the peripheral nerve, the nerve roots, or the spinal cord at that level. Hypoactive

(Text continues on page 208.)

Tracing the reflex arc

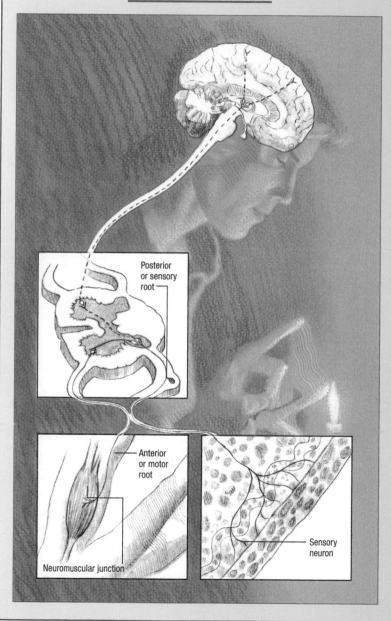

Sharply tapping a tendon initiates a sensory (afferent) impulse that travels along a peripheral nerve to a spinal nerve and then to the spinal cord. The impulse enters the spinal cord through the posterior root, synapses with a motor (efferent) neuron in the anterior horn on the same side of the spinal cord, and then is transmitted through a motor nerve fiber back to the muscle. When the impulse crosses the neuromuscular junction, the muscle contracts, completing the reflex arc.

BICEPS REFLEX
(C5-6 innervation)

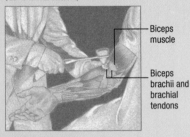

Biceps muscle

Biceps brachii and brachial tendons

TRICEPS REFLEX
(C7-8 innervation)

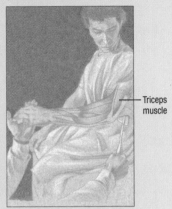

Triceps muscle

PATELLAR REFLEX
(L2, 3, 4 innervation)

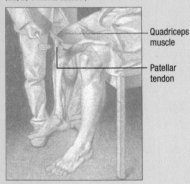

Quadriceps muscle

Patellar tendon

BRACHIORADIALIS REFLEX
(C5-6 innervation)

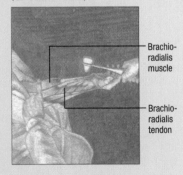

Brachio-radialis muscle

Brachio-radialis tendon

ACHILLES TENDON REFLEX
(S1-2 innervation)

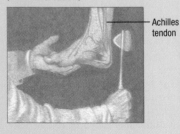

Achilles tendon

Documenting deep tendon reflexes

Record the patient's deep tendon reflex (DTR) scores by drawing a stick figure and entering the grades on this scale at the proper location. The figure shown here indicates hypoactive DTRs in the legs; other reflexes are normal.

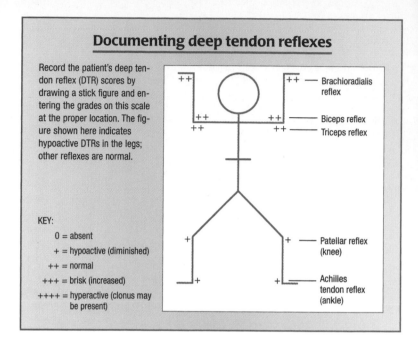

KEY:
    0 = absent
    + = hypoactive (diminished)
    ++ = normal
    +++ = brisk (increased)
    ++++ = hyperactive (clonus may be present)

DTRs are an important sign of many disorders, especially when they appear with other neurologic signs and symptoms. (See *Documenting deep tendon reflexes*.)

Assessment

After eliciting hypoactive DTRs, obtain a thorough history from the patient or a family member. Have him describe current signs and symptoms in detail. Then take a family and drug history.

Next, evaluate the patient's level of consciousness. Test motor function in his limbs. Palpate for muscle atrophy or increased mass. Test sensory function, including pain, touch, temperature, and vibration sense. Ask about paresthesia. To check for Romberg's sign, ask him to stand with his feet together and his eyes closed. During conversation, evaluate his speech. Check for signs of vision or hearing loss.

Check the patient's vital signs and monitor for increased heart rate and blood pressure. Inspect the skin for pallor, dryness, flushing, or diaphoresis. Auscultate for hypoactive bowel sounds, and palpate for bladder distention.

Causes

◆ *Botulism.* With botulism, generalized hypoactive DTRs accompany progressive descending muscle weakness. Initially, the patient usually complains of blurred and double vision and, occasionally, anorexia, nausea, and vomiting. Other early findings include vertigo, hearing loss, dysarthria, and dysphagia.
◆ *Eaton-Lambert syndrome.* Eaton-Lambert syndrome produces generalized hypoactive DTRs. Early signs include difficulty rising from a chair, climbing stairs, and walking. The pa-

tient may complain of achiness, paresthesia, and muscle weakness that are most severe in the morning.

◆ *Guillain-Barré syndrome.* Guillain-Barré syndrome causes bilateral hypoactive DTRs that progress rapidly from hypotonia to areflexia within several days. This disorder typically causes muscle weakness that begins in the legs and then extends to the arms and, possibly, to the trunk and neck muscles. Other signs and symptoms include cranial nerve palsies, pain, paresthesia, flushing, fluctuating blood pressure, and anhidrosis or episodic diaphoresis.

◆ *Peripheral neuropathy.* Peripheral neuropathy is characteristic of end-stage diabetes mellitus, renal failure, and alcoholism and as an adverse effect of various medications. It results in progressive hypoactive DTRs. Other effects include motor weakness, sensory loss, paresthesia, tremors, orthostatic hypotension, and incontinence.

◆ *Polymyositis.* With polymyositis, hypoactive DTRs accompany muscle weakness, pain, stiffness, spasms and, possibly, increased size or atrophy.

◆ *Spinal cord lesions.* Spinal cord injury produces spinal shock, resulting in hypoactive DTRs below the level of the lesion. Associated signs and symptoms include quadriplegia or paraplegia, flaccidity, a loss of sensation below the level of the lesion, and dry, pale skin.

◆ *Syringomyelia.* Permanent bilateral hypoactive DTRs occur early in syringomyelia, a slowly progressive disorder in which cavities lined with dense tissue develop in the spinal cord. Other signs and symptoms include muscle weakness and atrophy, scoliosis of the spine, and loss of sensation, usually extending in a capelike fashion over the arms, shoulders, neck, back and, occasionally, the legs.

Diaphoresis

Diaphoresis is profuse sweating and represents an autonomic nervous system response to physical or psychogenic stress, fever, or high environmental temperature. When caused by stress, diaphoresis may be generalized or limited to the palms, soles, and forehead. When caused by fever or environmental temperature, it's usually generalized.

Diaphoresis usually begins abruptly and may be accompanied by other signs, such as tachycardia and increased blood pressure. (See *When diaphoresis spells crisis,* page 210.) This sign varies with age because sweat glands function immaturely in infants and are less active in elderly patients. Intermittent diaphoresis may accompany chronic disorders characterized by recurrent fever; isolated diaphoresis may mark an episode of acute pain or fever.

When caused by a high external temperature, diaphoresis is a normal response. Diaphoresis also commonly occurs during menopause and is preceded by a sensation of intense heat. Other normal causes include exertion that accelerates metabolism and mild to moderate anxiety that helps initiate the fight-or-flight response. (See *Understanding diaphoresis,* pages 212 and 213.)

Assessment

If the patient is diaphoretic, begin the history by having the patient describe his chief complaint. Then explore associated signs and symptoms. Does the patient have insomnia, headache, or changes in vision or hearing? Does he have palpitations? Ask about pleuritic pain, a cough, difficulty breathing, paresthesia, muscle cramps or stiffness,

EMERGENCY INTERVENTIONS

When diaphoresis spells crisis

Diaphoresis is an early sign of life-threatening disorders. These guidelines will help you promptly detect such disorders and intervene to minimize any harm to the patient.

Hypoglycemia

If you observe diaphoresis in a patient who complains of blurred vision, suspect hypoglycemia.
◆ Ask the patient about increased irritability and anxiety.
◆ Ask if he has been unusually hungry lately.
◆ Assess the patient for tremors.
◆ Check the patient's vital signs, noting hypotension and tachycardia.
◆ Ask about a history of type 2 diabetes or antidiabetic therapy.
◆ Evaluate the patient's blood glucose level.
◆ Administer I.V. glucose 50%, as ordered, to return the patient's glucose level to normal.
◆ Monitor the patient's vital signs and cardiac rhythm.
◆ Ensure a patent airway, and be prepared to assist with breathing and circulation if necessary.

Heatstroke

If you observe profuse diaphoresis in a weak, tired, and apprehensive patient, suspect heatstroke, which can progress to circulatory collapse.
◆ Ask whether the patient was exposed to high temperature and humidity.
◆ Take the patient's vital signs, noting a normal or subnormal temperature.
◆ Check for ashen gray skin and dilated pupils.
◆ Take the patient to a cool room.
◆ Remove the patient's clothes.
◆ Use a fan to direct cool air over the patient's body.
◆ Insert an I.V. catheter, and prepare for electrolyte and fluid replacement.

◆ Monitor the patient for signs of shock.
◆ Check the patient's urine output along with other sources of output, such as tubes, drains, and ostomies.

Autonomic hyperreflexia

If you observe diaphoresis in a patient with a spinal cord injury above T6 or T7, ask if he has a pounding headache, restlessness, blurred vision, or nasal congestion.
◆ Take the patient's vital signs, noting bradycardia and extremely elevated blood pressure.
◆ Examine the patient for eye pain associated with intraocular hemorrhage and for facial paralysis, slurred speech, or limb weakness associated with intracerebral hemorrhage.
◆ Reposition the patient to remove pressure stimuli.
◆ Check for bladder distention or fecal impaction. Remove kinks in the urinary catheter tubing, if necessary. Administer a suppository or manually remove impacted feces.
◆ Insert an I.V. catheter, and prepare to administer hydralazine (Apresoline) if you can't locate and relieve a causative stimulus.

Myocardial infarction or heart failure

If the diaphoretic patient complains of chest pain and dyspnea or has arrhythmias or electrocardiogram changes, suspect a myocardial infarction or heart failure.
◆ Connect the patient to a cardiac monitor.
◆ Ensure a patent airway and administer supplemental oxygen.
◆ Insert an I.V. catheter, and administer an analgesic.
◆ Be prepared to begin emergency resuscitation if cardiac or respiratory arrest occurs.

joint pain, nausea, vomiting, and abdominal pain. Ask the female patient about amenorrhea and changes in her menstrual cycle. Complete the history by asking about travel to tropical countries. Did the patient recently experience an insect bite that may have transmitted a disease such as typhoid fever? Finally, obtain a thorough drug history.

Next, perform a physical examination. Determine the extent of diaphoresis by inspecting the trunk and extremities as well as the palms, soles, and forehead. Note whether diaphoresis occurs during the day or at night. Note poor skin turgor and dry mucous membranes. Check for splinter hemorrhages and Plummer's nails. Check the patient's vital signs. Examine the eyes for pupillary abnormalities, exophthalmos, and excessive tearing.

Causes

◆ *Acquired immunodeficiency syndrome (AIDS).* Night sweats may be an early finding with AIDS, occurring either as a manifestation of the disease itself or secondary to an opportunistic infection. The patient also displays a fever, fatigue, lymphadenopathy, anorexia, dramatic and unexplained weight loss, diarrhea, and a persistent cough.

◆ *Acromegaly.* With acromegaly, diaphoresis is a sensitive gauge of disease activity, which involves the hypersecretion of growth hormone and an increased metabolic rate. The patient has a hulking appearance with an enlarged supraorbital ridge and thickened ears and nose.

◆ *Anxiety disorders.* Acute anxiety characterizes panic, whereas chronic anxiety characterizes phobias, conversion disorders, obsessions, and compulsions. Both types of anxiety may cause diaphoresis. It's most dramatic

on the patient's palms, soles, and forehead and is accompanied by palpitations, tachycardia, tachypnea, tremors, and GI distress.

◆ *Autonomic hyperreflexia.* Occurring after resolution of spinal shock in a spinal cord injury above T6, hyperreflexia causes profuse diaphoresis, a pounding headache, blurred vision, and dramatically elevated blood pressure.

◆ *Drug and alcohol withdrawal syndromes.* Withdrawal from alcohol or an opioid analgesic may cause generalized diaphoresis, dilated pupils, tachycardia, tremors, and an altered mental status.

◆ *Drugs.* Sympathomimetics, certain antipsychotics, thyroid hormones, corticosteroids, and antipyretics may cause diaphoresis. Aspirin and acetaminophen (Tylenol) poisoning also cause this sign.

◆ *Empyema.* Pus accumulation in the pleural space leads to drenching night sweats and fever. The patient also complains of chest pain, cough, and weight loss.

◆ *Heart failure.* Typically, diaphoresis follows fatigue, dyspnea, orthopnea, and tachycardia in patients with left-sided heart failure. It follows jugular vein distention and a dry cough in patients with right-sided heart failure.

◧ *Heat exhaustion.* Although heat exhaustion is marked by failure of heat to dissipate, it initially may cause profuse diaphoresis, fatigue, weakness, and anxiety. Heat exhaustion may eventually progress to shock and circulatory collapse.

◆ *Hodgkin's disease.* Early findings of Hodgkin's disease may include night sweats, fever, fatigue, pruritus, and weight loss. Usually, this disease initially causes painless swelling of a cervical lymph node.

◧ *Hypoglycemia.* Rapidly induced hypoglycemia may cause diaphoresis accompanied by irritability, tremors, hy-

Understanding diaphoresis

potension, blurred vision, tachycardia, hunger, and loss of consciousness.
◆ *Infective endocarditis (subacute).* Generalized night sweats occur early with infective endocarditis. Accompanying signs and symptoms include an intermittent low-grade fever, weakness, fatigue, weight loss, anorexia, and arthralgia.
◆ *Lung abscess.* Drenching night sweats are common with lung abscess. Its chief sign, however, is a cough that produces copious purulent, foul-smelling, and typically bloody sputum.
◆ *Malaria.* Profuse diaphoresis marks the third stage of paroxysmal malaria. Chills mark the first stage; high fever, the second stage. Headache, arthralgia,

and hepatosplenomegaly may also occur.
◆ *Myocardial infarction (MI).* Diaphoresis usually accompanies acute, substernal, radiating chest pain with MI. Other findings include dyspnea, nausea, vomiting, tachycardia, an irregular pulse, pallor, and clammy skin.
◆ *Pesticide poisoning.* Diaphoresis is one of the toxic effects of pesticides. Others include nausea, vomiting, diarrhea, blurred vision, miosis, excessive lacrimation and salivation, muscle weakness, and flaccid paralysis.
◆ *Pheochromocytoma.* Pheochromocytoma commonly produces diaphoresis, but its cardinal sign is hypertension.
◆ *Pneumonia.* Intermittent, generalized diaphoresis accompanies fever

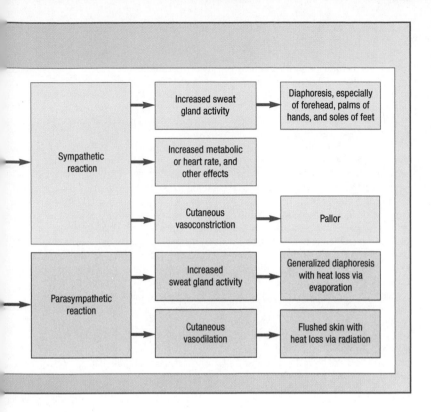

and chills in patients with pneumonia. Other findings are pleuritic chest pain that increases with deep inspiration, tachypnea, dyspnea, a productive cough, headache, fatigue, myalgia, abdominal pain, anorexia, and cyanosis.

◆ *Tetanus.* Tetanus commonly causes profuse sweating accompanied by a low-grade fever, tachycardia, and hyperactive deep tendon reflexes.

◆ *Thyrotoxicosis.* Thyrotoxicosis commonly produces diaphoresis accompanied by heat intolerance, weight loss despite increased appetite, tachycardia, palpitations, an enlarged thyroid, dyspnea, diarrhea, and Plummer's nails.

◆ *Tuberculosis (TB).* TB may cause night sweats, a low-grade fever, fatigue, weakness, anorexia, and weight loss.

In TB reactivation, a productive cough with mucopurulent sputum, occasional hemoptysis, and chest pain may be present.

Diarrhea

Usually a chief sign of an intestinal disorder, diarrhea is an abnormal frequency and liquidity of fecal discharges compared with the patient's normal bowel habits. It varies in severity and may be acute or chronic. Acute diarrhea may result from infection, stress, fecal impaction, or the effect of a drug. Chronic diarrhea may result from bowel disease, malabsorption syndrome, an endocrine disorder, or GI surgery. Periodic diarrhea may result from food intolerance or from ingestion of spicy or high-fiber foods or caffeine. (See *What causes diarrhea?*) The fluid and electrolyte imbalances that diarrhea produces may precipitate arrhythmias or hypovolemic shock.

Assessment

Initially, explore signs and symptoms associated with diarrhea. Does the patient have abdominal pain and cramps or difficulty breathing? Is he weak or fatigued? Find out about his drug history. Has he had GI surgery or radiation therapy recently? Ask the patient to briefly describe his diet. Does he have known food allergies? Inquire about unusual stress. Then proceed with a physical examination. Evaluate hydration and check skin turgor and mucous membranes. Take his blood pressure with the patient lying, sitting, and standing. Inspect the abdomen for distention, and palpate for tenderness. Auscultate bowel sounds. Check for tympany over the abdomen. Take the patient's temperature, and note any chills. Also, look for a rash.

Causes

◆ *Anthrax (GI).* Anthrax manifests after the patient has eaten contaminated meat from an animal infected with *Bacillus anthracis.* Severe bloody diarrhea is a late sign of infection.
◆ *Carcinoid syndrome.* In carcinoid syndrome, severe diarrhea occurs with flushing—usually of the head and neck—that's commonly caused by emotional stimuli or the ingestion of food, hot water, or alcohol.
◆ *Cholera.* After ingesting water or food contaminated by the bacterium *Vibrio cholerae,* the patient experiences abrupt watery diarrhea and vomiting. Other findings include thirst, weak-

ness, muscle cramps, decreased skin turgor, oliguria, tachycardia, and hypotension. Without treatment, death can occur within hours.
◆ Clostridium difficile *infection.* With *C. difficile* infection, the patient may have soft, unformed stools or watery diarrhea that may be foul smelling or grossly bloody.
◆ *Crohn's disease.* Crohn's disease is a recurring inflammatory disorder that produces diarrhea accompanied by abdominal pain and nausea. The patient may also display fever, chills, weakness, anorexia, and weight loss.
◆ *Drugs.* Diarrhea is an adverse effect of many drugs, including antibiotics, magnesium-containing antacids and, in high doses, cardiac glycosides and quinidine (Quinalan) among others. Laxative abuse can also cause diarrhea.
◆ *Escherichia coli O157:H7.* Watery or bloody diarrhea, nausea, vomiting, fever, and abdominal cramps occur after the patient eats undercooked beef or other foods contaminated with *E. coli* O157:H7.
◆ *Infections.* Acute viral, bacterial, and protozoal infections cause the sudden onset of watery diarrhea as well as abdominal pain, cramps, nausea, vomiting, and fever. Significant fluid and electrolyte loss may cause signs of dehydration and shock. Chronic tuberculosis and fungal and parasitic infections may produce less severe but more persistent diarrhea, accompanied by epigastric distress, vomiting, and weight loss.
◆ *Intestinal obstruction.* Partial intestinal obstruction increases intestinal motility, resulting in diarrhea, abdominal pain with tenderness and guarding, nausea and, possibly, distention.
◆ *Irritable bowel syndrome (IBS).* With IBS, diarrhea alternates with constipation or normal bowel function. Related findings include abdominal pain,

What causes diarrhea?

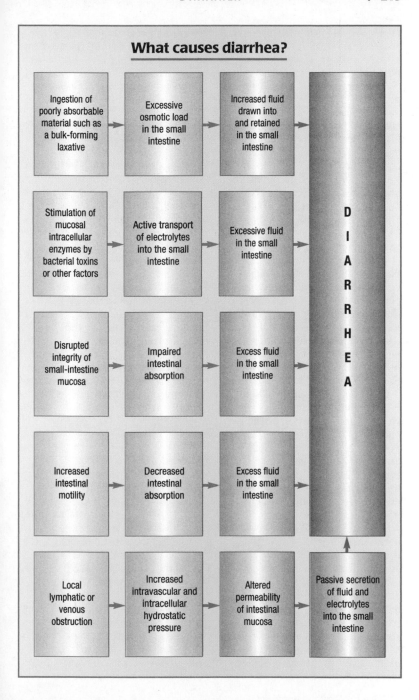

tenderness, and distention; dyspepsia; and nausea.

◆ *Ischemic bowel disease.* Ischemic bowel disease is a disorder that causes bloody diarrhea with abdominal pain.

◆ *Lactose intolerance.* With lactose intolerance, diarrhea occurs within several hours of ingesting milk or milk products. It's accompanied by cramps, abdominal pain, borborygmi, bloating, nausea, and flatus.

◆ *Listeriosis.* With listeriosis, diarrhea occurs along with fever, myalgia, abdominal pain, nausea, and vomiting. This infection primarily affects pregnant women, neonates, and those with weakened immune systems.

◆ *Pseudomembranous enterocolitis.* Pseudomembranous enterocolitis is a disorder that commonly follows antibiotic administration. It produces copious watery, green, foul-smelling, bloody diarrhea. Other signs and symptoms include colicky abdominal pain, distention, fever, and dehydration.

◆ *Q Fever.* Q Fever is caused by the bacterium *Coxiella burnetii* and causes diarrhea along with fever, chills, severe headache, malaise, chest pain, and vomiting. In severe cases, hepatitis or pneumonia may follow.

◆ *Rotavirus gastroenteritis.* Rotavirus gastroenteritis commonly starts with a fever, nausea, and vomiting followed by diarrhea. The illness can range from mild to severe and lasts from 3 to 9 days.

◆ *Thyrotoxicosis.* With thyrotoxicosis, nervousness, tremors, diaphoresis, weight loss despite increased appetite, dyspnea, palpitations, tachycardia, an enlarged thyroid, and heat intolerance accompany diarrhea.

◆ *Ulcerative colitis.* The hallmark of ulcerative colitis is recurrent bloody diarrhea with pus or mucus. Other signs and symptoms include tenesmus (a painful spasm of the anal sphincter that's accompanied by an urgent desire to evacuate the bowel or bladder), hyperactive bowel sounds, cramping lower abdominal pain, a low-grade fever, anorexia and, at times, nausea and vomiting. Weight loss, anemia, and weakness are late findings.

Diplopia

Diplopia is double vision—seeing one object as two. This symptom results when extraocular muscles fail to work together, causing images to fall on noncorresponding parts of the retinas. Orbital lesions, the effects of surgery, or impaired function of cranial nerves may be responsible. (See *Testing extraocular muscles*.)

Diplopia usually begins intermittently and affects near or far vision exclusively. Binocular diplopia may result from ocular deviation or displacement, extraocular muscle palsies, or psychoneurosis. Monocular diplopia may result from an early cataract, retinal edema or scarring, iridodialysis, a subluxated lens, or an uncorrected refractive error.

Assessment

If the patient complains of double vision, first check his neurologic status. Evaluate motor and sensory function and pupil size, equality, and response to light. Then check his vital signs. Ask about associated symptoms, especially severe headache, because diplopia can accompany serious disorders. Find out when the patient first noticed diplopia. Ask if it has worsened, remained the same, or subsided. Does its severity change throughout the day? Ask about the patient's medical history and note a history of extraocular muscle disorders, trauma, or eye surgery. Observe the patient for ocular deviation, ptosis, proptosis (protrusion of the eyeball),

Testing extraocular muscles

The coordinated action of six muscles controls eyeball movements. To test the function of each muscle and the cranial nerve (CN) that innervates it, ask the patient to look in the direction controlled by that muscle. The six directions you can test make up the cardinal fields of gaze. The patient's inability to turn the eye in the designated direction indicates muscle weakness or paralysis.

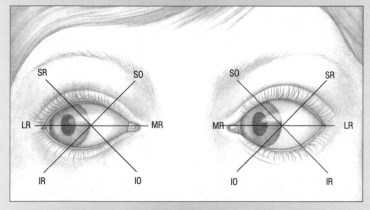

SR = superior rectus (CN III)   IR = inferior rectus (CN III)   MR = medial rectus (CN III)
LR = lateral rectus (CN VI)   IO = inferior oblique (CN III)   SO = superior oblique (CN IV)

lid edema, and conjunctival injection. Distinguish monocular from binocular diplopia by asking the patient to occlude one eye at a time. If he still sees double out of one eye, he has monocular diplopia. Test his visual acuity and extraocular muscles.

Causes

◆ *Alcohol intoxication.* Diplopia is a common symptom of alcohol intoxication.
◆ *Botulism.* Hallmark signs of botulism include diplopia, dysarthria, dysphagia, and ptosis. Early findings include dry mouth, sore throat, vomiting, and diarrhea.
◆ *Brain tumor.* Diplopia may be an early symptom of a brain tumor. Other

findings vary with the tumor's size and location.
◆ *Cavernous sinus thrombosis.* Cavernous sinus thrombosis may produce diplopia and limited eye movement. Other findings include orbital and lid edema, abnormal pupillary responses, impaired visual acuity, papilledema, and fever.
◆ *Diabetes mellitus.* Among the long-term effects of diabetes mellitus may be diplopia due to isolated cranial nerve III palsy. Diplopia typically begins suddenly and may be accompanied by pain.
◆ *Head injury.* Head injuries may cause diplopia, depending on the site and extent of the injury. Other findings include eye deviation, pupillary changes, altered vital signs, nausea,

vomiting, and motor weakness or paralysis.

◢ *Intracranial aneurysm.* Intracranial aneurysm is a disorder that initially produces diplopia and eye deviation. The patient complains of a recurrent, severe, unilateral, frontal headache.

◆ *Multiple sclerosis (MS).* Blurred vision and paresthesia usually accompany diplopia, an early symptom in MS.

◆ *Myasthenia gravis.* Myasthenia gravis initially produces diplopia and ptosis, which worsen throughout the day. It progressively involves other muscles, resulting in a blank facial expression and difficulty chewing, swallowing, and making fine hand movements.

◆ *Ophthalmologic migraine.* Most common in young adults, ophthalmologic migraine results in diplopia that persists for days after the headache. Other findings include ptosis, extraocular muscle palsies, and severe, unilateral pain.

◆ *Orbital blowout fracture.* An orbital blowout fracture usually causes monocular diplopia affecting the upward gaze. However, with marked periorbital edema, diplopia may affect other directions of gaze.

◆ *Orbital cellulitis.* Inflammation of the orbital tissues and eyelids causes sudden diplopia. Other findings are eye deviation and pain, purulent drainage, lid edema, chemosis and redness, proptosis, nausea, and fever.

◆ *Orbital tumor.* An enlarging orbital tumor can cause diplopia. Proptosis and blurred vision may also occur.

◢ *Stroke.* Diplopia characterizes stroke when it affects the vertebrobasilar artery. Other findings include unilateral motor weakness or paralysis, visual field deficits, circumoral numbness, slurred speech, dysphagia, and amnesia.

◆ *Thyrotoxicosis.* Diplopia occurs when exophthalmos is associated with thyrotoxicosis. It usually begins in the upper field of gaze. It's accompanied by impaired eye movement, excessive tearing, and lid edema.

◆ *Transient ischemic attack (TIA).* Diplopia, dizziness, tinnitus, hearing loss, and numbness generally accompany a TIA. It can last for a few seconds or up to 24 hours and may be a warning sign of a future stroke.

Dizziness

Dizziness is a sensation of imbalance or faintness, sometimes associated with weakness, confusion, and blurred or double vision. It's a common symptom. Episodes of dizziness are usually brief. They may be mild or severe with an abrupt or gradual onset. Dizziness may be aggravated by standing up quickly and alleviated by lying down or by rest.

Dizziness typically results from inadequate blood flow and oxygen supply to the cerebrum and spinal cord. It's commonly confused with vertigo—a sensation of revolving in space or of surroundings revolving about oneself. However, unlike dizziness, vertigo is commonly accompanied by nausea, vomiting, nystagmus, a staggering gait, and tinnitus or hearing loss. Dizziness and vertigo may occur together such as in postconcussion syndrome.

Assessment

Ask the patient if he has a history of diabetes or cardiovascular disease. Is he taking antihypertensive medications? If so, when did he take his last dose? If the patient's blood pressure is normal, obtain a more complete medical history, including a complete drug history. Then explore the patient's dizziness. How often does it occur? How long does each episode last? Does the dizziness abate spontaneously? Does it lead to loss of consciousness? Find out if sitting or standing up suddenly or stooping over triggers dizziness. Also ask about palpitations, chest pain, diaphoresis, shortness of breath, and chronic cough.

Next, perform a physical examination. Begin with a quick neurologic assessment, checking the patient's level of consciousness, motor and sensory functions, and reflexes. Inspect for poor skin turgor and dry mucous membranes. Auscultate heart rate and rhythm. Inspect for barrel chest, clubbing, cyanosis, and accessory muscle use. Also auscultate breath sounds. Take the patient's blood pressure while he's lying down, sitting, and standing to check for orthostatic hypotension. Test capillary refill time in the extremities and palpate for edema.

Causes

◆ *Anemia.* Typically, anemia causes dizziness that's aggravated by postural changes or exertion. Other signs and symptoms include pallor, dyspnea, fatigue, tachycardia, and a bounding pulse. Capillary refill time is increased.

◪ *Cardiac arrhythmias.* With arrhythmias, dizziness lasts for several seconds or longer and may precede fainting. The patient may experience palpitations, weakness, blurred vision, paresthesia, or an irregular pulse.

◆ *Drugs.* Anxiolytics, central nervous system depressants, opioids, decongestants, antihistamines, antihypertensives, and vasodilators commonly cause dizziness. Herbal remedies, such as St. John's wort, can also produce dizziness.

◆ *Emphysema.* Dizziness may follow exertion or the chronic, productive cough in patients with emphysema. Other findings include dyspnea, accessory muscle use, pursed-lip breathing, tachypnea, and peripheral cyanosis.

◆ *Generalized anxiety disorder.* Generalized anxiety disorder produces continuous dizziness that may intensify as the disorder worsens. Associated signs and symptoms are persistent anxiety (for at least 1 month), insomnia, difficulty concentrating, irritability, twitching or fidgeting, muscle aches, a furrowed brow, and a tendency to be startled.

◆ *Hypertension.* With hypertension, dizziness may precede fainting, but it may also be relieved by rest. Other common signs and symptoms include headache and blurred vision.

◆ *Hyperventilation syndrome.* Episodes of hyperventilation cause dizziness that usually last a few minutes; however, if episodes of hyperventilation occur frequently, dizziness may persist between them.

◪ *Hypovolemia.* With hypovolemia, dizziness is caused by a lack of circulating volume and may be accompanied by dry mucous membranes, decreased blood pressure, or increased heart rate.

◆ *Orthostatic hypotension.* Orthostatic hypotension produces dizziness that may end with fainting or disappear with rest. Other findings include dim vision, spots before the eyes, pallor, diaphoresis, hypotension, and tachycardia.

◆ *Postconcussion syndrome.* Occurring 1 to 3 weeks after a head injury, postconcussion syndrome is marked by dizziness, headache, emotional lability, fatigue, anxiety and, possibly, vertigo.

◆ *Transient ischemic attack (TIA).* Dizziness of varying severity is typically present during a TIA. Lasting from a few seconds to 24 hours, a TIA commonly signals an impending stroke.

Doll's eye sign, absent

An indicator of brain stem dysfunction, the absence of the doll's eye sign is detected by rapid, gentle turning of the patient's head from side to side. The eyes remain fixed in midposition instead of the normal response of moving laterally toward the side opposite the direction the head is turned. (See *Testing for absent doll's eye sign.*)

The absence of doll's eye sign indicates injury to the midbrain or pons, involving cranial nerves III and VI. It typically accompanies coma caused by lesions of the cerebellum and brain stem. This sign isn't usually reliable in a conscious patient because he can control eye movements voluntarily. Absent doll's eye sign is necessary for a diagnosis of brain death.

A variant of absent doll's eye sign that develops gradually is known as *abnormal doll's eye sign.* Because conjugate eye movement is lost, one eye may move laterally while the other remains fixed or moves in the opposite direction. An abnormal doll's eye sign usually accompanies metabolic coma or increased intracranial pressure (ICP). Associated brain stem dysfunction may be reversible or may progress to deeper coma with absent doll's eye sign.

Assessment

After detecting an absent doll's eye sign, perform a neurologic examination. Evaluate the patient's level of consciousness, using the Glasgow Coma Scale. Note decerebrate or decorticate posture. Examine the pupils for size, equality, and response to light. Check for signs of increased ICP.

Testing for absent doll's eye sign

To evaluate the patient's oculocephalic reflex, hold her upper eyelids open and quickly but gently turn her head from side to side, noting eye movements with each head turn.

With absent doll's eye sign, the eyes remain fixed in midposition.

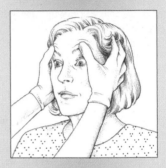

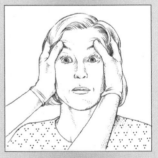

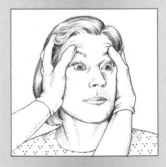

Causes

◈ *Brain stem infarction.* Brain stem infarction causes absent doll's eye sign with coma. It also causes limb paralysis, cranial nerve palsies, variable sensory loss, a positive Babinski's reflex, decerebrate posture, and muscle flaccidity.

◈ *Brain stem tumor.* Absent doll's eye sign accompanies coma in a brain stem tumor. This sign may be preceded by hemiparesis, nystagmus, extraocular nerve palsies, diminished corneal reflex, dysphagia, and drooling.

◈ *Central midbrain infarction.* Accompanying absent doll's eye sign are coma, Weber's syndrome (oculomotor palsy with contralateral hemiplegia), contralateral ataxic tremor, nystagmus, and pupillary abnormalities.

◈ *Pontine hemorrhage.* Absent doll's eye sign and coma develop within minutes with pontine hemorrhage. Other signs include complete paralysis, decerebrate posture, a positive Babinski's reflex, and small, reactive pupils.

◈ *Posterior fossa hematoma.* A subdural hematoma at the posterior fossa typically causes absent doll's eye sign and coma. These signs may be preceded by headache, vomiting, drowsiness, confusion, unequal pupils, dysphagia, cranial nerve palsies, a stiff neck, and cerebellar ataxia.

Drooling

Drooling—the flow of saliva from the mouth—results from a failure to swallow or retain saliva or from excess salivation. Drooling may stem from facial muscle paralysis or weakness that prevents mouth closure, from neuromuscular disorders or local pain that causes dysphagia or, less commonly, from the effects of drugs or toxins that induce salivation. Because it signals an inability to handle secretions, drooling warns of potential aspiration.

Assessment

If you observe the patient drooling, first determine the amount. Is it scant or copious? When did it begin? Ask the patient if his pillow is wet in the morning. Ask about sore throat and difficulty swallowing, chewing, speaking, or breathing. Have the patient describe pain or stiffness in the face and neck and muscle weakness in the face and extremities. Ask about changes in vision, hearing, and sense of taste. Has the patient recently had a cold or other infection? Was he recently bitten by an animal or exposed to pesticides? Obtain a complete drug history.

Next, perform a physical examination. Take the patient's vital signs. Inspect for circumoral irritation, signs of facial paralysis or abnormal expression, mouth and neck swelling, throat edema and redness, and tonsil exudate. Note foul breath odor. Examine the tongue for bilateral furrowing. Look for frontal baldness. Carefully assess any bite or puncture marks. Observe the patient's ability to swallow. Assess his gag reflex and speech.

Causes

◆ *Bell's palsy.* With Bell's palsy, drooling accompanies the gradual onset of facial hemiplegia. The affected side of the face sags and is expressionless, the nasolabial fold flattens, and the palpebral fissure widens. The patient usually complains of pain in or behind the ear. Other cardinal signs and symptoms include unilateral diminished or absent corneal reflex, Bell's phenomenon (upward deviation of the eye with attempt at lid closure), and partial loss of taste or abnormal taste sensation.

◆ *Esophageal tumor.* With an esophageal tumor, weight loss and progressively severe dysphagia typically precede copious and persistent drooling.

◆ *Ludwig's angina.* In Ludwig's angina, moderate to copious drooling stems from dysphagia and local swelling of the floor of the mouth, causing tongue displacement. Submandibular swelling of the neck may also occur.

◆ *Myotonic dystrophy.* Facial weakness and a sagging jaw account for constant drooling with myotonic dystrophy. Other findings include myotonia (delayed relaxation of a muscle after strong contraction), muscle wasting, cataracts, testicular atrophy, frontal baldness, ptosis, and a nasal, monotone voice.

◆ *Peritonsillar abscess.* A severe sore throat causes dysphagia with moderate to copious drooling with a peritonsillar abscess. Other findings include high fever, rancid breath, and enlarged, reddened, edematous tonsils that may be covered by a soft, gray exudate. Palpation may reveal cervical lymphadenopathy.

◼ *Pesticide poisoning.* Toxic effects of pesticides may include excess salivation with drooling. Other effects are diaphoresis, nausea and vomiting, involuntary urination and defecation, blurred vision, miosis, increased lacrimation, fasciculations, weakness, flaccid paralysis, signs of respiratory distress, and coma.

◼ *Rabies.* When rabies advances to the brain stem, it produces drooling or "foaming at the mouth." Drooling stems from excessive salivation, facial palsy, or extremely painful pharyngeal spasms that prohibit swallowing. Rabies is accompanied by hydrophobia in about 50% of cases.

◆ *Seizures (generalized).* Generalized seizures are tonic-clonic muscular reactions that cause excessive salivation. They are accompanied by loss of consciousness and cyanosis. The patient may also drool during the postictal state.

Dysarthria

Dysarthria (poorly articulated speech) is characterized by slurring and labored, irregular rhythm. It may be accompanied by a nasal voice tone caused by palate weakness and results from degenerative neurologic and cerebellar disorders and damage to the brain stem that affects cranial nerves IX, X, or XII. Asking the patient to produce a few simple sounds and words, such as "ba," "sh," and "cat," will confirm dysarthria.

Assessment

Explore the patient's dysarthria completely. When did it begin? Has it gotten better? Ask if dysarthria worsens during the day. Ask about difficulty swallowing, double vision, and a history of seizures. Then obtain a drug and alcohol history.

Check the patient's vital signs, especially noting respiratory rate and depth. Compare muscle strength and tone in the limbs and evaluate tactile sensation. Test deep tendon reflexes (DTRs) and note gait ataxia. Assess cerebellar function by observing rapid alternating movement, which should be smooth and coordinated. Then test visual fields and check for signs of facial weakness such as ptosis.

Causes

◆ *Alcoholic cerebellar degeneration.* Alcoholic cerebellar degeneration commonly causes chronic, progressive dysarthria along with ataxia, diplopia, ophthalmoplegia (paralysis of one or more of the ocular muscles), hypotension, and an altered mental status.

◆ *Amyotrophic lateral sclerosis (ALS).* Dysarthria occurs when ALS affects the bulbar nuclei. It may worsen as the disease progresses. Other findings include dysphagia, difficulty breathing, muscle atrophy and weakness, fasciculations, spasticity, hyperactive DTRs in the legs and, occasionally, excessive drooling.

◆ *Basilar artery insufficiency.* Basilar artery insufficiency causes random, brief episodes of dysarthria. Other findings include diplopia, vertigo, facial numbness, ataxia, paresis, and visual field loss. Any of these findings may last for minutes or hours.

◆ *Botulism.* The hallmark of botulism is acute cranial nerve dysfunction causing dysarthria, dysphagia, diplopia, and ptosis. Early findings include dry mouth, sore throat, weakness, vomiting, and diarrhea.

◆ *Mercury poisoning.* Chronic mercury poisoning causes progressive dysarthria accompanied by weakness, fatigue, depression, lethargy, irritability, confusion, ataxia, and tremors.

◆ *Multiple sclerosis (MS).* The patient with MS displays dysarthria accompanied by blurred or double vision, dysphagia, ataxia, and intention tremor. Exacerbations and remissions of these signs and symptoms are common.

◆ *Myasthenia gravis.* Myasthenia gravis causes dysarthria associated with a nasal voice tone. Typically, the dysarthria worsens during the day and may temporarily improve with short rest periods. Other findings include dysphagia, drooling, facial weakness, diplopia, ptosis, dyspnea, and muscle weakness.

◆ *Olivopontocerebellar degeneration.* With olivopontocerebellar degeneration, dysarthria accompanies cerebellar ataxia and spasticity.

◆ *Parkinson's disease.* Parkinson's disease produces dysarthria and a monotone voice. It also produces muscle rigidity, bradykinesia, involuntary tremor usually beginning in the fingers, difficulty walking, muscle weakness, and a stooped posture. Other findings include masklike facies, dysphagia and, occasionally, drooling.

◆ *Shy-Drager syndrome.* Marked by chronic orthostatic hypotension, Shy-Drager syndrome eventually causes dysarthria as well as cerebellar ataxia, bradykinesia, masklike facies, and dementia.

◪ *Stroke (brain stem).* A brain stem stroke is characterized by the triad of dysarthria, dysphonia, and dysphagia. Dysarthria is most severe at the stroke's onset. It may lessen or disappear with rehabilitation and training.

◪ *Stroke (cerebral).* A massive bilateral stroke causes dysarthria that's most severe at onset. Dysarthria is accompanied by dysphagia, drooling, dysphonia, bilateral hemianopsia, and aphasia.

Dysmenorrhea

Dysmenorrhea (painful menstruation) affects more than 50% of menstruating women; in fact, it's the leading cause of lost time from school and work among women of childbearing age. Dysmenorrhea may involve sharp, intermittent pain or dull, aching pain. It's usually characterized by mild to severe cramping or colicky pain in the pelvis or lower abdomen. The pain may radiate to the thighs and lower sacrum. It may precede menstruation by several days or may accompany it. The pain gradually subsides as bleeding tapers off. (See *Relief for dysmenorrhea,* page 224.)

Dysmenorrhea commonly results from endometriosis and other pelvic

Relief for dysmenorrhea

To relieve cramping and other symptoms caused by primary dysmenorrhea or an intrauterine device, the patient may receive a prostaglandin inhibitor, such as aspirin, ibuprofen (Motrin), indomethacin (Indocin), or naproxen (Naprosyn). These nonsteroidal anti-inflammatory drugs block prostaglandin synthesis early in the inflammatory reaction, thereby inhibiting prostaglandin action at receptor sites. These drugs also have analgesic and antipyretic effects.

Make sure that you and the patient are informed about the adverse effects and cautions associated with these drugs.

Adverse effects

Alert the patient to possible adverse effects of prostaglandin inhibitors. Central nervous system effects include dizziness, headache, and vision disturbances. GI effects include nausea, vomiting, heartburn, and diarrhea.

Advise the patient to take the drug with milk or after meals to reduce gastric irritation.

Contraindications

Because prostaglandin inhibitors are potentially teratogenic, be sure to rule out the possibility of pregnancy before starting therapy. Advise the patient who suspects she's pregnant to delay therapy until menses begins.

Other cautions

If the patient has cardiac decompensation, hypertension, renal dysfunction, an ulcer, or a coagulation defect (and is receiving ongoing anticoagulant therapy), use caution when administering a prostaglandin inhibitor. Because a patient who's hypersensitive to aspirin may also be hypersensitive to other prostaglandin inhibitors, watch for signs of gastric ulceration and bleeding.

disorders. Stress and poor health may aggravate dysmenorrhea; rest and mild exercise may relieve it.

Assessment

If the patient complains of dysmenorrhea, have her describe it fully. Is it intermittent or continuous? Sharp, cramping, or aching? Ask where the pain is located and whether it's bilateral. When does the pain begin and end? When is it severe? Does it radiate to the back? How long has she been experiencing the pain? Ask about nausea and vomiting, altered bowel or urinary habits, bloating, water retention, pelvic or rectal pressure, and unusual fatigue, irritability, or depression. Obtain a menstrual and sexual history. Note her method of contraception, and ask about a history of pelvic infection.

Does she have signs and symptoms of urinary system obstruction or a sexually transmitted disease?

Next, perform a focused physical examination. Check the patient's vital signs, noting fever and accompanying chills. Inspect the abdomen for distention. Palpate for tenderness and masses. Note costovertebral angle tenderness.

Causes

◆ *Adenomyosis.* In adenomyosis, endometrial tissue invades the myometrium, resulting in severe dysmenorrhea with pain radiating to the back or rectum, menorrhagia, and a symmetrically enlarged, globular uterus.
◆ *Cervical stenosis.* Cervical stenosis causes dysmenorrhea and scant or absent menstrual flow.

◆ *Endometriosis.* Endometriosis typically produces steady, aching pain that begins before menses and peaks at the height of menstrual flow; however, the pain may also occur between menstrual periods. Other findings include premenstrual spotting, dyspareunia, infertility, and painful defecation.

◆ *Pelvic inflammatory disease.* Pelvic inflammatory disease produces dysmenorrhea accompanied by fever; malaise; foul smelling, purulent vaginal discharge; menorrhagia; dyspareunia; severe abdominal pain; and diarrhea.

◆ *Premenstrual syndrome (PMS).* The cramping pain of PMS usually begins with menstrual flow and persists for several hours or days, diminishing with decreasing flow.

◆ *Uterine leiomyomas.* Uterine leiomyomas may cause constant or intermittent lower abdominal pain that worsens with menses. Other findings include backache, constipation, menorrhagia, and urinary frequency or retention.

Dyspepsia

Dyspepsia refers to an uncomfortable fullness after meals that's associated with nausea, belching, heartburn and, possibly, cramping and abdominal distention. Frequently aggravated by spicy, fatty, or high-fiber foods and by excessive caffeine intake, dyspepsia without other pathology indicates impaired digestive function. Other causes include emotional upset and cardiac, pulmonary, and renal disorders. It usually occurs a few hours after eating. Its severity depends on the amount and type of food eaten and on GI motility.

Assessment

If the patient complains of dyspepsia, ask him to describe it in detail. How often and when does it occur? Do drugs or activities relieve or aggravate it? Has he had nausea, vomiting, melena, hematemesis, a cough, or chest pain? Ask if he's taking prescription drugs and if he has recently had surgery. Does he have a history of renal, cardiovascular, or pulmonary disease? Ask if he's experiencing an unusual or overwhelming amount of emotional stress.

Focus the physical examination on the abdomen. Inspect for distention, ascites, scars, obvious hernias, jaundice, and bruising. Auscultate for bowel sounds and palpate and percuss the abdomen, noting tenderness, pain, organ enlargement, or tympany. Finally, examine other body systems.

Causes

◆ *Cholelithiasis.* Dyspepsia may occur with gallstones, usually after eating fatty foods.

◆ *Cirrhosis.* With cirrhosis, dyspepsia varies in intensity and duration and is relieved by taking an antacid. Other GI findings include anorexia, flatulence, abdominal distention, and epigastric or right upper quadrant pain. Skin changes include severe pruritus, extreme dryness, easy bruising, and lesions, such as telangiectasis and palmar erythema.

◆ *Duodenal ulcer.* A primary symptom of a duodenal ulcer, dyspepsia ranges from a vague feeling of fullness or pressure to a boring or aching sensation in the middle or right epigastrium. It usually occurs 1½ to 3 hours after a meal and is relieved by eating food or taking an antacid.

◆ *Gastric dilation (acute).* Epigastric fullness is an early symptom of gastric dilation. Other findings include nausea, vomiting, upper abdominal distention, and signs and symptoms of dehydration and electrolyte imbalance.

◆ *Gastric ulcer.* Typically, dyspepsia and heartburn after eating occur early in a patient with a gastric ulcer. However, the cardinal symptom is epigastric pain that may not be relieved by eating food.

◆ *Gastritis (chronic).* With chronic gastritis, dyspepsia is aggravated by spicy foods or excessive caffeine. It's relieved by antacids and lessened by smaller, more frequent meals.

◆ *GI cancer.* GI cancer usually produces chronic dyspepsia. Other findings include anorexia, fatigue, jaundice, melena, hematemesis, constipation, and abdominal pain.

◆ *Heart failure.* Common with right-sided heart failure, transient dyspepsia may occur with chest tightness and a constant ache or sharp pain in the right upper quadrant.

◆ *Hepatitis.* Dyspepsia occurs with hepatitis during the preicteric and icteric phases. Jaundice marks the onset of the icteric phase. As jaundice clears, dyspepsia and other GI effects also diminish.

◆ *Hiatal hernia.* With hiatal hernia, dyspepsia is a result of the lower portion of the esophagus and the upper portion of the stomach rising into the chest when abdominal pressure increases.

◼ *Pulmonary embolism.* With pulmonary embolism, dyspepsia may occur as an oppressive, severe, substernal discomfort. Other findings include hemoptysis, syncope, cyanosis, jugular vein distention, and hypotension.

◆ *Pulmonary tuberculosis (TB).* Vague dyspepsia may occur with pulmonary TB along with anorexia, malaise, and weight loss. Other common findings include high fever, night sweats, and a productive cough.

◆ *Uremia.* Of the many GI complaints associated with uremia, dyspepsia may be the earliest and most important. Others include anorexia, nausea, vomiting, bloating, diarrhea, abdominal cramps, epigastric pain, and weight gain.

Dysphagia

Dysphagia—difficulty swallowing—is classified by the phase of swallowing it affects. (See *Classifying dysphagia.*) It's the most common—and sometimes the only—symptom of esophageal disorders. Dysphagia increases the risk of choking and aspiration and may lead to malnutrition and dehydration.

Assessment

If the patient's dysphagia suggests an airway obstruction, institute emergency procedures. Otherwise, begin a health history. Ask the patient if swallowing is painful. Have him point to where dysphagia feels most intense. Are solids or liquids more difficult to swallow? Is swallowing easier if he changes position? Ask if he has recently experienced vomiting, anorexia, regurgitation, weight loss, hoarseness, dyspnea, or a cough.

To evaluate the patient's swallowing reflex, place your finger along his thyroid notch and instruct him to swallow. If you feel his larynx rise, the reflex is intact. Check his gag reflex and assess the patient's mouth for dry mucous membranes and thick, sticky secretions. Also assess the patient for disorientation, which may make him neglect to swallow.

Causes

◆ *Achalasia.* Most common in patients ages 20 to 40, achalasia produces phase 3 dysphagia for solids and liquids. The dysphagia develops gradually and may be precipitated or exacerbated by stress.

Classifying dysphagia

Because swallowing occurs in three distinct phases, dysphagia can be classified by the phase that it affects. Each phase suggests a specific pathology for dysphagia.

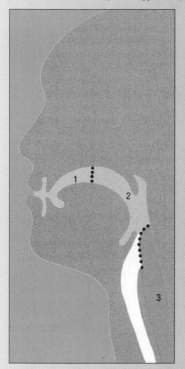

Phase 1

Swallowing begins in the transfer phase with chewing and moistening of food with saliva. The tongue presses against the hard palate to transfer the chewed food to the back of the throat; cranial nerve V then stimulates the swallowing reflex. Phase 1 dysphagia typically results from a neuromuscular disorder.

Phase 2

In the transport phase, the soft palate closes against the pharyngeal wall to prevent nasal regurgitation. At the same time, the larynx rises and the vocal cords close to keep food out of the lungs; breathing stops momentarily as the throat muscles constrict to move food into the esophagus. Phase 2 dysphagia usually indicates spasm or cancer.

Phase 3

Peristalsis and gravity work together in the entrance phase to move food through the esophageal sphincter and into the stomach. Phase 3 dysphagia results from lower esophageal narrowing by diverticula, esophagitis, and other disorders.

◈ *Airway obstruction.* Signs of respiratory distress, such as crowing and stridor, mark upper airway obstruction. Phase 2 dysphagia occurs with gagging and dysphonia. When hemorrhage obstructs the trachea, dysphagia is usually painless and rapid in onset. When inflammation causes the obstruction, dysphagia may be painful and develop slowly.

◆ *Amyotrophic lateral sclerosis (ALS).* ALS causes dysphagia, muscle weakness and atrophy, dysarthria, dyspnea, shallow respirations, slurred speech, and emotional lability.

◆ *Bulbar paralysis.* With bulbar paralysis, phase 1 dysphagia occurs along with drooling, difficulty chewing, dysarthria, and nasal regurgitation. Dysphagia for solids and liquids is painful and progressive.

◆ *Esophageal cancer.* Phase 2 and 3 dysphagia is the earliest and most common symptom of esophageal cancer. Typically, the cancer begins painlessly, accompanied by rapid weight loss. As it advances, the cancer becomes painful and constant.

◆ *Esophageal diverticulum.* Esophageal diverticulum causes phase 3 dysphagia when the diverticulum obstructs the esophagus. Other findings include food regurgitation, a chronic cough, hoarseness, chest pain, and halitosis.

◆ *Esophageal obstruction by a foreign body.* This condition causes a sudden onset of phase 2 or 3 dysphagia, gagging, coughing, and esophageal pain. Dyspnea may occur if the obstruction compresses the trachea.

◆ *Esophageal spasm.* The most striking symptoms of esophageal spasm are phase 2 dysphagia for solids and liquids and dull or squeezing substernal chest pain. Drinking a glass of water may relieve the pain.

◆ *Esophageal stricture.* Usually caused by chemical ingestion or scar tissue, esophageal stricture causes phase 3 dysphagia. Drooling, tachypnea, and gagging may also be evident.

◆ *Esophagitis.* Corrosive esophagitis, resulting from ingestion of alkali or acids, causes severe phase 3 dysphagia that's aggravated by swallowing. Candidal esophagitis causes phase 2 dysphagia and a sore throat. With reflux esophagitis, phase 3 dysphagia is a late symptom that usually occurs with stricture development.

◆ *Gastric carcinoma.* Infiltration of the cardia or esophagus by gastric carcinoma causes phase 3 dysphagia.

◆ *Laryngeal cancer (extrinsic).* Phase 2 dysphagia and dyspnea develop late in laryngeal cancer.

◆ *Lead poisoning.* Painless, progressive dysphagia may result from lead poisoning. Related findings include a lead line on the gums, a metallic taste, papilledema, ocular palsy, footdrop or wristdrop, and signs of hemolytic anemia.

◆ *Myasthenia gravis.* Fatigue and progressive muscle weakness characterize myasthenia gravis and account for painless phase 1 dysphagia and, possibly, choking.

◆ *Oral cavity tumor.* Painful phase 1 dysphagia develops along with hoarseness and ulcerating lesions.

◆ *Plummer-Vinson syndrome.* Plummer-Vinson syndrome causes phase 3 dysphagia for solids in some women with severe iron deficiency anemia.

◆ *Rabies.* Severe phase 2 dysphagia for liquids results from pharyngeal muscle spasms occurring late with rabies.

◆ *Tetanus.* With tetanus, phase 1 dysphagia usually develops about 1 week after the patient receives a puncture wound.

Dyspnea

Dyspnea is the sensation of difficult or uncomfortable breathing and is typically a symptom of cardiopulmonary dysfunction. Its severity varies greatly and may be unrelated to the severity of the underlying cause. Most people normally experience dyspnea when they exert themselves with the severity depending on their physical condition. In a healthy person, rest quickly relieves dyspnea. Pathologic causes of dyspnea include pulmonary, cardiac, neuromuscular, and allergic disorders. It may also be caused by anxiety.

Assessment

If the patient complains of shortness of breath, quickly look for signs of respiratory distress, such as tachypnea, cyanosis, restlessness, and accessory muscle use. Prepare to administer oxygen by nasal cannula, mask, or endotracheal tube.

If the patient can answer questions without increasing his distress, take a complete history. Ask if the shortness of breath began suddenly or gradually. Is it constant or intermittent? Does it occur during activity or while at rest? Can he identify what aggravates or alleviates the dyspnea? Does he have a productive or nonproductive cough or chest pain? Ask about recent trauma and note a history of upper respiratory tract infection, deep vein phlebitis, or other disorders. Ask the patient if he smokes or is exposed to toxic fumes or irritants at work. Find out if he also has orthopnea, paroxysmal nocturnal dyspnea, or progressive fatigue.

During the physical examination, look for signs of chronic dyspnea such as accessory muscle hypertrophy (especially in the shoulders and neck). Also look for pursed-lip exhalation, clubbing, peripheral edema, barrel chest, diaphoresis, and jugular vein distention. Check the patient's vital signs and auscultate for crackles, abnormal heart sounds or rhythms, egophony, bronchophony, and whispered pectoriloquy. Finally, palpate the abdomen for hepatomegaly and assess the patient for edema.

Causes

◤ *Acute respiratory distress syndrome (ARDS).* ARDS is a form of noncardiogenic pulmonary edema that usually produces acute dyspnea as the first complaint, then develops into progressive respiratory distress with restlessness, anxiety, decreased mental acuity, tachycardia, and crackles and rhonchi in both lung fields.

◆ *Amyotrophic lateral sclerosis (ALS).* ALS causes the slow onset of dyspnea that worsens with time. Other findings include dysphagia, dysarthria, muscle weakness and atrophy, tachypnea, and emotional lability.

◤ *Anthrax (inhalation).* Dyspnea is a symptom of the second stage of anthrax, along with fever, stridor, and hypotension (death usually occurs within 24 hours).

◤ *Aspiration of a foreign body.* Acute dyspnea marks aspiration of a foreign body, along with paroxysmal intercostal, suprasternal, and substernal retractions.

◆ *Asthma.* Acute dyspneic attacks occur with asthma, along with audible wheezing, accessory muscle use, nasal flaring, intercostal and supraclavicular retractions, tachypnea, prolonged expiration, and flushing or cyanosis.

◆ *Cor pulmonale.* With cor pulmonale, chronic dyspnea begins gradually with exertion and progressively worsens until it occurs even at rest. Underlying cardiac or pulmonary disease is usually present.

◆ *Emphysema.* Emphysema is a chronic disorder that gradually causes progressive exertional dyspnea. The patient usually has a history of smoking, an alpha$_1$-antitrypsin deficiency, or exposure to an occupational irritant.

◤ *Flail chest.* With flail chest, sudden dyspnea results from multiple rib fractures and is accompanied by paradoxical chest movement, severe chest pain, hypotension, tachypnea, tachycardia, and cyanosis.

◆ *Heart failure.* Dyspnea usually develops gradually in patients with heart failure. Chronic paroxysmal nocturnal dyspnea, orthopnea, tachypnea, dependent peripheral edema, a dry cough, and loss of mental acuity may occur.

◤ *Inhalation injury.* Dyspnea may develop suddenly or gradually after the inhalation of chemicals or hot gases. Increasing hoarseness, a persistent cough, sooty or bloody sputum, and oropharyngeal edema may also be present.

◆ *Myasthenia gravis.* Myasthenia gravis causes bouts of dyspnea as the respiratory muscles weaken.

◼ *Myocardial infarction (MI).* With MI, sudden dyspnea occurs with crushing substernal chest pain that may radiate to the back, neck, jaw, and arms.

◆ *Plague* (Yersinia pestis). Among the symptoms of the pneumonic form of plague are dyspnea, a productive cough, chest pain, tachypnea, hemoptysis, increasing respiratory distress, and cardiopulmonary insufficiency.

◆ *Pleural effusion.* Dyspnea develops slowly and becomes progressively worse with pleural effusion. Initial findings include a pleural friction rub accompanied by pleuritic pain that worsens with coughing or deep breathing.

◆ *Pneumonia.* With pneumonia, dyspnea occurs suddenly, usually accompanied by fever, shaking chills, pleuritic chest pain that worsens with deep inspiration, and a productive cough.

◆ *Pneumothorax.* Pneumothorax causes acute dyspnea unrelated to the severity of the pain. Sudden, stabbing chest pain may radiate to the arms, face, back, or abdomen.

◼ *Pulmonary edema.* Pulmonary edema causes acute dyspnea and is commonly preceded by signs of heart failure, such as jugular vein distention and orthopnea.

◼ *Pulmonary embolism.* Acute dyspnea that's usually accompanied by sudden pleuritic chest pain characterizes pulmonary embolism. Related findings include tachycardia, a pleural friction rub, diffuse wheezing, and diaphoresis.

◼ *Severe acute respiratory syndrome (SARS).* SARS generally begins with a fever and its severity is highly variable. Symptoms include headache; malaise; a dry, nonproductive cough; and dyspnea.

◼ *Shock.* Dyspnea arises suddenly and worsens progressively in shock. Related findings include severe hypotension, tachypnea, tachycardia, decreased peripheral pulses, restlessness, anxiety, and cool, clammy skin.

◆ *Tuberculosis (TB).* With TB, dyspnea commonly occurs with chest pain, crackles, and a productive cough. Other findings include night sweats, fever, anorexia, weight loss, vague dyspepsia, and palpitations on mild exertion.

◆ *Tularemia.* Also known as *rabbit fever,* tularemia causes dyspnea along with fever, chills, headache, generalized myalgia, a nonproductive cough, pleuritic chest pain, and empyema.

Dysuria

Dysuria—painful or difficult urination—is commonly accompanied by urinary frequency, urgency, or hesitancy. This symptom usually reflects lower urinary tract infection—a common disorder, especially in women. The onset of pain provides clues to its cause. For example, pain just before voiding usually indicates bladder irritation or distention, whereas pain at the start of urination typically results from bladder outlet irritation. Pain at the end of voiding may signal bladder spasms. Dysuria in women may indicate vaginal candidiasis.

Assessment

If the patient complains of dysuria, have him describe its severity and location. When did he first notice it? Did anything precipitate it? Does anything aggravate or alleviate it? Next, ask about previous urinary or genital tract infections. Also ask if he has a history of intestinal disease. Ask the female patient about menstrual disorders and the use of products, such as bubble bath salts, feminine deodorants, contraceptive gels, or perineal lotions that irritate the urinary tract. Also ask her about vaginal discharge or pruritus.

During the physical examination, inspect the urethral meatus for discharge, irritation, or other abnormalities. A pelvic or rectal examination may be necessary.

Causes

◆ *Appendicitis.* Occasionally, appendicitis causes dysuria that persists throughout voiding and is accompanied by bladder tenderness.

◆ *Bladder cancer.* Bladder cancer, a predominantly male disorder, causes dysuria throughout voiding. It's a late symptom associated with urinary frequency and urgency, nocturia, and hematuria and perineal, back, or flank pain.

◆ *Cystitis.* Dysuria throughout voiding is common in all types of cystitis, as are urinary frequency, nocturia, straining to void, and hematuria.

◆ *Paraurethral gland inflammation.* Dysuria throughout voiding occurs with urinary frequency and urgency, a diminished urine stream, mild perineal pain and, occasionally, hematuria.

◆ *Prostatitis.* Acute prostatitis commonly causes dysuria throughout or toward the end of voiding as well as diminished urine stream, urinary frequency and urgency, hematuria, and suprapubic fullness. With chronic prostatitis, urethral narrowing causes dysuria throughout voiding.

◆ *Pyelonephritis (acute).* Pyelonephritis causes dysuria throughout voiding as well as hematuria, urinary urgency, and frequency. Other findings include a persistent high fever with chills, costovertebral angle tenderness, and unilateral or bilateral flank pain.

◆ *Reiter syndrome.* Reiter syndrome is a predominantly male disorder in which dysuria occurs 1 to 2 weeks after sexual contact. Initially, the patient

has a mucopurulent discharge, urinary urgency and frequency, meatal swelling and redness, suprapubic pain, anorexia, weight loss, and a low-grade fever.

◆ *Urinary obstruction.* Outflow obstruction by urethral strictures or calculi produces dysuria throughout voiding. Other findings include a diminished urine stream, frequency, urgency, and a sensation of fullness or bloating in the lower abdomen or groin.

◆ *Vaginitis.* Characteristically, dysuria occurs throughout voiding with vaginitis, as urine touches inflamed or ulcerated labia. Other findings in vaginitis include urinary frequency and urgency, nocturia, hematuria, perineal pain, and vaginal discharge and odor.

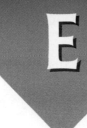

Earache

Earaches usually result from disorders of the external and middle ear associated with infection, obstruction, or trauma. Their severity ranges from a feeling of fullness or blockage to deep, boring pain. Earaches can be intermittent or continuous and may develop suddenly or gradually.

Assessment

Ask the patient to characterize his earache. How long has he had it? Is it intermittent or continuous? Is it painful or slightly annoying? Can he localize the site of ear pain? Does he have pain in other areas such as the jaw? Does he experience hearing loss? Ask about recent ear injury or other trauma. Does swimming or showering trigger ear discomfort? Is discomfort associated with itching? If so, find out where the itching is most intense and when it began. Ask about ear drainage and, if present, have the patient characterize it. Does he hear noise in his ears? Ask about dizziness or vertigo. Does the dizziness or vertigo worsen when he changes position? Does he have difficulty swallowing, hoarseness, neck pain, or pain when he opens his mouth? Ask if he has had a head cold or recent problems with his eyes, mouth, teeth, jaw,

sinuses, or throat. Find out if he has flown in an airplane, been to a high-altitude location, or been scuba diving.

Begin your physical examination by inspecting the external ear for redness, drainage, swelling, or deformity. Then apply pressure to the mastoid process and tragus to elicit tenderness. Using an otoscope, examine the external auditory canal for lesions, bleeding or discharge, impacted cerumen, foreign bodies, tenderness, or swelling. Examine the tympanic membrane. Look for tympanic membrane landmarks: the cone of light, umbo, pars tensa, and the handle and short process of the malleus. (See *Using an otoscope correctly*.) Perform the watch tick, whispered voice, Rinne, and Weber's tests to assess for hearing loss.

Causes

◆ *Abscess (extradural)*. Severe earache accompanied by persistent ipsilateral headache, malaise, and a recurrent mild fever characterize an abscess, which is a serious complication of middle ear infection.

◆ *Barotrauma (acute)*. Earache associated with barotrauma ranges from mild pressure to severe pain. Tympanic membrane ecchymosis or bleeding into the tympanic cavity may occur. The eardrum usually isn't perforated.

Using an otoscope correctly

When the patient reports an earache, use an otoscope to inspect ear structures closely. Follow these techniques to obtain the best view and ensure patient safety.

Child younger than age 3

To inspect an infant's or a young child's ear, grasp the lower part of the auricle and pull it down and back to straighten the upward S-curve of the external canal. Then gently insert the speculum into the canal no more than ½" (1.3 cm).

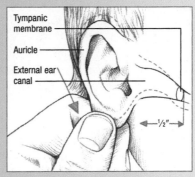

Tympanic membrane
Auricle
External ear canal
½"

Adult

To inspect an adult's ear, grasp the upper part of the auricle and pull it up and back to straighten the external canal. Then insert the speculum about 1" (2.5 cm). Also use this technique for children ages 3 and older.

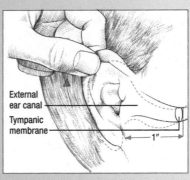

External ear canal
Tympanic membrane
1"

◆ *Cerumen impaction.* Impacted cerumen may cause a sensation of blockage or fullness in the ear. Additional findings include partial hearing loss, itching and, possibly, dizziness.

◆ *Herpes zoster oticus (Ramsay Hunt syndrome).* Herpes zoster oticus causes burning or stabbing ear pain commonly associated with ear vesicles. The patient also complains of hearing loss and vertigo.

◆ *Keratosis obturans.* Mild ear pain along with otorrhea and tinnitus is common with keratosis obturans. Inspection reveals a white glistening plug obstructing the external meatus.

◆ *Mastoiditis (acute).* Mastoiditis causes a dull ache behind the ear accompanied by a low-grade fever. The eardrum appears dull and edematous and may perforate. A purulent discharge may be seen in the external canal.

◆ *Ménière's disease.* Ménière's disease is an inner ear disorder that can produce a sensation of fullness in the affected ear. Its classic effects, however, include severe vertigo, tinnitus, and sensorineural hearing loss.

◆ *Otitis externa.* Earache characterizes acute and malignant otitis externa. Acute otitis externa begins with mild to moderate ear pain that occurs with tragus manipulation. Malignant otitis externa abruptly causes ear pain that's aggravated by moving the auricle or tragus.

◆ *Otitis media (acute).* Otitis media is middle ear inflammation that may be serous or suppurative. Acute serous otitis media may cause a feeling of fullness in the ear, hearing loss, and a vague sensation of top-heaviness. Severe, deep, throbbing ear pain along with hearing loss and fever characterize acute suppurative otitis media. The pain increases steadily over several hours or days and may be aggravated by pressure on the mastoid antrum. Chronic otitis media usually isn't painful except during exacerbations. Persistent pain and discharge from the ear suggest osteomyelitis of the skull base or cancer.

Edema, generalized

A common sign in severely ill patients, generalized edema is the excessive accumulation of interstitial fluid throughout the body. Its severity varies widely. Slight edema may be difficult to detect, especially if the patient is obese, whereas massive edema is immediately apparent. Generalized edema is typically chronic and progressive. It may result from cardiac, renal, endocrine, or hepatic disorders or from severe burns, malnutrition, or the effects of certain drugs and treatments. Common factors responsible for edema are hypoalbuminemia and excess sodium ingestion or retention, both of which influence plasma osmotic pressure. (See *Understanding fluid balance.*) Cyclic edema

associated with increased aldosterone secretion may occur in premenopausal women.

Assessment

Determine the location and severity of edema including the degree of pitting. (See *Edema: Pitting or nonpitting?* page 236.) Obtain a complete medical history. Note when the edema began. Does it move throughout the course of the day—for example, from the upper extremities to the lower? Is the edema worse in the morning or at the end of the day? Is it affected by position changes? Is it accompanied by shortness of breath or pain in the arms or legs? Find out how much weight the patient has gained. Has his urine output changed? Next, ask about the patient's medical history. Have him describe his diet so you can determine whether he suffers from protein malnutrition.

Begin the physical examination by comparing the patient's arms and legs for symmetrical edema. Also note ecchymoses and cyanosis. Next, assess the back, sacrum, and hips of the bedridden patient for dependent edema. Palpate peripheral pulses, noting whether the hands and feet feel cold. Finally, perform a complete cardiac and respiratory assessment.

Causes

◆ *Angioneurotic edema or angioedema.* Angioneurotic edema and angioedema are recurrent attacks of acute, painless, nonpitting edema involving the skin and mucous membranes. These attacks are caused by a food or drug allergy or emotional stress. They may also be hereditary.

▪ *Burns.* Edema and associated tissue damage vary with the severity of the burn. Severe generalized edema (4 +)

Understanding fluid balance

Normally, fluid moves freely between the interstitial and intravascular spaces to maintain homeostasis. Four basic pressures control fluid shifts across the capillary membrane that separates these spaces:
◆ capillary hydrostatic pressure (the internal fluid pressure on the capillary membrane)
◆ interstitial fluid pressure (the external fluid pressure on the capillary membrane)
◆ osmotic pressure (the fluid-attracting pressure from protein concentration within the capillary)
◆ interstitial osmotic pressure (the fluid-attracting pressure from protein concentration outside the capillary).

Here's how these pressures maintain homeostasis. Normally, capillary hydrostatic pressure is greater than plasma osmotic pressure at the capillary's arterial end, forcing fluid out of the capillary. At the capillary's venous end, the reverse is true: The plasma osmotic pressure is greater than the capillary hydrostatic pressure, drawing fluid into the capillary. Normally, the lymphatic system transports excess interstitial fluid back to the intravascular space.

Edema results when this balance is upset by increased capillary permeability, lymphatic obstruction, persistently increased capillary hydrostatic pressure, decreased plasma osmotic or interstitial fluid pressure, or dilation of precapillary sphincters.

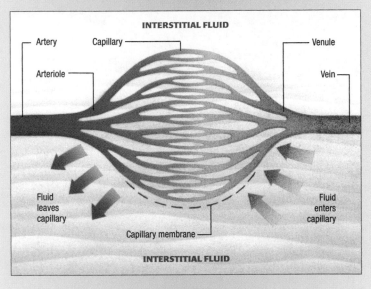

may occur within 2 days of a major burn; localized edema may occur with a less severe burn.
◆ *Drugs.* Drugs that cause sodium retention may aggravate or cause generalized edema. Examples include anti-hypertensives, corticosteroids, androgenic and anabolic steroids, and nonsteroidal anti-inflammatory drugs.
◆ *Heart failure.* Severe, generalized pitting edema—occasionally anasarca—may follow leg edema late in heart fail-

Edema: Pitting or nonpitting?

To differentiate pitting from nonpitting edema, press your finger against a swollen area for 5 seconds and then quickly remove it.

With pitting edema, pressure forces fluid into the underlying tissues, causing an indentation that slowly fills. To determine the severity of pitting edema, estimate the in-

dentation's depth in centimeters: 1+ (1 cm), 2+ (2 cm), 3+ (3 cm), or 4+ (4 cm).

With nonpitting edema, pressure leaves no indentation because fluid has coagulated in the tissues. Typically, the skin feels unusually tight and firm.

PITTING EDEMA (4+)

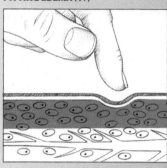

NONPITTING EDEMA

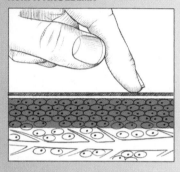

ure. The edema may improve with exercise or by elevating the limbs. Typically, it's worse at the end of the day.

◆ *Malnutrition.* Anasarca in malnutrition may mask dramatic muscle wasting. Malnutrition also typically causes muscle weakness, lethargy, anorexia, diarrhea, apathy, signs of anemia, and dry, wrinkled skin.

◆ *Myxedema.* With myxedema (a severe form of hypothyroidism), generalized nonpitting edema is accompanied by a puffy face, upper eyelid droop, and dry, flaky, inelastic, waxy, pale skin.

◆ *Nephrotic syndrome.* Nephrotic syndrome is characterized by generalized pitting edema; however, it's initially localized around the eyes. With severe cases, anasarca develops, increasing body weight by up to 50%.

◆ *Pericardial effusion.* With pericardial effusion, generalized pitting edema may be most prominent in the arms and legs. It may be accompanied by chest pain, dyspnea, orthopnea, jugular vein distention, dysphagia, and fever.

◆ *Pericarditis (chronic constrictive).* Resembling right-sided heart failure, pericarditis usually begins with pitting edema of the arms and legs that may progress to generalized edema.

◆ *Renal failure.* With acute renal failure, generalized pitting edema occurs as a late sign. With chronic renal failure, edema is less likely to become generalized; its severity depends on the degree of fluid overload.

Edema of the arm

Arm edema signals a localized fluid imbalance between the vascular and interstitial spaces. (See *Understanding fluid balance*, page 235.) It may be unilateral or bilateral and may develop gradually or abruptly. It may be aggravated by immobility and alleviated by arm elevation and exercise. It commonly results from trauma, venous disorders, or toxins.

Assessment

Begin by taking the patient's history. Ask how long his arm has been swollen. Then find out if he also has arm pain, numbness, or tingling. Does exercise or elevating the arm decrease the edema? Ask about any recent arm injury. Also, note recent I.V. therapy, surgery, or radiation therapy for breast cancer.

Determine the edema's severity by comparing the size and symmetry of both arms. Use a tape measure to determine the exact girth. Mark the location where the measurement was obtained to make comparative measurements later. Be sure to note whether the edema is unilateral or bilateral. Test for pitting. (See *Edema: Pitting or nonpitting?*) Examine and compare the color and temperature of both arms. Palpate and compare radial and brachial pulses. Finally, look for arm injuries, tenderness, and decreased sensation or mobility.

Causes

◆ *Arm trauma.* Shortly after a crush injury, severe edema may affect the entire arm. Ecchymoses or superficial bleeding, pain, numbness, and paralysis may occur.

◪ *Burns.* Two days or less after injury, arm burns may cause mild to severe edema, pain, and tissue damage.

◆ *Envenomation.* Envenomation by snakes, aquatic animals, or insects may initially cause edema around the bite or sting that quickly spreads to the entire arm. Pain, erythema, and pruritus at the site are common.

◆ *Superior vena cava syndrome.* Bilateral arm edema usually progresses slowly and is accompanied by facial and neck edema. Dilated veins mark the edematous areas. The patient also complains of headache, vertigo, and vision disturbances.

◆ *Thrombophlebitis.* Thrombophlebitis, which can result from I.V. therapy, may cause arm edema, pain, and warmth. Deep vein thrombophlebitis can also produce cyanosis, fever, chills, and malaise. Superficial thrombophlebitis causes redness, tenderness, and induration along the vein.

◆ *Treatments.* A radical or modified radical mastectomy or axillary lymph node dissection that disrupts lymphatic drainage may cause edema of the entire arm. Radiation therapy for breast cancer may also produce arm edema either immediately after treatment or months later.

Edema of the face

Facial edema refers to either localized swelling—for example, around the eyes—or more generalized swelling that may extend to the neck and upper arms. Occasionally painful, this sign may develop gradually or abruptly. Sometimes, it precedes the onset of peripheral or generalized edema. Facial edema results from disruption of the hydrostatic and osmotic pressures that govern fluid movement among the arteries, veins, and lymphatics. (See *Understanding fluid balance*, page 235.) It

Recognizing angioneurotic edema

Most dramatic in the lips, eyelids, and tongue, angioneurotic edema commonly results from an allergic reaction. It's characterized by the rapid onset of painless, nonpitting, subcutaneous swelling that usually resolves in 1 to 2 days. This type of edema may also involve the hands, feet, genitalia, and viscera; laryngeal edema may cause life-threatening airway obstruction.

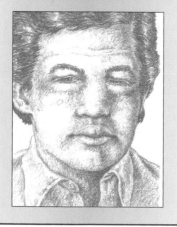

may result from venous, inflammatory, and certain systemic disorders; trauma; allergy; malnutrition; or the effects of certain drugs, tests, and treatments.

Assessment

If the patient has facial edema associated with burns or if he reports recent exposure to an allergen, quickly evaluate his respiratory status. Edema may also affect his upper airway, causing life-threatening obstruction. Assess the patient's respiratory status if you detect audible wheezing, inspiratory stridor,

or other signs of distress. Report your findings immediately.

If the patient isn't in severe distress, take his health history. Ask if facial edema developed suddenly or gradually. Is it more prominent in early morning, or does it worsen through the day? Has the patient gained weight? Has he noticed a change in his urine color or output? His appetite? Take a drug history. Ask about recent facial trauma.

Begin the physical examination by characterizing the edema. Is it localized to one part of the face, or does it affect the entire face or other parts of the body? Is the edema pitting or nonpitting? Grade its severity. (See *Edema: Pitting or nonpitting?* page 236.) Finally, check the patient's vital signs and assess his neurologic status.

Causes

◆ *Allergic reaction.* Facial edema may characterize local allergic reactions and anaphylaxis. With life-threatening anaphylaxis, angioneurotic facial edema may occur with urticaria and flushing. (See *Recognizing angioneurotic edema.*) Airway edema causes hoarseness, stridor, and bronchospasm with dyspnea and tachypnea. A localized reaction produces facial edema, erythema, and urticaria.
◆ *Cavernous sinus thrombosis.* Cavernous sinus thrombosis may begin with unilateral edema that quickly progresses to bilateral edema of the forehead, base of the nose, and eyelids.
◆ *Chalazion.* A chalazion causes localized swelling and tenderness of the affected eyelid, accompanied by a small red lump on the conjunctival surface.
◆ *Conjunctivitis.* Conjunctivitis causes eyelid edema, excessive tearing, and itchy, burning eyes. Inspection reveals a thick purulent discharge, crusty eyelids, and conjunctival injection.

◆ *Dacryoadenitis.* Severe periorbital swelling characterizes dacryoadenitis, which may also cause conjunctival injection, purulent discharge, and temporal pain.

◆ *Dacryocystitis.* Lacrimal sac inflammation causes prominent eyelid edema and constant tearing. In acute cases, pain and tenderness near the tear sac accompany purulent discharge.

◆ *Facial burns.* Burns may cause extensive edema that impairs respiration. Additional findings include singed nasal hairs, red mucosa, sooty sputum, and signs of respiratory distress such as inspiratory stridor.

◆ *Facial trauma.* The extent of edema with facial trauma varies with the type of injury. For example, a contusion may cause localized edema; a nasal or maxillary fracture causes more generalized edema.

◆ *Herpes zoster ophthalmicus (shingles).* With shingles, excessive tearing and a serous discharge usually accompany edematous, red eyelids. Severe unilateral facial pain may occur several days before vesicles erupt.

◆ *Myxedema.* Myxedema eventually causes generalized facial edema, hair loss or coarsening, and waxy, dry skin.

◆ *Nephrotic syndrome.* Periorbital edema is commonly the first sign of nephrotic syndrome and precedes dependent and abdominal edema. Associated findings include weight gain, nausea, anorexia, lethargy, fatigue, and pallor.

◆ *Orbital cellulitis.* The sudden onset of periorbital edema marks orbital cellulitis. Other findings include a purulent discharge, exophthalmos, conjunctival injection, impaired extraocular movements, fever, and extreme orbital pain.

◆ *Preeclampsia.* Edema of the face, hands, and ankles is an early sign of preeclampsia. Other characteristics include excessive weight gain, severe headache, blurred vision, hypertension, and midepigastric pain.

◆ *Rhinitis (allergic).* With rhinitis, paroxysmal sneezing, itchy nose and eyes, and profuse, watery rhinorrhea accompany red, edematous eyelids.

◆ *Sinusitis.* Frontal sinusitis causes edema of the forehead and eyelids. Maxillary sinusitis produces edema in the maxillary area as well as malaise, gingival swelling, and trismus.

◆ *Superior vena cava syndrome.* Superior vena cava syndrome gradually produces facial and neck edema accompanied by thoracic or jugular vein distention. It also causes central nervous system symptoms.

◆ *Trachoma.* With trachoma, edema affects the eyelid and conjunctiva and is accompanied by eye pain, excessive tearing, photophobia, and eye discharge.

◆ *Trichinosis.* Trichinosis is a relatively rare infectious disorder that causes the sudden onset of eyelid edema accompanied by fever, conjunctivitis, muscle pain, itching and burning skin, sweating, skin lesions, and delirium.

Edema of the leg

Leg edema is a common sign that results when excess interstitial fluid accumulates in one or both legs. It may affect just the foot and ankle or extend to the thigh. It may be slight or dramatic, pitting or nonpitting. Leg edema may result from venous disorders, nephrotic syndrome, cirrhosis, cellulitis, trauma, drugs, and certain bone and cardiac disorders that disturb normal fluid balance. (See *Understanding fluid balance,* page 235.) However, several nonpathologic mechanisms may also cause leg edema. For example, prolonged sitting, standing, or immobility may cause bilateral orthostatic edema. Increased venous pressure late in pregnancy may cause ankle edema.

Assessment

To evaluate the patient, first ask how long he has had the edema. Did it develop suddenly or gradually? Does it decrease if he elevates his legs? Is it painful when touched or when he walks? Is it worse in the morning, or does it get progressively worse during the day? Ask about a recent leg injury, surgery, or illness that may have immobilized the patient. Does he have a history of cardiovascular disease? Finally, obtain a drug history.

Begin the physical examination by examining each leg for pitting edema. (See *Edema: Pitting or nonpitting?* page 236.) Because leg edema may compromise arterial blood flow, use a Doppler ultrasound blood flow detector to auscultate peripheral pulses to detect an insufficiency. Observe leg color and look for unusual vein patterns. Then gently palpate for warmth and tenderness. Gently squeeze the calf muscle against the tibia to check for deep pain. If leg edema is unilateral, dorsiflex the foot to look for Homans' sign. Finally, note skin thickening or ulceration in edematous areas.

Causes

◆ *Burns.* Two days or less after injury, leg burns may cause mild to severe edema, pain, and tissue damage.
◆ *Cellulitis.* Cellulitis causes pitting edema and orange peel skin that most commonly occurs in the lower extremities. It's typically caused by a streptococcal or staphylococcal infection.
◆ *Envenomation.* Mild to severe localized edema along with erythema, pain, urticaria, pruritus, and a burning sensation may develop suddenly at the site of a bite or sting.

◆ *Heart failure.* Bilateral leg edema is an early sign of right-sided heart failure. Other findings include weight gain, chest tightness, hypotension, pallor, orthopnea, and exertional and paroxysmal nocturnal dyspnea.
◆ *Leg trauma.* Mild to severe localized edema may form around a trauma site.
◆ *Osteomyelitis.* When osteomyelitis affects the lower leg, it usually produces localized edema, which may spread to the adjacent joint. Edema typically follows fever, localized tenderness, and pain that increases with leg movement.
◆ *Thrombophlebitis.* Deep and superficial vein thrombosis may cause unilateral mild to moderate edema. Deep vein thrombophlebitis may also cause warmth and cyanosis in the affected leg. Superficial thrombophlebitis typically causes pain, warmth, redness, tenderness, and induration along the affected vein.
◆ *Venous insufficiency (chronic).* Moderate to severe unilateral or bilateral leg edema occurs in patients with venous insufficiency. Initially, the edema is soft and pitting. Later, it becomes hard as tissues thicken. Other signs include darkened skin and painless, easily infected stasis ulcers around the ankle.

Enuresis

Enuresis usually refers to nighttime urinary incontinence in girls age 5 and older and in boys age 6 and older. It's most common in boys and rarely continues into adulthood; however, it may occur in some adults with sleep apnea. Primary enuresis describes a child who has never achieved bladder control; secondary enuresis describes a child who achieved bladder control for at least 3 months but later lost it.

Factors that may contribute to enuresis include delayed development of detrusor muscle control, unusually deep or sound sleep, organic disorders, and psychological stress. Psychological stress, probably the most important factor, commonly results from the birth of a sibling, the death of a parent or loved one, divorce, or premature, rigorous toilet training. The child may be too embarrassed or ashamed to discuss his bed-wetting, which intensifies psychological stress and makes enuresis more likely, thus creating a vicious cycle.

Assessment

When taking a history, include the parents as well as the child. First, determine the number of nights each week or month that the child wets the bed. Is there a family history of enurèsis? Ask about the child's daily fluid intake. Does he drink much after supper? What are his typical sleep and voiding patterns? Then find out if the child has ever achieved bladder control. If so, try to pinpoint what factor, such as an organic disorder or psychological stress, may have precipitated enuresis. Does the bed-wetting occur at home and away from home? Ask the parents how they've tried to manage the problem. Have them describe the child's toilet training. Observe the child's and parents' attitudes toward bed-wetting. Finally, ask the child if it hurts when he urinates.

Next, perform a physical examination to detect signs of neurologic or urinary tract disorders. Observe the child's gait to check for motor dysfunction, and test sensory function in the legs. Inspect the urethral meatus for erythema. Obtain a urine specimen.

Causes

◆ *Detrusor muscle hyperactivity.* Involuntary detrusor muscle contractions may cause primary or secondary enuresis associated with urinary urgency, frequency, and incontinence.
◆ *Urinary tract infection (UTI).* In children, most UTIs produce secondary enuresis. Associated findings include urinary frequency and urgency, dysuria, and hematuria. Lower back pain and suprapubic discomfort may also occur.
◆ *Urinary tract obstruction.* Urinary tract obstruction may produce primary or secondary enuresis. It may also cause flank and lower back pain; upper abdominal distention; urinary frequency, urgency, hesitancy, and dribbling; dysuria; a diminished urine stream; hematuria; and variable urine output.

Epistaxis

Epistaxis, a common sign, ranges from mild oozing to severe blood loss. It can be spontaneous or induced from the front or back of the nose. Most nosebleeds occur in the anterior-inferior nasal septum, but they may also occur at the point where the inferior turbinates meet the nasopharynx. Usually unilateral, they appear bilateral when blood runs from the bleeding side behind the nasal septum and out the opposite side.

A rich supply of fragile blood vessels makes the nose particularly vulnerable to bleeding. Air moving through the nose can dry and irritate the mucous membranes, forming crusts that bleed when they're removed. Dry mucous membranes are also more susceptible to infection, which can also produce epistaxis. Trauma is another common cause of epistaxis.

Assessment

If the patient has severe epistaxis, quickly check his vital signs. Assess for tachypnea, hypotension, and other signs of hypovolemic shock. Monitor airway patency. (See *Controlling epistaxis*.)

If the patient isn't in distress, take a complete history. Does he have a history of recent trauma? How often has he had nosebleeds in the past? Have the nosebleeds been long or unusually severe? Ask about a history of hypertension, bleeding or liver disorders, and other recent illnesses. Ask if the patient bruises easily. Find out what drugs he uses, especially anti-inflammatories and anticoagulants. Ask about a history of cocaine use.

Begin the physical examination by inspecting the patient's skin for other signs of bleeding, such as ecchymoses and petechiae, and by noting jaundice, pallor, or other abnormalities. When examining a trauma patient, look for associated injuries, such as eye trauma or facial fractures.

Causes

◆ *Aplastic anemia.* Aplastic anemia develops insidiously, eventually producing nosebleeds as well as ecchymoses, retinal hemorrhages, menorrhagia, petechiae, bleeding from the mouth, and signs of GI bleeding.

◆ *Barotrauma.* Commonly seen in airline passengers and scuba divers, barotrauma (injury to the middle ear or paranasal sinuses that results from an imbalance between ambient pressure and pressure within the affected cavity) can cause severe, painful epistaxis when the patient has an upper respiratory tract infection.

◆ *Chemical irritants.* Some chemicals—including phosphorus, sulfuric acid, ammonia, printer's ink, and chromates—irritate the nasal mucosa, producing epistaxis.

◆ *Coagulation disorders.* Such coagulation disorders as hemophilia and thrombocytopenic purpura can cause epistaxis along with ecchymoses, petechiae, and bleeding from the gums, mouth, and I.V. puncture sites.

◆ *Drugs.* Anticoagulants and anti-inflammatories can cause epistaxis. Cocaine use, especially if frequent, can also cause epistaxis.

◆ *Glomerulonephritis (chronic).* Glomerulonephritis produces nosebleeds as well as hypertension, proteinuria, hematuria, headache, edema, oliguria, hemoptysis, nausea, vomiting, pruritus, dyspnea, malaise, and fatigue.

◆ *Hepatitis.* When hepatitis interferes with the clotting mechanism, epistaxis and abnormal bleeding tendencies can result.

◆ *Hypertension.* Severe hypertension can produce extreme epistaxis, usually in the posterior nose, with pulsation above the middle turbinate.

◆ *Leukemia.* In patients with acute leukemia, sudden epistaxis is accompanied by a high fever and other types of abnormal bleeding, such as bleeding gums, ecchymoses, petechiae, easy bruising, and prolonged menses. These may follow less noticeable signs and symptoms, such as weakness, pallor, chills, recurrent infections, and a low-grade fever.

◆ *Maxillofacial injury.* With a maxillofacial injury, a pumping arterial bleed usually causes severe epistaxis.

◆ *Nasal fracture.* Unilateral or bilateral epistaxis occurs with nasal swelling, periorbital ecchymoses and edema, pain, nasal deformity, and crepitation of the nasal bones.

◆ *Nasal tumor.* Blood may ooze from the nose when a tumor disrupts the nasal vasculature. Benign tumors usually bleed when touched, but malignant tumors produce spontaneous uni-

EMERGENCY INTERVENTIONS

Controlling epistaxis

If the patient with epistaxis is hypovolemic, have him lie down and turn his head to the side to prevent blood from draining down the back of his throat, which could cause aspiration or vomiting of swallowed blood. If the patient isn't hypovolemic, have him sit upright and tilt his head forward. If direct pressure and cautery fail to control epistaxis, the patient may require nasal packing. Anterior packing may be used if the patient has severe bleeding in the anterior nose. Horizontal layers of petroleum jelly gauze strips are inserted into the nostrils near the turbinates.

Posterior packing may be needed if the patient has severe bleeding in the posterior nose or if blood from anterior bleeding starts flowing backward. This type of packing consists of a gauze pack secured by three strong silk sutures. After the nose is anesthetized, sutures are pulled through the nostrils with a soft catheter and the pack is positioned behind the soft palate. Two of the sutures are tied to a gauze roll under the patient's nose, which keeps the pack in place. The third suture is taped to his cheek. Instead of a gauze pack, an indwelling urinary or nasal epistaxis catheter may be in-

serted through the nose into the area behind the soft palate and inflated with 10 ml of water to compress the bleeding point.

Interventions

If the patient has nasal packing, follow these guidelines:
◆ Watch for signs of respiratory distress, such as dyspnea, which may occur if the packing slips and obstructs the airway.
◆ Keep emergency equipment (flashlights, scissors, and a hemostat) at the patient's bedside. Expect to cut the cheek suture (or deflate the catheter) and remove the pack at the first sign of airway obstruction.
◆ Avoid tension on the cheek suture, which could cause the posterior pack to slip out of place.
◆ Keep the call bell within easy reach.
◆ Monitor the patient's vital signs frequently. Watch for signs of hypoxia, such as tachycardia and restlessness.
◆ Elevate the head of the patient's bed, and remind him to breathe through his mouth.
◆ Administer humidified oxygen as needed.
◆ Instruct the patient not to blow his nose for 48 hours after the packing is removed.

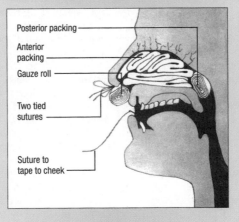

Posterior packing

Anterior packing

Gauze roll

Two tied sutures

Suture to tape to cheek

lateral epistaxis, along with a foul discharge.

◆ *Polycythemia vera.* A common sign of polycythemia vera, spontaneous epistaxis may be accompanied by bleeding gums, ecchymoses, and ruddy cyanosis of the face, nose, ears, and lips.

◆ *Sarcoidosis.* Oozing epistaxis may occur in sarcoidosis, along with a nonproductive cough, substernal pain, malaise, and weight loss.

◆ *Scleroma.* In scleroma, oozing epistaxis occurs with a watery nasal discharge that becomes foul-smelling and crusty. Progressive anosmia and turbinate atrophy may also occur.

◆ *Sinusitis (acute).* Patients with sinusitis may experience a bloody or blood-tinged nasal discharge that may become purulent and copious after 24 to 48 hours. Other findings include nasal congestion, tenderness, headache, and red, edematous nasal mucosa.

▧ *Skull fracture.* Depending on the type of fracture, epistaxis can be direct (when blood flows directly down the nares) or indirect (when blood drains through the eustachian tube into the nose). Abrasions, contusions, lacerations, or avulsions are common. A basilar fracture may also cause bleeding from the pharynx, ears, and conjunctiva as well as raccoon eyes and Battle's sign.

◆ *Systemic lupus erythematosus (SLE).* SLE causes oozing epistaxis. More characteristic findings include butterfly rash, lymphadenopathy, joint pain and stiffness, anorexia, nausea, vomiting, myalgia, and weight loss.

◆ *Typhoid fever.* Oozing epistaxis and a dry cough are common with typhoid fever. It may also cause an abrupt onset of chills and a high fever, "rosespot" rash, jaundice, anorexia, weight loss, and profound fatigue.

Erythema

Dilated or congested blood vessels produce red skin, or erythema, the most common sign of skin inflammation or irritation. Erythema may be localized or generalized and may occur suddenly or gradually. Skin color can range from bright red in patients with acute conditions to pale violet or brown in those with chronic problems. Erythema must be differentiated from purpura, which causes redness from bleeding into the skin. When pressure is applied directly to the skin, erythema blanches momentarily, but purpura doesn't.

Erythema usually results from changes in the arteries, veins, and small vessels that lead to increased small-vessel perfusion. Drugs and neurogenic mechanisms can allow extra blood to enter the small vessels. Erythema can also result from trauma and tissue damage, changes in supporting tissues that increase vessel visibility, and many rare disorders. (See *Rare causes of erythema*.)

Assessment

If the patient's condition permits, obtain a detailed health history. Ask how long he has had the erythema and where it first began. Has he had associated pain or itching? Has he recently had a fever, upper respiratory tract infection, or joint pain? Does he have a history of skin disease or other illness? Find out if he has been exposed to someone who has had a similar rash or who's now ill. Did he have a recent fall or injury that may have caused the erythema?

Obtain a complete drug history, including recent immunizations. Ask about food intake and exposure to chemicals.

Begin the physical examination by assessing the extent, distribution, and intensity of erythema. Look for edema and other skin lesions, such as hives, scales, papules, and purpura. Examine the affected area for warmth, and gently palpate it to check for tenderness or crepitus.

Causes

◼ *Allergic reactions.* Foods, drugs, chemicals, and other allergens can cause an allergic reaction and erythema. A localized allergic reaction also produces hivelike eruptions and edema. Anaphylaxis produces relatively sudden erythema in the form of urticaria.

◆ *Burns.* With thermal burns, erythema and swelling appear first, possibly followed by deep or superficial blisters and other signs of damage that vary with the burn's severity.

◆ *Candidiasis.* When candidiasis affects the skin, it produces erythema and a scaly, papular rash—also known as *intertrigo*—under the breasts and at the axillae, neck, umbilicus, and groin.

◆ *Cellulitis.* Cellulitis is a bacterial infection of the skin and subcutaneous tissue and causes erythema, tenderness, and edema.

◆ *Dermatitis.* Erythema commonly occurs in dermatitis, a family of inflammatory disorders. With atopic dermatitis, erythema and intense pruritus precede the development of small papules that may redden, weep, scale, and lichenify. Contact dermatitis occurs after exposure to an irritant. It quickly produces erythema and vesicles, blisters, or ulcerations on exposed skin. With seborrheic dermatitis, erythema appears with dull red or yellow lesions that usually occur on the scalp, eyebrows, ears, and nasolabial folds.

◆ *Dermatomyositis.* Dermatomyositis, most common in women age 50 or older, produces a dusky lilac rash on the face, neck, upper torso, and nail beds. Gottron's papules (violet, flat-topped lesions) may appear on finger joints.

◆ *Drugs.* Many drugs commonly cause erythema. (See *Drugs associated with erythema,* page 246.)

◆ *Erythema annulare centrifugum.* Erythema annulare centrifugum causes small, pink infiltrated papules to appear on the trunk, buttocks, and inner thighs. They slowly spread at the margins and clear in the center.

◆ *Erythema marginatum rheumaticum.* Associated with rheumatic fever, erythema marginatum rheumaticum causes erythematous lesions that are

---

Rare causes of erythema

In exceptional cases, a patient's erythema may be caused by one of these rare disorders:

◆ acute febrile neutrophilic dermatosis, which produces erythematous lesions on the face, neck, and extremities after a high fever

◆ erythema abigne, which produces lacy erythema and telangiectases after exposure to radiant heat

◆ erythema chronicum migrans, which produces erythematous macules and papules on the trunk, upper arms, or thighs after a tick bite

◆ erythema gyratum repens, which produces wavy bands of erythema and is commonly associated with internal malignancy

◆ toxic epidermal necrolysis, which causes severe, widespread erythema, tenderness, bullae formation, and exfoliation and is most commonly caused by medications; it may be fatal due to epidermal destruction and its consequences.

Drugs associated with erythema

Suspect drug-induced erythema in a patient who develops this sign within 1 week of starting a drug. Erythematous lesions can vary in size, shape, type, and amount, but they almost always appear suddenly and symmetrically on the trunk and inner arms. These drugs can produce erythematous lesions:

- ◆ allopurinol (Zyloprim)
- ◆ anticoagulants
- ◆ antimetabolites
- ◆ barbiturates
- ◆ cephalosporins
- ◆ chlordiazepoxide (Librium)
- ◆ codeine
- ◆ corticosteroids
- ◆ co-trimoxazole (Bactrim)
- ◆ diazepam (Valium)

- ◆ erythromycin (E-Mycin)
- ◆ gentamicin (Garamycin)
- ◆ gold
- ◆ griseofulvin (Grispeg)
- ◆ hormonal contraceptives
- ◆ indomethacin (Indocin)
- ◆ iodide bromides
- ◆ isoniazid (Laniazid)
- ◆ lithium (Lithonate)
- ◆ nitrofurantoin (Macrodantin)

- ◆ penicillin
- ◆ phenothiazines
- ◆ phenytoin (Dilantin)
- ◆ quinidine (Quinora)
- ◆ salicylates
- ◆ sulfonamides
- ◆ sulfonylureas
- ◆ tetracyclines
- ◆ thiazides

Some drugs—particularly barbiturates, hormonal contraceptives, salicylates, sulfonamides, and tetracyclines—can cause a "fixed" drug eruption. In this type of reaction, lesions can appear on any body part and flake off after a few days, leaving a brownish purple pigmentation. Repeated drug administration causes the original lesions to recur and new ones to develop.

superficial, flat, and slightly hardened. They shift, spread rapidly, and may last for hours or days, recurring after a time.

◆ *Erythema multiforme.* Erythema multiforme is an acute inflammatory skin disease that develops as a result of drug sensitivity after infection (most commonly herpes simplex and *Mycoplasma*), allergies, and pregnancy. One-half of the cases are of idiopathic origin. Erythema multiforme minor has typical urticarial red-pink iris-shaped localized lesions with little or no mucous membrane involvement. Erythema multiforme major usually occurs as a drug reaction and includes erosions

of the mucous membranes with widespread symmetrical, bullous lesions that may become confluent. The maximal variant of this disease is Stevens-Johnson syndrome, a multisystem disorder that can occasionally be fatal. The patient develops exfoliation of the skin from disruptions of bullae and may experience tachypnea, chest pain, malaise, muscle or joint pain, and a weak, rapid pulse.

◆ *Erythema nodosum.* Sudden bilateral eruption of tender erythematous nodules characterizes erythema nodosum. These firm, round, protruding lesions usually appear in crops on the shins, knees, and ankles but may occur on the buttocks, arms, calves, and trunk as well. Erythema nodosum is associated with various diseases, most notably inflammatory bowel disease, sarcoidosis, tuberculosis, and streptococcal and fungal infections.

◆ *Gout.* Gout is characterized by tight and erythematous skin over an inflamed, edematous joint.

◆ *Lupus erythematosus.* Discoid and systemic lupus erythematosus can produce a characteristic butterfly rash. This erythematous eruption may range from a blush with swelling to a scaly, sharply demarcated, macular rash with plaques that may spread to the forehead, chin, ears, chest, and other sun-exposed parts of the body.

◆ *Psoriasis.* Silvery white scales over a thickened erythematous base usually affect the elbows, knees, chest, scalp, and intergluteal folds. The fingernails may become thick and pitted.

◆ *Raynaud's disease.* Typically, the skin on the hands and feet blanches and cools after exposure to cold and stress. Later, it becomes warm and purplish red.

◆ *Rosacea.* Scattered erythema initially develops across the center of the face, followed by superficial telangiectases, papules, pustules, and nodules. Rhinophyma may occur on the lower half of the nose.

◆ *Rubella.* With rubella, flat solitary lesions typically join to form a blotchy pink erythematous rash that spreads rapidly to the trunk and extremities.

Exophthalmos

Exophthalmos—the abnormal protrusion of one or both eyeballs—may result from hemorrhage, edema, or inflammation behind the eye; extraocular muscle relaxation; or space-occupying intraorbital lesions and metastatic tumors. This sign may occur suddenly or

gradually, causing mild to dramatic protrusion. Occasionally, the affected eye also pulsates. The most common cause of exophthalmos in adults is dysthyroid eye disease.

Exophthalmos is usually easily observed. However, lid retraction may mimic exophthalmos even when protrusion is absent. Similarly, ptosis in one eye may make the other eye appear exophthalmic by comparison. An exophthalmometer can differentiate these signs by measuring ocular protrusion.

Assessment

Begin by asking when the patient first noticed exophthalmos. Is it associated with pain in or around the eye? If so, ask him how severe the pain is and how long he has had it. Then ask about recent sinus infection or vision problems. Check the patient's vital signs. Next, evaluate the severity of exophthalmos with an exophthalmometer. (See *Detecting unilateral exophthalmos,* page 248.) If the eyes bulge severely, look for cloudiness on the cornea, which may indicate ulcer formation. Describe any eye discharge and observe for ptosis. Then check visual acuity with and without correction and evaluate extraocular movements. Palpate the patient's thyroid for enlargement or goiter.

Causes

◆ *Cavernous sinus thrombosis.* Usually, cavernous sinus thrombosis causes the sudden onset of pulsating, unilateral exophthalmos. Eyelid edema, decreased or absent pupillary reflexes, and impaired extraocular movement and visual acuity may accompany it.

◆ *Dacryoadenitis.* Unilateral, slowly progressive exophthalmos is the most common sign of dacryoadenitis. Other

Detecting unilateral exophthalmos

If one of the patient's eyes seems more prominent than the other, examine both eyes from above the patient's head. Look down across his face, gently draw his lids up, and compare the relationship of the corneas to the lower lids. Abnormal protrusion of one eye suggests unilateral exophthalmos.

Remember: Don't perform this test if you suspect eye trauma.

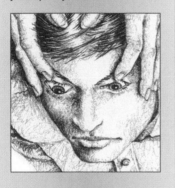

findings include limited extraocular movements, ptosis, eyelid edema and erythema, conjunctival injection, eye pain, and diplopia.

◆ *Foreign body in the eye.* When a foreign body enters the eye, exophthalmos may accompany other signs and symptoms of ocular trauma, including eye pain, redness, and tearing.

◆ *Hemangioma.* Most common in young adults, this orbital tumor produces progressive exophthalmos, which may be mild or severe, unilateral or bilateral. Other signs and symptoms include ptosis and blurred vision.

◆ *Lacrimal gland tumor.* Exophthalmos usually develops slowly in one

eye, causing the eye's downward displacement toward the nose. The patient may also have ptosis and eye deviation and pain.

◆ *Leiomyosarcoma.* Most common in people ages 45 and older, leiomyosarcoma is characterized by slowly developing, unilateral exophthalmos. Other effects include diplopia, impaired vision, and intermittent eye pain.

◆ *Orbital cellulitis.* Commonly the result of sinusitis, orbital cellulitis causes the sudden onset of unilateral exophthalmos, which may be mild or severe.

◆ *Orbital choristoma.* A common sign of orbital choristoma (a benign tumor), progressive exophthalmos may be associated with diplopia and blurred vision.

◆ *Orbital emphysema.* Air leaking from the sinus into the orbit usually causes unilateral exophthalmos. Palpation of the globe elicits crepitation.

◆ *Parasite infestation.* Usually, parasite infestation causes painless, progressive exophthalmos in one eye that may spread to the other eye.

◆ *Scleritis (posterior).* The gradual onset of mild to severe unilateral exophthalmos is common with scleritis. Other signs and symptoms include severe eye pain, diplopia, papilledema, and impaired visual acuity.

◆ *Thyrotoxicosis.* Although a classic sign of thyrotoxicosis, exophthalmos is absent in many patients. It's usually bilateral, progressive, and severe. Associated ocular findings include ptosis, increased tearing, lid lag and edema, photophobia, conjunctival injection, diplopia, and decreased visual acuity.

Eye discharge

Usually associated with conjunctivitis, eye discharge is the excretion of a substance other than tears. This common sign may occur in one or both eyes, producing scant to copious discharge.

The discharge may be purulent, frothy, mucoid, cheesy, serous, clear, or a stringy, white discharge. Sometimes, the discharge can be expressed by applying pressure to the tear sac, punctum, meibomian glands, or canaliculus.

Eye discharge commonly results from inflammatory and infectious eye disorders but may also occur in certain systemic disorders. (See *Sources of eye discharge*.) Because this sign may accompany a disorder that threatens vision, it must be assessed and treated immediately.

Assessment

Begin your evaluation by asking when the discharge began. Does it occur at certain times of the day or in connection with certain activities? If the patient complains of pain, ask him to describe it and to show you its exact location. Do his eyes itch or burn? Do they tear excessively? Are they sensitive to light? Does he feel like something is in them?

After checking the patient's vital signs, carefully inspect the eye discharge. Note its amount, color, and consistency. Then test his visual acuity

Sources of eye discharge

Eye discharge can come from the tear sac, punctum, meibomian glands, or canaliculi. If the patient reports a discharge that isn't immediately apparent, you can express a sample by pressing your fingertip lightly over these structures. Then characterize the discharge, and note its source.

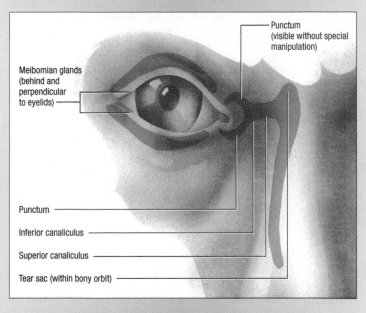

Meibomian glands (behind and perpendicular to eyelids)

Punctum (visible without special manipulation)

Punctum

Inferior canaliculus

Superior canaliculus

Tear sac (within bony orbit)

with and without correction. Examine external eye structures, beginning with the unaffected eye to prevent cross-contamination. Observe for eyelid edema, entropion, crusts, lesions, and trichiasis. Next, ask the patient to blink as you watch for impaired lid movement. Test the six cardinal fields of gaze. Examine his eyes for conjunctival injection and follicles and for corneal cloudiness or white lesions.

Causes

◆ *Conjunctivitis.* Five types of conjunctivitis may cause eye discharge with redness, hyperemia, foreign-body sensation, periocular edema, and tearing. With allergic conjunctivitis, a bilateral ropey discharge is accompanied by itching and tearing. Bacterial conjunctivitis causes a moderate, greenish white, purulent or mucopurulent discharge that may form sticky crusts on the eyelids during sleep. Viral conjunctivitis causes a serous, clear discharge and preauricular adenopathy. Fungal conjunctivitis produces a copious, thick, purulent discharge that makes the eyelids crusty and sticky. Inclusion conjunctivitis causes scant mucoid discharge—especially in the morning—in both eyes, accompanied by pseudoptosis and conjunctival follicles.

◆ *Corneal ulcers.* Bacterial and fungal corneal ulcers produce a copious, purulent unilateral eye discharge. Related findings include crusty, sticky eyelids and, possibly, severe pain, photophobia, and impaired visual acuity.

◆ *Herpes zoster ophthalmicus.* Herpes zoster ophthalmicus yields a moderate to copious serous eye discharge accompanied by excessive tearing, eyelid edema and erythema, conjunctival injection, and a white, cloudy cornea.

◆ *Keratoconjunctivitis sicca.* Keratoconjunctivitis sicca, better known as *dry eye syndrome,* typically causes excessive, continuous mucoid discharge and insufficient tearing.

◆ *Meibomianitis.* Meibomianitis may produce a continuous frothy eye discharge. Applying pressure on the meibomian glands yields a soft, foul-smelling, cheesy yellow discharge. The eyes also appear chronically red.

◆ *Orbital cellulitis.* Although exophthalmos is the most obvious sign of orbital cellulitis, a unilateral purulent eye discharge may also be present.

◆ *Psoriasis vulgaris.* Usually, psoriasis vulgaris causes a substantial mucus discharge in both eyes, accompanied by redness. The characteristic lesions it produces on the eyelids may extend into the conjunctiva.

◆ *Stevens-Johnson syndrome.* A purulent eye discharge characterizes Stevens-Johnson syndrome. Other ocular effects may include severe eye pain, trichiasis, photophobia, and decreased tear formation.

◆ *Trachoma.* A bilateral eye discharge occurs in trachoma along with severe pain, excessive tearing, photophobia, eyelid edema, redness, and visible conjunctival follicles.

Eye pain

Eye pain may be described as a burning, throbbing, aching, or stabbing sensation in or around the eye. It may also be characterized as a foreign-body sensation. The pain's duration and exact location provide clues to the causative disorder. Eye pain may result from disorders or trauma that stimulate nerve endings in the cornea or external eye.

Assessment

If the patient's condition permits, take a complete history. Have the patient describe the pain fully. How long does it last? Does burning, itching, or discharge accompany the pain? Is it worse in the morning or late evening? Ask about recent trauma or surgery, especially if the patient complains of sudden, severe pain. Does he have headaches?

Carefully assess the lids and conjunctiva for redness, inflammation, and swelling. (See *Examining the external eye*.) Then examine the eyes for ptosis or exophthalmos. During the physical examination, don't manipulate the eye

Examining the external eye

For patients with eye pain or other ocular symptoms, examining the external eye forms an important part of the ocular assessment. Here's how to do it.

Begin by inspecting the eyelids for ptosis and incomplete closure. Also, observe the lids for edema, erythema, cyanosis, hematoma, and masses. Evaluate skin lesions, growths, swelling, and tenderness by gross palpation. Are the lids everted or inverted? Do the eyelashes turn inward? Have some of them been lost? Do the lashes adhere to one another or contain a discharge? Next, examine the lid margins, noting especially debris, scaling, lesions, or unusual secretions. Also, watch for eyelid spasms.

Now gently retract the eyelid with your thumb and forefinger. Assess the conjunctiva for redness, cloudiness, follicles, and blisters or other lesions. Check for chemosis by pressing the lower lid against the eyeball and noting bulging above this compression point. Observe the sclera, noting a change from its normal white color.

Next, shine a light across the cornea to detect scars, abrasions, or ulcers. Note color changes, dots, or opaque or cloudy areas. Also, assess the anterior eye chamber, which should be clean, deep, shadow-free, and filled with clear aqueous humor.

Finally, inspect the color, shape, texture, and pattern of the iris. Then assess the pupils' size, shape, and equality. Evaluate their response to light. Are they sluggish, fixed, or unresponsive? Does pupil dilation or constriction occur only on one side?

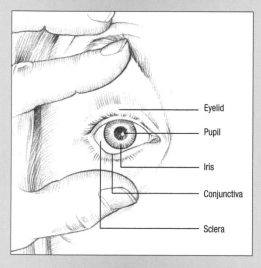

- Eyelid
- Pupil
- Iris
- Conjunctiva
- Sclera

if you suspect trauma. Finally, test visual acuity and assess extraocular movements. Characterize any discharge.

Causes

◆ *Acute angle-closure glaucoma.* Blurred vision and sudden, excruciating pain in and around the eye characterize acute angle-closure glaucoma. Pain may be so severe that it causes nausea, vomiting, and abdominal pain.

◆ *Blepharitis.* Itching, sticky discharge and conjunctival injection accompany burning pain in both eyelids. Related findings include a foreign-body sensation, lid ulcerations, and loss of eyelashes.

◆ *Burns.* With chemical burns, sudden and severe eye pain may occur with erythema and blistering of the face and lids, photophobia, miosis, conjunctival injection, blurring, and an inability to keep the eyelids open.

◆ *Chalazion.* A chalazion causes localized tenderness and swelling on the upper or lower eyelid. Eversion of the lid reveals conjunctival injection and a small red lump.

◆ *Conjunctivitis.* Some degree of eye pain and excessive tearing occurs with four types of conjunctivitis. Allergic conjunctivitis causes mild, burning, bilateral pain. Bacterial conjunctivitis causes pain only when it affects the cornea. If the cornea is affected, fungal conjunctivitis may cause pain and photophobia. Viral conjunctivitis produces itching, red eyes; a foreign-body sensation; visible conjunctival follicles; and eyelid edema.

◆ *Corneal abrasions.* With a corneal abrasion, eye pain is characterized by a foreign-body sensation. Excessive tearing, photophobia, and conjunctival injection are also common.

◆ *Corneal ulcers.* Bacterial and fungal corneal ulcers cause severe eye pain.

They may also cause a purulent eye discharge, sticky eyelids, photophobia, and impaired visual acuity.

◆ *Dacryocystitis.* Pain and tenderness near the tear sac characterize acute dacryocystitis.

◆ *Episcleritis.* Deep eye pain occurs as tissues over the sclera become inflamed. Related effects include photophobia, excessive tearing, conjunctival edema, and a red or purplish sclera.

◆ *Foreign bodies in the cornea and conjunctiva.* Sudden severe pain is common with foreign bodies in the eye. Other findings include excessive tearing and dramatic conjunctival injection.

◆ *Hordeolum (stye).* Hordeolum usually produces localized eye pain that increases as the stye grows. Eyelid erythema and edema are also common.

◆ *Iritis (acute).* Moderate to severe eye pain occurs with severe photophobia, dramatic conjunctival injection, and blurred vision. The constricted pupil may respond poorly to light.

◆ *Lacrimal gland tumor.* A lacrimal gland tumor is a neoplastic lesion that usually produces unilateral eye pain, impaired visual acuity, and some degree of exophthalmos.

◆ *Migraine headache.* Migraines can produce pain so severe that the eyes also ache. Additionally, nausea, vomiting, blurred vision, and light and noise sensitivity may occur.

◆ *Ocular laceration and intraocular foreign bodies.* Penetrating eye injuries usually cause mild to severe unilateral eye pain and impaired visual acuity.

◆ *Optic neuritis.* With optic neuritis, pain in and around the eye occurs with eye movement. Severe vision loss and tunnel vision develop but improve within 2 to 3 weeks. Pupils respond sluggishly to direct light.

◆ *Scleritis.* Scleritis produces severe eye pain and tenderness, along with conjunctival injection, a bluish purple sclera and, possibly, photophobia and excessive tearing.

◆ *Sclerokeratitis.* Inflammation of the sclera and cornea causes pain, burning, irritation, and photophobia.

◆ *Stevens-Johnson syndrome.* Stevens-Johnson syndrome commonly produces severe eye pain, entropion, trichiasis, purulent conjunctivitis, photophobia, and decreased tear formation.

◼ *Subdural hematoma.* After head trauma, a subdural hematoma commonly causes severe eye ache and headache. Related neurologic signs depend on the hematoma's location and size.

◆ *Trachoma.* Along with pain in the affected eye, trachoma causes excessive tearing, photophobia, eye discharge, eyelid edema and redness, and visible conjunctival follicles.

◆ *Uveitis.* Anterior uveitis causes the sudden onset of severe pain, dramatic conjunctival injection, photophobia, and a small, nonreactive pupil. Posterior uveitis causes an insidious onset of similar findings. Lens-induced uveitis causes moderate eye pain and severely impaired visual acuity. In most cases, the patient can perceive only light.

F

Fasciculations

Fasciculations are local involuntary muscle contractions representing the spontaneous discharge of a muscle fiber bundle innervated by a single motor nerve filament. These contractions cause visible dimpling or wave-like twitching of the skin, but they aren't strong enough to cause a joint to move. They occur irregularly at frequencies ranging from once every several seconds to two or three times per second. Infrequently, myokymia—continuous, rapid fasciculations that cause a rippling effect—may occur. Because fasciculations are brief and painless, they commonly go undetected or are ignored.

Benign, nonpathologic fasciculations are common and normal. They typically occur in tense, anxious, or overtired people and affect the eyelid, thumb, or calf. However, fasciculations may also indicate a severe neurologic disorder, most notably a diffuse motor neuron disorder that causes loss of control over muscle fiber discharge. They can also be an early sign of pesticide poisoning.

Assessment

If the patient isn't in severe distress, ask him if he has experienced sensory changes, such as paresthesia, or difficulty speaking, swallowing, breathing, or controlling bowel or bladder function. Ask him if he's in pain.

Explore the patient's medical history for neurologic disorders, cancer, and recent infections. Also, ask him about his lifestyle—especially stress at home, work, or school. Ask the patient about his dietary habits and for a recall of his food and fluid intake during the past few days because electrolyte imbalances may also cause muscle twitching.

Perform a physical assessment, looking for fasciculations while the affected muscle is at rest. Observe and test for motor and sensory abnormalities (particularly muscle atrophy and weakness) and decreased deep tendon reflexes. If you note these signs and symptoms, suspect motor neuron disease and perform a comprehensive neurologic examination.

Causes

◪ *Amyotrophic lateral sclerosis (ALS).* With ALS, coarse fasciculations usually begin in the small muscles of the hands and feet and then spread to the forearms and legs. Widespread, symmetrical muscle atrophy and weakness may result in dysarthria and difficulty chewing, swallowing, and breathing; occasionally, choking and drooling occur.

◆ *Bulbar palsy.* Fasciculations of the face and tongue commonly appear early with bulbar palsy. Progressive findings include dysarthria, dysphagia, hoarseness, and drooling. Eventually, weakness spreads to the respiratory muscles.

▧ *Pesticide poisoning.* Ingestion of organophosphate or carbamate pesticides commonly produces an acute onset of long, wavelike fasciculations and muscle weakness that rapidly progresses to flaccid paralysis. Other common effects include nausea, vomiting, diarrhea, loss of bowel and bladder control, hyperactive bowel sounds, and abdominal cramping.

◆ *Poliomyelitis (spinal paralytic).* Coarse fasciculations, usually transient but occasionally persistent, accompany progressive muscle weakness, spasms, and atrophy that characterize poliomyelitis.

◆ *Spinal cord tumors.* With spinal cord tumors, fasciculations may develop along with muscle atrophy and cramps. They appear asymmetrically at first and then bilaterally as cord compression progresses.

Fatigue

Fatigue is a feeling of excessive tiredness, a lack of energy, or exhaustion accompanied by a strong desire to rest or sleep. This common symptom is distinct from weakness, which involves the muscles; however, fatigue and weakness may occur together.

Fatigue is a normal and important response to physical overexertion, prolonged emotional stress, and sleep deprivation. However, it can also be a nonspecific symptom of a psychological or physiologic disorder—especially viral or bacterial infection and endocrine, cardiovascular, or neurologic disease.

Fatigue reflects hypermetabolic and hypometabolic states in which nutrients needed for cellular energy and growth are lacking because of overly rapid depletion, impaired replacement mechanisms, insufficient hormone production, or inadequate nutrient intake or metabolism.

Assessment

Obtain a careful history to identify the patient's fatigue pattern. Fatigue that worsens with activity and improves with rest generally indicates a physical disorder; the opposite pattern, a psychological disorder. Fatigue lasting longer than 4 months, constant fatigue that's unrelieved by rest, and transient exhaustion that quickly gives way to bursts of energy are other findings associated with psychological disorders.

Ask about related symptoms and recent viral or bacterial illness or stressful changes in lifestyle. Explore nutritional habits and appetite or weight changes. Carefully review the patient's medical and psychiatric history for chronic disorders that commonly produce fatigue. Ask about a family history of such disorders. Obtain a thorough drug history, noting the use of any drug with fatigue as an adverse effect. Ask about alcohol and drug use patterns. Determine if the patient is at risk for carbon monoxide poisoning.

Observe the patient's general appearance for overt signs of depression or organic illness. Is he unkempt or expressionless? Does he appear tired or sickly or have a slumped posture? If warranted, evaluate his mental status, noting especially mental clouding, attention deficits, agitation, or psychomotor retardation.

Causes

◆ *Acquired immunodeficiency syndrome (AIDS)*. In addition to fatigue, AIDS may cause fever, night sweats, weight loss, diarrhea, and cough, followed by several concurrent opportunistic infections.

◆ *Adrenocortical insufficiency*. Mild fatigue, the hallmark of adrenocortical insufficiency, initially appears after exertion and stress, but later becomes more severe and persistent. Weakness and weight loss typically accompany GI disturbances, such as nausea, vomiting, anorexia, abdominal pain, and chronic diarrhea.

◆ *Anemia*. Fatigue following mild activity is commonly the first symptom of anemia. Associated findings vary, but generally include pallor, tachycardia, and dyspnea.

◆ *Anxiety*. Chronic, unremitting anxiety invariably produces fatigue, typically characterized as nervous exhaustion. Other persistent findings include apprehension, indecisiveness, restlessness, insomnia, trembling, and increased muscle tension.

◆ *Cancer*. Unexplained fatigue is commonly the earliest sign of cancer. Related findings reflect the type, location, and stage of the tumor.

◼ *Carbon monoxide poisoning*. Fatigue occurs along with a headache, dyspnea, and confusion and can eventually progress to unconsciousness and apnea.

◆ *Chronic fatigue syndrome*. Chronic fatigue syndrome, whose cause is unknown, is characterized by incapacitating fatigue. Other findings are sore throat, myalgia, and cognitive dysfunction.

◆ *Chronic obstructive pulmonary disease (COPD)*. The earliest and most persistent symptoms of COPD are progressive fatigue and dyspnea.

◆ *Depression*. Persistent fatigue unrelated to exertion nearly always accompanies chronic depression. Associated complaints include headache, anorexia, constipation, insomnia, slowed speech, agitation or bradykinesia, irritability, loss of concentration, feelings of worthlessness, and persistent thoughts of death.

◆ *Diabetes mellitus*. Fatigue, the most common symptom in diabetes mellitus, may begin insidiously or abruptly. Related findings include weight loss, blurred vision, polyuria, polydipsia, and polyphagia.

◆ *Heart failure*. Persistent fatigue and lethargy characterize heart failure.

◆ *Hypercortisolism*. Hypercortisolism typically causes fatigue, related in part to accompanying sleep disturbances. Unmistakable signs include truncal obesity with slender extremities, buffalo hump, moon face, purple striae, acne, and hirsutism.

◆ *Hypothyroidism*. Fatigue occurs early in hypothyroidism, along with forgetfulness, cold intolerance, weight gain, metrorrhagia, and constipation.

◆ *Infection*. With chronic infection, fatigue is commonly the most prominent symptom—and sometimes the only one. A low-grade fever and weight loss may accompany signs and symptoms—such as burning upon urination or swollen, painful gums—that reflect the type and location of infection.

◆ *Lyme disease*. In addition to fatigue and malaise, signs and symptoms of Lyme disease include intermittent headache, fever, chills, an expanding red rash, and muscle and joint aches.

◆ *Malnutrition.* Easy fatigability, along with lethargy and apathy, is common in patients with protein-calorie malnutrition. Patients may also exhibit weight loss, muscle wasting, sensations of coldness, edema, and dry, flaky skin.

◆ *Myasthenia gravis.* The cardinal symptoms of myasthenia gravis are easy fatigability and muscle weakness, which worsen as the day progresses. They also worsen with exertion and abate with rest.

◆ *Renal failure.* Acute renal failure commonly causes sudden fatigue, drowsiness, and lethargy. With chronic renal failure, insidious fatigue and lethargy occur with marked changes in all body systems.

◆ *Systemic lupus erythematosus (SLE).* With SLE, fatigue usually occurs along with generalized aching, malaise, a low-grade fever, headache, and irritability.

◆ *Valvular heart disease.* All types of valvular heart disease commonly produce progressive fatigue and a cardiac murmur. Additional signs and symptoms vary, but generally include exertional dyspnea, cough, and hemoptysis.

Fecal incontinence

Fecal incontinence, the involuntary passage of feces, follows a loss or an impairment of external anal sphincter control. It can result from many GI, neurologic, and psychological disorders; the effects of drugs; or surgery. In some patients, it may even be a purposeful manipulative behavior.

Fecal incontinence may be temporary or permanent. Its onset may be gradual, such as in dementia, or sudden such as in spinal cord trauma. Although usually not a sign of severe illness, it can greatly affect the patient's physical and psychological well-being.

Assessment

Ask the patient with fecal incontinence about its onset, duration, and severity and about any discernible pattern; for example, does it occur at night or only with episodes of diarrhea? Note the frequency, consistency, and volume of stools passed within the past 24 hours. Obtain a stool sample. Focus your history taking on GI, neurologic, and psychological disorders.

Let the patient's history guide your physical examination. If you suspect a brain or spinal cord lesion, perform a complete neurologic examination. (See *Neurologic control of defecation,* page 258.) If a GI disturbance seems likely, inspect the abdomen for distention, auscultate for bowel sounds, and percuss and palpate for a mass. Inspect the anal area for signs of excoriation or infection. If not contraindicated, check for fecal impaction, which may be associated with incontinence.

Causes

◆ *Dementia.* Any chronic degenerative brain disease can produce fecal as well as urinary incontinence. Associated signs and symptoms include impaired judgment and abstract thinking, amnesia, emotional lability, hyperactive deep tendon reflexes, aphasia or dysarthria and, possibly, diffuse choreoathetoid movements.

◆ *Drugs.* Chronic laxative abuse may cause insensitivity to a fecal mass or loss of the colonic defecation reflex.

◼ *Head trauma.* Disruption of the neurologic pathways that control defecation can cause fecal incontinence. Additional findings depend on the location and severity of the injury.

Neurologic control of defecation

Three neurologic mechanisms normally regulate defecation: the intrinsic defecation reflex in the colon, the parasympathetic defecation reflex involving sacral segments of the spinal cord, and voluntary control. Here's how they interact.

Fecal distention of the rectum activates the relatively weak intrinsic reflex, causing afferent impulses to spread through the myenteric plexus, initiating peristalsis in the descending and sigmoid colon and rectum. Subsequent movement of stools toward the anus causes receptive relaxation of the internal anal sphincter.

To ensure defecation, the parasympathetic reflex magnifies the intrinsic reflex. Stimulation of afferent nerves in the rectal wall propels impulses through the spinal cord and back to the descending and sigmoid colon, rectum, and anus to intensify peristalsis (see illustration).

However, fecal movement and internal sphincter relaxation cause immediate contraction of the external anal sphincter and temporary fecal retention. At this point, conscious control of the external sphincter either prevents or permits defecation. Except in infants or neurologically impaired patients, this voluntary mechanism further contracts the sphincter to prevent defecation at inappropriate times or relaxes it and allows defecation to occur.

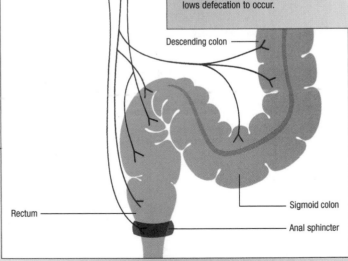

From conscious cortex

Afferent nerves

Skeletal motor nerve

Parasympathetic nerves

Descending colon

Sigmoid colon

Anal sphincter

Rectum

◆ *Inflammatory bowel disease.* With inflammatory bowel disease, nocturnal fecal incontinence occurs occasionally with diarrhea. Other findings include abdominal pain, weight loss, blood in the stools, and hyperactive bowel sounds.

◆ *Rectovaginal fistula.* With rectovaginal fistula, fecal incontinence occurs with uninhibited passage of flatus.

◆ *Spinal cord lesions.* Any lesion that causes compression or transsection of sensorimotor spinal tracts can lead to fecal incontinence. Incontinence may be permanent, especially with severe lesions of the sacral segments.

Fetor hepaticus

Fetor hepaticus—a distinctive musty, sweet breath odor—characterizes hepatic encephalopathy, a life-threatening complication of severe liver disease. The odor results from the damaged liver's inability to metabolize and detoxify mercaptans produced by bacterial degradation of methionine, a sulfurous amino acid. These substances circulate in the blood, are expelled by the lungs, and flavor the breath.

Assessment

If the patient is conscious, closely observe him for signs of impending coma. Evaluate deep tendon reflexes and test for asterixis and Babinski's sign. Stay alert for signs of GI bleeding and shock; both are common complications of end-stage liver failure. Also, watch for increased anxiety, restlessness, tachycardia, tachypnea, hypotension, oliguria, hematemesis, melena, or cool, moist, pale skin.

Place the patient in a supine position with the head of the bed at 30 degrees or greater. Administer oxygen if necessary. Determine the patient's need for I.V. fluids or albumin replacement. Draw blood samples for liver function tests, serum electrolyte levels, hepatitis panel, blood alcohol content, a complete blood count, typing and crossmatching, a clotting profile, and ammonia level. Intubation, ventilation, or cardiopulmonary resuscitation may be necessary. Evaluate the degree of jaundice and abdominal distention, and palpate the liver to assess the degree of enlargement.

Obtain a complete medical history, relying on information from the patient's family if necessary. Focus on factors that may have precipitated hepatic disease or coma. These factors could include a recent severe infection; overuse of sedatives, analgesics, alcohol, or diuretics; excessive protein intake; or recent blood transfusion, surgery, or GI bleeding.

Causes

◆ *Hepatic encephalopathy.* Fetor hepaticus usually occurs in the final, comatose stage of hepatic encephalopathy but may occur earlier. Tremors progress to asterixis in the impending stage. Lethargy, aberrant behavior, and apraxia also occur. Hyperventilation and stupor mark the stuporous stage, during which the patient acts agitated when aroused.

Fever

Fever is a common sign that can arise from many disorders. Because these disorders can affect virtually any body system, fever in the absence of other signs usually has little diagnostic significance, although persistent high fever represents an emergency.

Fever can be classified as low (oral reading of 99° to 100.4° F [37.2° to 38° C]), moderate (100.5° to 104° F [38.1° to 40° C]), or high (above 104° F). Fever greater than 106° F (41.1° C) causes unconsciousness and, if sustained, leads to permanent brain damage.

Fever may also be classified as remittent, intermittent, sustained, relapsing, or undulant. Remittent fever, the most common type, is characterized by daily temperature fluctuations above the normal range. Intermittent fever is marked by a daily temperature drop into the normal range and then a rise in temperature to above normal. An intermittent fever is one that fluctuates widely and typically produces chills and sweating; it's called hectic, or septic, fever. Sustained fever involves persistent temperature elevation with little fluctuation. Relapsing fever consists of alternating feverish and afebrile periods. Undulant fever refers to a gradual increase in temperature that stays high for a few days and then decreases gradually.

Further classification involves duration—either brief (less than 3 weeks) or prolonged. Prolonged fever includes fever of unknown origin, a classification used when careful examination fails to detect an underlying cause.

Assessment

If the patient's fever is only mild to moderate, ask him when it began and how high his temperature reached. Did the fever disappear only to reappear later? Did he experience other symptoms, such as chills, fatigue, or pain?

Obtain a complete medical history, making special note of immunosuppressive treatments or disorders, infection, trauma, surgery, diagnostic testing, and the use of medications. Ask about recent travel because certain diseases are endemic.

Let the history findings direct your physical examination. Because a fever can accompany diverse disorders, the examination may range from a brief evaluation of one body system to a comprehensive review of all systems. (See *How fever develops.*)

Causes

◆ *Anthrax (cutaneous).* With cutaneous anthrax, the patient may experience fever along with lymphadenopathy, malaise, and headache.
◆ *Anthrax (GI).* GI anthrax follows the ingestion of contaminated meat from an infected animal. The patient experiences fever, loss of appetite, nausea, and vomiting.
◣ *Anthrax (inhalation).* The initial signs and symptoms of inhalation anthrax are flulike, including fever, chills, weakness, cough, and chest pain.
◆ *Drugs.* Fever and rash commonly result from hypersensitivity to antifungals, sulfonamides, penicillins, cephalosporins, tetracyclines, barbiturates, phenytoin (Dilantin), quinidine (Cardioquin), iodides, methyldopa (Aldomet), procainamide (Pronestyl), and some antitoxins. Fever can accompany chemotherapy, especially with bleomycin (Blenoxane), vincristine (Oncovin), and asparaginase (Elspar). It can result from drugs that impair sweating, such as anticholinergics, phenothiazines, and monoamine oxidase inhibitors. Fever can also stem from toxic doses of salicylates, amphetamines, and tricyclic antidepressants. Inhaled anesthetics and muscle relaxants can trigger malignant hyperthermia in patients with this inherited trait.
◆ *Escherichia coli O157:H7.* Fever, bloody diarrhea, nausea, vomiting, and abdominal cramps occur after eating

How fever develops

Body temperature is regulated by the hypothalamic thermostat, which has a specific set point under normal conditions. Fever can result from a resetting of this set point or from an abnormality in the thermoregulatory system itself, as shown in this flowchart.

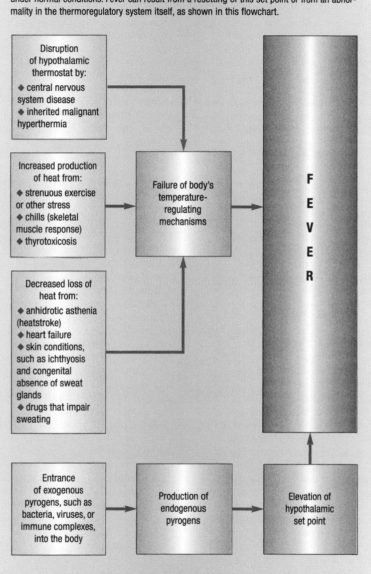

undercooked beef or other foods contaminated with *E. coli* O157:H7. In children younger than age 5 and in elderly patients, hemolytic uremic syndrome may develop, which may ultimately lead to acute renal failure.

◆ *Immune complex dysfunction.* When present with immune complex dysfunction, fever usually remains low, although moderate elevations may accompany erythema multiforme. Fever may be remittent or intermittent, such as in acquired immunodeficiency syndrome (AIDS) or systemic lupus erythematosus, or sustained such as in polyarteritis. As one of several vague, prodromal complaints (such as fatigue, anorexia, and weight loss), fever produces nocturnal diaphoresis and accompanies such associated signs and symptoms as diarrhea and a persistent cough (with AIDS) or morning stiffness (with rheumatoid arthritis). Other disease-specific findings include headache and vision loss (temporal arteritis); pain and stiffness in the neck, shoulders, back, or pelvis (ankylosing spondylitis and polymyalgia rheumatica); skin and mucous membrane lesions (erythema multiforme); and urethritis with urethral discharge and conjunctivitis (Reiter syndrome).

◆ *Infectious and inflammatory disorders.* Fever ranges from low (in patients with Crohn's disease or ulcerative colitis) to extremely high (in those with bacterial pneumonia, necrotizing fasciitis, or *Ebola* or *Hantavirus*). It may be remittent, such as in those with infectious mononucleosis or otitis media; hectic (recurring daily with sweating, chills, and flushing), such as in those with lung abscess, influenza, or endocarditis; sustained, such as in those with meningitis; or relapsing such as in those with malaria. Fever may arise abruptly, such as in those with toxic shock syndrome or Rocky Mountain spotted fever, or insidiously such as in those with mycoplasmal pneumonia. In patients with hepatitis, fever may represent a disease prodrome; in those with appendicitis, it follows the acute stage. Its sudden, late appearance with tachycardia, tachypnea, and confusion heralds life-threatening septic shock in patients with peritonitis or gram-negative bacteremia.

◆ *Listeriosis.* Signs and symptoms of listeriosis include fever, myalgia, abdominal pain, nausea, vomiting, and diarrhea. If the infection spreads to the nervous system, meningitis may develop.

◆ *Neoplasms.* Primary neoplasms and metastases can produce prolonged fever of varying elevations.

◆ *Plague* (Yersinia pestis). The bubonic form of plague (transmitted via bites by infected fleas) causes fever, chills, and swollen, inflamed, and tender lymph nodes near the bite site. The septicemic form of plague develops as a fulminant illness generally with the bubonic form. The pneumonic form manifests as a sudden onset of chills, fever, headache, and myalgia after person-to-person transmission via the respiratory tract.

◆ *Q fever.* Q fever is a rickettsial disease caused by *Coxiella burnetii* infection. It causes fever, chills, severe headache, malaise, chest pain, nausea, vomiting, and diarrhea. The fever may last up to 2 weeks.

◆ *Rhabdomyolysis.* Rhabdomyolysis results in muscle breakdown and release of muscle cell contents (myoglobin) into the bloodstream. Its signs and symptoms include fever, muscle weakness or pain, nausea, vomiting, malaise, and dark urine.

◤ *Severe acute respiratory syndrome (SARS).* SARS is an acute infectious disease of unknown etiology; however, a novel coronavirus has been implicated as a possible cause. The incubation period is 2 to 7 days. In most cases, SARS begins with fever (usually greater than 100.4° F [38° C]).

◆ *Smallpox (variola major).* Initial signs and symptoms of smallpox include a high fever, malaise, prostration, severe headache, backache, and abdominal pain. A maculopapular rash develops on the mucosa of the mouth, pharynx, face, and forearms and then spreads to the trunk and legs.

◤ *Thermoregulatory dysfunction.* Thermoregulatory dysfunction is marked by a sudden onset of fever that rises rapidly and remains as high as 107° F (41.7° C). It occurs in such life-threatening disorders as heatstroke, thyroid storm, neuroleptic malignant syndrome, and malignant hyperthermia and in central nervous system lesions. A low or moderate fever appears in dehydrated patients.

◆ *Tularemia.* Tularemia, also known as *rabbit fever,* causes an abrupt onset of fever, chills, headache, generalized myalgia, a nonproductive cough, dyspnea, pleuritic chest pain, and empyema.

◆ *Typhus.* Typhus is a rickettsial disease. Initially, the patient experiences headache, myalgia, arthralgia, and malaise followed by an abrupt onset of fever, chills, nausea, and vomiting.

◤ *West Nile encephalitis.* West Nile encephalitis is a brain infection caused by West Nile virus—a mosquito-borne flavivirus. Mild infection is common. Signs and symptoms include fever, headache, and body aches, usually with a skin rash and swollen lymph glands. More severe infection is marked by high fever.

Flank pain

Pain in the flank, the area extending from the ribs to the ilium, is a leading indicator of renal and upper urinary tract disease or trauma. Depending on the cause, this symptom may vary from a dull ache to severe stabbing or throbbing pain. It may be unilateral or bilateral and constant or intermittent. It's aggravated by costovertebral angle (CVA) percussion and, in patients with renal or urinary tract obstruction, by increased fluid intake and ingestion of alcohol, caffeine, or diuretics. Unaffected by position changes, flank pain typically responds only to analgesics or to treatment of the underlying disorder.

Assessment

If the patient has suffered trauma, quickly look for a visible or palpable flank mass, associated injuries, CVA pain, hematuria, Turner's sign, and signs of shock. (See *Responding when flank pain is associated with trauma,* page 264.)

If the patient's condition isn't critical, take a thorough history. Ask about the pain's onset and apparent precipitating events. Have the patient describe the pain's location, intensity, pattern, and duration. Find out if anything aggravates or alleviates it. Ask the patient about changes in his normal pattern of fluid intake and urine output. Explore his history for a urinary tract infection or obstruction, renal disease, or recent streptococcal infection.

During the physical examination, palpate the patient's flank area and percuss the CVA to determine the extent of pain.

EMERGENCY INTERVENTIONS

Responding when flank pain is associated with trauma

If your patient has suffered trauma and develops flank pain, associated injuries, a flank mass, costovertebral angle pain, hematuria, Turner's sign, or signs of shock, be sure to:
◆ immediately notify the practitioner
◆ insert an I.V. catheter

◆ prepare to administer fluid or drug infusion, as prescribed
◆ insert an indwelling urinary catheter, as prescribed, to monitor urine output and evaluate hematuria
◆ obtain blood samples for typing and crossmatching, a complete blood count, and electrolyte levels.

Causes

◆ *Calculi.* Renal and ureteral calculi produce intense unilateral, colicky flank pain. Typically, initial CVA pain radiates to the flank, suprapubic region, and perhaps the genitalia.

◆ *Cortical necrosis (acute).* Unilateral flank pain is usually severe with cortical necrosis. Accompanying findings include gross hematuria, anuria, leukocytosis, and fever.

◆ *Obstructive uropathy.* With acute obstruction, flank pain may be excruciating; with gradual obstruction, it's typically a dull ache. In either case, the pain may also localize in the upper abdomen and radiate to the groin.

◆ *Papillary necrosis (acute).* With papillary necrosis, intense bilateral flank pain occurs along with renal colic, CVA tenderness, and abdominal pain and rigidity.

◆ *Perirenal abscess.* With perirenal abscess, intense unilateral flank pain and CVA tenderness accompany dysuria, a persistent high fever, chills and, in some patients, a palpable abdominal mass.

◆ *Polycystic kidney disease.* Dull, aching, bilateral flank pain is commonly the earliest symptom of polycystic kidney disease. The pain can become severe and colicky if cysts rupture and clots migrate or cause obstruction.

◆ *Pyelonephritis (acute).* With pyelonephritis, intense, constant, and unilateral or bilateral flank pain develops over a few hours or days. Pain is accompanied by typical urinary findings that include dysuria, nocturia, hematuria, urgency, frequency, and tenesmus (a painful spasm of the anal sphincter that's accompanied by an urgent desire to evacuate the bowel or bladder).

◆ *Renal cancer.* Unilateral flank pain, gross hematuria, and a palpable flank mass form the classic clinical triad of renal cancer. Flank pain is usually dull and vague, although severe colicky pain can occur during bleeding or passage of clots.

◆ *Renal infarction.* With renal infarction, unilateral constant severe flank pain and tenderness typically accompany persistent severe upper abdominal pain.

◆ *Renal trauma.* Variable bilateral or unilateral flank pain is a common symptom of renal trauma. A visible or palpable flank mass may also exist, along with CVA or abdominal pain, which may be severe and radiate to the groin.

◆ *Renal vein thrombosis.* Severe unilateral flank and lower back pain with CVA and epigastric tenderness typify the rapid onset of venous obstruction. Other findings include fever, hematuria, and leg edema. Bilateral flank pain, oliguria, and other uremic signs and symptoms typify bilateral obstruction.

Fontanel, bulging

In a normal infant, the anterior fontanel, or "soft spot," is flat, soft yet firm, and well demarcated against surrounding skull bones. The posterior fontanel shouldn't be fused at birth, but may be overriding following the birthing process. This fontanel usually closes by age 3 months. (See *Locating fontanels.*) Subtle pulsations may be visible, reflecting the arterial pulse.

A bulging fontanel—widened, tense, and with marked pulsations—is a cardinal sign of meningitis associated with increased intracranial pressure (ICP), a

Locating fontanels

The anterior fontanel lies at the junction of the sagittal, coronal, and frontal sutures. Normally, it measures about 2.5 × 5 cm at birth and closes by age 18 to 20 months.

The posterior fontanel lies at the junction of the sagittal and lambdoidal sutures. It measures 1 to 2 cm around and normally closes by age 3 months.

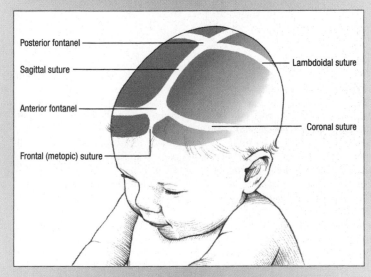

EMERGENCY INTERVENTIONS

Responding to increased ICP

If an infant with bulging fontanels shows signs of increased intracranial pressure (ICP), act quickly.
◆ Maintain a patent airway.
◆ Administer supplemental oxygen or assist with endotracheal intubation and mechanical ventilation if necessary.

◆ Institute and maintain seizure precautions.
◆ Insert an I.V. catheter.
◆ Prepare to administer an anticonvulsant, as prescribed.
◆ Administer an osmotic diuretic, as prescribed, to help reduce cerebral edema.

medical emergency. It can also be an indication of encephalitis or fluid overload. Because prolonged coughing, crying, or lying down can cause transient, physiologic bulging, the infant's head should be observed and palpated while the infant is upright and relaxed to detect pathologic bulging.

Assessment

If you detect a bulging fontanel, measure its size and the infant's head circumference and note the overall shape of the head. Check the infant's vital signs and determine his level of consciousness (LOC) by observing spontaneous activity, postural reflex activity, and sensory responses. Note whether the infant assumes a normal, flexed posture or one of extreme extension, opisthotonos (a tetanic spasm in which the spine and extremities are convexly bent forward, with the body resting on the head and heels), or hypotonia. Observe arm and leg movements; excessive tremulousness or frequent twitching may herald the onset of a seizure. Look for other signs of increased ICP, including abnormal respiratory patterns and a distinctive, high-pitched cry. (See *Responding to increased ICP.*)

When the infant's condition is stabilized, you can begin investigating the underlying cause of increased ICP. Obtain the child's medical history from a parent or caretaker, paying particular attention to a recent infection or trauma, including birth trauma. Has the infant or a family member had a recent rash or fever? Ask about changes in the infant's behavior, such as frequent vomiting, lethargy, or disinterest in feeding.

Causes

◼ *Increased ICP.* Besides a bulging fontanel and increased head circumference, other early signs and symptoms are usually subtle and difficult to discern. They may include behavioral changes, irritability, fatigue, and vomiting. As ICP rises, the infant's pupils may dilate and his LOC may decrease to drowsiness and eventual coma. Seizures commonly occur.

Fontanel depression

Depression of the anterior fontanel below the surrounding bony ridges of the skull is a sign of dehydration. A common disorder of infancy and early childhood, dehydration can result from insufficient fluid intake, but typically reflects excessive fluid loss from severe vomiting or diarrhea. It may also reflect insensible water loss, pyloric stenosis, or tracheoesophageal fistula. It's best to assess the fontanel when the infant is in an upright position and isn't crying.

Assessment

If you detect a markedly depressed fontanel, check the infant's vital signs, weigh him, and assess for signs of shock. If these signs are present, prepare to insert an I.V. catheter and administer fluids, as prescribed. Obtain a thorough patient history from a parent or caretaker, focusing on recent fever, vomiting, diarrhea, and behavioral changes. Monitor the infant's fluid intake and urine output over the past 24 hours, including the number of wet diapers during that time. Ask about the child's weight before he became ill and compare it to his current weight; weight loss in an infant reflects water loss.

Causes

◼ *Dehydration.* With mild dehydration (5% weight loss), the anterior fontanel appears slightly depressed. The infant has pale, dry skin and mucous membranes, decreased urine output, a normal or slightly elevated pulse rate and, possibly, irritability. Moderate dehydration (10% weight loss) causes slightly more pronounced fontanel depression, along with gray skin with poor turgor, dry mucous membranes, decreased tears, and decreased urine output. The infant has normal or decreased blood pressure, an increased pulse rate and, possibly, lethargy. Severe dehydration (15% or greater weight loss) may result in a markedly sunken fontanel, along with extremely poor skin turgor, parched mucous membranes, marked oliguria or anuria, lethargy, and signs of shock.

G

Gag reflex abnormalities

The gag reflex—a protective mechanism that prevents aspiration of food, fluid, and vomitus—normally can be elicited by touching the posterior wall of the oropharynx with a tongue depressor or by suctioning the throat. Prompt elevation of the palate, constriction of the pharyngeal musculature, and a sensation of gagging indicate a normal gag reflex. An abnormal gag reflex (either decreased or absent) interferes with the ability to swallow and, more important, increases susceptibility to life-threatening aspiration.

An impaired gag reflex can result from a lesion that affects its mediators—cranial nerves (CNs) IX (glossopharyngeal) and X (vagus) or the pons or medulla. An impaired gag reflex can also occur in a patient who's in a coma, in muscle diseases such as severe myasthenia gravis, or as a temporary result of anesthesia.

Assessment

Ask the patient (or a family member if the patient can't communicate) about the onset and duration of swallowing difficulties, if applicable. Are liquids more difficult to swallow than solids? Is swallowing more difficult at certain times of the day? If the patient also has trouble chewing, suspect more widespread neurologic involvement because chewing involves different cranial nerves. Explore the patient's medical history for vascular and degenerative disorders. Then assess his respiratory status for evidence of aspiration and perform a neurologic examination. If you detect an abnormal gag reflex, stop the patient's oral intake to prevent aspiration. If his level of consciousness (LOC) is decreased, place him in a side-lying position to prevent aspiration; if not, place him in Fowler's position.

Causes

◆ *Basilar artery occlusion.* Basilar artery occlusion may suddenly diminish or obliterate the gag reflex. It also causes diffuse sensory loss, dysarthria, facial weakness, extraocular muscle palsies, quadriplegia, and a decreased LOC.

◆ *Brain stem glioma.* Brain stem glioma causes a gradual loss of the gag reflex. Related symptoms include diplopia and facial weakness that reflect bilateral brain stem involvement.

◆ *Bulbar palsy.* In bulbar palsy, the loss of the gag reflex reflects temporary or permanent paralysis of muscles supplied by CNs IX and X. Other indicators of bulbar palsy include jaw and facial muscle weakness, dysphagia, loss of sensation at the base of the tongue, increased salivation, possible difficulty articulating and breathing, and fasciculations.

♦ *Wallenberg syndrome.* With Wallenberg syndrome, paresis of the palate and an impaired gag reflex usually develop within hours to days of thrombosis. The patient may experience analgesia and thermanesthesia, occurring ipsilaterally on the face and contralaterally on the body.

Gait, bizarre

A bizarre gait has no obvious organic basis; rather, it's produced unconsciously by a person with a somatoform disorder (hysterical neurosis) or consciously by a malingerer. The gait has no consistent pattern. It may mimic an organic impairment. Characteristically, a bizarre gait has a more theatrical or bizarre quality with key elements missing, such as a spastic gait without hip circumduction or leg "paralysis" with normal reflexes and motor strength. Its manifestations may include wild gyrations, exaggerated stepping, leg dragging, or mimicking unusual walks such as that of a tightrope walker.

Assessment

If you suspect that the patient's gait impairment has no organic cause, investigate other possibilities. Ask the patient when he first developed the impairment and whether it coincided with a stressful period or event. Also ask about associated symptoms. Explore reports of frequent unexplained illnesses and multiple physician visits.

Subtly try to determine if the patient can gain anything from malingering; for example, added attention or an insurance settlement.

Begin your assessment by testing the patient's reflexes and sensorimotor function, noting abnormal response patterns. To quickly check his reports of leg weakness or paralysis, perform a test for Hoover's sign: Place the patient in the supine position and stand at his feet. Cradle a heel in each of your palms and then rest your hands on the table. Ask the patient to raise the affected leg. In true motor weakness, the heel of the other leg will press downward; in hysteria, this movement will be absent.

Causes

♦ *Conversion disorder.* Conversion disorder is a rare somatoform disorder in which a bizarre gait or paralysis may develop after severe stress and isn't accompanied by other symptoms.
♦ *Malingering.* Malingering is a rare cause of a bizarre gait in which the patient may also complain of a headache and chest and back pain.
♦ *Somatization disorder.* Bizarre gait is one of many possible somatic complaints with somatization disorder. The patient may exhibit any combination of pseudoneurologic signs and symptoms, including fainting, weakness, memory loss, dysphagia, vision problems, seizures, and bladder dysfunction. He may also report pain in the back, joints, and extremities and complaints in almost any body system.

Gait, propulsive

A propulsive gait is characterized by a stooped, rigid posture. The patient's head and neck are bent forward. His

Identifying gait abnormalities

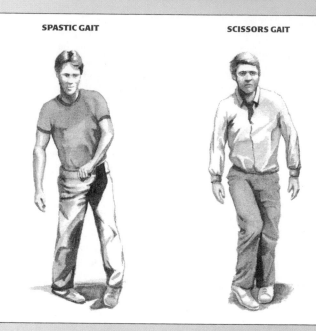

SPASTIC GAIT   SCISSORS GAIT

flexed, stiffened arms are held away from the body. His fingers are extended, and his knees and hips are stiffly bent. During ambulation, this posture results in a forward shifting of the body's center of gravity and consequent impairment of balance, causing increasingly rapid short shuffling steps with involuntary acceleration and lack of control over forward or backward motion. (See *Identifying gait abnormalities*.)

A propulsive gait is a cardinal sign of advanced Parkinson's disease. It results from progressive degeneration of the ganglia, which are primarily responsible for smooth muscle movement. Because a propulsive gait develops gradually and its accompanying effects are usually wrongly attributed to aging, it commonly goes unnoticed or unreported until severe disability results.

Assessment

Ask the patient when his gait impairment first developed and whether it has recently worsened. Because he may have difficulty remembering, you may be able to gain information from family members or friends, especially those who see the patient only sporadically. Also obtain a thorough drug his-

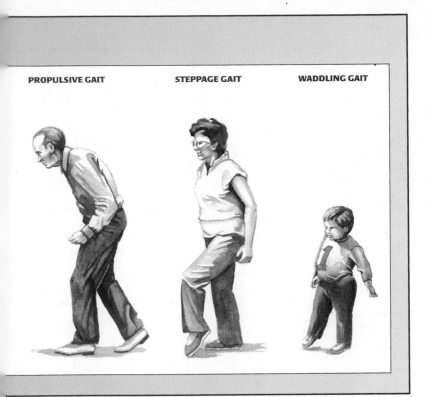

PROPULSIVE GAIT **STEPPAGE GAIT** **WADDLING GAIT**

tory, including medication type and dosage. Ask the patient if he has been taking tranquilizers, especially phenothiazines. If he knows he has Parkinson's disease and has been taking levodopa (Larodopa), pay particular attention to the dosage because an overdose can cause an acute exacerbation of signs and symptoms. If Parkinson's disease isn't a known or suspected diagnosis, ask the patient if he has been acutely or routinely exposed to carbon monoxide or manganese.

Begin your assessment by testing the patient's reflexes and sensorimotor function, noting abnormal response patterns.

Causes

◤ *Carbon monoxide poisoning.* A propulsive gait commonly appears several weeks after acute carbon monoxide intoxication.

◆ *Drugs.* A propulsive gait and possibly other extrapyramidal effects can result from the use of phenothiazines, other antipsychotics (notably haloperidol [Haldol], thiothixene [Navane], and loxapine [Loxitane]) and, infrequently, metoclopramide (Reglan) and metyrosine (Demser). Such effects are usually temporary.

◆ *Manganese poisoning.* Chronic overexposure to manganese can cause an insidious, usually permanent, propulsive gait. Typical early findings include fatigue, muscle weakness and rigidity, dystonia, resting tremor, choreoathetoid movements, masklike facies, and personality changes. Those at risk for manganese poisoning include welders, railroad workers, miners, steelworkers, and those who handle pesticides.

◆ *Parkinson's disease.* The characteristic propulsive gait with Parkinson's disease begins as a shuffle. As the disease progresses, the gait slows. Cardinal signs of the disease are progressive muscle rigidity, which may be uniform or jerky; akinesia; and an insidious tremor that begins in the fingers, increases during stress or anxiety, and decreases with purposeful movement and sleep.

Gait, scissors

Resulting from bilateral spastic paresis, a scissors gait affects both legs and has little or no effect on the arms. The patient's legs flex slightly at the hips and knees, so he looks like he's crouching. With each step, his thighs adduct and his knees hit or cross in a scissorslike movement. (See *Identifying gait abnormalities,* pages 270 and 271.) His steps are short, regular, and laborious, as if he were wading through waist-deep water. His feet may be plantar flexed and turned inward with a shortened Achilles tendon. As a result, he may walk on his toes or on the balls of his feet and scrape his toes on the ground.

Assessment

Ask the patient (or a family member, if the patient can't answer) about the on-

set and duration of the gait. Has it remained constant or progressively worsened? Ask about a history of trauma, including birth trauma, and neurologic disorders. Thoroughly evaluate motor and sensory function and deep tendon reflexes (DTRs) in the legs.

Causes

◆ *Cerebral palsy.* In the spastic form of cerebral palsy, patients walk on their toes with a scissors gait. Other findings include hyperactive DTRs, increased stretch reflexes, rapid alternating muscle contraction and relaxation, muscle weakness, underdevelopment of affected limbs, and a tendency toward contractures.

◆ *Cervical spondylosis with myelopathy.* A scissors gait develops in the late stages of cervical spondylosis with myelopathy and steadily worsens.

◆ *Multiple sclerosis (MS).* With MS, a progressive scissors gait usually develops gradually, with infrequent remissions. Characteristic muscle weakness, usually in the legs, ranges from minor fatigability to paraparesis with urinary urgency and constipation.

◆ *Spinal cord tumor.* A scissors gait can develop gradually from a thoracic or lumbar tumor. Other findings reflect the location of the tumor.

◆ *Syringomyelia.* A scissors gait usually occurs late in syringomyelia, with analgesia and thermanesthesia, muscle atrophy and weakness, and Charcot's joint.

Gait, spastic

A spastic gait—sometimes referred to as a *paretic* or *weak gait*—is a stiff, foot-dragging walk caused by unilateral leg muscle hypertonicity. This gait indicates focal damage to the corticospinal tract. The affected leg becomes rigid, with a marked decrease in flexion at the hip and knee and possibly plantar flexion and equinovarus deformity of the foot. Because the patient's leg doesn't swing normally at the hip or knee, his foot tends to drag or shuffle, scraping his toes on the ground. (See *Identifying gait abnormalities*, pages 270 and 271.) To compensate, the pelvis of the affected side tilts upward in an attempt to lift the toes, causing the patient's leg to abduct and circumduct. Also, arm swing is hindered on the same side as the affected leg. A spastic gait usually develops after a period of flaccidity (hypotonicity) in the affected leg. Whatever the cause, the gait is usually permanent after it develops.

Assessment

Determine when the patient first noticed the gait impairment. Did it develop suddenly or gradually? Ask him if it waxes and wanes or if it has worsened progressively. Does fatigue, hot weather, or warm baths or showers worsen the gait? (Such exacerbation typically occurs in multiple sclerosis [MS].) Focus your medical history questions on neurologic disorders, recent head trauma, and degenerative diseases.

During the physical examination, test and compare strength, range of motion, and sensory function in all limbs. Also, observe and palpate for muscle flaccidity or atrophy.

Causes

◆ *Brain abscess.* In brain abscess, a spastic gait generally develops slowly after a period of muscle flaccidity and fever. Early signs and symptoms of abscess reflect increased intracranial pressure (ICP). Later, site-specific findings may include hemiparesis, tremors, vision disturbances, nystagmus, and pupillary inequality.

◆ *Brain tumor.* Depending on the site and type of tumor, a spastic gait usually develops gradually and worsens over time. Accompanying effects may include signs of increased ICP, papilledema, sensory loss on the affected side, dysarthria, ocular palsies, aphasia, and personality changes.

◼ *Head trauma.* A spastic gait typically follows the acute stage of head trauma. The patient may also experience focal or generalized seizures, personality changes, headache, and focal neurologic signs.

◆ *MS.* A spastic gait begins insidiously and follows MS's characteristic cycle of exacerbation and remission. The gait commonly worsens in warm weather or after a warm bath or shower.

◼ *Stroke.* With a stroke, a spastic gait usually appears after a period of muscle weakness and hypotonicity on the affected side.

Gait, steppage

A steppage gait typically results from footdrop caused by weakness or paralysis of pretibial and peroneal muscles, usually from lower motor neuron lesions. Footdrop causes the foot to hang with the toes pointing down, so the toes scrape the ground during ambulation. To compensate, the hip rotates outward and the hip and knee flex in an exaggerated fashion to lift the advancing leg off the ground. The foot is thrown forward and the toes hit the ground first, producing an audible slap.

(See *Identifying gait abnormalities*, pages 270 and 271.) The rhythm of the gait is usually regular, with even steps and normal upper body posture and arm swing. A steppage gait can be unilateral or bilateral and permanent or transient, depending on the site and type of neural damage.

Assessment

Begin by asking the patient about the onset of the gait and recent changes in its character. Does a family member have a similar gait? Inquire about traumatic injury to the buttocks, hips, legs, or knees. Ask about a history of chronic disorders that may be associated with polyneuropathy, such as diabetes mellitus, polyarteritis nodosa, and alcoholism. While you're taking the history, observe whether the patient crosses his legs while sitting because this may put pressure on the peroneal nerve.

Inspect and palpate the patient's calves and feet for muscle atrophy and wasting. Using a pin, test for sensory deficits along the entire length of both legs.

Causes

◆ *Guillain-Barré syndrome.* A steppage gait typically occurs after recovery from the acute stage of Guillain-Barré syndrome. It can be mild or severe, unilateral or bilateral. Invariably, it's permanent. Muscle weakness usually begins in the legs and then extends to the arms and face within 72 hours.
◆ *Herniated lumbar disk.* With a herniated lumbar disk, a unilateral steppage gait and footdrop commonly occur with late-stage weakness and atrophy of leg muscles. However, the most pronounced symptom is severe low back pain, which may radiate to the buttocks, legs, and feet, usually unilaterally.
◆ *Multiple sclerosis (MS).* A steppage gait and footdrop typically fluctuate in severity with MS's characteristic cycle of exacerbation and remission.
◆ *Peroneal muscle atrophy.* A bilateral steppage gait and footdrop begin insidiously in peroneal muscle atrophy. Foot, peroneal, and ankle dorsiflexor muscles are affected first.
◆ *Peroneal nerve trauma.* A temporary ipsilateral steppage gait occurs suddenly but resolves with the release of peroneal nerve pressure. The gait is associated with footdrop and muscle weakness and sensory loss over the lateral surface of the calf and foot.

Gait, waddling

A waddling gait, a distinctive ducklike walk, is an important sign of muscular dystrophy, spinal muscle atrophy or, rarely, congenital hip displacement. It may be present when a child begins to walk or may appear only later in life. The gait results from deterioration of the pelvic girdle muscles—primarily the gluteus medius, hip flexors, and hip extensors. Weakness in these muscles hinders stabilization of the weight-bearing hip during walking, causing the opposite hip to drop and the trunk to lean toward that side in an attempt to maintain balance. (See *Identifying gait abnormalities*, pages 270 and 271.) Typically, the legs assume a wide stance and the trunk is thrown back to further improve stability, exaggerating lordosis and abdominal protrusion. In severe cases, leg and foot muscle contractures may cause equinovarus deformity of the foot combined with circumduction or bowing of the legs.

Assessment

Ask the patient (or a family member, if the patient is a young child) when the gait first appeared and if it has recently worsened. To determine the extent of pelvic girdle and leg muscle weakness, ask if the patient falls frequently or has difficulty when climbing stairs, rising from a chair, or walking. Also, find out if he was late in learning to walk or holding his head upright. Obtain a family history, focusing on problems of muscle weakness and gait and on congenital motor disorders.

Inspect and palpate leg muscles, especially the calves, for size and tone. Check for a positive Gowers' sign, which indicates pelvic muscle weakness. (See *Identifying Gowers' sign.*) Next, assess motor strength and function in the shoulders, arms, and hands, noting weakness or asymmetrical movements.

Causes

◆ *Congenital hip dysplasia.* Bilateral hip dislocation produces a waddling gait with lordosis and pain.
◆ *Muscular dystrophy (Duchenne's).* With Duchenne's muscular dystrophy, a waddling gait becomes clinically evident from ages 3 to 5. The gait worsens as the disease progresses until the child loses the ability to walk and requires a wheelchair, usually from ages 10 to 12. Early signs are usually sub-

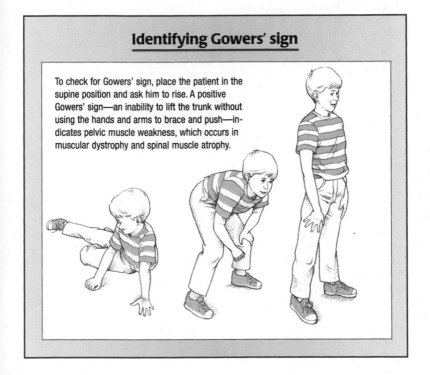

Identifying Gowers' sign

To check for Gowers' sign, place the patient in the supine position and ask him to rise. A positive Gowers' sign—an inability to lift the trunk without using the hands and arms to brace and push—indicates pelvic muscle weakness, which occurs in muscular dystrophy and spinal muscle atrophy.

tle—a delay in learning to walk, frequent falls, gait or posture abnormalities, and intermittent calf pain. A positive Gowers' sign appears later.

◆ *Muscular dystrophy (Becker's)*. With Becker's muscular dystrophy, a waddling gait typically becomes apparent in late adolescence, slowly worsens during the third decade, and culminates in total loss of ambulation. Progressive wasting with selected muscle hypertrophy produces a positive Gowers' sign.

◆ *Muscular dystrophy (facioscapulohumeral)*. With facioscapulohumeral muscular dystrophy, which usually occurs late in childhood and during adolescence, a waddling gait appears after muscle wasting has spread downward from the face and shoulder girdle to the pelvic girdle and legs.

◆ *Spinal muscle atrophy*. With Kugelberg-Welander syndrome, a waddling gait occurs early, usually after age 2, and typically progresses slowly, culminating in the total loss of ambulation up to 20 years later. With Werdnig-Hoffmann disease, a waddling gait typically begins when the child learns to walk. Reflexes may be absent. The gait progressively worsens, culminating in complete loss of ambulation by adolescence.

Gallop, atrial

An atrial or presystolic gallop is an extra heart sound (known as S_4) that's heard or typically palpated immediately before the first heart sound (S_1), late in diastole. This low-pitched sound is heard best with the bell of the stethoscope pressed lightly against the cardiac apex. Some clinicians say that an S_4 has the cadence of the "Ten" in Tennessee (Ten = S_4; nes = S_1; see = S_2).

This gallop typically results from hypertension, conduction defects, valvular disorders, or other problems such as ischemia. Occasionally, it helps differentiate angina from other causes of chest pain. It results from abnormal forceful atrial contraction caused by augmented ventricular filling or by decreased left ventricular compliance. An atrial gallop usually originates from left atrial contraction, is heard at the apex, and doesn't vary with inspiration. A left-sided S_4 can occur in hypertensive heart disease, coronary artery disease, aortic stenosis, and cardiomyopathy. It may also originate from right atrial contraction. A right-sided S_4 indicates pulmonary hypertension and pulmonary stenosis; it's heard best at the lower left sternal border and intensifies with inspiration.

An atrial gallop seldom occurs in normal hearts; however, it may occur in elderly people and in athletes with physiologic hypertrophy of the left ventricle.

Assessment

Suspect myocardial ischemia if you auscultate an atrial gallop in a patient with chest pain. Check the patient's vital signs and assess for signs of heart failure. If you detect these signs, attach the patient to a cardiac monitor and obtain an electrocardiogram to assess the patient's cardiac status. When the patient's condition permits, ask about a history of hypertension, angina, valvular stenosis, or cardiomyopathy. If appropriate, have him describe the frequency and severity of anginal attacks. (See *Responding when you suspect myocardial ischemia*. See also *Interpreting heart sounds*, pages 278 and 279.)

EMERGENCY INTERVENTIONS

Responding when you suspect myocardial ischemia

If you suspect myocardial ischemia, you need to respond quickly. Be sure to:
◆ connect the patient to a cardiac monitor
◆ obtain an electrocardiogram
◆ administer an antianginal, as prescribed
◆ administer supplemental oxygen, as ordered
◆ elevate the head of the bed if the patient has dyspnea

◆ auscultate for abnormal breath sounds
◆ insert an I.V. catheter, as ordered
◆ prepare to administer a diuretic, as prescribed, if you detect coarse crackles
◆ apply a transcutaneous pacemaker if the patient develops symptomatic bradycardia and prepare to administer atropine.

Causes

◆ *Angina.* An intermittent atrial gallop characteristically occurs during an anginal attack and disappears when angina subsides. A paradoxical S_2 or a new murmur may accompany the gallop. Typically, the patient complains of anginal chest pain that usually radiates from the retrosternal area to the neck, jaws, left shoulder, and arm.
◆ *Aortic insufficiency (acute).* Acute aortic insufficiency causes an atrial gallop accompanied by a soft, short diastolic murmur along the left sternal border. S_2 may be soft or absent. Sometimes a soft, short midsystolic murmur may be heard over the second right intercostal space.
◆ *Aortic stenosis.* Aortic stenosis usually causes an atrial gallop, especially when valvular obstruction is severe. Auscultation reveals a harsh, crescendo-decrescendo, systolic ejection murmur that's loudest at the right sternal border near the second intercostal space.
◆ *Atrioventricular (AV) block.* First-degree AV block may cause an atrial gallop accompanied by a faint S_1.

Although the patient may have bradycardia, he's usually asymptomatic. In second-degree AV block, an atrial gallop is easily heard. An atrial gallop is also common in third-degree AV block. It varies in intensity with S_1 and is loudest when atrial systole coincides with early, rapid ventricular filling during diastole.
◆ *Cardiomyopathy.* An atrial gallop is a sign associated with cardiomyopathy, regardless of the type: dilated (most common), hypertrophic, or restrictive (least common).
◆ *Hypertension.* One of the earliest findings in systemic arterial hypertension is an atrial gallop. The patient may be asymptomatic or he may experience headache, weakness, epistaxis, tinnitus, dizziness, and fatigue.
◆ *Myocardial infarction (MI).* An atrial gallop is a classic sign of an MI; in fact, it may persist even after the infarction heals. Typically, the patient reports crushing substernal chest pain that may radiate to the back, neck, jaw, shoulder, and left arm.
◆ *Pulmonary embolism.* Pulmonary embolism causes a right-sided atrial

Interpreting heart sounds

Detecting subtle variations in heart sounds requires concentration and practice. When you can recognize normal heart sounds, the abnormal sounds become more obvious.

HEART SOUND AND CAUSE	TIMING AND CADENCE
First heart sound (S_1) Vibrations associated with mitral and tricuspid valve closure	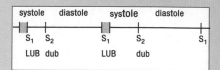
Second heart sound (S_2) Vibrations associated with aortic and pulmonic valve closure	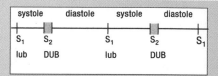
Ventricular gallop (S_3) Vibrations produced by rapid blood flow into the ventricles	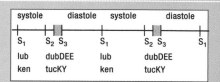
Atrial gallop (S_4) Vibrations produced by an increased resistance to sudden, forceful ejection of atrial blood	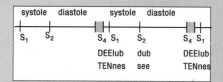
Summation gallop Vibrations produced in mid-diastole by a simultaneous S_3 and S_4, usually caused by tachycardia	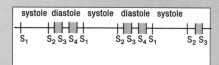

gallop that's usually heard along the lower left sternal border with a loud pulmonic closure sound.

◆ *Thyrotoxicosis.* An atrial gallop and an S_3 may be auscultated in thyroid hormone overproduction.

Gallop, ventricular

A ventricular gallop is a heart sound (known as S_3) associated with rapid ventricular filling in early diastole. Usually palpable, this low-frequency sound occurs about 0.15 second after the second heart sound (S_2). It may originate in either the left or right ventricle. A right-sided gallop usually sounds louder on inspiration and is heard best along the lower left sternal border or over the xiphoid region. A left-sided gallop usually sounds louder on expiration and is heard best at the apex.

Ventricular gallops are easily overlooked because they're usually faint. Fortunately, certain techniques make their detection more likely. These include auscultating in a quiet environment; examining the patient in the supine, left lateral, and semi-Fowler's positions; and having the patient cough or raise his legs to augment the sound.

A physiologic ventricular gallop normally occurs in children and adults younger than age 40 (most people lose this third heart sound by age 40). This gallop may also occur during the third trimester of pregnancy. Abnormal S_3 (in adults older than age 40) can be a sign of decreased myocardial contractility, myocardial failure, and volume overload of the ventricle such as in mitral and tricuspid valve regurgitation. Although the physiologic S_3 has the same timing as the pathologic S_3, its intensity waxes and wanes with respi-

Summation gallop: Two gallops in one

When atrial and ventricular gallops occur simultaneously, they produce a short, low-pitched sound known as a *summation gallop*. This relatively uncommon sound occurs during mid-diastole (between S_2 and S_1) and is best heard with the bell of the stethoscope pressed lightly against the cardiac apex. A summation gallop may be louder than either S_1 or S_2 and may cause visible apical movement during diastole.

Causes

A summation gallop may result from tachycardia or from delayed or blocked atrioventricular (AV) conduction. Tachycardia shortens ventricular filling time during diastole, causing it to coincide with atrial contraction.

When the heart rate slows, the summation gallop is replaced by separate atrial and ventricular gallops, producing a quadruple rhythm much like the canter of a horse. Delayed AV conduction also brings atrial contraction closer to ventricular filling, creating a summation gallop.

A summation gallop usually results from heart failure or dilated congestive cardiomyopathy. It may also accompany other cardiac disorders. Occasionally, it signals further cardiac deterioration. For example, consider the hypertensive patient with a chronic atrial gallop who develops tachycardia and a superimposed ventricular gallop. If this patient abruptly displays a summation gallop, heart failure is the likely cause.

ration. It's also heard more faintly if the patient is sitting or standing.

A pathologic ventricular gallop may be one of the earliest signs of ventricular failure and may result from one of two mechanisms: rapid deceleration of blood entering a stiff, noncompliant ventricle or rapid acceleration of blood associated with increased flow into the ventricle. A gallop that persists despite therapy indicates a poor prognosis.

Patients with cardiomyopathy or heart failure may develop a ventricular and an atrial gallop—a condition known as a summation gallop. (See *Summation gallop: Two gallops in one*.)

Assessment

After auscultating a ventricular gallop, focus your history and examination on the cardiovascular system. Begin by asking the patient if he has had chest pain. If so, have him describe its char-

acter, location, frequency, duration, and alleviating or aggravating factors. Also, ask about palpitations, dizziness, or syncope. Does he have difficulty breathing after exertion? At rest? Does he have a cough? Ask about a history of cardiac disorders. Is he currently receiving treatment for heart failure? If so, which medications is he taking?

During the physical examination, carefully auscultate for murmurs or abnormalities in S_1 and S_2. Then listen for pulmonary crackles. Next, assess peripheral pulses, noting an alternating strong and weak pulse. Finally, assess for jugular vein distention and peripheral edema.

Causes

◆ *Aortic insufficiency.* Acute and chronic aortic insufficiency may produce an S_3. Typically, acute aortic insufficiency also causes an atrial gallop and a soft, short diastolic murmur over the left sternal border. S_2 may be soft or absent. At times, a soft, short mid-systolic murmur may be heard over the second right intercostal space. Chronic aortic insufficiency produces a ventricular gallop and a high-pitched, blowing, decrescendo diastolic murmur that's best heard over the second or third right intercostal space or the left sternal border. An Austin Flint murmur (an apical, rumbling, mid- to late-diastolic murmur) may also occur.

◆ *Cardiomyopathy.* A ventricular gallop is characteristic in cardiomyopathy. When accompanied by an alternating pulse and altered S_1 and S_2, this gallop usually signals advanced heart disease.

◆ *Heart failure.* A cardinal sign of heart failure is a ventricular gallop. When it's loud and accompanied by sinus tachycardia, this gallop may indicate severe heart failure.

◆ *Mitral insufficiency.* Acute and chronic mitral insufficiency may produce a ventricular gallop. In acute mitral insufficiency, auscultation may also reveal an early or holosystolic decrescendo murmur at the apex, an atrial gallop, and a widely split S_2. In chronic mitral insufficiency, a progressively severe ventricular gallop is typical. Auscultation also reveals a holosystolic, blowing, high-pitched apical murmur.

◆ *Thyrotoxicosis.* Thyrotoxicosis may produce ventricular and atrial gallops.

Genital lesions in the male

Among the diverse lesions that may affect the male genitalia are warts, papules, ulcers, scales, and pustules. These common lesions may be painful or painless, singular or multiple. They may be limited to the genitalia or may also occur elsewhere on the body. (See *Recognizing common male genital lesions,* page 282.) Genital lesions may result from infection, neoplasms, parasites, allergy, or the effects of drugs. They can profoundly affect the patient's self-image and relationships. In fact, the patient may hesitate to seek medical attention because he fears cancer or a sexually transmitted disease (STD).

Genital lesions that arise from an STD could mean that the patient is at risk for human immunodeficiency virus (HIV). Genital ulcers make HIV transmission between sexual partners more likely.

Assessment

Begin by asking the patient when he first noticed the lesion. Was it after he began taking a new drug or after a trip out of the country? Has he had similar lesions before? Has he been treating the lesion himself? If so, how? Does the lesion itch? Note whether the lesion is painful. Ask for a description of any drainage from the lesion. Next, take a complete sexual history, noting the frequency of relations, number of partners, and pattern of condom use.

Before you examine the patient, observe his clothing. Do his pants fit properly? Tight pants or underwear, especially those made of nonabsorbent fabrics, can promote the growth of bacteria and fungi. Examine the entire skin surface, noting the location, size, color, and pattern of the lesions. Do genital lesions resemble lesions on other parts of the body? Palpate for nodules, masses, and tenderness. Also, look for bleeding, edema, or signs of infection, such as purulent drainage or

Recognizing common male genital lesions

Many lesions may affect the male genitalia. Some of the more common ones and their causes appear here.

Penile cancer causes a painless ulcerative lesion on the glans or foreskin, possibly accompanied by a foul-smelling discharge.

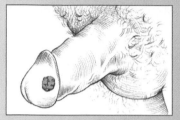

A fixed drug eruption causes a bright red to purplish lesion on the glans penis.

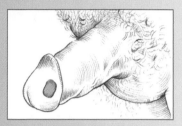

Genital warts are marked by clusters of flesh-colored papillary growths; they may be barely visible or several inches in diameter.

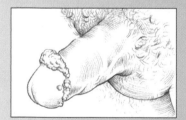

Genital herpes begins as a swollen, slightly pruritic wheal and later becomes a group of small vesicles or blisters on the foreskin, glans, or penile shaft.

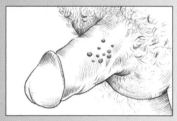

Tinea cruris (commonly known as *jock itch*) produces itchy patches of well-defined, slightly raised, scaly lesions that usually affect the inner thighs and groin.

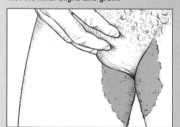

Chancroid causes a painful ulcer that's usually less than 2 cm in diameter and bleeds easily. The lesion may be deep and covered by a gray or yellow exudate at its base.

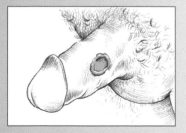

erythema. Finally, check the patient's vital signs.

Causes

◆ *Balanitis and balanoposthitis.* Typically, balanitis (glans infection) and posthitis (prepuce infection) occur together (balanoposthitis), causing painful ulceration on the glans, foreskin, or penile shaft. Ulceration is usually preceded by 2 to 3 days of prepuce irritation and soreness followed by a foul discharge and edema. Without treatment, the ulcers may deepen and multiply. The entire penis and scrotum may become gangrenous, resulting in life-threatening sepsis.

◆ *Bowen's disease.* Bowen's disease is a painless, premalignant lesion that commonly occurs on the penis or scrotum, but may also appear elsewhere. It appears as a brownish red, raised scaly indurated plaque with well-defined borders, which may ulcerate at its center.

◆ *Chancroid.* Chancroid is an STD that's characterized by the eruption of one or more lesions, usually on the groin, inner thigh, or penis. Within 24 hours, the lesion changes from a reddened area to a small papule. It then becomes an inflamed pustule that rapidly ulcerates. This painful ulcer bleeds easily and commonly has a purulent gray or yellow exudate covering its base. Rarely more than 2 cm in diameter, it's typically irregular in shape.

◆ *Folliculitis and furunculosis.* Folliculitis is an inflammatory reaction in hair follicles that may cause red, sharply pointed lesions that are tender and swollen with central pustules. If folliculitis progresses to furunculosis (localized infection deep in the hair follicle), these lesions become hard, painful nodules that may gradually enlarge and rupture, discharging pus and necrotic material.

◆ *Genital herpes.* Genital herpes is an STD. It's caused by herpesvirus type 1 or 2, which produces fluid-filled vesicles on the glans penis, foreskin, or penile shaft and, occasionally, on the mouth or anus. Usually painless at first, these vesicles may rupture and become extensive shallow painful ulcers accompanied by redness, marked edema, and tender, inguinal lymph nodes.

◆ *Genital warts.* Most common in sexually active males, genital warts initially develop on the subpreputial sac or urethral meatus and less commonly on the penile shaft; from there, they spread to the perineum and perianal area. These painless warts start as tiny red or pink swellings that may grow to 10 cm and become pedunculated. Multiple swellings are common, giving the warts a cauliflower appearance. Infected warts are also malodorous.

◆ *Leukoplakia.* Leukoplakia is a precancerous disorder that's characterized by white, scaly patches on the glans and prepuce accompanied by skin thickening and, occasionally, fissures.

◆ *Pediculosis pubis.* Pediculosis pubis is a parasitic infestation that's characterized by erythematous, itching papules in the pubic area and around the anus, abdomen, and thigh. Inspection may detect grayish white specks (lice eggs) attached to hair shafts.

◆ *Penile cancer.* Penile cancer usually produces a painless, enlarging wartlike lesion on the glans or foreskin. However, if the foreskin becomes unretractable, the patient may experience localized pain. Examination may reveal a foul-smelling discharge from the prepuce, a firm lump in the glans, and enlarged lymph nodes.

◆ *Scabies.* Mites that burrow under the skin in scabies may cause crusted lesions or large papules on the glans and shaft of the penis and on the scrotum. They're usually raised, threadlike, and have a swollen nodule or red papule that contains the mite.

◆ *Syphilis.* Two to 4 weeks after exposure to the spirochete *Treponema pallidum,* one or more primary lesions, or chancres, may erupt on the genitalia; occasionally, they also erupt elsewhere on the body, typically on the mouth or perianal area. The chancre usually starts as a small, red, fluid-filled papule and then erodes to form a painless, firm, and indurated shallow ulcer with a clear base and a scant yellow serous discharge or less commonly a hard papule.

◆ *Tinea cruris.* Also called *jock itch,* tinea cruris is a superficial fungal infection that usually causes sharply defined, slightly raised, scaling patches on the inner thigh or groin and less commonly on the scrotum and penis. Pruritus may be severe.

◆ *Urticaria.* Urticaria is a common allergic reaction that's characterized by intensely pruritic hives, which may appear on the genitalia, especially on the foreskin or shaft of the penis.

Gum bleeding

Bleeding gums usually result from dental disorders; less commonly, they may stem from a blood dyscrasia or the effects of certain drugs. Physiologic causes of this common sign include pregnancy, atmospheric pressure changes, and oral trauma. Bleeding ranges from slight oozing to life-threatening hemorrhage. It may be spontaneous or may follow trauma.

Assessment

If gum bleeding isn't an emergency, obtain a history. Find out when the bleeding began. Has it been continuous or intermittent? Does it occur spontaneously or when the patient brushes his teeth or flosses? Find out if the patient or any family members have bleeding tendencies. Ask about easy bruising and frequent nosebleeds. Next, check the patient's dental history. Has he seen a dentist recently? To evaluate nutritional status, have the patient describe his normal diet and alcohol intake. Finally, note any prescription and over-the-counter drugs he takes.

Then perform a complete oral examination. If the patient wears dentures, have him remove them. Examine the gums to determine the site and amount of bleeding. Gums normally appear pink and rippled with their margins snugly against the teeth. Check for inflammation, pockets around the teeth, swelling, retraction, hypertrophy, discoloration, and gum hyperplasia. Note obvious decay, discoloration, foreign material such as food, and absence of teeth.

Causes

◆ *Agranulocytosis.* Spontaneous gum bleeding and other systemic hemorrhages may occur in agranulocytosis. Inspection may reveal oral and perianal lesions, which are usually rough edged with a gray or black membrane.

◆ *Aplastic anemia.* In aplastic anemia, profuse or scant gum bleeding may follow trauma. Other signs of bleeding, such as epistaxis and ecchymoses, are also characteristic.

◆ *Ehlers-Danlos syndrome.* In Ehlers-Danlos syndrome, gums bleed easily after toothbrushing. Easy bruising and other signs of abnormal bleeding are also typical. The skin is fragile and hyperelastic; joints are hyperextendible.

◆ *Gingivitis.* Reddened and edematous gums are characteristic of gingivitis. The gingivae between the teeth become bulbous and bleed easily with slight trauma. With acute necrotizing ulcerative gingivitis, bleeding is spontaneous and the gums become so painful that the patient may be unable to eat. A characteristic grayish yellow pseudomembrane develops over punched-out gum erosions.

◆ *Hemophilia.* With hemophilia, hemorrhage occurs from many sites in the oral cavity, especially the gums.

◆ *Hereditary hemorrhagic telangiectasia.* Hereditary hemorrhagic telangiectasia is characterized by red to violet spiderlike hemorrhagic areas on the gums, which blanch on pressure and bleed spontaneously.

◼ *Leukemia.* Easy gum bleeding, which is an early sign of acute monocytic, lymphocytic, or myelocytic leukemia, is accompanied by gum swelling, necrosis, and petechiae. The soft, tender gums appear glossy and bluish.

◆ *Pemphigoid (benign mucosal).* Most common in women ages 40 to 50, pemphigoid typically causes thick-walled gum lesions that rupture, desquamate, and then bleed easily. Extensive scars form with healing; the gums remain red for months.

◆ *Periodontal disease.* Gum bleeding typically occurs after chewing, toothbrushing, or gum probing, but may also occur spontaneously. As gingivae separate from the bone, pus-filled pockets develop around the teeth.

◆ *Polycythemia vera.* In polycythemia vera, engorged gums ooze blood after even slight trauma. This disorder usually turns the oral mucosa—especially the gums and tongue—a deep red-violet.

◆ *Thrombocytopenia.* Blood usually oozes between the teeth and gums; however, severe bleeding may follow minor trauma.

◼ *Thrombocytopenic purpura (idiopathic).* Profuse gum bleeding occurs in idiopathic thrombocytopenic purpura. Its classic feature, however, is spontaneous hemorrhagic skin lesions that range from pinpoint petechiae to massive hemorrhages.

◆ *Vitamin K deficiency.* In most cases, the first sign of vitamin K deficiency is gums that bleed when the teeth are brushed.

Gynecomastia

Occurring only in males, gynecomastia refers to increased breast size due to excessive mammary gland development. This change in breast size is usually bilateral and may be barely palpable or immediately obvious. Gynecomastia may be associated with breast tenderness and milk secretion.

Normally, several hormones regulate breast development. Estrogens, growth hormone, and corticosteroids stimulate ductal growth, while progesterone and prolactin stimulate growth of the alveolar lobules. Although the pathophysiology of gynecomastia isn't fully understood, a hormonal imbalance—particularly a change in the estrogen-androgen ratio and an increase in prolactin—is a likely contributing factor. Gynecomastia may also result from hormone-secreting tumors and from endocrine, genetic, hepatic, or adrenal disorders. Physiologic gynecomastia may occur in neonatal, pubertal, and elderly males because of normal fluctuations in hormone levels.

Assessment

Begin the history by asking the patient when he first noticed his breast enlargement. How old was he at the time? Have his breasts gotten progressively larger, smaller, or stayed the same? Does he also have breast tenderness or discharge? Ask him if he's ever had his nipples pierced. Next, take a thorough drug history, including prescription, over-the-counter, herbal, and illicit drugs. Explore associated signs and symptoms, such as testicular mass or pain, loss of libido, decreased potency, and loss of chest, axillary, or facial hair.

Focus the physical examination on the breasts, testicles, and penis. As you examine the breasts, note asymmetry, dimpling, abnormal pigmentation, or ulceration. Observe the testicles for size and symmetry. Then palpate them to detect nodules, tenderness, or unusual consistency. Look for normal penile development after puberty and note hypospadias.

Causes

◆ *Adrenal carcinoma.* Estrogen production by an adrenal tumor may produce a feminizing syndrome in males characterized by bilateral gynecomastia, loss of libido, impotence, testicular atrophy, and reduced facial hair growth.

◆ *Breast cancer.* Painful unilateral gynecomastia develops rapidly in males with breast cancer. Palpation may reveal a hard or stony breast lump suggesting a malignant tumor.

◆ *Drugs.* When gynecomastia is an effect of drugs, it's typically painful and unilateral. Estrogens used to treat prostate cancer and drugs that have an estrogen-like effect, such as cardiac glycosides and human chorionic gonadotropin, directly affect the estrogen-androgen ratio. Regular use of alcohol, marijuana, or heroin reduces plasma testosterone levels and also causes gynecomastia. Other drugs, such as flutamide (Eulexin), spironolactone (Aldactone), cimetidine (Tagamet), and ketoconazole (Nizoral), produce this sign by interfering with androgen production or action. Some common drugs, including phenothiazines, tricyclic antidepressants, and antihypertensives, produce gynecomastia in an unknown way.

◆ *Hypothyroidism.* Typically, hypothyroidism produces bilateral gynecomastia along with bradycardia, cold intolerance, weight gain despite anorexia, and mental dullness.

◆ *Klinefelter's syndrome.* In Klinefelter's syndrome, a genetic disorder, painless bilateral gynecomastia first appears during adolescence. Before puberty, symptoms also include abnormally small testicles and a slight mental deficiency; after puberty, symptoms include sparse facial hair, a small penis, decreased libido, and impotence.

◆ *Liver cancer.* Liver cancer may produce bilateral gynecomastia and other characteristics of feminization, such as testicular atrophy, impotence, and reduced facial hair growth. The patient may complain of severe epigastric or right upper quadrant pain associated with a right upper quadrant mass.

◆ *Pituitary tumor.* A pituitary tumor that secretes hormones may cause bilateral gynecomastia accompanied by galactorrhea, impotence, and decreased libido.

◆ *Reifenstein's syndrome.* Reifenstein's syndrome is a genetic disorder that produces painless bilateral gynecomastia at puberty. Associated signs may include hypospadias, testicular atrophy, and an underdeveloped penis.

H

Halo vision

When light passes through water, it breaks up into spectral colors. Similarly, when light passes through excess fluid in the eye—such as tears or various cells within the retina—rainbow-colored rings appear around lights or bright objects. Known as halo vision, this condition typically accompanies disorders that produce excessive tearing or corneal epithelial edema.

Halo vision usually develops suddenly; its duration depends on the cause. The most common—and most significant—cause is acute angle-closure glaucoma. In this disorder, increased intraocular pressure (IOP) forces fluid into corneal tissues anterior to Bowman's membrane, causing edema. Halo vision may also be an early symptom of cataracts, resulting when light is dispersed by abnormal opacities on the lens.

Nonpathologic causes of excessive tearing and resultant halo vision include poorly fitted or worn contact lenses, laughing, crying, and exposure to intense light such as snow blindness.

Assessment

First, ask the patient how long he has been seeing halos around lights and the time of day it usually occurs. (Patients with glaucoma usually see halos in the morning, when IOP is most elevated.) Next, ask the patient if light bothers his eyes. Does he have eye pain? If so, ask him to describe it. (Halos associated with excruciating eye pain or a severe headache may point to acute angle-closure glaucoma, an ocular emergency.) Inquire about a history of glaucoma or cataracts.

Next, examine the patient's eyes, noting conjunctival injection, excessive tearing, and lens changes. Examine pupil size, shape, and response to light. Then test visual acuity by performing an ophthalmoscopic examination.

Causes

◆ *Cataract.* Halo vision may be an early symptom of painless, progressive cataract formation. The glare of headlights may blind the patient, making nighttime driving impossible. Other findings include blurred vision, impaired visual acuity, and lens opacity, all of which develop gradually.
◆ *Corneal endothelial dystrophy.* Typically, halo vision is a late symptom. Impaired visual acuity may also occur.

◆

◆ *Glaucoma.* Halo vision characterizes all types of glaucoma. Acute angle-closure glaucoma also causes blurred vision, followed by a severe headache or excruciating pain in and around the affected eye. Examination reveals a moderately dilated fixed pupil that doesn't respond to light, conjunctival injection, a cloudy cornea, and impaired visual acuity. Chronic angle-closure glaucoma usually produces no symptoms until pain and blindness occur in advanced disease. Halo vision is a late symptom with this disorder, which also produces a mild eyeache, peripheral vision loss, and impaired visual acuity.

Headache

The most common neurologic symptom, headaches may be localized or generalized, producing mild to severe pain. About 90% of all headaches are benign and can be described as vascular, muscle-contraction, or a combination of both. (See *Clinical features of headaches,* page 290.) Occasionally, however, headaches indicate a severe neurologic disorder associated with intracranial inflammation, increased intracranial pressure (ICP), or meningeal irritation. They may also result from an ocular or sinus disorder, diagnostic tests, drugs, or other treatments. Other causes of headache include fever, eyestrain, dehydration, and systemic febrile illnesses. Some individuals develop headaches after seizures, coughing or sneezing, heavy lifting, or stooping.

Assessment

If the patient reports a headache, ask him to describe its characteristics and location. How often does he get a headache? How long does a typical headache last? Try to identify precipitating factors, such as certain foods or exposure to bright lights. Ask what helps to relieve it. Is the patient under stress? Has he had trouble sleeping?

Take a drug and alcohol history, and ask about head trauma within the past 4 weeks. Has the patient recently experienced nausea, vomiting, photophobia, or vision changes? Does he feel drowsy, confused, or dizzy? Does he have a history of seizures?

Begin the physical examination by evaluating the patient's level of consciousness (LOC). Then check his vital signs. Stay alert for signs of increased ICP. Check pupil size and response to light, and note neck stiffness.

Causes

◆ *Anthrax (cutaneous).* Headache, lymphadenopathy, fever, and malaise may occur with cutaneous anthrax, along with a maculopapular lesion that develops into a vesicle and, finally, a painless ulcer.

◆ *Arteriovenous malformations.* Less common than cerebral aneurysms, arteriovenous malformations usually result from developmental defects of the cerebral veins and arteries. Although many are present from birth, they manifest in adulthood with a triad of symptoms: headache, hemorrhage, and seizures.

◆ *Brain abscess.* With brain abscess, the headache is localized to the abscess site. Usually, it intensifies over a few days and is aggravated by straining. Accompanying the headache may be nausea, vomiting, and focal or generalized seizures. Other findings vary, depending on the abscess site.

◆ *Brain tumor.* Initially, a brain tumor causes a localized headache near the tumor site; as the tumor grows, the headache becomes generalized. The

Clinical features of headaches

Headaches include migraines, tension-type headaches, and cluster headaches. The International Headache Society classifies migraines as occurring with or without an aura. The differentiating characteristics of each type are listed here.

Migraines without an aura

Previously called *common migraines* or *hemicrania simplex,* migraine headaches without an aura are diagnosed when the patient has five attacks that:
◆ last 4 to 72 hours (whether untreated or unsuccessfully treated)
◆ include two of the following: pain that's unilateral, pulsating, moderate or severe in intensity, or aggravated by activity
◆ include at least one of the following: nausea, vomiting, photophobia, or phonophobia
◆ can't be attributed to another disorder.

Migraines with an aura

Previously called *classic, classical, ophthalmic, hemiplegic, or aphasic migraines,* migraine headaches with an aura are diagnosed when the patient has at least two attacks with three of the following characteristics:
◆ one or more reversible aura symptoms (which indicates focal cerebral cortical or brain stem dysfunction)
◆ one or more aura symptoms that develop over more than 4 minutes or two or more symptoms that occur in succession
◆ an aura symptom that lasts less than 60 minutes (per symptom)
◆ a headache that begins before, occurs with, or follows an aura with a free interval of less than 60 minutes.

To be classified as a typical aura, migraines with an aura must also have one of the following:
◆ homonymous vision disturbance
◆ unilateral paresthesia, numbness, or both
◆ unilateral weakness
◆ aphasia or other speech difficulty.

To be classified as a migraine, the patient's history and physical and neurologic examination must either:
◆ be negative for a disorder
◆ suggest a disorder that's ruled out by appropriate investigation
◆ reveal a disorder that has no relation to the onset of the migraines.

Tension-type headaches

In contrast to migraines, episodic tension-type headaches are diagnosed when the headache occurs on fewer than 180 days per year or the patient has fewer than 15 headaches per month. Tension-type headaches:
◆ last from 30 minutes to 7 days
◆ cause pain that's pressing or tightening in quality, mild to moderate, bilateral, and not aggravated by activity
◆ may be accompanied by photophobia or phonophobia, but usually not nausea or vomiting.

Cluster headaches

Cluster headaches are a treatable type of vascular headache syndrome that may be either episodic (most common) or chronic. Characteristics of cluster headaches include:
◆ unilateral pain occurring without warning, reaching a crescendo within 5 minutes, and described as excruciating and deep
◆ associated symptoms, such as tearing, reddening of the eye, nasal stuffiness, and ptosis ipsilateral to the pain.

Episodic cluster headaches:
◆ produce at least five attacks of periorbital pain, each lasting 15 to 180 minutes (if untreated)
◆ occur at a frequency of one every other day to eight per day
◆ must occur in at least two cluster periods lasting 7 days to 1 year, followed by a pain-free interval of at least 1 month.

Chronic cluster headaches:
◆ cause attacks for more than 1 year without a pain-free interval lasting at least 1 month.

pain is usually intermittent, deep seated, dull, and most intense in the morning. It's aggravated by coughing, stooping, Valsalva's maneuver, and changes in head position.

◢ *Cerebral aneurysm (ruptured).* A ruptured cerebral aneurysm is characterized by a sudden, excruciating headache, which may be unilateral and usually peaks within minutes of the rupture. The patient may lose consciousness immediately or display a variably altered LOC.

◆ *Drugs.* Many drugs can cause headaches. For example, indomethacin (Indocin) produces headaches—usually in the morning—in many patients. Vasodilators and drugs with a vasodilation effect, such as nitrates, typically cause a throbbing headache. Headaches may also follow withdrawal from vasopressors, such as caffeine, ergotamine (Ergomar), and sympathomimetics.

◢ *Ebola virus.* A headache is usually abrupt in onset, commonly occurring on the 5th day of illness. Additionally, the patient has a history of malaise, myalgia, a high fever, diarrhea, abdominal pain, dehydration, and lethargy. Death usually occurs in the 2nd week of the illness, preceded by severe blood loss and shock.

◢ *Encephalitis.* A severe, generalized headache is characteristic with encephalitis. Within 48 hours, the patient's LOC typically deteriorates. Associated findings include fever, nuchal rigidity, irritability, seizures, nausea and vomiting, photophobia, cranial nerve palsies, and focal neurologic deficits.

◢ *Epidural hemorrhage (acute).* Head trauma and a sudden, brief loss of consciousness usually precede acute epidural hemorrhage, which causes a progressively severe headache that's accompanied by nausea and vomiting, bladder distention, confusion, and then a rapid decrease in the patient's LOC.

◆ *Glaucoma (acute angle-closure).* Glaucoma may cause an excruciating headache as well as acute eye pain, blurred vision, halo vision, and nausea and vomiting. Assessment reveals conjunctival injection, a cloudy cornea, and a moderately dilated, fixed pupil.

◆ *Hantavirus pulmonary syndrome.* Noncardiogenic pulmonary edema distinguishes Hantavirus pulmonary syndrome, a viral disease. Common reasons for seeking treatment include flu-like signs and symptoms—headache, myalgia, fever, nausea, vomiting, and a cough—followed by respiratory distress.

◆ *Hypertension.* Hypertension may cause a slightly throbbing occipital headache on awakening that decreases in severity during the day. However, if the patient's diastolic blood pressure exceeds 120 mm Hg, the headache remains constant.

◆ *Influenza.* A severe generalized or frontal headache usually begins suddenly with the flu. Accompanying signs and symptoms include stabbing retro-orbital pain, weakness, diffuse myalgia, fever, chills, coughing, and rhinorrhea.

◆ *Listeriosis.* When listeriosis spreads to the nervous system, meningitis may develop, causing headache, nuchal rigidity, fever, and a change in the patient's LOC.

◆ *Meningitis.* Meningitis is marked by the sudden onset of a severe, constant, generalized headache that worsens with movement. Associated signs include nuchal rigidity, positive Kernig's and Brudzinski's signs, hyperreflexia and, possibly, opisthotonos.

◢ *Plague* (Yersinia pestis). The pneumonic form of the plague causes a sudden onset of headache, chills, fever, myalgia, a productive cough, chest pain, tachypnea, dyspnea, hemoptysis, respiratory distress, and cardiopulmonary insufficiency.

◆ *Postconcussion syndrome.* A generalized or localized headache may develop 1 to 30 days after head trauma and last for 2 to 3 weeks. This characteristic symptom may be described as an aching, pounding, pressing, stabbing, or throbbing pain. The patient's neurologic examination is typically normal; however, he may experience dizziness, blurred vision, fatigue, insomnia, an inability to concentrate, and noise and alcohol intolerance.

◆ *Q Fever.* Signs and symptoms of Q fever include a severe headache, fever, chills, malaise, chest pain, nausea, vomiting, and diarrhea. Fever may last up to 2 weeks.

◼ *Severe acute respiratory syndrome (SARS).* SARS is an acute infectious disease that causes headache, malaise, dyspnea, and a dry, nonproductive cough.

◆ *Smallpox (variola major).* Initial signs and symptoms of smallpox include a severe headache, backache, abdominal pain, a high fever, prostration, and a maculopapular rash on the mucosa of the mouth, pharynx, face, and forearms.

◼ *Subarachnoid hemorrhage.* Subarachnoid hemorrhage commonly produces a sudden, violent headache along with nuchal rigidity, nausea and vomiting, seizures, dizziness, ipsilateral pupil dilation, and an altered LOC. The patient also exhibits positive Kernig's and Brudzinski's signs, photophobia, and blurred vision.

◼ *Subdural hematoma.* Typically associated with head trauma, acute and chronic subdural hematomas may cause headache and a decreased LOC. With acute subdural hematoma, head trauma also produces drowsiness, confusion, and agitation that may progress to a coma. Chronic subdural hematoma produces a dull, pounding headache that fluctuates in severity and is located over the hematoma. Weeks or months after the initial head trauma, the patient may experience giddiness, personality changes, confusion, seizures, and a progressively worsening LOC.

◆ *Tularemia.* Signs and symptoms following inhalation of the bacterium *Francisella tularensis* include an abrupt onset of headache, fever, chills, generalized myalgia, a nonproductive cough, dyspnea, chest pain, and empyema.

◆ *Typhus.* Initial symptoms of typhus include headache, myalgia, arthralgia, and malaise followed by an abrupt onset of chills, fever, and nausea and vomiting. A maculopapular rash may be present in some cases.

◆ *West Nile encephalitis.* The signs and symptoms of West Nile encephalitis include fever, headache, and body aches, commonly with a skin rash and swollen lymph glands.

Hearing loss

Affecting nearly 16 million Americans, hearing loss may be temporary or permanent and partial or complete. This common symptom may involve reception of low-, middle-, or high-frequency tones. If the hearing loss doesn't affect speech frequencies, the patient may be unaware of it.

Normally, sound waves enter the external auditory canal, and then travel to the middle ear's tympanic membrane and ossicles and into the inner ear's cochlea. The cochlear division of cranial nerve (CN) VIII carries the sound impulse to the brain. This type of sound transmission, called *air conduction,* is normally better than bone conduction—sound transmission through bone to the inner ear.

Hearing loss can be classified as conductive, sensorineural, mixed, or functional. Conductive hearing loss results from external or middle ear disorders that block sound transmission. Sensorineural hearing loss results from disorders of the inner ear or of CN VIII. Mixed hearing loss combines aspects of conductive and sensorineural hearing loss. Functional hearing loss results from psychological factors rather than identifiable organic damage.

In most cases, hearing loss results from presbycusis, a type of sensorineural hearing loss that usually affects people older than age 50. Other causes include trauma, infection, allergy, tumors, certain systemic and hereditary disorders, and the effects of ototoxic drugs and treatments. Other physiologic causes of hearing loss include cerumen impaction, barotitis media, and chronic exposure to noise over 90 decibels, which can occur at work, with certain hobbies, or from listening to live or recorded music.

Assessment

If the patient reports hearing loss, ask him to describe it. Is it unilateral or bilateral? Continuous or intermittent? Then obtain the patient's medical history, noting chronic ear infections, ear surgery, and ear or head trauma. Has the patient recently had an upper respiratory tract infection? After taking a drug history, have the patient describe his occupation and work environment. Next, explore associated signs and symptoms. Does the patient have ear pain? Ask the patient if he has noticed discharge from his ears. Does he hear ringing, buzzing, hissing, or other noises in his ears? Does he experience dizziness? If so, when did he first notice it?

Begin the physical examination by inspecting the external ear for inflammation, boils, foreign bodies, and discharge. Then apply pressure to the tragus and mastoid to elicit tenderness. If you detect tenderness or external ear

abnormalities, notify the physician to discuss whether an otoscopic examination should be done. (See *Using an otoscope correctly,* page 233.) During the otoscopic examination, note color change, perforation, bulging, or retraction of the tympanic membrane, which normally looks like a shiny, pearl gray cone.

Next, evaluate the patient's hearing acuity, using the ticking watch and whispered voice tests. Then perform Weber's and the Rinne tests to obtain a preliminary evaluation of the type and degree of hearing loss. (See *Differentiating conductive from sensorineural hearing loss,* page 294.)

Causes

◆ *Acoustic neuroma.* Acoustic neuroma, which is a CN VIII tumor, causes unilateral, progressive, sensorineural hearing loss. The patient may also develop tinnitus, vertigo and, with cranial nerve compression, facial paralysis.

◆ *Adenoid hypertrophy.* Adenoid hypertrophy may obstruct the eustachian tube, causing gradual conductive hearing loss accompanied by intermittent ear discharge. The patient tends to breathe through his mouth and may complain of ear fullness.

◆ *Aural polyps.* If a polyp occludes the external auditory canal, partial hearing loss may occur. The polyp typically bleeds easily and is covered by a purulent discharge.

◆ *Cholesteatoma.* Gradual hearing loss is characteristic with cholesteatoma. It can be accompanied by vertigo and, at times, facial paralysis. Examination reveals eardrum perforation and pearly white balls in the ear canal.

◆ *Cyst.* Ear canal obstruction by a sebaceous or dermoid cyst causes progressive conductive hearing loss. On inspection, the cyst looks like a soft mass.

Differentiating conductive from sensorineural hearing loss

Weber's and the Rinne tests can help determine whether the patient's hearing loss is conductive or sensorineural. Weber's test evaluates bone conduction; the Rinne test, bone and air conduction. Using a 512 Hz tuning fork, perform these preliminary tests as described here.

Weber's test

Place the base of a vibrating tuning fork firmly against the midline of the patient's skull at the forehead. Ask her if she hears the tone equally well in both ears. If she does, Weber's test is graded midline—a normal finding. In an abnormal Weber's test (graded right or left), sound is louder in one ear, suggesting a conductive hearing loss in that ear, or a sensorineural loss in the opposite ear.

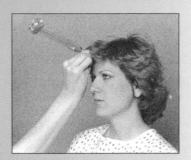

Rinne test

Hold the base of a vibrating tuning fork against the patient's mastoid process to test bone conduction. Then quickly move the vibrating fork in front of her ear canal to test air conduction. Ask her to tell you which location has the louder or longer sound. Repeat the procedure for the other ear. In a positive Rinne test, air conduction lasts longer or sounds louder than bone conduction—a normal finding. In a negative test, the opposite is true: Bone conduction lasts longer or sounds louder than air conduction.

After performing both tests, correlate the results with other assessment data.

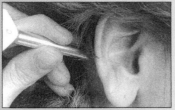

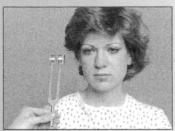

Implications of results

Conductive hearing loss produces:
◆ abnormal Weber's test result
◆ negative Rinne test result
◆ improved hearing in noisy areas
◆ normal ability to discriminate sounds
◆ difficulty hearing when chewing
◆ a quiet speaking voice.

Sensorineural hearing loss produces:
◆ positive Rinne test
◆ poor hearing in noisy areas
◆ difficulty hearing high-frequency sounds
◆ complaints that others mumble or shout
◆ tinnitus.

◆ *Drugs.* Ototoxic drugs typically produce ringing or buzzing tinnitus and a feeling of fullness in the ear. Chloroquine (Aralen), cisplatin (Platinol), vancomycin (Vancocin), and aminoglycosides may cause irreversible hearing loss. Loop diuretics, such as furosemide (Lasix), ethacrynic acid (Edecrin), and bumetanide (Bumex), and high doses of erythromycin (Erythrocin) or salicylates (such as aspirin) may also cause reversible hearing loss.

◆ *External ear canal tumor (malignant).* Progressive conductive hearing loss is characteristic with a tumor of the external ear canal and is accompanied by deep, boring ear pain, a purulent discharge and, eventually, facial paralysis.

◆ *Glomus jugulare tumor.* Initially, this benign tumor causes mild, unilateral conductive hearing loss that becomes progressively more severe. The patient may report tinnitus that sounds like his heartbeat. Although the tympanic membrane is normal, a reddened mass appears behind it.

◆ *Head trauma.* Sudden conductive or sensorineural hearing loss may result from ossicle disruption, ear canal fracture, tympanic membrane perforation, or cochlear fracture associated with head trauma. Typically, the patient reports a headache and exhibits bleeding from his ear.

◆ *Ménière's disease.* Initially, Ménière's disease produces intermittent, unilateral sensorineural hearing loss that involves only low tones. Later, hearing loss becomes constant and affects other tones. Other findings include intermittent severe vertigo, a feeling of fullness in the ear, and a roaring or hollow-seashell tinnitus.

◆ *Nasopharyngeal cancer.* Nasopharyngeal cancer causes mild unilateral conductive hearing loss when it compresses the eustachian tube. Inspection reveals a retracted tympanic membrane backed by fluid. When this tumor obstructs the nasal airway, the patient may exhibit nasal speech and a bloody nasal and postnasal discharge.

◆ *Otitis externa (acute).* Otitis externa is hearing loss that results from debris in the ear canal. With acute otitis externa, ear canal inflammation produces pain, itching, and a foul-smelling, sticky yellow discharge. Severe tenderness is typically elicited by chewing, opening the mouth, and pressing on the tragus or mastoid. Examination may reveal greenish white debris or edema in the canal.

◼ *Otitis externa (malignant).* Malignant otitis externa most commonly occurs in patients with diabetes and is a life-threatening disorder. It causes sensorineural hearing loss, pruritus, tinnitus, and severe ear pain.

◆ *Otitis media.* Otitis media is a middle ear inflammation that typically produces unilateral conductive hearing loss. In patients with acute suppurative otitis media, hearing loss develops gradually over a few hours and is usually accompanied by an upper respiratory tract infection. Rupture of the bulging, swollen tympanic membrane relieves the pain and produces a brief, bloody, purulent discharge. Hearing returns after the infection subsides. Hearing loss also develops gradually in patients with chronic otitis media. Assessment may reveal a perforated tympanic membrane, purulent ear drainage, an earache, nausea, and vertigo. Serous otitis media commonly produces a stuffy feeling in the ear and pain that worsens at night. Examination reveals a retracted—and perhaps discolored—tympanic membrane and possibly air bubbles behind the membrane.

◆ *Otosclerosis.* Otosclerosis is a hereditary disorder in which unilateral conductive hearing loss usually begins when the patient is in his early 20s and may gradually progress to bilateral mixed loss. The patient may report tinnitus and an ability to hear better in a noisy environment. The deafness is usually noticed from ages 11 to 30.

◆ *Skull fracture.* Auditory nerve injury causes sudden unilateral sensorineural hearing loss. Accompanying signs and symptoms include ringing tinnitus and blood behind the tympanic membrane.

◆ *Temporal bone fracture.* Temporal bone fracture can cause sudden unilateral sensorineural hearing loss accompanied by hissing tinnitus. The tympanic membrane may be perforated, depending on the fracture's location.

◆ *Tympanic membrane perforation.* Commonly caused by trauma from sharp objects or rapid pressure changes, tympanic membrane perforation causes abrupt hearing loss along with ear pain, tinnitus, vertigo, and a sensation of fullness in the ear.

Heat intolerance

Heat intolerance refers to the inability to withstand high temperatures or to maintain a comfortable body temperature. This symptom produces a continuous feeling of being overheated and, at times, profuse diaphoresis. It usually develops gradually and is chronic.

Assessment

Ask the patient when he first noticed his heat intolerance. Is it difficult for him to adjust to warm weather? Find out if his appetite or weight has changed. Also, ask about unusual nervousness or other personality changes. Then take a drug history, especially noting the use of thyroid drugs, amphetamines, or amphetamine-like drugs.

As you begin the examination, notice how much clothing the patient is wearing. After taking his vital signs, inspect his skin for flushing and diaphoresis. Also, note tremors and lid lag.

Causes

◆ *Hypothalamic disease.* With hypothalamic disease, body temperature fluctuates dramatically, causing alternating heat and cold intolerance. Related findings include amenorrhea, disturbed sleep patterns, increased thirst and urination, increased appetite with weight gain, impaired visual acuity, headache, and personality changes.

◆ *Thyrotoxicosis.* With thyrotoxicosis, excess thyroid hormone stimulates peripheral tissues, increasing basal metabolism and producing excess heat. A classic symptom of this disorder, heat intolerance may be accompanied by an enlarged thyroid, nervousness, weight loss despite increased appetite, diaphoresis, diarrhea, tremor, and palpitations. Some common associated findings include irritability, fatigue, lid lag, tachycardia, amenorrhea, and gynecomastia. Typically, the patient's skin is warm and flushed; premature graying and alopecia occur in both sexes.

Hematemesis

Hematemesis, the vomiting of blood, usually indicates GI bleeding above the ligament of Treitz, which suspends the duodenum at its junction with the jejunum. Bright red or blood-streaked vomitus indicates fresh or recent bleeding. Dark red, brown, or black vomitus (the color and consistency of coffee grounds) indicates that blood has been retained in the stomach and partially digested.

Although hematemesis usually results from a GI disorder, it may stem from a coagulation disorder or a treatment that irritates the GI tract. Esophageal varices may also cause hematemesis. Swallowed blood from epistaxis or oropharyngeal erosion may also cause bloody vomitus. (See *Rare causes of hematemesis.*)

Hematemesis is always an important sign, but its severity depends on the amount, source, and rapidity of the bleeding. Massive hematemesis (vomiting 500 to 1,000 ml of blood) may be life-threatening. (See *Responding to hematemesis* and *Managing hematemesis with intubation,* page 298.)

Assessment

If the patient's hematemesis isn't immediately life-threatening, begin with a thorough history. First, have the patient describe the amount, color, and consistency of the vomitus. Has he ever had hematemesis before? Find out if he also has bloody or black, tarry stools. Note whether nausea, flatulence, diarrhea, or weakness usually precede the hematemesis. Has he recently had bouts of retching with or without vomiting? Next, ask about a history of ulcers or of liver or coagulation disorders. Find out how much alcohol the patient drinks, if any. Does he regularly take aspirin or other nonsteroidal anti-inflammatory drugs (NSAIDs)? Does he take warfarin (Coumadin) or other drugs with anticoagulant properties?

Rare causes of hematemesis

Two rare disorders commonly cause hematemesis: malaria and yellow fever. Malaria produces hematemesis and other GI signs, but its most characteristic effects are chills, fever, headache, muscle pain, and splenomegaly. Yellow fever also causes hematemesis as well as a sudden fever, bradycardia, jaundice, and severe prostration.

Two relatively common disorders may cause hematemesis in rare cases such as acute diverticulitis and secondary syphilis. When acute diverticulitis affects the duodenum, GI bleeding and resultant hematemesis occur with abdominal pain and fever. With GI involvement, secondary syphilis can cause hematemesis; more characteristic signs and symptoms include a primary chancre, a rash, fever, weight loss, malaise, anorexia, and headache.

 EMERGENCY INTERVENTIONS

Responding to hematemesis

If your patient has massive hematemesis, immediately check his vital signs. If you detect signs of shock, take the following steps:
◆ Place the patient in a supine position.
◆ Elevate his feet 20 to 30 degrees.
◆ Insert a large-bore I.V. catheter for emergency fluid replacement.
◆ Obtain a blood sample for typing and crossmatching, hemoglobin level, and hematocrit.
◆ Administer oxygen, as prescribed.
◆ Prepare to insert a nasogastric tube for suction or iced lavage. (A Sengstaken-Blakemore tube may be used to compress esophageal varices.)

Managing hematemesis with intubation

A patient with hematemesis will need to have a GI tube inserted to allow blood drainage, aspirate gastric contents, or facilitate gastric lavage, if necessary. Here are the most common tubes and their uses.

Nasogastric tubes

The Salem-Sump tube (at right), a double-lumen nasogastric (NG) tube, is used to remove stomach fluid and gas or to aspirate gastric contents. It may also be used for gastric lavage, drug administration, or feeding. Its main advantage over the Levin tube—a single-lumen NG tube—is that it allows atmospheric air to enter the patient's stomach so the tube can float freely instead of risking adhesion and damage to the gastric mucosa.

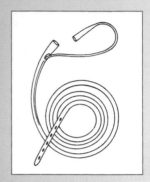

Wide-bore gastric tubes

The Edlich tube (at right) has one wide-bore lumen with four openings near the closed distal tip. A funnel or syringe can be connected at the proximal end. Like the other tubes, the Edlich tube can aspirate a large volume of gastric contents quickly.

The Ewald tube, a wide-bore tube that allows quick passage of a large amount of fluid and clots, is especially useful for gastric lavage in patients with profuse GI bleeding and in those who have ingested poison. Another wide-bore tube, the double-lumen Levacuator, has a large lumen for evacuation of gastric contents and a small one for lavage.

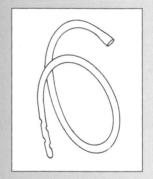

Esophageal tubes

The Sengstaken-Blakemore tube (at right), a triple-lumen double-balloon esophageal tube, provides a gastric aspiration port that allows drainage from below the gastric balloon. It can also be used to instill medication. A similar tube, the Linton shunt, can aspirate esophageal and gastric contents without risking necrosis because it has no esophageal balloon. The Minnesota esophagogastric tamponade tube, which has four lumens and two balloons, provides pressure-monitoring ports for both balloons without the need for Y-connectors.

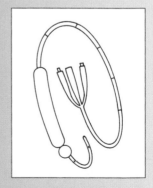

Begin the physical examination by checking for orthostatic hypotension, an early warning sign of hypovolemia. Take blood pressure and pulse with the patient supine, sitting, and standing. After obtaining other vital signs, inspect the mucous membranes, nasopharynx, and skin for signs of bleeding or other abnormalities. Finally, perform a GI assessment. Note abdominal tenderness, pain, or masses. While palpating the patient's abdomen, check for lymphadenopathy.

Causes

◆ *Anthrax (GI)*. Initial signs and symptoms after eating contaminated meat from an animal infected with the gram-positive, spore-forming bacterium *Bacillus anthracis* include a loss of appetite, nausea, vomiting, and fever. Signs and symptoms may progress to hematemesis, abdominal pain, and severe, bloody diarrhea.

◆ *Coagulation disorders*. Coagulation disorders disrupt normal clotting and may result in GI bleeding and moderate to severe hematemesis.

◆ *Esophageal cancer*. A late sign of esophageal cancer, hematemesis may be accompanied by steady chest pain that radiates to the back. Other findings include substernal fullness, severe dysphagia, hiccups, melena, and halitosis.

◼ *Esophageal rupture*. The severity of hematemesis depends on the cause of the rupture. Rupture due to Boerhaave's syndrome (spontaneous rupture of the lower esophagus) or other esophageal disorders typically causes more severe hematemesis. Rupture may also produce severe retrosternal, epigastric, neck, or scapular pain accompanied by chest and neck edema.

◼ *Esophageal varices (ruptured)*. Ruptured esophageal varices may produce coffee-ground or massive, bright red vomitus. Signs of shock may follow or even precede hematemesis if the stomach fills with blood before vomiting occurs.

◆ *Gastric cancer*. Painless bright red or dark brown vomitus is a late sign of gastric cancer, which usually begins insidiously with upper abdominal discomfort. The patient then develops anorexia, mild nausea, and chronic dyspepsia unrelieved by antacids and exacerbated by food.

◆ *Gastritis (acute)*. Hematemesis and melena are the most common signs of acute gastritis. They may even be the only signs, although mild epigastric discomfort, nausea, fever, and malaise may also occur. Typically, the patient has a history of alcohol abuse. Gastritis may also occur secondary to *Helicobacter pylori* infection.

◆ *Mallory-Weiss syndrome*. Characterized by a tear of the mucous membrane at the junction of the esophagus and stomach, Mallory-Weiss syndrome may produce hematemesis and melena. It's commonly triggered by severe vomiting, retching, or straining, most commonly in alcoholics or in people with an obstructed pylorus.

◆ *Peptic ulcer*. Hematemesis may occur when a peptic ulcer penetrates an artery, a vein, or highly vascular tissue. Other findings include melena or hematochezia, chills, fever, and signs and symptoms of shock and dehydration. The patient may also have a history of habitually using tobacco, alcohol, or NSAIDs.

Hematochezia

The passage of bloody stools, known as hematochezia, usually indicates— and may be the first sign of—GI bleeding below the ligament of Treitz. However, this sign—usually preceded by hematemesis—may also accompany rapid hemorrhage of 1 L or more from the upper GI tract.

Hematochezia ranges from formed, blood-streaked stools to liquid, bloody stools that may be bright red, dark mahogany, or maroon in color. This sign usually develops abruptly and is heralded by abdominal pain.

Although hematochezia is commonly associated with GI disorders, it may also result from a coagulation disorder, exposure to toxins, or certain diagnostic tests. Always a significant sign, hematochezia may precipitate life-threatening hypovolemia. (See *Responding to hematochezia*.)

Assessment

If hematochezia isn't immediately life-threatening, ask the patient to fully describe the amount, color, and consistency of his bloody stools. (If possible, also inspect and characterize the stools yourself.) How long have the stools been bloody? Does the amount of blood seem to vary? Ask about other signs and symptoms. Next, explore the patient's medical history, focusing on GI and coagulation disorders. Ask about the use of GI irritants, such as alcohol, aspirin, and other nonsteroidal anti-inflammatory drugs (NSAIDs).

Begin the physical examination by checking for orthostatic hypotension, an early sign of shock. Take the patient's blood pressure and pulse while he's lying down, sitting, and standing. Examine the skin for petechiae or spider angiomas. Then perform a GI assessment, checking for abdominal tenderness, pain, or masses. While palpating the patient's abdomen, check for lymphadenopathy. Finally, a digital rectal examination must be done to rule out rectal masses or hemorrhoids.

Causes

◆ *Anal fissure.* Slight hematochezia characterizes anal fissure; blood may streak the stools or appear on toilet tissue. Other findings include severe rectal pain that may make the patient reluctant to defecate, causing constipation.

◆ *Angiodysplastic lesions.* Most common in elderly patients, these arteriovenous lesions of the ascending colon typically cause chronic, bright red rectal bleeding.

◼ *Coagulation disorders.* Patients with a coagulation disorder may experience GI bleeding marked by moderate to severe hematochezia. Bleeding may also occur in other body systems.

◆ *Colitis.* Ischemic colitis commonly causes bloody diarrhea, especially in elderly patients. Hematochezia may be slight or massive and is usually accompanied by severe, cramping lower abdominal pain and hypotension. Ulcerative colitis typically causes bloody diarrhea that may also contain mucus. Hematochezia is preceded by mild to severe abdominal cramps and may cause slight to massive blood loss. Severe colitis may cause hypovolemic shock and peritonitis.

◆ *Colon cancer.* Bright red rectal bleeding with or without pain is a telling sign of colon cancer, especially in cancer of the left colon. Usually, a left colon tumor causes early signs of obstruction, such as rectal pressure, bleeding, and intermittent fullness or cramping. Early tumor growth in the right colon may cause melena, abdominal aching, pressure, and dull cramps.

◆ *Colorectal polyps.* Colorectal polyps are the most common cause of intermittent hematochezia in adults younger than age 60; however, sometimes such polyps produce no symptoms. When located high in the colon, polyps may cause blood-streaked stools. If the polyps are located closer to the rectum, they may bleed freely.

◆ *Diverticulitis.* Most common in the elderly patient, diverticulitis can suddenly cause rectal bleeding after the patient feels the urge to defecate. Other findings include left lower quadrant pain that's relieved by defecation, alternating episodes of constipation and diarrhea, anorexia, nausea and vomiting, and rebound tenderness.

◆ *Dysentery.* Bloody diarrhea is common in infection with *Shigella, Amoeba,* and *Campylobacter,* but rare with *Salmonella.* Abdominal pain or cramps,

tenesmus, fever, and nausea may also occur.

◾ *Esophageal varices (ruptured).* In esophageal varices, painless hematochezia may range from slight rectal oozing to grossly bloody stools and may be accompanied by mild to severe hematemesis or melena.

◆ *Food poisoning (staphylococcal).* The patient may have bloody diarrhea 1 to 6 hours after ingesting food toxins. Other findings include severe, cramping abdominal pain, nausea and vomiting, and prostration.

◆ *Hemorrhoids.* Hematochezia may accompany external hemorrhoids, which typically cause painful defecation, resulting in constipation. Less painful internal hemorrhoids usually produce chronic bleeding with bowel movements.

◆ *Leptospirosis.* The severe form of leptospirosis—Weil's syndrome—produces hematochezia or melena along with other signs of bleeding, such as epistaxis and hemoptysis. The bleeding is typically preceded by a sudden frontal headache and severe thigh and lumbar myalgia that may be accompanied by cutaneous hyperesthesia.

◆ *Peptic ulcer.* Upper GI bleeding is a common complication in a peptic ulcer. The patient may display hematochezia, hematemesis, or melena, depending on the rapidity and amount of bleeding. The patient typically has a history of epigastric pain that's relieved by foods or antacids; he may also have a history of habitually using tobacco, alcohol, or NSAIDs.

◆ *Ulcerative proctitis.* Ulcerative proctitis typically causes an intense urge to defecate, but the patient passes only bright red blood, pus, or mucus. Other common signs and symptoms include acute constipation and tenesmus.

Hematuria

A cardinal sign of renal and urinary tract disorders, hematuria is the abnormal presence of blood in urine. Microscopic hematuria is confirmed by an occult blood test, whereas macroscopic hematuria is immediately visible. However, macroscopic hematuria must be distinguished from pseudohematuria. (See *Confirming hematuria.*) Macroscopic hematuria may be continuous or intermittent, is commonly accompanied by pain, and may be aggravated by prolonged standing or walking.

Hematuria may be classified by the stage of urination it predominantly affects. Bleeding at the start of urination—*initial hematuria*—usually indicates a urethral disorder; bleeding at the end of urination—*terminal hematuria*—usually indicates disease of the bladder neck, posterior urethra, or prostate; bleeding throughout urination—*total hematuria*—usually indicates a disorder above the bladder neck.

Hematuria may result from one of two mechanisms—rupture or perforation of vessels in the renal system or urinary tract, or impaired glomerular filtration, which allows red blood cells to seep into the urine. The color of the bloody urine provides a clue to the source of bleeding. Generally, dark or brownish blood indicates renal or upper urinary tract bleeding, whereas bright red blood indicates lower urinary tract bleeding.

Although hematuria usually results from renal and urinary tract disorders, it may also result from certain GI, prostate, vaginal, or coagulation disorders or from the effects of certain drugs. Invasive therapy and diagnostic tests that involve manipulative instrumentation of the renal and urologic systems may also cause hematuria.

Hematuria not related to a specific disorder may result from fever and hypercatabolic states. Transient hematuria may follow strenuous exercise.

Assessment

After detecting hematuria, take a pertinent health history. If hematuria is macroscopic, ask the patient when he first noticed blood in his urine. Does it vary in severity between voidings? Is it worse at the beginning, middle, or end of urination? Has it occurred before? Is the patient passing clots? Ask if there's pain or burning with hematuria.

Ask about recent abdominal or flank trauma. Has the patient been exercising strenuously? Note a history of renal, urinary, prostate, or coagulation disorders. Then obtain a drug history, noting anticoagulants or aspirin.

Begin the physical examination by palpating and percussing the abdomen and flanks. Next, percuss the costovertebral angle (CVA) to elicit tenderness. Check the urinary meatus for bleeding or other abnormalities. Using a chemical reagent strip, test a urine specimen for protein. A vaginal or digital rectal examination may be necessary.

Causes

◆ *Bladder cancer.* A primary cause of gross hematuria in men, bladder cancer may also produce pain in the bladder, rectum, pelvis, flank, back, or leg.
◆ *Bladder trauma.* Gross hematuria is characteristic in traumatic rupture or perforation of the bladder. Typically, hematuria is accompanied by lower abdominal pain and, occasionally, anuria despite a strong urge to void. The patient may also develop swelling of the scrotum, buttocks, or perineum and signs of shock.
◆ *Calculi.* Bladder and renal calculi produce hematuria, which may be as-

sociated with signs of a urinary tract infection (UTI). Bladder calculi usually cause gross hematuria, referred pain to the lower back or penile or vulvar area and, in some patients, bladder distention. Renal calculi may produce microscopic or gross hematuria. The cardinal symptom, however, is colicky pain that travels from the CVA to the flank, suprapubic region, and external genitalia when a calculus is passed.

◣ *Coagulation disorders.* Macroscopic hematuria is usually the first sign of hemorrhage in coagulation disorders, such as thrombocytopenia or disseminated intravascular coagulation.

◆ *Cortical necrosis (acute).* Accompanying gross hematuria in acute cortical necrosis are intense flank pain, anuria, leukocytosis, and fever.

◆ *Cystitis.* Bacterial cystitis usually produces macroscopic hematuria with urinary urgency and frequency, dysuria, nocturia, and tenesmus. Chronic interstitial cystitis occasionally causes grossly bloody hematuria. Microscopic and macroscopic hematuria may occur with tubercular cystitis, which may also cause urinary urgency and frequency, dysuria, tenesmus, flank pain, fatigue, and anorexia. Viral cystitis usually produces hematuria, urinary urgency and frequency, dysuria, nocturia, tenesmus, and fever.

◆ *Diverticulitis.* When diverticulitis involves the bladder, it usually causes microscopic hematuria, urinary frequency and urgency, dysuria, and nocturia.

◆ *Glomerulonephritis.* Acute glomerulonephritis usually begins with gross hematuria that tapers off to microscopic hematuria and red cell casts, which may persist for months. It may also produce proteinuria, a mild fever, fatigue, flank and abdominal pain, increased blood pressure, and signs of lung congestion. Chronic glomerulonephritis usually causes microscopic

Confirming hematuria

If the patient's urine appears blood tinged, be sure to rule out pseudohematuria: red or pink urine caused by urinary pigments. First, carefully observe the urine specimen. If it contains red sediment, it's probably true hematuria.

Next, check the patient's history for the use of drugs associated with pseudohematuria, including rifampin (Rifadin), chlorzoxazone (Parafon Forte), phenazopyridine (Pyridium), phenothiazines, doxorubicin (Adriamycin), phenytoin (Dilantin), daunomycin (Cerubidine), and laxatives with phenolphthalein.

Ask about the patient's intake of beets, berries, or foods with red dyes that may color the urine red. Be aware that porphyrinuria and excess urate excretion can also cause pseudohematuria.

Finally, test the urine using a chemical reagent strip. This test can confirm even microscopic hematuria and can also estimate the amount of blood present.

hematuria accompanied by proteinuria, generalized edema, and increased blood pressure.

◆ *Nephritis (interstitial).* Typically, nephritis causes microscopic hematuria. However, the patient with acute interstitial nephritis may develop gross hematuria. In chronic interstitial nephritis, the patient has dilute—almost colorless—urine that may be accompanied by polyuria and increased blood pressure.

◆ *Nephropathy (obstructive).* Obstructive nephropathy may cause microscopic or macroscopic hematuria, but urine is rarely grossly bloody. The patient may report colicky flank and abdominal pain, CVA tenderness, and anuria or oliguria that alternates with polyuria.

◆ *Polycystic kidney disease.* Polycystic kidney disease may cause recurrent microscopic or gross hematuria. Although it commonly produces no symptoms before age 40, it may cause increased blood pressure, polyuria, dull flank pain, and signs of a UTI.

◆ *Prostatitis.* Whether acute or chronic, prostatitis may cause macroscopic hematuria, usually at the end of urination. It may also produce urinary frequency and urgency and dysuria followed by visible bladder distention.

◆ *Pyelonephritis (acute).* Acute pyelonephritis typically produces microscopic or macroscopic hematuria that progresses to grossly bloody hematuria. Microscopic hematuria may persist for a few months after the infection resolves. Other common symptoms include urinary urgency and frequency, burning on urination, fever, chills, anorexia, flank pain, and general fatigue.

◆ *Renal cancer.* The classic triad of signs and symptoms of renal cancer includes grossly bloody hematuria; dull, aching flank pain; and a smooth, firm, palpable flank mass. Colicky pain may accompany the passage of clots.

◆ *Renal infarction.* Typically, renal infarction produces gross hematuria. The patient may complain of constant, severe flank and upper abdominal pain accompanied by CVA tenderness, anorexia, and nausea and vomiting.

◆ *Renal papillary necrosis (acute).* Acute renal papillary necrosis usually produces grossly bloody hematuria, which may be accompanied by intense flank pain, CVA tenderness, abdominal rigidity and colicky pain, oliguria or anuria, pyuria, fever, chills, vomiting, and hypoactive bowel sounds. Arthralgia and hypertension are common.

◆ *Renal trauma.* About 80% of patients with renal trauma have hematuria. Other findings may include flank pain, oliguria, hematoma or ecchymoses over the upper abdomen or flank, and hypoactive bowel sounds.

◆ *Renal tuberculosis (TB).* Gross hematuria is commonly the first sign of renal TB. It may be accompanied by urinary frequency, dysuria, pyuria, tenesmus, colicky abdominal pain, lumbar pain, and proteinuria.

◆ *Renal vein thrombosis.* Grossly bloody hematuria usually occurs in renal vein thrombosis. In abrupt venous obstruction, the patient experiences severe flank and lumbar pain as well as epigastric and CVA tenderness. Gradual venous obstruction causes signs of nephrotic syndrome, proteinuria and, occasionally, peripheral edema.

◆ *Schistosomiasis.* Schistosomiasis usually causes intermittent hematuria at the end of urination. It may be accompanied by dysuria, colicky renal and bladder pain, and palpable lower abdominal masses.

◆ *Sickle cell anemia.* Sickle cell anemia causes gross hematuria that may result from congestion of the renal papillae. Other signs and symptoms include chronic fatigue, unexplained dyspnea, joint swelling, aching bones, ischemic leg ulcers, and increased susceptibility to infection.

◆ *Systemic lupus erythematosus (SLE).* Gross hematuria and proteinuria may occur when SLE involves the kidneys. It may be accompanied by fever, anorexia, weight loss, fatigue, abdominal pain, nausea, vomiting, diarrhea or constipation, rash, and polyarthralgia.

◆ *Urethral trauma.* With urethral trauma, initial hematuria may occur, possibly with blood at the urinary meatus, local pain, and penile or vulvar ecchymoses.

◆ *Vasculitis.* Hematuria is usually microscopic in vasculitis. Other findings include malaise, myalgia, polyarthralgia, fever, increased blood pressure, pallor and, occasionally, anuria.

Hemianopsia

A vision loss involving half the normal visual field in one or both eyes is called hemianopsia. This visual field defect usually results from a lesion on the optic pathway in the parietal or temporal lobe. However, if the visual field defects are identical in both eyes but affect less than half the field of vision (incomplete homonymous hemianopsia), the lesion may be in the occipital lobe. (See *Recognizing types of hemianopsia,* page 306.)

Assessment

Suspect a visual field defect if the patient seems startled when you approach him from one side or if he fails to see objects placed directly in front of him. To help determine the type of defect, compare the patient's visual fields with your own—assuming that yours are normal. First, ask the patient to cover his right eye while you cover your left eye. Then move a pen or similarly shaped object from the periphery of his (and your) uncovered eye into his field of vision. Ask the patient to indicate when he first sees the object. Does he see it at the same time you do? After you do? Repeat this test in each quadrant of both eyes. Then, for each eye, plot the defect by shading the area of a circle that corresponds to the area of vision loss.

Next, evaluate the patient's level of consciousness, take his vital signs, and check pupillary reaction and motor response. Ask if he has recently experienced headache, dysarthria, or seizures. Does he have ptosis or facial or extremity weakness? Hallucinations or loss of color vision? When did neurologic symptoms start? Obtain a medical history, noting especially eye disorders, hypertension, diabetes mellitus, and recent head trauma.

Causes

◼ *Carotid artery aneurysm.* An aneurysm in the internal carotid artery can cause contralateral or bilateral defects in the visual fields. It can also cause hemiplegia, headache, aphasia, behavior disturbances, and unilateral hypoesthesia.

◆ *Occipital lobe lesion.* The most common symptoms arising from a lesion of one occipital lobe are incomplete homonymous hemianopsia, scotomas (areas within the visual field in which vision is absent or depressed), and impaired color vision. The patient may also experience visual hallucinations— flashes of light or color or visions of objects, people, animals, or geometric forms.

◆ *Parietal lobe lesion.* A parietal lobe lesion produces homonymous hemianopsia and sensory deficits, such as an inability to perceive body position or passive movement or to localize tactile, thermal, or vibratory stimuli.

◆ *Pituitary tumor.* A tumor that compresses nerve fibers supplying the nasal half of both retinas causes complete or partial bitemporal hemianopsia that first occurs in the upper visual fields but later can progress to blindness. Patients may also experience frontal headaches, amenorrhea, decreased libido, impotence, lethargy, weakness, increased fatigability, sensitivity to cold, constipation, and seizures.

◼ *Stroke.* Hemianopsia can result when a hemorrhagic, thrombotic, or embolic stroke affects part of the optic pathway. Associated signs and symp-

Recognizing types of hemianopsia

Lesions of the optic pathways cause visual field defects. The lesion's site determines the type of defect. For example, a lesion of the optic chiasm involving only those fibers that cross over to the opposite side causes bitemporal hemianopsia—vision loss in the temporal half of each field. However, a lesion of the optic tract or a complete lesion of the optic radiation produces vision loss in the same half of each field—either left or right homonymous hemianopsia.

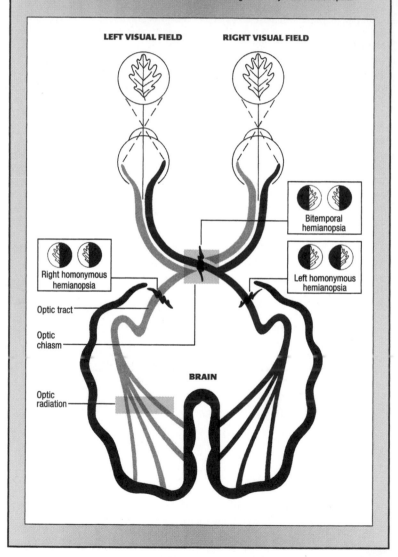

toms vary according to the location and size of the stroke.

Hemoptysis

Hemoptysis is the expectoration of blood or bloody sputum from the lungs or tracheobronchial tree. It's sometimes confused with bleeding from the mouth, throat, nasopharynx, or GI tract. (See *Identifying hemoptysis*.)

Hemoptysis may result from inflammatory, infectious, cardiovascular, or coagulation disorders and, rarely, from a ruptured aortic aneurysm. The most common causes of massive hemoptysis are lung cancer, bronchiectasis, active tuberculosis (TB), and cavitary pulmonary disease from necrotic infections or TB. Several pathophysiologic processes can cause hemoptysis. (See *Responding to hemoptysis* and *What happens in hemoptysis,* page 308.)

Assessment

If the hemoptysis is mild, ask the patient when it began. Has he ever coughed up blood before? About how much blood is he coughing up now and about how often? Ask about a history of cardiac, pulmonary, or bleeding disorders. Is he taking prescription drugs? Does he smoke? Ask the patient if he has had a recent infection. Has he been exposed to TB?

Take the patient's vital signs and examine his nose, mouth, and pharynx for sources of bleeding. Inspect the configuration of his chest and look for abnormal movement during breathing. Observe his respiratory rate, depth, and rhythm. Next, palpate the patient's chest for diaphragm level and for tenderness, respiratory excursion, fremitus, and abnormal pulsations, and then percuss for flatness, dullness, resonance, hyperresonance, and tympany.

Identifying hemoptysis

These guidelines will help you distinguish hemoptysis from epistaxis, hematemesis, and brown, red, or pink sputum.

Hemoptysis

Usually frothy because it's mixed with air, hemoptysis is typically bright red with an alkaline pH (when tested with nitrazine paper). Respiratory signs and symptoms—including a cough, a tickling sensation in the throat, and blood produced from repeated coughing episodes—strongly suggest hemoptysis. Unlike epistaxis, the nasal passages and posterior pharynx usually remain free from blood.

Hematemesis

The patient with hematemesis vomits or regurgitates coffee-ground material that contains food particles, tests positive for occult blood, and has an acid pH. While the usual site of hematemesis is the GI tract, the patient may vomit bright red blood or swallowed blood from the oral cavity or nasopharynx. After an episode of hematemesis, he may complain of dyspepsia and pass stools containing traces of blood.

Brown, red, or pink sputum

Sputum that appears brown, red, or pink may result from oxidation of inhaled bronchodilators. Sputum that looks like old blood may occur after an amebic abscess ruptures into the bronchus. The enterobacterium *Serratia marcescens* may produce red or brown sputum in a patient with pneumonia.

EMERGENCY INTERVENTIONS

Responding to hemoptysis

Massive hemoptysis can cause airway obstruction and asphyxiation. If a patient coughs up copious amounts of blood, take the following steps:

◆ Suction frequently to remove blood.
◆ Insert an I.V. catheter for fluid replacement, drug administration, and blood transfusions, if needed.
◆ Monitor the patient's blood pressure and pulse to detect hypotension and tachycardia.

◆ Prepare to draw an arterial blood sample for laboratory analysis to monitor the patient's respiratory status.
◆ Be aware that endotracheal intubation may be required.

An emergency bronchoscopy may be performed to identify the bleeding site.

What happens in hemoptysis

Changes in vascular walls, or an alteration in blood-clotting mechanisms, can cause bronchial or pulmonary vessels to bleed into the respiratory tract, resulting in hemoptysis. Any of these pathophysiologic processes can trigger hemoptysis:

◆ hemorrhage and diapedesis of red blood cells from the pulmonary microvasculature into the alveoli
◆ necrosis of lung tissue, resulting in inflammation and rupture of blood vessels or hemorrhage into alveolar spaces
◆ rupture of an aortic aneurysm into the tracheobronchial tree
◆ rupture of distended endobronchial blood vessels from pulmonary hypertension due to mitral stenosis
◆ rupture of a pulmonary arteriovenous fistula, a bronchial or pulmonary artery, or a pulmonary venous collateral channel
◆ sloughing of a caseous lesion into the tracheobronchial tree
◆ ulceration and erosion of the bronchial epithelium.

Finally, auscultate the lungs, noting especially the quality and intensity of breath sounds. Obtain a sputum sample and examine it for overall quantity, for the amount of blood it contains, and for its color, odor, and consistency.

Causes

◆ *Bronchial adenoma.* Bronchial adenoma is an insidious disorder that causes recurring hemoptysis in up to 30% of patients, along with a chronic cough and local wheezing.
◆ *Bronchiectasis.* Inflamed bronchial surfaces and eroded bronchial blood vessels cause hemoptysis, which can vary from blood-tinged sputum to frank blood. The patient's sputum may also be copious, foul smelling, and purulent.
◆ *Bronchitis (chronic).* The first sign of chronic bronchitis is typically a productive cough that lasts at least 3 months. Eventually this leads to the production of blood-streaked sputum; massive hemorrhage is unusual.
◆ *Coagulation disorders.* Such disorders as thrombocytopenia and disseminated intravascular coagulation can cause hemoptysis. These disorders may

share such general signs as multisystem hemorrhaging and purpuric lesions.

◆ *Lung abscess.* In about 50% of patients, lung abscesses produce blood-streaked sputum resulting from bronchial ulceration, necrosis, and granulation tissue. Another common finding is a cough with large amounts of purulent, foul-smelling sputum.

◆ *Lung cancer.* Ulceration of the bronchus commonly causes recurring hemoptysis, which can vary from blood-streaked sputum to blood. Related findings include a productive cough, dyspnea, anorexia, weight loss, and wheezing.

◼ *Plague* (Yersinia pestis). The pneumonic form of this acute bacterial infection can produce hemoptysis, a productive cough, chest pain, tachypnea, dyspnea, increasing respiratory distress, and cardiopulmonary insufficiency.

◆ *Pneumonia.* In up to 50% of cases, *Klebsiella* pneumonia produces dark brown or red (currant jelly) sputum, which is so tenacious that the patient has difficulty expelling it from his mouth. This type of pneumonia begins abruptly with chills, fever, dyspnea, a productive cough, and severe pleuritic chest pain. Pneumococcal pneumonia causes pinkish or rusty mucoid sputum. It begins with sudden, shaking chills; a rapidly rising temperature; and, in over 80% of cases, tachycardia and tachypnea.

◼ *Pulmonary edema.* Severe pulmonary edema commonly causes frothy, blood-tinged pink sputum, which accompanies severe dyspnea, orthopnea, gasping, anxiety, cyanosis, diffuse crackles, a ventricular gallop, and cold, clammy skin.

◼ *Pulmonary embolism with infarction.* Hemoptysis is a common finding in pulmonary embolism with infarction, although massive hemoptysis is infrequent. Typical initial symptoms are dyspnea and anginal or pleuritic chest pain. Other common findings include tachycardia, tachypnea, a low-grade fever, and diaphoresis.

◆ *Pulmonary hypertension (primary).* Hemoptysis, exertional dyspnea, and fatigue are common with pulmonary hypertension. Angina-like pain usually occurs with exertion and may radiate to the neck but not to the arms.

◆ *Pulmonary TB.* Blood-streaked or blood-tinged sputum commonly occurs in pulmonary TB; massive hemoptysis may occur in advanced cavitary TB. Other findings include a chronic productive cough, fine crackles after coughing, dyspnea, dullness on percussion, increased tactile fremitus, and possible amphoric hollow breath sounds.

◆ *Systemic lupus erythematosus (SLE).* In 50% of patients with SLE, pleuritis and pneumonitis cause hemoptysis, a cough, dyspnea, pleuritic chest pain, and crackles.

◼ *Tracheal trauma.* Torn tracheal mucosa may cause hemoptysis, hoarseness, dysphagia, neck pain, airway occlusion, and respiratory distress.

Hepatomegaly

Hepatomegaly, an enlarged liver, indicates potentially reversible primary or secondary liver disease. This sign may stem from diverse pathophysiologic mechanisms, including dilated hepatic sinusoids, persistently high venous pressure leading to liver congestion, dysfunction and engorgement of hepatocytes, fatty infiltration of parenchymal cells causing fibrous tissue, distention of liver cells with glycogen, and infiltration of amyloid. Hepatomegaly may be confirmed by palpation, percussion, or radiologic tests.

Assessment

Hepatomegaly usually comes to light during palpation and percussion of the abdomen. If you suspect hepatomegaly, ask the patient about his use of alcohol and exposure to hepatitis. Also ask if he's currently ill or taking prescription drugs. If he complains of abdominal pain, ask him to locate and describe it.

Inspect the patient's skin and sclera for jaundice, dilated veins, scars from previous surgery, and spider angiomas. Next, inspect the contour of his abdomen. Is it protuberant over the liver or distended? Percuss the liver, but be careful to identify structures and conditions that can obscure dull percussion notes, such as the sternum, ribs, breast tissue, pleural effusions, and gas in the colon. (See *Percussing for liver size and position.*) Next, during deep inspiration, palpate the liver's edge; it's tender and rounded in hepatitis and cardiac decompensation, rocklike in carcinoma, and firm in cirrhosis. Take the patient's baseline vital signs, and assess his nutritional status. An enlarged liver that's functioning poorly causes muscle wasting, exaggerated skeletal prominences, weight loss, thin hair, and edema. Evaluate the patient's level of consciousness. When an enlarged liver loses its ability to detoxify waste products, the result is accumulation of metabolic substances toxic to brain cells.

Percussing for liver size and position

Place the patient in a supine position. Percuss along the right midclavicular line (MCL), beginning at the right iliac crest, as shown below. The percussion note becomes dull when you reach the liver's inferior border—usually at the costal margin, but sometimes at a lower point in a patient with liver disease. Mark this point. Next, percuss down from the right clavicle, again along the right MCL. The liver's superior border usually lies between the fifth and seventh intercostal spaces. Mark the superior border. The distance between the two marked points represents the approximate span of the liver's right lobe, which normally ranges from 2¼" to 4¾" (6 to 12 cm).

Next, assess the liver's left lobe. Similarly, percuss along the sternal midline, marking the points where you hear dull percussion notes. Measure the span of the left lobe, which normally ranges from 1½" to 3⅛" (4 to 8 cm). Record your findings for use as a baseline.

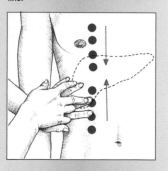

Causes

◆ *Amyloidosis.* Amyloidosis is a rare disorder that may cause hepatomegaly and mild jaundice as well as renal, cardiac, and other GI effects.
◆ *Cirrhosis.* The liver becomes enlarged, nodular, and hard late in cirrhosis. Other late signs and symptoms affect all body systems. The patient may also develop fetor hepaticus, enlarged superficial abdominal veins, muscle atrophy, right upper quadrant pain that worsens when sitting up or leaning forward, and a palpable spleen.

◆ *Diabetes mellitus.* Poorly controlled diabetes in overweight patients commonly produces fatty infiltration of the liver, hepatomegaly, and right upper quadrant tenderness along with polydipsia, polyphagia, and polyuria.

◆ *Granulomatous disorders.* Sarcoidosis, histoplasmosis, and other such disorders commonly produce a slightly enlarged, firm liver.

◆ *Hepatic abscess.* With hepatic abscess, hepatomegaly may accompany fever, nausea and vomiting, chills, weakness, diarrhea, anorexia, an elevated right hemidiaphragm, and right upper quadrant pain and tenderness.

◆ *Hepatitis.* In viral hepatitis, early signs and symptoms include nausea, anorexia, vomiting, fatigue, malaise, photophobia, sore throat, cough, and headache.

◆ *Leukemia and lymphomas.* Leukemia and lymphomas are proliferative blood cell disorders that typically cause moderate to massive hepatomegaly and splenomegaly as well as abdominal discomfort.

◆ *Liver cancer.* Primary tumors commonly cause irregular, nodular, firm hepatomegaly, with pain or tenderness in the right upper quadrant and a friction rub or bruit over the liver. When metastatic liver tumors cause hepatomegaly, the patient's accompanying signs and symptoms reflect his primary cancer.

◆ *Mononucleosis (infectious).* Occasionally, infectious mononucleosis causes hepatomegaly. Prodromal symptoms include headache, malaise, and fatigue.

◆ *Obesity.* Hepatomegaly can result from fatty infiltration of the liver. Weight loss reduces the liver's size.

◆ *Pancreatic cancer.* In pancreatic cancer, hepatomegaly accompanies such signs and symptoms as anorexia, weight loss, abdominal or back pain, and jaundice.

◆ *Pericarditis.* In chronic constrictive pericarditis, an increase in systemic venous pressure produces marked congestive hepatomegaly. Distended jugular veins (more prominent on inspiration) are a common finding.

Hoarseness

Hoarseness—a rough or harsh sound to the voice—can result from infections, inflammatory lesions, or exudates of the larynx; laryngeal edema; and compression or disruption of the vocal cords or recurrent laryngeal nerve. This common sign can also result from a thoracic aortic aneurysm, vocal cord paralysis, and systemic disorders such as rheumatoid arthritis. It's characteristically worsened by excessive alcohol intake, smoking, inhaling noxious fumes, excessive talking, and shouting. Hoarseness may also result from progressive atrophy of the laryngeal muscles and mucosa due to aging, which leads to diminished control of the vocal cords.

Assessment

Obtain a patient history. Be sure to ask about the onset of hoarseness. Has the patient been overusing his voice? Has he experienced shortness of breath, a sore throat, a dry mouth, a cough, or difficulty swallowing? Does the patient have a history of cancer, rheumatoid arthritis, or aortic aneurysm? Does he regularly drink alcohol or smoke?

Inspect the oral cavity and pharynx for redness or exudate. Palpate the neck for masses, the cervical lymph nodes and thyroid for enlargement, and the trachea for position. Examine the eyes for corneal ulcers and enlarged lacrimal ducts. Check for dilated jugular and chest veins, which may indicate compression by an aortic aneurysm. Take the patient's vital signs, noting especially a fever and bradycardia. Inspect for asymmetrical chest expansion or signs of respiratory distress. Then auscultate for crackles, rhonchi, wheezing, and tubular sounds, and percuss for dullness.

Causes

◆ *Gastroesophageal reflux.* With gastroesophageal reflux, retrograde flow of gastric juices into the esophagus may then spill into the hypopharynx. This, in turn, irritates the larynx, resulting in hoarseness.

◆ *Hypothyroidism.* With hypothyroidism, hoarseness may be an early sign. Other findings include fatigue, cold intolerance, weight gain despite anorexia, and menorrhagia.

◆ *Laryngeal cancer.* Hoarseness is an early sign of vocal cord cancer; however, it may not occur until later in cancer of other laryngeal areas. The patient usually has a long history of smoking.

◆ *Laryngeal leukoplakia.* Leukoplakia is a common cause of hoarseness, especially in smokers. Histologic examination from direct laryngoscopy usually reveals mild, moderate, or severe dysphagia.

◆ *Laryngitis.* Persistent hoarseness may be the only sign of chronic laryngitis. With acute laryngitis, hoarseness or a complete loss of voice develops suddenly.

◆ *Rheumatoid arthritis.* Hoarseness may signal laryngeal involvement in rheumatoid arthritis. Other findings include pain, dysphagia, a sensation of fullness or tension in the throat, dyspnea on exertion, and stridor.

◼ *Thoracic aortic aneurysm.* A thoracic aortic aneurysm typically produces no symptoms, but may cause hoarseness. Its most common symptom is penetrating pain that's especially severe when the patient is supine.

◼ *Tracheal trauma.* Torn tracheal mucosa may cause hoarseness, hemoptysis, dysphagia, neck pain, airway occlusion, and respiratory distress.

◆ *Vocal cord paralysis.* Unilateral vocal cord paralysis causes hoarseness and vocal weakness. Paralysis may accompany signs of trauma, such as pain and swelling of the head and neck.

◆ *Vocal cord polyps or nodules.* Raspy hoarseness, the chief complaint with vocal cord polyps, accompanies a chronic cough and a crackling voice.

Homans' sign

Homans' sign is positive when deep calf pain results from strong and abrupt dorsiflexion of the ankle. This pain results from venous thrombosis or inflammation of the calf muscles. However, because a positive Homans' sign appears in only 35% of patients with these conditions, it's an unreliable indicator. (See *Eliciting Homans' sign.*) Even when accurate, a positive Homans' sign doesn't indicate the extent of the venous disorder. This elicited sign may be confused with continuous calf pain, which can result from strains, contusions, cellulitis, or arterial occlusion or with pain in the posterior ankle or Achilles tendon.

Assessment

When you detect a positive Homans' sign, focus the patient history on signs and symptoms that accompany deep vein thrombosis (DVT) or thrombophlebitis. These include throbbing, aching, heavy, or tight sensations in the calf and leg pain during or after exercise or routine activity. Also, ask about shortness of breath or chest pain, which may indicate pulmonary

Eliciting Homans' sign

To elicit Homans' sign, first support the patient's thigh with one hand and his foot with the other, as shown below. Bend his leg slightly at the knee, and then firmly and abruptly dorsiflex the ankle. Resulting deep calf pain indicates a positive Homans' sign. (The patient may also resist ankle dorsiflexion or flex the knee involuntarily if Homans' sign is positive.)

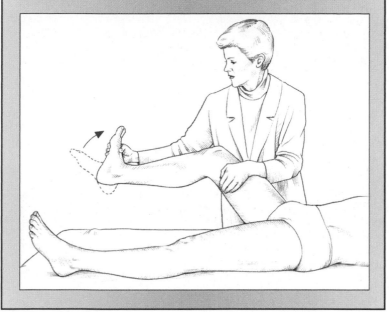

embolism. Be sure to ask about predisposing events, such as a leg injury, recent surgery, childbirth, use of hormonal contraceptives, and prolonged inactivity or bed rest.

Next, inspect and palpate the patient's calf for warmth, tenderness, redness, swelling, and the presence of a palpable vein. If you strongly suspect DVT, elicit Homans' sign very carefully to avoid dislodging the clot, which could cause pulmonary embolism, a life-threatening condition. In addition, measure the circumferences of the patient's calves. The calf with the positive Homans' sign may be larger because of edema and swelling.

Causes

◆ *Cellulitis (superficial).* Superficial cellulitis typically affects the legs, but can also affect the arms, producing pain, redness, tenderness, and edema.
◆ *Deep vein thrombophlebitis.* A positive Homans' sign and calf tenderness may be the only clinical findings of deep vein thrombophlebitis. However, the patient may also have severe pain, warmth, and swelling of the affected leg.
◆ *DVT.* DVT causes a positive Homans' sign along with tenderness over the deep calf veins, slight edema of the calves and thighs, a low-grade

fever, and tachycardia. If DVT affects the femoral and iliac veins, you'll notice marked local swelling and tenderness. If DVT causes venous obstruction, you'll notice cyanosis and possibly cool skin in the affected leg.

◆ *Popliteal cyst (ruptured)*. Rupture of this synovial cyst may produce a positive Homans' sign as well as a sudden onset of calf tenderness, swelling, and redness.

Hyperpnea

Hyperpnea indicates increased respiratory effort for a sustained period—a normal rate with increased depth, an increased rate with normal depth, or an increased rate and depth. This sign differs from sighing and may be associated with tachypnea. The typical patient with hyperpnea breathes at a normal or increased rate and inhales deeply, displaying marked chest expansion. He may complain of shortness of breath if a respiratory disorder is causing hypoxemia, or he may not be aware of his breathing if a metabolic, psychiatric, or neurologic disorder is causing involuntary hyperpnea. Hyperventilation, a consequence of hyperpnea, is characterized by alkalosis. In central neurogenic hyperventilation, brain stem dysfunction increases the rate and depth of respirations. In acute

Kussmaul's respirations: A compensatory mechanism

Kussmaul's respirations—fast, deep breathing without pauses—characteristically sound labored, with deep breaths that resemble sighs. This breathing pattern develops when respiratory centers in the medulla detect decreased blood pH, thereby triggering compensatory fast and deep breathing to remove excess carbon dioxide and restore pH balance.

Disorders (such as diabetes mellitus and renal failure), drug effects, and other conditions cause metabolic acidosis (loss of bicarbonate ions and retention of acid).

Disorders (such as diabetes mellitus and renal failure), drug effects, and other conditions cause metabolic acidosis (loss of bicarbonate ions and retention of acid).

↓

Blood pH decreases.

↓

Kussmaul's respirations develop to blow off excess carbon dioxide.

↓

Blood pH rises.

↓

Respiratory rate and depth decrease (corrected pH) in effective compensation.

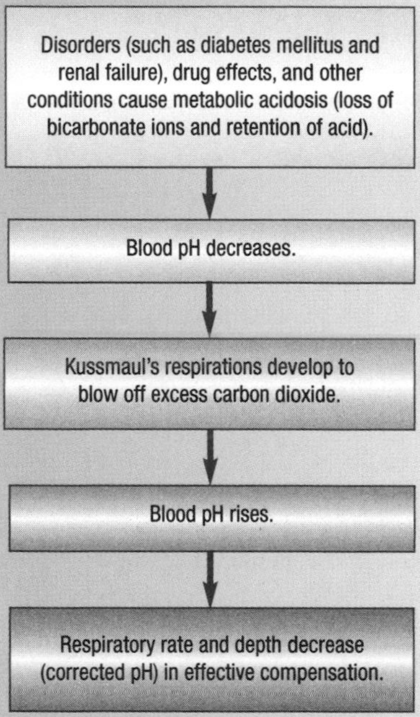

EMERGENCY INTERVENTIONS

Responding to hyperpnea

When the condition of a patient with hyperpnea begins to deteriorate, immediate intervention is necessary to prevent cardiovascular collapse. Institute the following measures:
◆ Insert an I.V. catheter for administration of fluid, blood, and vasopressors, as ordered.
◆ Prepare to administer ventilatory support, if needed.
◆ Prepare the patient for arterial blood gas analysis and blood chemistry studies.

intermittent hyperventilation, the respiratory pattern may be a response to hypoxemia, anxiety, fear, pain, or excitement. Hyperpnea may also be a compensatory mechanism to metabolic acidosis. Under these conditions, it's known as *Kussmaul's respirations.* (See *Kussmaul's respirations: A compensatory mechanism.*)

Assessment

If you observe hyperpnea in a patient whose other signs and symptoms signal a life-threatening emergency, you must intervene quickly and effectively. Monitor vital signs, including oxygen saturation, in every patient with hyperpnea, and observe for increasing respiratory distress, an irregular respiratory pattern, or hypoxia—all of which signal deterioration. (See *Responding to hyperpnea* and *Managing hyperpnea,* page 316.) If the patient's condition isn't grave, first determine his level of consciousness (LOC). If he's alert, ask about recent illnesses or infections and ingestion or inhalation of drugs or chemicals. Find out if the patient has diabetes mellitus, renal disease, or a pulmonary condition. Is he excessively thirsty or hungry? Has he recently had severe diarrhea or an upper respiratory tract infection?

Next, observe the patient for clues to his abnormal breathing pattern. Is his breathing abnormally rapid? Examine the patient for cyanosis, restlessness, and anxiety. In addition, observe the patient for intercostal and abdominal retractions, accessory muscle use, and diaphoresis. Then, inspect for draining wounds, and ask about nausea and vomiting. Examine his skin and mucous membranes for turgor, possibly indicating dehydration. Auscultate the patient's heart and lungs.

Causes

◆ Head injury. Hyperpnea that results from a severe head injury is called *central neurogenic hyperventilation.* Whether its onset is acute or gradual, this type of hyperpnea indicates damage to the lower midbrain or upper pons.
◆ *Hyperventilation syndrome.* Acute anxiety triggers episodic hyperpnea, resulting in respiratory alkalosis.
◆ Hypoxemia. Pulmonary disorders that cause hypoxemia—for example, pneumonia, pulmonary edema, chronic obstructive pulmonary disease, and pneumothorax—may cause hyperpnea with chest pain, dizziness, and paresthesia.

Managing hyperpnea

Carefully examine the patient with hyperpnea for signs of a life-threatening condition, such as increased intracranial pressure (ICP), metabolic acidosis, diabetic ketoacidosis (DKA), and uremia. Be prepared to intervene quickly.

Increased ICP

If an unconscious patient with signs of recent head trauma (soft-tissue injury, edema, or ecchymoses on the face or head) develops hyperpnea, act quickly to prevent further brain stem injury and irreversible deterioration. Take the patient's vital signs, noting bradycardia, increased systolic blood pressure, and widening pulse pressure—signs of increased ICP. Examine pupillary reactions.

Elevate the head of the bed 30 degrees (unless you suspect spinal cord injury). Insert an artificial airway and administer supplemental oxygen, as ordered. Attach the patient to a cardiac monitor and continuously monitor his cardiac rhythm and respiratory pattern. Watch for arrhythmias and irregular respirations, which signal deterioration. Keep emergency resuscitation equipment close by. Obtain a blood sample for arterial blood gas analysis to help guide treatment. Insert an I.V. catheter at a slow infusion rate, as ordered, and prepare to administer an osmotic diuretic, such as mannitol (Osmitrol), to decrease cerebral edema. Insert an indwelling urinary catheter, as ordered, to closely measure urine output.

Metabolic acidosis

In the absence of a head injury, hyperpnea is most likely the result of metabolic acidosis. If the patient has a decreased level of consciousness, check his history for clues as to the cause of metabolic acidosis, and intervene appropriately.

Suspect shock if the patient has cold, clammy skin. Palpate for a rapid, thready pulse and take his blood pressure, noting hypotension. Elevate the patient's legs 30 degrees. If the patient has an obvious hemorrhage, apply pressure dressings. Insert several large-bore I.V. catheters, as ordered, and prepare to administer fluids, vasopressors, and blood transfusions.

Other causes of metabolic acidosis include a history of alcohol abuse; profuse vomiting, diarrhea or abdominal drainage; aspirin overdose; and cachexia and starvation. Inspect the patient's skin for dryness and poor turgor, indicating dehydration. Take his vital signs, looking for a low-grade fever and hypotension. Insert an I.V. catheter for fluid replacement, as ordered, and prepare to administer sodium bicarbonate. Obtain blood samples for electrolyte studies, as ordered.

DKA

If the patient has a history of diabetes mellitus, is vomiting, and has a fruity breath odor (acetone breath), suspect DKA. Immediately perform a fingerstick to obtain a blood glucose level. Insert an I.V. catheter and begin an infusion of saline solution. Insert an indwelling urinary catheter to obtain a urine specimen to test for glucose and acetone and to closely monitor urine output. Obtain a blood sample for glucose and ketone levels. Administer I.V. fluids, insulin, potassium, and sodium bicarbonate, as ordered.

Uremia

If the patient has a history of renal disease, an ammonia breath odor (uremic fetor), and a fine, white powder on his skin (uremic frost), suspect uremia. Insert an I.V. catheter at a slow infusion rate, and prepare to administer sodium bicarbonate. Monitor the patient's electrocardiogram for arrhythmias due to hyperkalemia. Obtain blood samples for analysis of electrolytes, blood urea nitrogen, and creatinine. Prepare to begin hemodialysis or peritoneal dialysis.

◼ *Ketoacidosis.* Alcoholic ketoacidosis typically follows cessation of drinking after a marked increase in alcohol consumption has caused severe vomiting. Kussmaul's respirations begin abruptly and are accompanied by vomiting for several days, a fruity breath odor, slight dehydration, abdominal pain and distention, and absent bowel sounds.

Diabetic ketoacidosis typically produces Kussmaul's respirations. The patient usually experiences polydipsia, polyphagia, and polyuria before the onset of acidosis; he may or may not have a history of diabetes mellitus.

Starvation ketoacidosis can cause Kussmaul's respirations. Its onset is gradual; typical findings include signs of cachexia and dehydration, a decreased LOC, bradycardia, and a history of severely limited food intake.

◆ *Renal failure.* Acute or chronic renal failure can cause acidosis with Kussmaul's respirations. Signs and symptoms of severe renal failure include oliguria or anuria, uremic fetor, and yellow, dry, scaly skin.

◆ *Sepsis.* A severe infection may cause lactic acidosis, resulting in Kussmaul's respirations. Other findings include tachycardia, fever or low temperature, chills, headache, lethargy, profuse diaphoresis, anorexia, cough, wound drainage, burning on urination, confusion or a change in mental status, and other signs of local infection.

◼ *Shock.* Hyperpnea is a classic sign of shock. Other clinical findings may include external or internal bleeding (in hypovolemic shock), chest pain or arrhythmias and signs of heart failure (in cardiogenic shock), a high fever and chills (in septic shock), or stridor due to laryngeal edema (in anaphylactic shock). The onset is usually acute in hypovolemic, cardiogenic, or anaphylactic shock, but it may be gradual in septic shock.

Impotence

Impotence is the inability to achieve and maintain penile erection sufficient to complete satisfactory sexual intercourse; ejaculation may occur normally.

Impotence varies from occasional and minimal to permanent and complete. Occasional impotence occurs in about one-half of adult American men, whereas chronic impotence affects about 10 million American men.

Impotence can be classified as primary or secondary. A man with primary impotence has never been potent with a sexual partner, but may achieve normal erections in other situations. This uncommon condition is difficult to treat. Secondary impotence carries a more favorable prognosis because, despite the present erectile dysfunction, the patient has completed satisfactory intercourse in the past.

Penile erection involves increased arterial blood flow secondary to psychological, tactile, and other sensory stimulation. Trapping of blood within the penis produces increased length, circumference, and rigidity. Impotence results when any component of this process—psychological, vascular, neurologic, or hormonal—malfunctions.

Assessment

If the patient complains of impotence, allow him to describe his problem without interruption. Then begin your examination in a systematic way, moving from less sensitive to more sensitive matters. Begin with a psychosocial history. Is the patient married, single, or widowed? How long has he been married or had a sexual relationship? What's the age and health status of his sexual partner? Is he feeling stress or pressure from his partner to conceive a child? If you can do so discreetly, ask about sexual activity outside marriage or his primary sexual relationship. Also ask about his job history, his typical daily activities, and his living situation. How well does he get along with others in his household?

Focus your medical history on the causes of erectile dysfunction. Does the patient have type 2 diabetes mellitus, hypertension, or heart disease? If so, ask about its onset and treatment. Also ask about neurologic diseases such as multiple sclerosis (MS). Obtain a surgical history, emphasizing neurologic, vascular, and urologic surgery. If trauma may be causing the patient's impotence, find out the date of the injury as well as its severity, associated effects, and treatment. Ask about alcohol intake, drug use or abuse, smoking, diet, and exercise. Obtain a urologic history, including voiding problems and past injury. Next, ask the patient when his impotence began. How did it progress? What's its current status? Make your questions specific, but remember that he may have difficulty discussing sexual problems or may not understand the physiology involved.

These sample questions may yield helpful data: When was the first time you remember not being able to initiate or maintain an erection? How often do you wake in the morning or at night with an erection? Do you have wet dreams? Has your sexual drive changed? How often do you try to have intercourse with your partner? How often would you *like* to? Can you ejaculate with or without an erection? Do you experience orgasm with ejaculation? Ask the patient to rate the quality of a typical erection on a scale of 0 to 10, with 0 being completely flaccid and 10 being completely erect. Using the same scale, also ask him to rate his ability to ejaculate during sexual activity, with 0 being never and 10 being always.

Next, perform a brief physical examination. Inspect and palpate the genitalia for structural abnormalities. Assess the patient's sensory function, concentrating on the perineal area. Next, test motor strength and deep tendon reflexes in all extremities, and note other neurologic deficits. Take the patient's vital signs and palpate his pulses for quality. Note signs of peripheral vascular disease, such as cyanosis and cool extremities. Auscultate for abdominal aortic, femoral, carotid, or iliac bruits, and palpate for thyroid gland enlargement.

Drugs that may cause impotence

Many commonly used drugs—especially antihypertensives—can cause impotence. The impotence may resolve when the drug is discontinued or the dosage reduced. Here are some of the drugs that may cause impotence:

◆ amitriptyline (Elavil)
◆ atenolol (Tenormin)
◆ bicalutamide (Casodex)
◆ carbamazepine (Tegretol)
◆ cimetidine (Tagamet)
◆ clonidine (Catapres)
◆ desipramine (Norpramin)
◆ digoxin (Lanoxin)
◆ escitalopram (Lexapro)
◆ finasteride (Proscar)
◆ hydralazine (Apresoline)
◆ imipramine (Tofranil)
◆ methyldopa (Aldomet)
◆ nortriptyline (Pamelor)
◆ perphenazine (Trilafon)
◆ prazosin (Minipress)
◆ propranolol (Inderal)
◆ thiazide diuretics
◆ thioridazine (Mellaril)
◆ tranylcypromine (Parnate)

Causes

◆ *Alcohol and drugs.* Alcoholism and drug abuse are associated with impotence, as are many prescription drugs, especially antihypertensives. (See *Drugs that may cause impotence.*)
◆ *Central nervous system disorders.* Spinal cord lesions from trauma produce sudden impotence. A complete lesion above S2 disrupts descending motor tracts to the genital area, causing a loss of voluntary erectile control but not of reflex erection and reflex ejaculation. However, a complete lesion in

the lumbosacral spinal cord causes a loss of reflex ejaculation and reflex erection. Spinal cord tumors and degenerative diseases of the brain and spinal cord, such as MS and amyotrophic lateral sclerosis, cause progressive impotence.

◆ *Endocrine disorders.* Hypogonadism from testicular or pituitary dysfunction may lead to impotence from a deficient secretion of androgens (primarily testosterone). Adrenocortical and thyroid dysfunction and chronic hepatic disease may also cause impotence because these organs play a role (although minor) in sex hormone regulation.

◆ *Penile disorders.* Inflammatory, infectious, or destructive diseases of the penis may cause impotence. With Peyronie's disease, the penis is bent, making erection painful and penetration difficult and eventually impossible. Phimosis prevents erection until circumcision releases the constricted foreskin.

◆ *Psychological distress.* Impotence can result from diverse psychological causes, including depression, performance anxiety, memories of previous traumatic sexual experiences, moral or religious conflicts, and troubled emotional or sexual relationships.

◆ *Surgery.* Surgical injury to the prostate gland, penis, bladder neck, urinary sphincter, rectum, or perineum can cause impotence, as can injury to local nerves or blood vessels.

Insomnia

Insomnia is the inability to fall asleep, remain asleep, or feel refreshed by sleep. Acute and transient during periods of stress, insomnia may become chronic, causing constant fatigue, extreme anxiety as bedtime approaches, and psychiatric disorders. This common complaint is experienced occa-

sionally by about 25% of Americans and chronically by another 10%.

Pathophysiologic causes range from medical and psychiatric disorders to pain and adverse effects of a drug. Complaints of insomnia are subjective and require close investigation; for example, the patient may mistakenly attribute his fatigue to insomnia, when its etiology is actually from an organic cause such as anemia. Depending on the cause, comfort and relaxation techniques can help promote natural sleep. (See *Tips for relieving insomnia.*)

Assessment

Take a thorough sleep and health history. Find out when the patient's insomnia began and the circumstances surrounding it. Is the patient trying to stop using a sedative? Does he take a central nervous system stimulant, such as an amphetamine, pseudoephedrine (Sudafed), a theophylline derivative, cocaine, or a drug that contains caffeine? Does he drink caffeinated beverages?

Find out if the patient has a chronic or acute condition, the effects of which may be disturbing his sleep. Ask if he has an endocrine or neurologic disorder, or a history of drug or alcohol abuse. Does he use his legs a lot during the day and then feel restless at night? Ask about daytime fatigue and regular exercise. Also ask if he commonly finds himself gasping for air, experiencing apnea, or frequently repositioning his body. If possible, consult the patient's spouse or sleep partner because the patient may be unaware of his behavior. Ask how many pillows the patient uses to sleep.

Assess the patient's emotional status. Ask about personal and professional problems and psychological stress. After reviewing complaints that

Tips for relieving insomnia

COMMON CAUSES	DESCRIPTION	INTERVENTIONS
Acro-paresthesia	Improper positioning may compress superficial (ulnar, radial, and peroneal) nerves, disrupting circulation to the compressed nerve. This causes numbness, tingling, and stiffness in an arm or leg.	Teach the patient to assume a comfortable position in bed, with his limbs unrestricted. If he tends to awaken with a numb arm or leg, tell him to massage and move it until sensation returns completely and then to assume an unrestricted position.
Anxiety	Physical and emotional stress produces anxiety, which causes autonomic stimulation.	Encourage the patient to discuss his fears and concerns, and teach him relaxation techniques, such as guided imagery and deep breathing. If ordered, administer a mild sedative, such as temazepam (Restoril) or another sedative hypnotic, before bedtime. Emphasize that these medications are for short-term use only.
Dyspnea	With many cardiac and pulmonary disorders, a recumbent position and inactivity cause restricted chest expansion, secretion pooling, and pulmonary vascular congestion, leading to coughing and shortness of breath.	Elevate the head of the bed, or provide at least two pillows or a reclining chair to help the patient sleep. Suction him when he awakens, and encourage deep breathing and incentive spirometry every 2 to 4 hours. Also, provide supplementary oxygen by nasal cannula. If the patient is pregnant, encourage her to sleep on her left side at a comfortable elevation to ease dyspnea.
Pain	Chronic or acute pain from any cause can prevent or disrupt sleep.	Administer pain medication, as ordered, 20 minutes before bedtime, and teach deep, even, slow breathing to promote relaxation. If the patient has back pain, help him lie on his side with his legs flexed. If he has epigastric pain, encourage him to take an antacid before bedtime and to sleep with the head of the bed elevated. If he has incisions, instruct him to splint during coughing or movement.
Pruritus	A localized skin infection or a systemic disorder, such as liver failure, may produce intensely annoying itching, even during the night.	Wash the skin with a mild soap and water, and dry it thoroughly. Apply moisturizing lotion on dry, unbroken skin and an antipruritic, such as calamine lotion, on pruritic areas. Administer diphenhydramine (Benadryl) or hydroxyzine (Atarax) to help minimize itching.
Restless leg	Excessive exercise during the day may cause tired, aching legs at night, requiring movement for relief.	Help the patient exercise his legs gently by slowly walking with him around the room and down the hall. If ordered, administer a muscle relaxant such as diazepam (Valium).

suggest an undiagnosed disorder, perform a physical examination.

Causes

◆ *Alcohol withdrawal syndrome.* Abrupt cessation of alcohol intake after long-term use causes insomnia that may persist for up to 2 years. Other early effects of this acute syndrome include excessive diaphoresis, tachycardia, hypertension, tremors, restlessness, irritability, headache, nausea, flushing, and nightmares.

◆ *Generalized anxiety disorder.* Anxiety can cause chronic insomnia as well as symptoms of tension, such as fatigue and restlessness; signs of autonomic hyperactivity, such as diaphoresis, dyspepsia, and a high resting pulse and respiratory rate; and signs of apprehension.

◆ *Mood (affective) disorders.* Depression commonly causes chronic insomnia with difficulty falling asleep or waking and being unable to fall back to sleep. Related findings include dysphoria, changes in appetite, and psychomotor agitation or retardation. The patient experiences loss of interest in his usual activities, feelings of worthlessness and guilt, fatigue, difficulty concentrating, indecisiveness, and recurrent thoughts of death.

Manic episodes produce a decreased need for sleep with an elevated mood and irritability. Related findings include increased energy and activity, fast speech, speeding thoughts, inflated self-esteem, easy distractibility, and involvement in high-risk activities such as reckless driving.

◆ *Nocturnal myoclonus.* With nocturnal myoclonus, a seizure disorder, involuntary and fleeting muscle jerks of the legs occur every 20 to 40 seconds, disturbing sleep.

◆ *Sleep apnea syndrome.* Apneic periods begin with the onset of sleep, continue for 10 to 90 seconds, and end with a series of gasps and arousal. With central sleep apnea, respiratory movement ceases for the apneic period; with obstructive sleep apnea, upper airway obstruction blocks incoming air, although breathing movements continue. Other findings include a morning headache, daytime fatigue, hypertension, ankle edema, and personality changes.

◆ *Thyrotoxicosis.* Difficulty falling asleep and then sleeping for only a brief period is one of the characteristic symptoms of thyrotoxicosis. Cardiopulmonary features include dyspnea, tachycardia, palpitations, and an atrial or a ventricular gallop.

Intermittent claudication

Most common in the legs, intermittent claudication is cramping limb pain brought on by exercise and relieved by 1 to 2 minutes of rest. It's most common in men ages 50 to 60 with a history of diabetes mellitus, hyperlipidemia, hypertension, or tobacco use. Without treatment, it may progress to pain at rest.

With occlusive artery disease, intermittent claudication results from an inadequate blood supply. Pain in the calf (the most common area) or foot indicates disease of the femoral or popliteal arteries; pain in the buttocks and upper thigh, disease of the aortoiliac arteries. During exercise, the pain typically results from the release of lactic acid due to anaerobic metabolism in the ischemic segment, secondary to obstruction. When exercise stops, the lactic acid clears and the pain subsides. With chronic arterial occlusion, collateral circulation usually develops.

EMERGENCY INTERVENTIONS

Responding to acute arterial occlusion

If you suspect acute arterial occlusion in a patient with sudden intermittent claudication, take the following steps:
◆ Mark the area of pallor, cyanosis, or mottling; reassess it frequently, noting an increase in the affected area.
◆ Don't elevate the affected leg or allow anything to press on it.

◆ Prepare the patient for preoperative blood tests, urinalysis, electrocardiography, chest X-rays, lower-extremity Doppler studies, and angiography.
◆ Insert an I.V. catheter and administer an anticoagulant and analgesics, as ordered.

Intermittent claudication may also have a neurologic cause: narrowing of the vertebral column at the level of the cauda equina. This condition creates pressure on the nerve roots to the lower extremities. Walking stimulates circulation to the cauda equina, causing increased pressure on those nerves and resultant pain.

Assessment

If the patient has sudden intermittent claudication with severe or aching leg pain at rest, suspect acute arterial occlusion and prepare for emergency interventions. (See *Responding to acute arterial occlusion.*) If the patient has chronic intermittent claudication, gather history data first. Ask how far he can walk before pain occurs and how long he must rest before it subsides. Can he walk less far now than before, or does he need to rest longer? Has this symptom affected his lifestyle? Obtain a history of risk factors for atherosclerosis. Next, ask about associated signs and symptoms, such as paresthesia in the affected limb and visible changes in the color of the fingers (white to blue to pink) when he's smoking, exposed to cold, or under stress. If the

patient is male, does he experience impotence?

Focus the physical examination on the cardiovascular system. Palpate for femoral, popliteal, dorsalis pedis, and posterior tibial pulses. Note character, amplitude, and bilateral equality. Listen for bruits over the major arteries. Note color and temperature differences between the patient's legs or compared with his arms; also note where on his leg the changes in temperature and color occur. Elevate the affected leg for 2 minutes; if it becomes pale or white, blood flow is severely decreased. When lowered, how long does it take for color to return? (Thirty seconds or longer indicates severe disease.) Note if the patient's deep tendon reflexes (DTRs) diminish in his lower extremities after exercise.

Examine the patient's feet, toes, and fingers for ulceration, and inspect his hands and lower legs for small, tender nodules and erythema along blood vessels. Note the quality of his nails and the amount of hair on his fingers and toes.

If the patient has arm pain, inspect his arms for a change in color (to white) on elevation. Next, palpate for changes in temperature, muscle wasting, and a pulsating mass in the subclavian area. Palpate and compare the radial, ulnar, brachial, axillary, and subclavian pulses to identify obstructed areas.

Causes

◆ *Arterial occlusion (acute)*. Acute arterial occlusion produces intense intermittent claudication. A saddle embolus may affect both legs. Associated findings include paresthesia, paresis, and a sensation of cold in the affected limb. The limb is cool, pale, and cyanotic (mottled) with absent pulses below the occlusion. Capillary refill time is increased.

◆ *Arteriosclerosis obliterans*. Arteriosclerosis obliterans usually affects the femoral and popliteal arteries, causing intermittent claudication in the calf. Associated findings include diminished or absent popliteal and pedal pulses, coolness in the affected limb, pallor on elevation, and profound limb weakness with continuing exercise. Other possible findings include numbness and, in severe disease, pain in the toes or foot while at rest, ulceration, and gangrene.

◆ *Buerger's disease*. Buerger's disease typically produces intermittent claudication of the instep. Men are affected more than women; most of the affected men smoke and are ages 20 to 40. Early signs include migratory superficial nodules and erythema along extremity blood vessels as well as migratory venous phlebitis. With exposure to cold, the feet initially become cold, cyanotic, and numb; later, they redden, become hot, and tingle. Occasionally, Buerger's disease also affects the hands and can cause painful ulcerations on the fingertips.

◆ *Neurogenic claudication*. Neurospinal disease causes pain from neurogenic intermittent claudication that re-

quires a longer rest time than the 2 to 3 minutes needed in vascular claudication. Associated findings include paresthesia, weakness and clumsiness when walking, and hypoactive DTRs after walking. Pulses are unaffected.

J

Jaundice

Jaundice is a yellow discoloration of the skin, mucous membranes, or sclera of the eyes that indicates excessive levels of conjugated or unconjugated bilirubin in the blood. In fair-skinned patients, it's most noticeable on the face, trunk, and sclera; in dark-skinned patients, on the hard palate, sclera, and conjunctiva.

Jaundice is most apparent in natural sunlight and may be undetectable in artificial or poor light. It's commonly accompanied by pruritus, dark urine, and clay-colored stools. It may result from any of three pathophysiologic processes and may be the only warning sign of certain disorders such as pancreatic cancer. (See *Jaundice: Impaired bilirubin metabolism,* page 326.)

Assessment

Documenting a history of the patient's jaundice is critical in determining its cause. Begin by asking the patient when he first noticed the jaundice. Does he also have pruritus, clay-colored stools, or dark urine? Does he have nonspecific signs or symptoms, such as fatigue, fever, or chills; GI signs or symptoms, such as anorexia, abdominal pain, nausea, weight loss, or vomiting; or cardiopulmonary symptoms, such as shortness of breath or palpitations? Ask about alcohol use and a history of cancer or liver, pancreatic, or gallbladder disease. Has the patient lost weight recently? Also obtain a drug history.

Perform the physical examination in a room with natural light. Make sure that the orange-yellow hue is jaundice and not due to hypercarotenemia, which is more prominent on the palms and soles and doesn't affect the sclera. Inspect the patient's skin for texture and dryness and for hyperpigmentation and xanthomas. Look for spider angiomas or petechiae, clubbed fingers, and gynecomastia. If the patient has heart failure, auscultate for arrhythmias, murmurs, and gallops as well as crackles and abnormal bowel sounds. Palpate the lymph nodes for swelling and the abdomen for tenderness, pain, and swelling. Palpate and percuss the liver and spleen for enlargement, and test for ascites with the shifting dullness and fluid wave techniques. Obtain baseline data on the patient's mental status. Slight changes in sensorium may be an early sign of deteriorating hepatic function.

Jaundice: Impaired bilirubin metabolism

Jaundice occurs in three forms: prehepatic, hepatic, and posthepatic. In all three, bilirubin levels in the blood increase due to impaired metabolism.

With prehepatic jaundice, certain conditions and disorders, such as transfusion reactions and sickle cell anemia, cause massive hemolysis. Red blood cells rupture faster than the liver can conjugate bilirubin, so large amounts of unconjugated bilirubin pass into the blood. The intestines increase conversion of this bilirubin to water-soluble urobilinogen for excretion in urine and stools. (Unconjugated bilirubin is insoluble in water, so it can't be directly excreted in urine.)

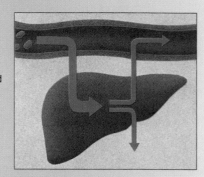

Hepatic jaundice results from the liver's inability to conjugate or excrete bilirubin, leading to increased blood levels of conjugated and unconjugated bilirubin. This occurs with such disorders as hepatitis, cirrhosis, and metastatic cancer and during the prolonged use of drugs metabolized by the liver.

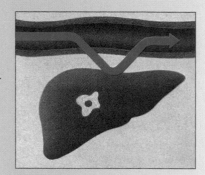

With posthepatic jaundice—which occurs in patients with a biliary or pancreatic disorder—bilirubin forms at its normal rate, but inflammation, scar tissue, a tumor, or gallstones block bile flow into the intestine. This causes an accumulation of conjugated bilirubin in the blood. Water-soluble, conjugated bilirubin is excreted in urine.

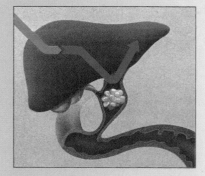

Causes

◆ *Carcinoma.* Cancer of the ampulla of Vater initially produces fluctuating jaundice, mild abdominal pain, a recurrent fever, and chills. Occult bleeding may be the first sign. Hepatic cancer may cause jaundice by causing bile duct obstruction. Even advanced cancer causes nonspecific signs and symptoms, such as right upper quadrant discomfort and tenderness, nausea, weight loss, and a slight fever. With pancreatic cancer, progressive jaundice—possibly with pruritus—may be the only sign. Related early findings include weight loss and back or abdominal pain. Other findings include anorexia, fever, steatorrhea, fatigue, weakness, diarrhea, and skin lesions (usually on the legs).

◆ *Cholangitis.* Obstruction and infection in the common bile duct cause Charcot's triad: jaundice, right upper quadrant pain, and a high fever with chills.

◆ *Cholecystitis.* Cholecystitis produces nonobstructive jaundice in about 25% of patients. Biliary colic typically peaks abruptly, persisting for 2 to 4 hours. The pain then localizes to the right upper quadrant and becomes constant. Local inflammation or passage of stones to the common bile duct causes jaundice. Other findings include nausea and vomiting, fever, diaphoresis, chills, tenderness on palpation, and a positive Murphy's sign.

◆ *Cholelithiasis.* Cholelithiasis commonly causes jaundice and biliary colic. It's characterized by severe, steady pain in the right upper quadrant or epigastrium that radiates to the right scapula or shoulder and intensifies over several hours. Other findings include nausea and vomiting, tachycardia, and restlessness.

◆ *Cirrhosis.* With Laënnec's cirrhosis, mild to moderate jaundice with pruritus usually signals hepatocellular necrosis or progressive hepatic insufficiency. Common early findings include ascites, weakness, leg edema, nausea and vomiting, diarrhea or constipation, anorexia, weight loss, and right upper quadrant pain. Massive hematemesis and other bleeding tendencies may also occur.

With primary biliary cirrhosis, fluctuating jaundice may appear years after the onset of other signs and symptoms, such as pruritus that worsens at bedtime, weakness, fatigue, weight loss, and vague abdominal pain.

◆ *Drugs.* Many drugs may cause hepatic injury and resultant jaundice. Examples include acetaminophen (Tylenol), isoniazid (INH), hormonal contraceptives, sulfonamides, mercaptopurine (Purinethol), erythromycin estolate (Ilosone), niacin (Nicobid), androgenic steroids, phenothiazines, ethanol, methyldopa (Aldomet), rifampin (Rifadin), and phenytoin (Dilantin).

◆ *Dubin-Johnson syndrome.* With Dubin-Johnson syndrome—a rare, chronic, inherited syndrome—fluctuating jaundice that increases with stress is the major sign, appearing as late as age 40. Related findings include slight hepatic enlargement and tenderness, upper abdominal pain, nausea, and vomiting.

◆ *Heart failure.* Jaundice due to liver dysfunction occurs in patients with severe right-sided heart failure. Other findings include jugular vein distention, cyanosis, dependent edema of the legs and sacrum, hepatomegaly, nausea and vomiting, abdominal discomfort, and anorexia due to visceral edema. Ascites is a late sign. If left-sided heart failure develops first, other findings may include fatigue, dyspnea, orthopnea, paroxysmal nocturnal dyspnea, tachypnea, arrhythmias, and tachycardia.

◆ *Hepatic abscess.* Multiple abscesses may cause jaundice, but the primary effects are a persistent fever with chills and sweating. Other findings include steady, severe pain in the right upper quadrant or midepigastrium that may be referred to the shoulder, nausea and vomiting, anorexia, hepatomegaly, an elevated right hemidiaphragm, and ascites.

◆ *Hepatitis.* Dark urine and clay-colored stools usually develop before jaundice in the late stages of acute viral hepatitis. Early systemic findings include fatigue, nausea and vomiting, malaise, arthralgia, myalgia, headache, anorexia, photophobia, pharyngitis, cough, and a low-grade fever associated with liver and lymph node enlargement.

◼ *Pancreatitis (acute).* Edema of the head of the pancreas and obstruction of the common bile duct may cause jaundice; however, the primary symptom of acute pancreatitis is usually severe epigastric pain that commonly radiates to the back.

◼ *Sickle cell anemia.* Hemolysis produces jaundice in the patient with sickle cell anemia. Other findings include increased susceptibility to infection, life-threatening thrombotic complications and, commonly, leg ulcers, swollen (painful) joints, fever, and chills. Severe hemolysis may cause hematuria, dyspnea, and tachycardia.

Jaw pain

Jaw pain may arise from either of the two bones that hold the teeth in the jaw—the maxilla (upper jaw) or the mandible (lower jaw). Jaw pain also includes pain in the temporomandibular joint (TMJ), where the mandible meets the temporal bone. It may develop gradually or abruptly and may range from barely noticeable to excruciating, depending on its cause. It usually results from disorders of the teeth, soft tissue, or glands of the mouth or throat or from local trauma or infection. Systemic causes include musculoskeletal, neurologic, cardiovascular, endocrine, immunologic, metabolic, and infectious disorders. Life-threatening disorders, such as a myocardial infarction (MI) and tetany, also produce jaw pain as well as certain drugs (especially phenothiazines) and dental or surgical procedures. It's seldom a primary indicator of any one disorder.

Assessment

Sudden severe jaw pain, especially when associated with chest pain, shortness of breath, or arm pain, requires prompt evaluation because it may herald a life-threatening MI. (See *Responding to jaw pain.*) Begin the patient history by asking him to describe the pain's character, intensity, and frequency. When did he first notice the jaw pain? Where on the jaw does he feel pain? Does the pain radiate to other areas? Sharp or burning pain arises from the skin or subcutaneous tissues. Causalgia, an intense burning sensation, usually results from damage to the fifth cranial, or trigeminal, nerve. This type of superficial pain is easily localized, unlike dull, aching, boring, or throbbing pain, which originates in muscle, bone, or joints. Ask about recent trauma, surgery, or procedures, especially dental work. Ask about other signs and symptoms, such as joint or chest pain, dyspnea, palpitations, fatigue, headache, malaise, anorexia, weight loss, intermittent claudication, diplopia, and hearing loss.

Focus your physical examination on the jaw. Inspect the painful area for

EMERGENCY INTERVENTIONS

Responding to jaw pain

If you suspect myocardial infarction in a patient complaining of jaw pain, immediately take the following steps:
◆ Perform an electrocardiogram.
◆ Obtain blood samples for analysis of cardiac enzyme levels.
◆ Administer oxygen, morphine, and a vasodilator, as ordered.

redness, and palpate for edema or warmth. Facing the patient directly, look for facial asymmetry that would indicate swelling. Check the TMJs by placing your fingertips just anterior to the external auditory meatus and asking the patient to open and close, and to thrust out and retract his jaw. Note the presence of crepitus, an abnormal scraping or grinding sensation in the joint. (Clicks heard when the jaw is widely spread apart are normal.) How wide can the patient open his mouth? Less than 1⅛″ (3 cm) or more than 2⅜″ (6 cm) between the upper and lower teeth is abnormal. Next, palpate the parotid area for pain and swelling, and inspect and palpate the oral cavity for lesions, elevation of the tongue, or masses.

Causes

◆ *Angina pectoris.* Angina may produce jaw pain (usually radiating from the substernal area) and left arm pain. Angina is less severe than the pain of an MI. It's commonly triggered by exertion, emotional stress, or ingestion of a heavy meal and usually subsides with rest and nitroglycerin administration.
◆ *Arthritis.* With osteoarthritis, which usually affects the small joints of the hand, aching jaw pain increases with activity and subsides with rest. Other

features are crepitus heard and felt over the TMJ, enlarged joints with a restricted range of motion (ROM), and stiffness on awakening that improves with a few minutes of activity.

Rheumatoid arthritis causes symmetrical pain in all joints (commonly affecting proximal finger joints first), including the jaw. The joints display limited ROM and are tender, warm, swollen, and stiff after inactivity, especially in the morning.
◆ *Head and neck cancer.* Many types of head and neck cancer, especially of the oral cavity and nasopharynx, produce aching jaw pain of insidious onset. Other findings include a history of leukoplakia; ulcers of the mucous membranes; palpable masses in the jaw, mouth, and neck; dysphagia; bloody discharge; drooling; lymphadenopathy; and trismus.
◼ *Hypocalcemic tetany.* Besides painful muscle contractions of the jaw and mouth, hypocalcemic tetany produces paresthesia and carpopedal spasms. The patient may complain of weakness, fatigue, and palpitations. Examination reveals hyperreflexia and positive Chvostek's and Trousseau's signs. With severe hypocalcemia, laryngeal spasm may occur with stridor, cyanosis, seizures, and cardiac arrhythmias.
◆ *Ludwig's angina.* Ludwig's angina is an acute streptococcal infection of

the sublingual and submandibular spaces that produces severe jaw pain in the mandibular area with tongue elevation, sublingual edema, and drooling. Fever is a common sign. Progressive disease produces dysphagia, dysphonia, and stridor and dyspnea due to laryngeal edema and obstruction by an elevated tongue.

◼ *MI.* Initially, MI causes intense, crushing substernal pain that's unrelieved by rest or nitroglycerin. The pain may radiate to the lower jaw, left arm, neck, back, or shoulder blades. Other findings include clammy skin, dyspnea, excessive diaphoresis, a feeling of impending doom, decreased or increased blood pressure, and arrhythmias.

◆ *Sinusitis.* Maxillary sinusitis produces intense boring pain in the maxilla and cheek that may radiate to the eye. This type of sinusitis also causes a feeling of fullness, increased pain on percussion of the first and second molars and, in those with nasal obstruction, the loss of the sense of smell.

◼ *Suppurative parotitis.* Bacterial infection of the parotid gland by *Staphylococcus aureus* tends to develop in debilitated patients with dry mouth or poor oral hygiene. Besides the abrupt onset of jaw pain, a high fever, and chills, findings include erythema and edema of the overlying skin; a tender, swollen gland; and pus at the second top molar.

◆ *Temporal arteritis.* Most common in women older than age 60, temporal arteritis produces sharp jaw pain after chewing or talking. Vascular lesions produce jaw pain; a throbbing, unilateral headache in the frontotemporal region; swollen, nodular, tender and, possibly, pulseless temporal arteries; and, at times, erythema of the overlying skin.

◆ *TMJ syndrome.* TMJ syndrome is a common syndrome that produces jaw pain at the TMJ; spasm and pain of the masticating muscle; clicking, popping, or crepitus of the TMJ; and restricted jaw movement. Unilateral, localized pain may radiate to other head and neck areas. The patient typically reports teeth clenching, bruxism, and emotional stress.

◼ *Tetanus.* A rare disorder caused by a bacterial toxin, tetanus produces stiffness and pain in the jaw and difficulty opening the mouth. Early nonspecific findings (commonly unnoticed or mistaken for influenza) include headache, irritability, restlessness, a low-grade fever, and chills. Examination reveals tachycardia, profuse diaphoresis, and hyperreflexia.

◆ *Trigeminal neuralgia.* Trigeminal neuralgia is marked by paroxysmal attacks of intense unilateral jaw pain (stopping at the facial midline) or rapid-fire shooting sensations in one division of the trigeminal nerve (usually the mandibular or maxillary division). This superficial pain, felt mainly over the lips and chin and in the teeth, lasts from 1 to 15 minutes. Mouth and nose areas may be hypersensitive.

Jugular vein distention

Jugular vein distention is the abnormal fullness and height of the pulse waves in the internal or external jugular veins. Engorged, distended veins reflect increased venous pressure in the right side of the heart, which, in turn, indicates increased central venous pressure. This common sign characteristically occurs in heart failure and other cardiovascular disorders, such as constrictive pericarditis, tricuspid stenosis, and obstruction of the superior vena cava. (See *Evaluating jugular vein distention.*)

Evaluating jugular vein distention

With the patient supine, turn his head so you can visualize jugular vein pulsations reflected from the right atrium. Elevate the head of the bed 45 to 90 degrees. (Normally, veins should only be distended when the patient is lying flat.)

The reference point for measuring venous pressure is the angle of Louis (sternal notch). To locate this point, palpate the clavicles where they join the sternum (the suprasternal notch). Place your first two fingers on the suprasternal notch. Then, without lifting them from the skin, slide them down the sternum until you feel a bony protuberance. This is the angle of Louis.

Now, find the internal jugular vein, which indicates venous pressure more reliably than the external jugular vein. Shine a flashlight across the patient's neck to create shadows highlighting his venous pulse. Be sure to distinguish jugular vein pulsations from carotid artery pulsations. One way to do this is to palpate the vessel: arterial pulsations continue, whereas venous pulsations disappear with light finger pressure. Also, venous pulsations increase or decrease with changes in body position; arterial pulsations remain constant.

Next, locate the highest point along the vein where you can see pulsations. Using a centimeter ruler, measure the distance between that high point and the sternal notch. Record this finding as well as the angle at which the patient was lying. A finding greater than 1⅛" to 1⅝" (3 to 4 cm) above the sternal notch, with the head of the bed at a 45-degree angle, indicates jugular vein distention.

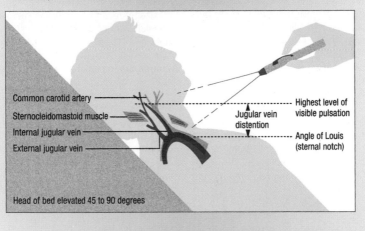

Common carotid artery
Sternocleidomastoid muscle
Internal jugular vein
External jugular vein

Jugular vein distention

Highest level of visible pulsation

Angle of Louis (sternal notch)

Head of bed elevated 45 to 90 degrees

Assessment

If you detect jugular vein distention in a patient with pale, clammy skin who suddenly appears anxious and dyspneic, take his blood pressure. If you note hypotension and a paradoxical pulse, suspect cardiac tamponade. (See *Responding to cardiac tamponade,* page 332.) If the patient isn't in severe distress, obtain a history. Has he recently gained weight? Are his ankles swollen? Ask about chest pain, shortness of breath, paroxysmal nocturnal dyspnea, anorexia, nausea or vomiting, and a history of cancer or cardiac, pulmonary, hepatic, or renal disease. Obtain

EMERGENCY INTERVENTIONS

Responding to cardiac tamponade

If you suspect that a patient with jugular vein distention has cardiac tamponade, take the following steps:
◆ Elevate the foot of the bed 20 to 30 degrees.
◆ Administer supplemental oxygen, as prescribed.
◆ Monitor the patient's cardiac status, including heart rhythm, oxygen saturation, and mental status.

◆ Insert an I.V. catheter for medication administration.
◆ Keep cardiopulmonary resuscitation equipment close by.
◆ Assemble the equipment needed to perform an emergency pericardiocentesis (performed to relieve pressure on the heart). Throughout the procedure, monitor the patient's blood pressure, heart rhythm, and respirations.

a drug history, noting diuretic use. Is the patient taking drugs as prescribed? Ask the patient about his regular diet patterns, noting a high sodium intake.

Next, perform a physical examination, beginning with the patient's vital signs. Tachycardia, tachypnea, and increased blood pressure indicate fluid overload that's stressing the heart. Inspect and palpate the patient's extremities and face for edema. Then weigh the patient and compare that weight to his baseline. Evaluating jugular vein distention involves visualizing and assessing venous pulsations. For a patient in a supine position with his head elevated 45 degrees, a pulse wave height greater than 1 1/8″ to 1 5/8″ (3 to 4 cm) above the angle of Louis indicates distention. Auscultate his lungs for crackles and his heart for gallops, a pericardial friction rub, and muffled heart sounds. Inspect his abdomen for distention, and palpate and percuss for an enlarged liver. Finally monitor urine output, noting any decrease.

Causes

▧ *Cardiac tamponade.* Cardiac tamponade produces jugular vein distention along with anxiety, restlessness, cyanosis, chest pain, dyspnea, hypotension, and clammy skin. It also causes tachycardia, tachypnea, muffled heart sounds, a pericardial friction rub, weak or absent peripheral pulses or pulses that decrease during inspiration, and hepatomegaly.
◆ *Heart failure.* Sudden or gradual development of right-sided heart failure commonly causes jugular vein distention, along with weakness and anxiety, cyanosis, dependent edema of the legs and sacrum, steady weight gain, confusion, and hepatomegaly. Massive right-sided heart failure may produce anasarca and oliguria.

If left-sided heart failure precedes right-sided heart failure, jugular vein distention is a late sign. Other signs and symptoms include orthopnea, paroxysmal nocturnal dyspnea, tachycardia, and arrhythmias. Auscultation reveals crackles and a ventricular gallop.

◆ *Hypervolemia.* Markedly increased intravascular fluid volume causes jugular vein distention, along with rapid weight gain, elevated blood pressure, bounding pulse, peripheral edema, dyspnea, and crackles.

◆ *Pericarditis (chronic constrictive).* Progressive signs and symptoms of restricted heart filling include jugular vein distention that's more prominent on inspiration (Kussmaul's sign). The patient usually complains of chest pain. Other signs and symptoms include fluid retention with dependent edema, hepatomegaly, ascites, and a pericardial friction rub.

◆ *Superior vena cava obstruction.* A tumor or, rarely, thrombosis may gradually lead to jugular vein distention when the veins of the head, neck, and arms fail to empty effectively, causing facial, neck, and upper arm edema. Metastasis of a malignant tumor to the mediastinum may cause dyspnea, cough, substernal chest pain, and hoarseness.

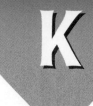

K

Kehr's sign

A cardinal sign of hemorrhage within the peritoneal cavity, Kehr's sign is referred left shoulder pain due to diaphragmatic irritation by intraperitoneal blood. The pain usually arises when the patient assumes the supine position or lowers his head. Such positioning increases the contact of free blood or clots with the left diaphragm, involving the phrenic nerve.

Kehr's sign usually develops right after the hemorrhage; however, its onset is sometimes delayed up to 48 hours. A classic symptom of a ruptured spleen, Kehr's sign also occurs in ruptured ectopic pregnancy. (See *Responding to Kehr's sign*.)

Assessment

Inspect the patient's abdomen for bruises and distention, and palpate for tenderness. Percuss for Ballance's sign—an indicator of massive perisplenic clotting and free blood in the peritoneal cavity from a ruptured spleen.

Causes

◼ *Intra-abdominal hemorrhage.* Kehr's sign usually accompanies intense abdominal pain, abdominal rigidity, and muscle spasm. Other findings vary with the cause of bleeding. Many patients have a history of blunt or penetrating abdominal injuries.

 EMERGENCY INTERVENTIONS

Responding to Kehr's sign

After you detect Kehr's sign, quickly take the patient's vital signs. If the patient shows signs of hypovolemia, take the following steps:
◆ Elevate the patient's feet 30 degrees.
◆ Insert a large-bore I.V. catheter for fluid and blood administration.

◆ Insert an indwelling urinary catheter and monitor intake and output.
◆ Obtain a blood sample for hematocrit analysis.
◆ Provide supplemental oxygen, as prescribed.

Kernig's sign

A reliable early indicator and tool used to diagnose meningeal irritation, Kernig's sign elicits resistance and hamstring muscle pain when the examiner attempts to extend the patient's knee while his hip and knee are flexed 90 degrees. However, when the patient's thigh isn't flexed on the abdomen, he can usually completely extend his leg. (See *Eliciting Kernig's sign*.) This sign is typically elicited in meningitis or subarachnoid hemorrhage. With these potentially life-threatening disorders, hamstring muscle resistance results from stretching the blood- or exudate-irritated meninges surrounding spinal nerve roots.

Kernig's sign can also indicate a herniated disk or spinal tumor. With these disorders, sciatic pain results from disk or tumor pressure on spinal nerve roots.

Assessment

If you elicit a positive Kernig's sign and suspect meningitis or subarachnoid hemorrhage, immediately prepare for emergency intervention. (See *When Kernig's sign signals CNS crisis*, page 336.)

If you don't suspect meningeal irritation, ask the patient if he feels back pain that radiates down one or both legs. Does he also feel leg numbness, tingling, or weakness? Ask about other signs and symptoms, and find out if he has a history of cancer or back injury.

Eliciting Kernig's sign

To elicit Kernig's sign, place the patient in a supine position. Flex her leg at the hip and knee, as shown here. Then try to extend the leg while you keep the hip flexed. If the patient experiences pain and possibly spasm in the hamstring muscle and resists further extension, you can assume that meningeal irritation has occurred.

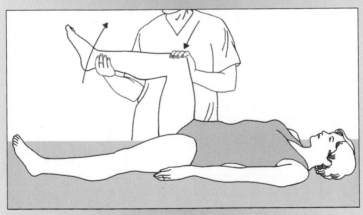

EMERGENCY INTERVENTIONS

When Kernig's sign signals CNS crisis

Because Kernig's sign may signal meningitis or subarachnoid hemorrhage—life-threatening central nervous system (CNS) disorders—take the patient's vital signs at once to obtain baseline information. Then test for Brudzinski's sign to obtain further evidence of meningeal irritation.

Next, ask the patient or his family to describe the onset of illness. Typically, the progressive onset of headache, fever, nuchal rigidity, and confusion suggests meningitis. Conversely, the sudden onset of a severe headache, nuchal rigidity, photophobia and, possibly, loss of consciousness usually indicates subarachnoid hemorrhage.

Meningitis

If a diagnosis of meningitis is suspected, ask about recent infections, especially tooth abscesses. Ask about exposure to infected persons or places where meningitis is endemic. Meningitis is usually a complication of another bacterial infection, so draw blood for culture studies to determine the causative organism. Prepare the patient for a lumbar puncture (if a tumor or abscess can be ruled out). Also, find out if the patient has a history of I.V. drug abuse, an open head injury, or endocarditis. Insert an I.V. catheter, and begin administering an antibiotic, as ordered.

Subarachnoid hemorrhage

If subarachnoid hemorrhage is the suspected diagnosis, ask about a history of hypertension, cerebral aneurysm, head trauma, or arteriovenous malformation. Also ask about sudden withdrawal of an antihypertensive.

Check the patient's pupils for dilation, and assess him for signs of increasing intracranial pressure, such as decreased level of consciousness, bradycardia, increased systolic blood pressure, and widened pulse pressure. Insert an I.V. catheter, and administer supplemental oxygen.

Then perform a physical examination, concentrating on motor and sensory function.

Causes

◆ *Lumbosacral herniated disk.* A positive Kernig's sign may be elicited in patients with a lumbosacral herniated disk, but the cardinal and earliest feature is sciatic pain on the affected side or on both sides. Associated findings include postural deformity (lumbar lordosis or scoliosis), paresthesia, hypoactive deep tendon reflexes in the involved leg, and dorsiflexor muscle weakness.

◆ *Meningitis.* A positive Kernig's sign usually occurs early with meningitis, along with fever and, possibly, chills. Other signs and symptoms of meningeal irritation include nuchal rigidity, hyperreflexia, Brudzinski's sign, and opisthotonos. As intracranial pressure (ICP) increases, headache and vomiting may occur. In severe meningitis, the patient may experience stupor, coma, and seizures. Cranial nerve involvement may produce ocular palsies, facial weakness, deafness, and photophobia. An erythematous maculopapular rash may occur in viral meningitis; a purpuric rash may be seen in meningococcal meningitis.

◆ *Spinal cord tumor.* Kernig's sign can be elicited occasionally in a spinal cord tumor, but the earliest symptom is typically pain felt locally or along the spinal nerve, commonly in the leg. Associated findings include weakness or paralysis distal to the tumor, paresthesia, urine retention, urinary or fecal incontinence, and sexual dysfunction.

◣ *Subarachnoid hemorrhage.* Kernig's and Brudzinski's signs can be elicited within minutes after the initial bleed. The patient experiences a sudden onset of a severe headache that begins in a localized area and then spreads, pupillary inequality, nuchal rigidity, and a decreased level of consciousness. Photophobia, fever, nausea and vomiting, dizziness, and seizures are possible. Focal signs include hemiparesis or hemiplegia, aphasia, and sensory or vision disturbances. Increasing ICP may produce bradycardia, increased blood pressure, respiratory pattern change, and rapid progression to coma.

L

Leg pain

Although leg pain commonly signifies a musculoskeletal disorder, it can also result from a more serious vascular or neurologic disorder. The pain may arise suddenly or gradually and may be localized or affect the entire leg. Constant or intermittent, it may feel dull, burning, sharp, shooting, or tingling. Leg pain may affect locomotion, limiting weight bearing. Severe leg pain that follows cast application for a fracture may signal limb-threatening compartment syndrome. The sudden onset of severe leg pain in a patient with underlying vascular insufficiency may signal acute deterioration, possibly requiring an arterial graft or amputation. (See *Highlighting causes of local leg pain.*)

Assessment

If the patient's condition permits, ask him when the pain began and have him describe its intensity, character, and pattern. Is the pain worse in the morning, at night, or with movement? If it doesn't prevent him from walking, must he rely on a crutch or other assistive device? Also ask him about the presence of other signs and symptoms.

Find out if the patient has a history of leg injury or surgery and if he has a history of joint, vascular, or back problems. Also ask which medications he's taking and whether they have helped to relieve his leg pain.

Begin the physical examination by watching the patient walk, if his condition permits. Observe how he holds his leg while standing and sitting. Palpate the legs, buttocks, and lower back to determine the extent of pain and tenderness. If a fracture has been ruled out, test the patient's range of motion (ROM) in the hip and knee. Also check reflexes with the patient's leg straightened and raised, noting action that causes pain. Then compare both legs for symmetry, movement, and active ROM. Additionally, assess sensation and strength. If the patient wears a leg cast, splint, or restrictive dressing, carefully check distal circulation, sensation, and mobility, and stretch his toes to elicit associated pain.

Causes

◆ *Bone cancer*. Continuous deep or boring pain, commonly worse at night, may be the first symptom of bone cancer. Later, skin breakdown and impaired circulation may occur, along with cachexia, fever, and impaired mobility.

◆

Highlighting causes of local leg pain

Various disorders cause hip, knee, ankle, or foot pain, which may radiate to surrounding tissues and be reported as leg pain. Local pain is commonly accompanied by tenderness, swelling, and deformity in the affected area. See below for some common causes of local leg pain.

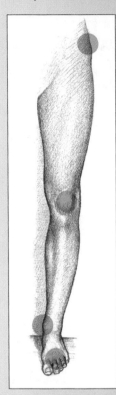

Hip pain
Arthritis
Avascular necrosis
Bursitis
Dislocation
Fracture
Sepsis
Tumor

Knee pain
Arthritis
Bursitis
Chondromalacia
Contusion
Cruciate ligament injury
Dislocation
Fracture
Meniscal injury
Osteochondritis dissecans
Phlebitis
Popliteal cyst
Radiculopathy
Ruptured extensor
   mechanism
Sprain

Ankle pain
Achilles tendon contracture
Arthritis
Dislocation
Fracture
Sprain
Tenosynovitis

Foot pain
Arthritis
Bunion
Callus or corn
Dislocation
Flatfoot
Fracture
Gout
Hallux rigidus
Hammer toe
Ingrown toenail
Köhler's bone disease
Morton's neuroma
Occlusive vascular disease
Plantar fasciitis
Plantar wart
Radiculopathy
Tabes dorsalis
Tarsal tunnel syndrome

◆ *Compartment syndrome.* Progressive, intense lower leg pain that increases with passive muscle stretching is a cardinal sign of compartment syndrome. Restrictive dressings or traction may aggravate the pain, which typically worsens despite analgesic administration. Other findings include muscle weakness and paresthesia, but apparently normal distal circulation. With irreversible muscle ischemia, paralysis and an absent pulse also occur.

◆ *Fracture.* Severe, acute pain accompanies swelling and ecchymosis in a fractured leg. Movement produces extreme pain, and the leg may be unable to bear weight. Neurovascular status distal to the fracture may be impaired, causing paresthesia, an absent pulse, mottled cyanosis, and cool skin. Deformity, muscle spasms, and bony crepitation may also occur.

◆ *Infection.* Local leg pain, erythema, swelling, streaking, and warmth characterize soft-tissue and bone infections. Fever and tachycardia may be present with other systemic signs.

◆ *Occlusive vascular disease.* With occlusive vascular disease, continuous cramping pain in the legs and feet may worsen with walking, inducing claudication. The patient may report increased pain at night, cold feet, cold intolerance, numbness, and tingling. Examination may reveal ankle and lower leg edema, decreased or absent pulses, and increased capillary refill time.

◆ *Sciatica.* Pain, described as shooting, aching, or tingling, radiates down the back of the leg along the sciatic nerve. Typically, activity exacerbates the pain and rest relieves it. The patient may have difficulty moving from a sitting to a standing position.

◆ *Strain or sprain.* Acute strain causes sharp, transient pain and rapid swelling, followed by leg tenderness and ecchymosis. Chronic strain produces stiffness, soreness, and generalized leg tenderness several hours after the injury; active and passive motion may be painful or impossible. A sprain causes local pain, especially during joint movement; ecchymosis and, possibly, local swelling and loss of mobility may develop.

◆ *Thrombophlebitis.* Discomfort may range from calf tenderness to severe pain accompanied by swelling, warmth, and a feeling of heaviness in the affected leg. The patient may also develop fever, chills, malaise, muscle cramps, and a positive Homans' sign.

◆ *Varicose veins.* Mild to severe leg symptoms may develop with varicose veins, including nocturnal cramping; a feeling of heaviness; diffuse, dull aching after prolonged standing or walking; and aching during menses. Assess-

ment may reveal palpable nodules, orthostatic edema, and stasis pigmentation of the calves and ankles.

◆ *Venous stasis ulcer.* Localized pain and bleeding arise from infected ulcerations on the lower extremities. Mottled, bluish pigmentation is characteristic, and local edema may occur.

Level of consciousness, decreased

A decrease in the level of consciousness (LOC), from lethargy to stupor to coma, usually results from a neurologic disorder and may signal a life-threatening complication, such as hemorrhage, trauma, or cerebral edema. However, this sign can also result from a metabolic, GI, musculoskeletal, urologic, or cardiopulmonary disorder; severe nutritional deficiency; the effects of toxins; or drug use. LOC can deteriorate suddenly or gradually and can remain altered temporarily or permanently. (See *Responding to a decreased level of consciousness.*)

Consciousness is affected by the reticular activating system (RAS), an intricate network of neurons with axons extending from the brain stem, thalamus, and hypothalamus to the cerebral cortex. A disturbance in any part of this integrated system prevents the intercommunication that makes consciousness possible. Loss of consciousness can result from a bilateral cerebral disturbance, an RAS disturbance, or both. Cerebral dysfunction characteristically produces the least dramatic decrease in a patient's LOC. In contrast, dysfunction of the RAS produces the most dramatic decrease in LOC—coma.

The most sensitive indicator of a decreased LOC is a change in the patient's mental status. The Glasgow

EMERGENCY INTERVENTIONS

Responding to a decreased level of consciousness

If the patient's score on the Glasgow Coma Scale is 13 or less, emergency surgery may be necessary. In this instance, take the following steps:

◆ Prepare to insert an artificial airway.
◆ Elevate the head of the bed 30 degrees.
◆ If spinal cord injury has been ruled out, turn the patient's head to the side.
◆ Suction the patient, as needed.

◆ Be prepared to hyperventilate the patient, as ordered, to reduce carbon dioxide levels and decrease intracranial pressure.

If the patient's Glasgow Coma Scale score is less than 9, implement the following:

◆ Prepare for possible intubation and resuscitation.
◆ Monitor the patient's vital signs for bradycardia and widening pulse pressure.

Coma Scale, which measures a patient's ability to respond to verbal, sensory, and motor stimulation, can be used to quickly evaluate a patient's LOC. Use this scale after evaluating the patient's airway, breathing, and circulation, to obtain baseline data. (See *Glasgow Coma Scale,* page 342.)

Assessment

Try to obtain history information from the patient, if he's lucid, or from his family. Did the patient complain of headache, dizziness, nausea, vision or hearing disturbances, weakness, fatigue, or other problems before his LOC decreased? Has his family noticed changes in the patient's behavior, personality, memory, or temperament? Also ask about a history of neurologic disease, cancer, or recent trauma or infections; drug and alcohol use; and the development of other signs and symptoms.

Because a decreased LOC can result from a disorder affecting virtually any body system, tailor the remainder of

your evaluation according to the patient's associated symptoms.

Causes

◼ *Adrenal crisis.* A decreased LOC, ranging from lethargy to coma, may develop within 8 to 12 hours of the onset of adrenal crisis. Early associated findings include progressive weakness, irritability, anorexia, headache, nausea and vomiting, diarrhea, abdominal pain, and fever. The patient with chronic adrenocortical hypofunction may have hyperpigmented skin and mucous membranes.

◆ *Brain abscess.* A decreased LOC varies from drowsiness to deep stupor, depending on the abscess size and site. Early signs and symptoms—a constant intractable headache, nausea, vomiting, and seizures—reflect increasing intracranial pressure. Other findings may include dizziness, aphasia, ataxia, tremor, and hemiparesis.

◆ *Brain tumor.* With a brain tumor, the patient's LOC decreases slowly, from lethargy to coma. He may also experience apathy, behavior changes,

Glasgow Coma Scale

You've probably heard such terms as lethargic, obtunded, and stuporous used to describe a progressive decrease in a patient's level of consciousness (LOC). However, the Glasgow Coma Scale—which grades consciousness in relation to eye opening and motor and verbal responses—provides a more accurate, less subjective method of recording such changes.

To use the Glasgow Coma Scale, test the patient's ability to respond to verbal, motor, and sensory stimulation. The scoring system doesn't determine the patient's exact LOC, but it does provide an easy way to describe his basic status and helps to detect and interpret changes from baseline findings. A decreased reaction score in one or more categories may signal an impending neurologic crisis. A score less than 9 indicates severe neurologic damage.

TEST	REACTION	SCORE
Eye opening response	Open spontaneously	4
	Open to verbal command	3
	Open to pain	2
	No response	1
Best motor response	Obeys verbal command	6
	Localizes painful stimulus	5
	Flexion—withdrawal	4
	Flexion—abnormal (decorticate rigidity)	3
	Extension (decerebrate rigidity)	2
	No response	1
Best verbal response	Oriented and conversable	5
	Disoriented and conversable	4
	Inappropriate words	3
	Incomprehensible sounds	2
	No response	1
Total		3 to 15

memory loss, a decreased attention span, a morning headache, dizziness, vision loss, ataxia, and sensorimotor disturbances. Signs and symptoms vary according to the location and size of the tumor.

◼ *Cerebral aneurysm (ruptured).* Somnolence, confusion and, at times, stupor characterize a moderate bleed; deep coma occurs with severe bleeding, which can be fatal. The onset is usually abrupt, with a sudden, severe headache and nausea and vomiting. Nuchal rigidity, restlessness, irritability, occasional seizures, and blurred vision point to meningeal irritation. The type and severity of other findings vary with

the site and severity of the hemorrhage.

◼ *Diabetic ketoacidosis (DKA).* DKA
produces a rapid decrease in the patient's LOC, ranging from lethargy to
coma, commonly preceded by polydipsia, polyphagia, and polyuria. He may
exhibit orthostatic hypotension; a fruity
breath odor; Kussmaul's respirations;
warm, dry skin; and a rapid, thready
pulse. Untreated, this condition invariably leads to coma and death.

◆ *Encephalitis.* Within 24 to 48 hours
after the onset of encephalitis, the patient may develop changes in his LOC
ranging from lethargy to coma. Other
possible findings include an abrupt onset of fever, headache, nuchal rigidity,
nausea and vomiting, seizures, aphasia, ataxia, hemiparesis, nystagmus,
myoclonus, and cranial nerve palsies.

◼ *Encephalomyelitis (postvaccinal).*
Postvaccinal encephalomyelitis is a disorder that produces rapid deterioration
in the patient's LOC, from drowsiness
to coma. He also experiences a rapid
onset of fever, headache, nuchal rigidity, back pain, vomiting, and seizures.

◼ *Encephalopathy.* With hepatic encephalopathy, signs and symptoms develop in four stages: in the prodromal
stage, slight personality changes and
slight tremor; in the impending stage,
tremor progressing to asterixis, lethargy, and apraxia; in the stuporous stage,
stupor and hyperventilation, with the
patient noisy and abusive when
aroused; and in the comatose stage,
coma with decerebrate posture, hyperactive reflexes, positive Babinski's reflex, and fetor hepaticus.

With life-threatening hypertensive
encephalopathy, the patient's LOC progressively decreases from lethargy to
stupor to coma. Besides markedly elevated blood pressure, he may experience a severe headache, vomiting,
seizures, vision disturbances, transient

paralysis and, eventually, Cheyne-
Stokes respirations.

With hypoglycemic encephalopathy,
the patient's LOC rapidly deteriorates
from lethargy to coma. Early signs and
symptoms include nervousness, restlessness, agitation, and confusion;
hunger; alternate flushing and cold
sweats; and headache, trembling, and
palpitations.

Depending on its severity, hypoxic
encephalopathy produces a sudden or
gradual decrease in the patient's LOC,
leading to coma and brain death. Early
on, he appears confused and restless,
with cyanosis and increased heart and
respiratory rates and blood pressure.
Later, his respiratory pattern becomes
abnormal, and assessment reveals a
decreased pulse, blood pressure, and
deep tendon reflexes (DTRs); a positive
Babinski's reflex; an absent doll's eye
sign; and fixed pupils.

With uremic encephalopathy, the
patient's LOC decreases gradually from
lethargy to coma. Early on, he may appear apathetic, inattentive, confused,
and irritable and may complain of
headache, nausea, fatigue, and anorexia. Other findings include vomiting,
tremors, edema, papilledema, hypertension, cardiac arrhythmias, dyspnea,
crackles, oliguria, and Kussmaul's and
Cheyne-Stokes respirations.

◼ *Heatstroke.* As body temperature increases, the patient's LOC gradually decreases from lethargy to coma. Early
signs and symptoms include malaise,
tachycardia, tachypnea, orthostatic hypotension, muscle cramps, rigidity, and
syncope. At the onset of heatstroke,
the patient's skin is hot, flushed, and
diaphoretic with blotchy cyanosis; later, when his fever exceeds 105° F
(40.6° C), his skin becomes anhidrotic.
Pulse and respiratory rate increase
markedly, and blood pressure drops
precipitously.

◆ *Hypernatremia.* Hypernatremia, life threatening if acute, causes the patient's LOC to deteriorate from lethargy to coma. He's irritable and exhibits twitches progressing to seizures. Other associated signs and symptoms include a weak, thready pulse, nausea, malaise, fever, thirst, flushed skin, and dry mucous membranes.

◳ *Hyperosmolar hyperglycemic nonketotic syndrome.* The patient's LOC decreases rapidly from lethargy to coma. Early findings include polyuria, polydipsia, weight loss, and weakness. Later, he may develop hypotension, poor skin turgor, dry skin and mucous membranes, tachycardia, tachypnea, oliguria, and seizures.

◆ *Hypokalemia.* LOC gradually decreases to lethargy; coma is rare. Other findings include confusion, polyuria, weakness, decreased reflexes, hypotension, arrhythmias, and abnormal electrocardiogram results.

◆ *Hyponatremia.* Hyponatremia, life threatening if acute, produces a decreased LOC in late stages. Early nausea and malaise may progress to behavior changes, confusion, lethargy, incoordination and, eventually, seizures and coma.

◳ *Hypothermia.* With severe hypothermia (temperature below 90° F [32.2° C]), the patient's LOC decreases from lethargy to coma. DTRs disappear, and ventricular fibrillation occurs, possibly followed by cardiopulmonary arrest. With mild to moderate hypothermia, the patient may experience memory loss and slurred speech as well as shivering, weakness, fatigue, and apathy.

◳ *Intracerebral hemorrhage.* Intracerebral hemorrhage produces a rapid, steady loss of consciousness within hours, commonly accompanied by a severe headache, dizziness, and nausea and vomiting. Associated signs and symptoms vary and may include increased blood pressure, irregular respirations, a positive Babinski's reflex, seizures, aphasia, decreased sensations, hemiplegia, decorticate or decerebrate posture, and dilated pupils.

◆ *Listeriosis.* If listeriosis spreads to the nervous system and causes meningitis, signs and symptoms include a decreased LOC, fever, headache, and nuchal rigidity. Early signs and symptoms include fever, myalgia, abdominal pain, nausea and vomiting, and diarrhea.

◳ *Meningitis.* Stupor, coma, and seizures may occur in the patient with severe meningitis. A fever develops early, possibly accompanied by chills. Associated findings include a severe headache, nuchal rigidity, hyperreflexia, Kernig's and Brudzinski's signs and, possibly, opisthotonos.

◳ *Pontine hemorrhage.* A sudden, rapid decrease in the patient's LOC to the point of coma occurs within minutes and death within hours. The patient may also exhibit total paralysis, decerebrate posture, a positive Babinski's reflex, an absent doll's eye sign, and bilateral miosis (however, the pupils remain reactive to light).

◆ *Seizure disorders.* A complex partial seizure produces a decreased LOC, manifested as a blank stare, purposeless behavior, and unintelligible speech. The seizure may be heralded by an aura and followed by several minutes of mental confusion.

An absence seizure usually involves a brief change in the patient's LOC, indicated by blinking or eye rolling, a blank stare, and slight mouth movements.

A generalized tonic-clonic seizure typically begins with a loud cry and sudden loss of consciousness. Muscle spasm alternates with relaxation. Tongue biting, incontinence, labored breathing, apnea, and cyanosis may also occur. Consciousness returns after the seizure, but the patient remains confused and may have difficulty talking. He may complain of drowsiness, fatigue, headache, muscle aching, and weakness and may fall into a deep sleep.

An atonic seizure produces sudden unconsciousness for a few seconds.

Status epilepticus, rapidly recurring seizures without intervening periods of physiologic recovery and return of consciousness, can be life threatening.

◼ *Shock.* A decreased LOC—lethargy progressing to stupor and coma—occurs late in shock. Associated findings include confusion, anxiety, and restlessness; hypotension; tachycardia; a weak pulse with narrowing pulse pressure; dyspnea; oliguria; and cool, clammy skin.

Hypovolemic shock is generally the result of massive or insidious bleeding, either internally or externally. Cardiogenic shock may produce chest pain or arrhythmias and signs of heart failure, such as dyspnea, cough, edema, jugular vein distention, and weight gain. Septic shock may be accompanied by a high fever and chills. Anaphylactic shock usually involves stridor.

◼ *Stroke.* With stroke, changes in the patient's LOC vary in degree and onset, depending on the lesion's size and location and the presence of edema. A thrombotic stroke usually follows multiple transient ischemic attacks (TIAs). Changes in the patient's LOC may be abrupt or take several minutes, hours, or days. An embolic stroke occurs suddenly, and deficits reach their peak almost at once. Deficits associated with a hemorrhagic stroke usually develop over minutes or hours. Associated findings vary with the stroke type and severity and may include disorientation; intellectual deficits, such as memory loss and poor judgment; personality changes; and emotional lability.

◼ *Subdural hemorrhage (acute).* With acute subdural hemorrhage, agitation and confusion are followed by a progressively decreasing LOC from somnolence to coma. The patient may also experience headache, unilateral pupil dilation, decreased pulse and respiratory rates, seizures, and a positive Babinski's reflex.

◼ *Thyroid storm.* With thyroid storm, the patient's LOC decreases suddenly and can progress to coma. Irritability, restlessness, confusion, and psychotic behavior precede the deterioration. Associated signs and symptoms include tremors and weakness; vision disturbances; tachycardia, arrhythmias, angina, and acute respiratory distress; and fever—possibly as high as 105° F (40.6° C).

◆ *TIA.* The patient's LOC decreases abruptly (with varying severity) and gradually returns to normal within 24 hours of a TIA. Site-specific findings may include vision loss, nystagmus, aphasia, dizziness, dysarthria, unilateral hemiparesis or hemiplegia, tinnitus, paresthesia, dysphagia, and a staggering or an uncoordinated gait.

◆ *West Nile encephalitis.* West Nile encephalitis is a brain infection that's caused by the West Nile virus. Mild infection is common. Signs and symptoms include fever, headache, and body aches, commonly with a skin rash and swollen lymph glands. More severe infection is marked by a high fever, headache, neck stiffness, stupor, disorientation, coma, tremors, paralysis and, rarely, death.

Light flashes

A cardinal symptom of vision-threatening retinal detachment, light flashes can occur locally or throughout the visual field. The patient usually reports seeing spots, stars, or lightning-type streaks. Flashes can occur suddenly or gradually and can indicate temporary or permanent vision impairment.

In most cases, light flashes signal the splitting of the posterior vitreous membrane into two layers; the inner layer detaches from the retina, and the outer layer remains fixed to it. The sensation of light flashes may result from vitreous traction on the retina, hemorrhage caused by a tear in the retinal capillary, or strands of solid vitreous floating in a local pool of liquid vitreous. Until retinal detachment is ruled out, restrict the patient's eye and body movement.

Assessment

Ask the patient when the light flashes began. Can he pinpoint their location, or do they occur throughout the visual field? If the patient is experiencing eye pain or headache, have him describe it. Ask if the patient wears or has ever worn corrective lenses and if he has a history of eye or vision problems. Also ask if the patient has other medical problems—especially hypertension or diabetes mellitus, which can cause retinopathy and, possibly, retinal detachment. Obtain an occupational history because light flashes may be related to job stress or eye strain.

Next, perform a complete eye and vision examination. Begin by inspecting the external eye, lids, lashes, and tear puncta for abnormalities and the iris and sclera for signs of bleeding. Observe pupillary size and shape and check for reaction to light, accommodation, and consensual light response. Then test visual acuity in each eye. Also test visual fields; document any light flashes that the patient reports during this test.

Causes

◆ *Head trauma.* A patient who has sustained minor head trauma may report "seeing stars" when the injury occurs. He may also complain of localized pain at the injury site, a generalized headache, and dizziness.

◆ *Migraine headache.* Light flashes—possibly accompanied by an aura—may herald a classic migraine headache. As these symptoms subside, the patient typically experiences a severe, throbbing, unilateral headache that usually lasts 1 to 12 hours and may be accompanied by slight confusion, photophobia, nausea and vomiting, and paresthesia of the lips, face, or hands.

◆ *Retinal detachment.* Light flashes described as floaters or spots are localized in the portion of the visual field where the retina is detaching. With macular involvement, the patient may experience painless vision impairment resembling a curtain covering the visual field.

◆ *Vitreous detachment.* Visual floaters may accompany a sudden onset of light flashes. Usually, one eye is affected at a time.

Low birth weight

Two groups of neonates are born weighing less than the normal minimum birth weight of 5½ lb (2,500 g)—those who are born prematurely (before 37 weeks' gestation) and those who are small for gestational age (SGA). Premature neonates weigh an appropriate amount for their gestational age and probably would have matured normally if carried to term. Conversely, SGA neonates weigh less than the normal amount for their age; however, their organs are mature. Differen-

Maternal causes of low birth weight

If the neonate is small for his gestational age, consider these possible maternal causes:
◆ acquired immunodeficiency syndrome
◆ alcohol or opioid abuse
◆ chronic maternal illness
◆ cigarette smoking
◆ hypertension
◆ hypoxemia
◆ malnutrition
◆ toxemia.

If the neonate is born prematurely, consider these common maternal causes:
◆ abruptio placentae
◆ amnionitis
◆ cocaine or crack use
◆ incompetent cervix
◆ placenta previa
◆ polyhydramnios
◆ preeclampsia
◆ premature rupture of membranes
◆ severe maternal illness
◆ urinary tract infection.

tiating between the two groups helps direct the search for a cause.

In the premature neonate, low birth weight usually results from a disorder that prevents the uterus from retaining the fetus, interferes with the normal course of pregnancy, causes premature separation of the placenta, or stimulates uterine contractions before term. In the SGA neonate, intrauterine growth may be retarded by a disorder that interferes with placental circulation, fetal development, or maternal health. (See *Maternal causes of low birth weight.*)

Regardless of the cause, low birth weight is associated with higher neonate morbidity and mortality; in fact, these neonates are 20 times more likely to die within the first month of life. Because it's commonly associated with poorly developed body systems, particularly the respiratory system, low birth weight can also signal a life-threatening emergency. (See *Responding to low birth weight.*)

EMERGENCY INTERVENTIONS

Responding to low birth weight

If you detect signs of distress in a neonate with low birth weight, take the following steps:
◆ Prepare to provide respiratory support as needed; this may include endotracheal intubation or the administration of supplemental oxygen through an oxygen hood.
◆ Monitor the neonate's axillary temperature. (A drop below 97.8° F [36.6° C] causes

increased oxygen consumption and exacerbates respiratory distress.)
◆ Cover the neonate's head to prevent heat loss.
◆ Use an overbed warmer or an Isolette, as ordered. (If these are unavailable, use a wrapped, rubber water bottle filled with warm water to provide warmth, being careful to avoid hyperthermia.)

Ballard Scale for calculating gestational age

NEUROMUSCULAR MATURITY

NEUROMUSCULAR MATURITY SIGN	SCORE							RECORD SCORE HERE
	-1	0	1	2	3	4	5	
POSTURE	–						–	
SQUARE WINDOW (Wrist)	>90°	90°	60°	45°	30°	0°	–	
ARM RECOIL	–	180°	140° to 180°	110° to 140°	90° to 100°	<90°		
POPLITEAL ANGLE	180°	160°	140°	120°	100°	90°	<90°	
SCARF SIGN							–	
HEEL TO EAR							–	

TOTAL NEUROMUSCULAR MATURITY SCORE

PHYSICAL MATURITY

PHYSICAL MATURITY SIGN	SCORE							RECORD SCORE HERE
	-1	0	1	2	3	4	5	
SKIN	Sticky, friable, transparent	Gelatinous, red, translucent	Smooth, pink; visible vessels	Superficial peeling or rash; few visible vessels	Cracking; pale areas; rare visible vessels	Parchment-like; deep cracking; no visible vessels	Leathery, cracked, wrinkled	
LANUGO	None	Sparse	Abundant	Thinning	Bald areas	Mostly bald	–	
PLANTAR SURFACE	Heel-toe 40 to 50 mm: –1; <40 mm: –2	>50 mm; no crease	Faint red marks	Anterior transverse crease only	Creases over anterior two-thirds	Creases over entire sole	–	
BREAST	Imperceptible	Barely perceptible	Flat areola, no bud	Stippled areola; 1- to 2-mm bud	Raised areola; 3- to 4-mm bud	Full areola; 5- to 10-mm bud	–	
EYE AND EAR	Lids fused, loosely: –1; tightly: –2	Lids open; pinna flat, stays folded	Slightly curved pinna; soft, slow recoil	Well-curved pinna; soft but ready recoil	Formed and firm; instant recoil	Thick cartilage; ear stiff	–	
GENITALIA, (Male)	Scrotum flat, smooth	Scrotum empty; faint rugae	Testes in upper canal; rare rugae	Testes descending; few rugae	Testes down; good rugae	Testes pendulous; deep rugae	–	
GENITALIA, (Female)	Clitoris prominent; labia flat	Prominent clitoris; small labia minora	Prominent clitoris; enlarging minora	Majora and minora equally prominent	Majora large; minora small	Majora cover clitoris and minora	–	

TOTAL PHYSICAL MATURITY SCORE

Reprinted from Ballard, J.L., "New Ballard Score Expanded to Include Extremely Premature Infants," *Journal of Pediatrics* 119 (3):417-23, 1991, with permission from Elsevier.

SGA neonates who will demonstrate catch-up growth do so by 8 to 12 months. Some SGA neonates will remain below the 10th percentile. Weight of the premature neonate should be corrected for gestational age by approximately 24 months.

Assessment

Stay alert for signs of distress, such as apnea, grunting respirations, intercostal or xiphoid retractions, or a respiratory rate exceeding 60 breaths/minute after the 1st hour of life. As soon as possible, evaluate the neonate's neuromuscular and physical maturity to determine gestational age. (See *Ballard Scale for calculating gestational age.*) Follow with a routine neonatal examination.

Causes

◆ *Chromosomal aberrations.* Abnormalities in the number, size, or configuration of chromosomes can cause low birth weight and possibly multiple congenital anomalies in a premature or SGA neonate. For example, a neonate with trisomy 21 (Down syndrome) may be SGA and have prominent epicanthal folds, a flat-bridged nose, a protruding tongue, palmar simian creases, muscular hypotonia, and an umbilical hernia.
◆ *Cytomegalovirus (CMV) infection.* Although low birth weight in CMV infection is usually associated with premature birth, the neonate may be SGA. Assessment at birth may reveal these classic signs: petechiae and ecchymoses, jaundice, and hepatosplenomegaly, which increases for several days. The neonate may also have a high fever, lymphadenopathy, tachypnea, and dyspnea, along with prolonged bleeding at puncture sites.
◆ *Placental dysfunction.* Low birth weight and a wasted appearance occur in an SGA neonate. He may be sym-

metrically short or may appear relatively long for his low weight. Additional findings reflect the underlying cause. For example, if maternal hyperparathyroidism caused placental dysfunction, the neonate may exhibit muscle jerking and twitching, carpopedal spasm, ankle clonus, vomiting, tachycardia, and tachypnea.

◆ *Rubella (congenital).* Usually, the low-birth-weight neonate with congenital rubella is born at term but is SGA. A characteristic "blueberry muffin" rash accompanies cataracts, purpuric lesions, hepatosplenomegaly, and a large anterior fontanel. Abnormal heart sounds, if present, vary with the type of associated congenital heart defect.

◆ *Varicella (congenital).* Cataracts and skin vesicles accompany low birth weight with varicella.

Lymphadenopathy

Lymphadenopathy—enlargement of one or more lymph nodes—may result from increased production of lymphocytes or reticuloendothelial cells or from infiltration of cells that aren't normally present. This sign may be generalized (involving three or more node groups) or localized. Generalized lymphadenopathy may be caused by an inflammatory process, such as bacterial or viral infection, connective tissue disease, an endocrine disorder, or a neoplasm. Localized lymphadenopathy most commonly results from infection or trauma affecting a specific area. (See *Areas of localized lymphadenopathy* and *Causes of localized lymphadenopathy,* page 352.)

Normally, lymph nodes are discrete, mobile, soft, nontender and, except in children, nonpalpable. (However, palpable nodes may be normal in adults.) Nodes that are more than $3/8''$ (1 cm) in diameter are cause for concern. They may be tender, and the skin overlying the lymph node may be erythematous, suggesting a draining lesion. Alternatively, they may be hard and fixed, tender or nontender, suggesting a malignant tumor.

Assessment

Ask the patient when he first noticed the swelling and whether it's located on one side of his body or both. Are the swollen areas sore, hard, or red? Ask the patient if he has recently had an infection or other health problem. Also ask if a biopsy has ever been done on any node because this may indicate a previously diagnosed cancer. Find out if the patient has a family history of cancer.

Palpate the entire lymph node system to determine the extent of lymphadenopathy and to detect other areas of local enlargement. Use the pads of your index and middle fingers to move the skin over underlying tissues at the nodal area. If you detect enlarged nodes, note their size in centimeters and whether they're fixed or mobile, tender or nontender, and erythematous or not. Note their texture: Is the node discrete, or does the area feel matted? If you detect tender, erythematous lymph nodes, check the area drained by that part of the lymph system for signs of infection, such as erythema and swelling. Also, gently palpate for and percuss the spleen.

Causes

◆ *Acquired immunodeficiency syndrome (AIDS).* Besides lymphadenopathy, findings of AIDS include a history of fatigue, night sweats, diarrhea, weight loss, and a cough with several

Areas of localized lymphadenopathy

When you detect an enlarged lymph node, palpate the entire lymph node system to determine the extent of lymphadenopathy. Include the lymph nodes indicated here in your assessment.

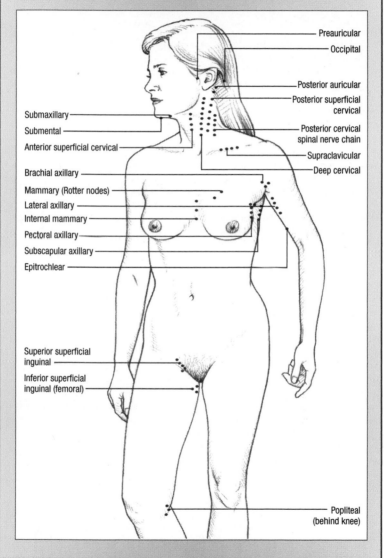

Preauricular
Occipital
Posterior auricular
Posterior superficial cervical
Posterior cervical spinal nerve chain
Supraclavicular
Deep cervical

Submaxillary
Submental
Anterior superficial cervical
Brachial axillary
Mammary (Rotter nodes)
Lateral axillary
Internal mammary
Pectoral axillary
Subscapular axillary
Epitrochlear

Superior superficial inguinal
Inferior superficial inguinal (femoral)

Popliteal (behind knee)

Causes of localized lymphadenopathy

Various disorders can cause localized lymphadenopathy, but this sign usually results from infection or trauma affecting the specific area. Here you'll find some common causes of lymphadenopathy listed according to the areas affected.

Auricular
◆ Erysipelas
◆ Herpes zoster ophthalmicus
◆ Infection
◆ Rubella
◆ Squamous cell carcinoma
◆ Styes or chalazion
◆ Tularemia

Axillary
◆ Breast cancer
◆ Infection
◆ Lymphoma
◆ Mastitis

Cervical
◆ Cat-scratch fever
◆ Facial or oral cancer
◆ Infection
◆ Mononucleosis
◆ Mucocutaneous lymph node syndrome
◆ Rubella
◆ Rubeola
◆ Thyrotoxicosis
◆ Tonsillitis
◆ Tuberculosis
◆ Varicella

Inguinal and femoral
◆ Carcinoma
◆ Chancroid
◆ Infection
◆ Lymphogranuloma venereum
◆ Syphilis

Occipital
◆ Infection
◆ Roseola
◆ Scalp infection
◆ Seborrheic dermatitis
◆ Tick bite
◆ Tinea capitis

Popliteal
◆ Infection

Submaxillary and submental
◆ Cystic fibrosis
◆ Dental infection
◆ Gingivitis
◆ Glossitis
◆ Infection

Supraclavicular
◆ Infection
◆ Neoplastic disease

concurrent infections appearing soon afterward.

◆ *Anthrax (cutaneous)*. With cutaneous anthrax, lymphadenopathy, malaise, headache, and fever may develop along with a lesion that progresses into a painless, necrotic-centered ulcer.

◆ *Brucellosis*. With brucellosis, generalized lymphadenopathy usually affects cervical and axillary lymph nodes, making them tender. It usually begins insidiously with easy fatigability, headache, backache, anorexia, weight loss, and arthralgia; it may also begin abruptly with fever that rises in the morning and subsides during the day.

◆ *Cytomegalovirus infection*. With cytomegalovirus infection, generalized lymphadenopathy occurs in the immunocompromised patient and is accompanied by fever, malaise, a rash, and hepatosplenomegaly.

◆ *Hodgkin's disease.* The extent of lymphadenopathy reflects the stage of malignancy in Hodgkin's disease—from stage I involvement of a single lymph node region to stage IV generalized lymphadenopathy. Common early signs and symptoms include pruritus and, in older patients, fatigue, weakness, night sweats, malaise, weight loss, and an unexplained fever.

◆ *Leukemia.* With acute lymphocytic leukemia, generalized lymphadenopathy is accompanied by fatigue, malaise, pallor, and a low-grade fever. The patient also experiences prolonged bleeding time, swollen gums, weight loss, bone or joint pain, and hepatosplenomegaly.

With chronic lymphocytic leukemia, generalized lymphadenopathy appears early, along with fatigue, malaise, and fever. As the disease progresses, hepatosplenomegaly, severe fatigue, and weight loss occur.

◆ *Lyme disease.* Spread by the bite of certain ticks, Lyme disease begins with a skin lesion called *erythema chronicum migrans.* As the disease progresses, the patient may suffer from lymphadenopathy, constant malaise and fatigue, an intermittent headache, fever, chills, and aches.

◆ *Mononucleosis (infectious).* Characteristic, painful lymphadenopathy involves cervical, axillary, and inguinal nodes in patients with infectious mononucleosis. Posterior cervical adenopathy is also common. Typically, prodromal symptoms—such as headache, malaise, and fatigue—occur 3 to 5 days before the appearance of the classic triad of lymphadenopathy, sore throat, and temperature fluctuations with an evening peak of about 102° F (38.9° C). Hepatosplenomegaly may develop, along with findings of stomatitis, exudative tonsillitis, or pharyngitis.

◆ *Mycosis fungoides.* Lymphadenopathy occurs in stage III of mycosis fungoides, a rare, chronic malignant lymphoma. It's accompanied by ulcerated brownish red tumors that are painful and itchy.

◆ *Non-Hodgkin's lymphoma.* Painless enlargement of one or more peripheral lymph nodes is the most common sign of non-Hodgkin's lymphoma, with generalized lymphadenopathy characterizing stage IV. Dyspnea, cough, and hepatosplenomegaly occur, along with systemic complaints of a fever of up to 101° F (38.3° C), night sweats, fatigue, malaise, and weight loss.

◆ *Rheumatoid arthritis.* Lymphadenopathy is an early, nonspecific finding in rheumatoid arthritis. Other associated findings include fatigue, malaise, a continuous low-grade fever, weight loss, and vague arthralgia and myalgia. Later, the patient develops joint tenderness, swelling, warmth, and stiffness after inactivity (especially in the morning).

◆ *Sarcoidosis.* Generalized, bilateral hilar and right paratracheal forms of lymphadenopathy (seen on chest X-ray) with splenomegaly are common with sarcoidosis. Initial findings are arthralgia, fatigue, malaise, weight loss, and pulmonary symptoms. Other findings vary with the site and extent of fibrosis.

◆ *Sjögren's syndrome.* Lymphadenopathy of the parotid and submaxillary nodes may occur in Sjögren's syndrome, a rare disorder. Assessment reveals cardinal signs of dry mouth, eyes, and mucous membranes, which may be accompanied by photosensitivity, poor vision, eye fatigue, nasal crusting, and epistaxis.

◆ *Syphilis (secondary).* Generalized lymphadenopathy occurs in the second stage of syphilis and may be accompanied by a macular, papular, pustular, or nodular rash on the arms, trunk, palms, soles, face, and scalp. A palmar rash is a significant diagnostic sign.

◆ *Systemic lupus erythematosus (SLE).* With SLE, generalized lymphadenopathy typically accompanies the hallmark butterfly rash, photosensitivity, Raynaud's phenomenon, and joint pain and stiffness. Pleuritic chest pain and a cough may appear with systemic findings, such as fever, anorexia, and weight loss.

◆ *Tuberculous lymphadenitis.* With tuberculous lymphadenitis, lymphadenopathy may be generalized or restricted to superficial lymph nodes. Affected lymph nodes may become fluctuant and drain to surrounding tissue. They may be accompanied by fever, chills, weakness, and fatigue.

◆ *Waldenström's macroglobulinemia.* With Waldenström's macroglobulinemia, lymphadenopathy may appear along with hepatosplenomegaly. Associated findings include retinal hemorrhage, pallor, and signs of heart failure. The patient shows a decreased level of consciousness, abnormal reflexes, and signs of peripheral neuritis. Circulatory impairment occurs because of increased blood viscosity.

M

McBurney sign

A telltale indicator of localized peritoneal inflammation in acute appendicitis, McBurney sign is tenderness elicited by palpating the right lower quadrant over McBurney point. McBurney point is about 2″ (5 cm) above the anterior superior spine of the ilium, on the line between the spine and the umbilicus.

Assessment

Ask the patient to describe the abdominal pain. When did it begin? Does coughing, movement, eating, or elimination worsen or help relieve it? Also ask about the development of other signs and symptoms, such as vomiting and a low-grade fever. Ask the patient to point with a finger to the spot where the pain is worst.

Before you attempt to elicit McBurney sign, inspect the abdomen for distention, auscultate for hypoactive or absent bowel sounds, and test for tympany. Continue light palpation of the patient's abdomen to detect additional tenderness, rigidity, guarding, or pain. Observe the patient's facial expression for signs of pain, such as grimacing or wincing. (See *Eliciting McBurney sign.*)

Eliciting McBurney sign

To elicit McBurney sign, help the patient into a supine position, with his knees slightly flexed and his abdominal muscles relaxed. Then, palpate deeply and slowly in the right lower quadrant over McBurney point—located about 2″ (5 cm) from the right anterior superior spine of the ilium, on a line between the spine and the umbilicus. Point pain and tenderness, a positive McBurney sign, indicates appendicitis.

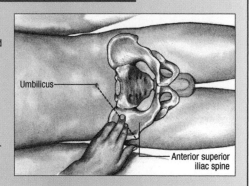

Umbilicus

Anterior superior iliac spine

Causes

◆ *Appendicitis.* McBurney sign appears within the first 2 to 12 hours after the onset of appendicitis, after initial pain in the epigastric and periumbilical area shifts to the right lower quadrant (McBurney point). This persistent pain increases with walking or coughing. Nausea and vomiting may occur from the start. Boardlike abdominal rigidity and rebound tenderness that worsen as the condition progresses accompany cutaneous hyperalgia, fever, constipation or diarrhea, tachycardia, retractive respirations, anorexia, and moderate malaise.

Rupture of the appendix causes sudden cessation of pain. Then, signs and symptoms of peritonitis develop, such as severe abdominal pain, pallor, hypoactive or absent bowel sounds, diaphoresis, and a high fever.

McMurray's sign

Commonly an indicator of medial meniscal injury, McMurray's sign is a palpable, audible click or pop elicited by rotating the tibia on the femur. It re-

Eliciting McMurray's sign

Eliciting McMurray's sign requires special training and gentle manipulation of the patient's leg to avoid extending a meniscal tear or locking the knee. If you've been trained to elicit McMurray's sign, place the patient in a supine position and flex his affected knee until his heel nearly touches his buttock. Place your thumb and index finger on either side of the knee joint space and grasp his heel with your other hand. Then rotate the foot and lower leg laterally to test the posterior aspect of the medial meniscus.

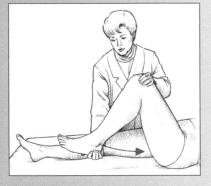

Keeping the patient's foot in a lateral position, extend the knee to a 90-degree angle to test the anterior aspect of the medial meniscus. A palpable or audible click—a positive McMurray's sign—indicates injury to meniscal structures.

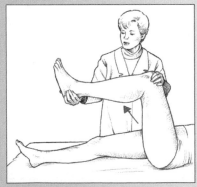

sults when gentle manipulation of the leg traps torn cartilage and then lets it snap free. Because eliciting McMurray's sign forces the surface of the tibial plateau against the femoral condyles, such manipulation is contraindicated in patients with suspected fractures of the tibial plateau or femoral condyles.

A positive McMurray's sign augments other findings commonly associated with meniscal injury, such as severe joint line tenderness, locking or clicking of the joint, and a decreased range of motion (ROM).

Assessment

After McMurray's sign has been elicited, find out if the patient is experiencing acute knee pain. Then ask him to describe a recent knee injury. For example, did his injury place twisting external or internal force on the knee, or did he experience blunt knee trauma from a fall? Also, ask about previous knee injury, surgery, prosthetic replacement, or other joint problems, such as arthritis, that could have weakened the knee. Ask if anything aggravates or relieves the pain and if he needs assistance to walk.

Have the patient point to the exact area of pain. Assess the leg's ROM, both passive and with resistance. Next, check for cruciate ligament stability by noting anterior or posterior movement of the tibia on the femur (drawer sign). Finally, measure the quadriceps muscles in both legs for symmetry. (See *Eliciting McMurray's sign.*)

Causes

◆ *Meniscal tear.* McMurray's sign can usually be elicited with a meniscal tear injury. Associated signs and symptoms include acute knee pain at the medial or lateral joint line (depending on the injury site) and decreased ROM or locking of the knee joint. Quadriceps weakening and atrophy may also occur.

Melena

A common sign of upper GI bleeding, melena is the passage of black, tarry stools containing blood that has been acted upon by digestive enzymes. The characteristic color results from bacterial degradation and hydrochloric acid acting on the blood as it travels through the GI tract. At least 60 ml of blood is needed to produce this sign. (See *Comparing melena to hematochezia,* page 358.)

Severe melena can signal acute bleeding and life-threatening hypovolemic shock. Usually, melena indicates bleeding from the esophagus, stomach, or duodenum, although it can also indicate bleeding from the jejunum, ileum, or ascending colon. This sign can also result from swallowing blood, such as in epistaxis; from taking certain drugs; or from ingesting alcohol. Because false melena may be caused by ingestion of lead, iron, bismuth, or licorice (which produces black stools without the presence of blood), all black stools should be tested for occult blood.

Assessment

If the patient is experiencing severe melena, quickly take his orthostatic vital signs to detect hypovolemic shock. A decline of 10 mm Hg or more in systolic pressure or an increase of 10 beats/minute or more in the pulse rate may indicate volume depletion. Quickly examine the patient for other signs of shock, such as tachycardia, tachypnea, and cool, clammy skin, and institute emergency interventions as needed. (See *Responding to melena,* page 359.)

Comparing melena to hematochezia

With GI bleeding, the site, amount, and rate of blood flow through the GI tract determine if a patient will develop melena (black, tarry stools) or hematochezia (bright red, bloody stools). Usually, melena indicates *upper* GI bleeding, and hematochezia indicates *lower* GI bleeding. However, with some disorders, melena may alternate with hematochezia. This chart helps differentiate these two commonly related signs.

SIGN	SITES	CHARACTERISTICS
Melena	◆ Esophagus, stomach, duodenum ◆ Rarely, jejunum, ileum, ascending colon	◆ Black, loose, tarry stools ◆ Reflects delayed or minimal passage of blood through the GI tract
Hematochezia	◆ Usually distal to or affecting the colon ◆ Esophagus, stomach, or duodenum with rapid hemorrhage of 1 L or more	◆ Bright red or dark, mahogany-colored stools; pure blood; blood mixed with formed stool; or bloody diarrhea ◆ Reflects passage of undigested blood through the GI tract from lower GI bleeding or rapid blood loss

If the patient's condition permits, ask when he discovered that his stools were black and tarry. Ask about the frequency and quantity of bowel movements. Has he had melena before? Ask about other signs and symptoms, notably hematemesis or hematochezia, and about the use of anti-inflammatories, aspirin, alcohol, or other GI irritants. Also, find out if he has a history of GI lesions. Ask if the patient takes iron supplements, which may also cause black stools. Obtain a drug history, noting the use of warfarin (Coumadin) or other anticoagulants.

Next, inspect the patient's mouth and nasopharynx for evidence of bleeding. Perform an abdominal examination that includes auscultation, palpation, and percussion.

Causes

◆ *Colon cancer.* On the right side of the colon, early tumor growth may cause melena accompanied by abdominal aching, pressure, or cramps. With a tumor on the left side, melena is a rare sign until late in the disease. Early tumor growth commonly causes rectal bleeding with intermittent abdominal fullness or cramping and rectal pressure.

◆ *Esophageal cancer.* Melena is a late sign of esophageal cancer, a malignant neoplastic disease that's three times more common in men than in women. Increasing obstruction first produces painless dysphagia and then rapid weight loss. The patient may experience steady chest pain with substernal fullness, nausea, vomiting, and hematemesis.

◆ *Esophageal varices (ruptured).* Ruptured esophageal varices can produce

EMERGENCY INTERVENTIONS

Responding to melena

If a patient with melena displays signs of shock, take the following steps:
◆ Insert a large-bore I.V. catheter for the administration of fluids and blood.
◆ Obtain a blood sample for analysis of hematocrit, prothrombin time, International

Normalized Ratio, and partial thromboplastin time.
◆ Place the patient in a flat position with his head turned to one side and his feet elevated.
◆ Administer supplemental oxygen, as prescribed.

---

melena, hematochezia, and hematemesis. Signs of shock precede melena.

◆ *Gastritis.* Melena and hematemesis are common with gastritis. The patient may also experience mild epigastric or abdominal discomfort that's exacerbated by eating, belching, nausea, and vomiting.

◆ *Mallory-Weiss syndrome.* Mallory-Weiss syndrome is characterized by massive bleeding from the upper GI tract due to a tear in the mucous membrane of the esophagus or the junction of the esophagus and the stomach. Melena and hematemesis follow vomiting. The patient may also report epigastric or back pain.

◆ *Mesenteric vascular occlusion.* Mesenteric vascular occlusion produces slight melena with 2 to 3 days of persistent, mild abdominal pain. Later, abdominal pain becomes severe and may be accompanied by tenderness, distention, guarding, and rigidity.

◆ *Peptic ulcer.* Melena may signal life-threatening hemorrhage from vascular penetration. The patient may also develop decreased appetite, nausea, vomiting, hematemesis, hematochezia, and left epigastric pain.

◆ *Small-bowel tumors.* Small-bowel tumors may bleed and produce melena. Other signs and symptoms include abdominal pain, distention, and an in-

creasing frequency and pitch of bowel sounds.

◆ *Thrombocytopenia.* Melena or hematochezia may accompany other manifestations of bleeding tendency: hematemesis, epistaxis, petechiae, ecchymoses, hematuria, vaginal bleeding, and blood-filled oral bullae.

Menorrhagia

Abnormally heavy or prolonged menstrual bleeding, menorrhagia may occur as a single episode or a chronic sign. In menorrhagia, bleeding is heavier than the patient's normal menstrual flow; menstrual blood loss is 80 ml or more per monthly period. A form of dysfunctional uterine bleeding, menorrhagia can result from endocrine and hematologic disorders, stress, and certain drugs and procedures.

Assessment

If the patient has severe bleeding, evaluate her hemodynamic status by taking orthostatic vital signs. If she shows an increase of 10 beats/minute in pulse rate, a decrease of 10 mm Hg in systolic blood pressure, pallor, tachycardia, tachypnea, or cool, clammy skin, suspect hypovolemic shock. Use menstrual pads to obtain information related to the quality and quantity of bleeding. When the patient's condition permits, obtain a history. Determine her age at menarche, the duration of menstrual periods, and the interval between them. Establish the date of the patient's last menses, and ask about recent changes in her normal menstrual pattern. Have the patient describe the character and amount of bleeding. For example, how many pads or tampons does the patient use? Has she noted clots or tissue in the blood? Also ask about the development of other signs and symptoms before and during her period.

Next, ask if the patient is sexually active. Does she use a method of birth control? If so, what kind? Could the patient be pregnant? Be sure to note the number of pregnancies, the outcome of each, and any pregnancy-related complications. Find out the dates of her most recent pelvic examination and Papanicolaou smear and the details of any previous gynecologic infections or neoplasms. Also, be sure to ask about previous episodes of abnormal bleeding and the outcome of treatment. If possible, obtain a pregnancy history of the patient's mother, and determine if the patient was exposed in utero to diethylstilbestrol. (This drug has been linked to vaginal adenosis.)

Be sure to ask the patient about her general health and medical history. Note particularly if the patient or her family has a history of thyroid, adrenal, or hepatic disease; blood dyscrasias; or tuberculosis because these may predispose the patient to menorrhagia. Also, ask about the patient's past surgical procedures and recent emotional stress. Find out if the patient has undergone X-ray or other radiation therapy, because this may indicate previous treatment for menorrhagia. Obtain a thorough drug and alcohol history, noting the use of anticoagulants or aspirin. Then prepare the patient for a pelvic examination to help determine the cause of bleeding, and obtain blood samples and urine specimens for pregnancy testing.

Causes

◆ *Blood dyscrasias.* Menorrhagia is one of several possible signs of a bleeding disorder. Other possible associated findings include epistaxis, bleeding gums, purpura, hematemesis, hematuria, and melena.

◆ *Hypothyroidism.* Menorrhagia is a common early sign of hypothyroidism and is accompanied by such nonspecific findings as fatigue, cold intolerance, constipation, and weight gain despite anorexia. As hypothyroidism progresses, intellectual and motor activity decrease; the skin becomes dry, pale, cool, and doughy; the hair becomes dry and sparse; and the nails become thick and brittle.

◆ *Uterine fibroids.* Menorrhagia is the most common sign of uterine fibroids; however, other forms of abnormal uterine bleeding as well as dysmenorrhea or leukorrhea can also occur. Related findings may include abdominal pain, a feeling of abdominal heaviness, backache, constipation, urinary urgency or frequency, and an enlarged uterus, which is usually nontender.

Metrorrhagia

Metrorrhagia—uterine bleeding that occurs irregularly between menstrual periods—is usually light, although it can range from staining to hemorrhage. Usually, this common sign reflects slight physiologic bleeding from the endometrium during ovulation. However, metrorrhagia may be the only indication of an underlying gynecologic disorder and can also result from stress, drugs, treatments, and intrauterine devices.

Assessment

Begin your evaluation by obtaining a thorough menstrual history. Ask the patient when she began menstruating and about the duration of menstrual periods, the interval between them, and the average number of tampons or pads she uses. When does metrorrhagia usually occur in relation to her period? Does she experience other signs or symptoms? Find out the date of her last menses, and ask about other recent changes in her normal menstrual pattern. Get details of previous gynecologic problems. If applicable, obtain a contraceptive and obstetric history. Record the dates of her last Papanicolaou smear and pelvic examination. Ask the patient when she last had sex and whether it was protected. Next, ask about her general health and any recent changes. Is she under emotional stress? If possible, obtain a pregnancy history of the patient's mother. Was the patient exposed in utero to diethylstilbestrol? (This drug has been linked to vaginal adenosis.)

Perform a pelvic examination if indicated, and obtain blood samples and urine specimens for pregnancy testing.

Causes

◆ *Abortion (incomplete).* A missed or incomplete abortion may cause metrorrhagia. Metrorrhagia may be accompanied by abdominal cramping and lower back or pelvic pain.
◆ *Cervicitis.* Cervicitis is a nonspecific infection that may cause spontaneous bleeding, spotting, or posttraumatic bleeding. Assessment reveals red, granular, irregular lesions on the external cervix. Purulent vaginal discharge (with or without odor), lower abdominal pain, and fever may occur.
◆ *Dysfunctional uterine bleeding.* Abnormal uterine bleeding not caused by major gynecologic disorders usually occurs as metrorrhagia, although menorrhagia is possible. Bleeding may be profuse or scant, intermittent or constant.
◆ *Endometrial polyps.* In most patients, endometrial polyps cause abnormal bleeding, usually intermenstrual or postmenopausal; however, some patients do remain asymptomatic.
◆ *Endometriosis.* Metrorrhagia (usually premenstrual) may be the only indication of endometriosis or it may accompany cyclical pelvic discomfort, infertility, and dyspareunia.
◆ *Endometritis.* Endometritis causes metrorrhagia, purulent vaginal discharge, and enlargement of the uterus. It also produces fever, lower abdominal pain, and abdominal muscle spasm.
◆ *Gynecologic cancer.* Metrorrhagia is commonly an early sign of cervical or uterine cancer. Later, the patient may experience weight loss, pelvic pain, fatigue and, possibly, an abdominal mass.
◆ *Uterine leiomyomas.* Besides metrorrhagia, uterine leiomyomas may cause increasing abdominal girth and heaviness in the abdomen, constipation, and urinary frequency or urgency. The patient may report pain if the uterus attempts to expel the tumor through contractions and if the tumors twist or necrose after circulatory occlusion or infection; however, the patient with leiomyomas is usually asymptomatic.
◆ *Vaginal adenosis.* Vaginal adenosis commonly produces metrorrhagia. Palpation reveals roughening or nodules in affected vaginal areas.

Miosis

Miosis—pupillary constriction caused by contraction of the sphincter muscle in the iris—occurs normally as a response to fatigue, increased light, or administration of a miotic; as part of the eye's accommodation reflex; and as part of the aging process (pupil size steadily decreases from adolescence to about age 60). However, it can also stem from an ocular or neurologic disorder, trauma, use of a systemic drug, or contact lens overuse. A rare form of miosis—Argyll Robertson pupils—can stem from tabes dorsalis and diverse neurologic disorders. Occurring bilaterally, these miotic (usually pinpoint), unequal, and irregularly shaped pupils don't dilate properly with mydriatic use and fail to react to light, although they constrict on accommodation.

Assessment

Begin by asking the patient if he has experienced other ocular symptoms, and have him describe their onset, duration, and intensity. Be sure to ask about trauma, serious systemic disease, and the use of contact lenses and drugs.

Next, perform a thorough eye examination. Test visual acuity in each eye, with and without correction, paying particular attention to blurred or decreased vision in the miotic eye. Examine and compare the pupils for size (many people have a normal discrepancy), color, shape, accommodation, and consensual light response. Evaluate extraocular muscle function by assessing the six cardinal fields of gaze. (See *Testing extraocular muscles*, page 217.)

Causes

◆ *Cerebrovascular arteriosclerosis.* With cerebrovascular arteriosclerosis, miosis is usually unilateral, depending on the site and extent of vascular damage. Other findings include blurred vision, slurred speech or possibly aphasia, vertigo, and headache.
◆ *Cluster headache.* Ipsilateral miosis, tearing, conjunctival injection, and ptosis commonly accompany a severe cluster headache, along with facial flushing and sweating, bradycardia, and nasal stuffiness or rhinorrhea.
◆ *Corneal foreign body.* Miosis in the affected eye occurs with pain, a foreign-body sensation in the cornea, slight vision loss, conjunctival injection, photophobia, and profuse tearing.
◆ *Corneal ulcer.* With a corneal ulcer, miosis in the affected eye appears with moderate pain, blurred vision, and diffuse conjunctival injection.
◆ *Horner syndrome.* Moderate miosis is common in Horner syndrome and occurs ipsilaterally to the spinal cord lesion. Related findings include a sluggish pupillary reflex, moderate ptosis, facial anhidrosis, transient conjunctival injection, and a vascular headache. When the syndrome is congenital, the iris on the affected side may appear lighter.
◆ *Iritis (acute).* Miosis typically occurs in the affected eye along with a decreased pupillary reflex, severe eye pain, photophobia, blurred vision, conjunctival injection and, possibly, pus accumulation in the anterior chamber. The eye appears cloudy, the iris bulges, and the pupil is constricted on ophthalmic examination.
◆ *Parry-Romberg syndrome.* Parry-Romberg syndrome is a facial hemiatrophy that typically produces miosis, sluggish pupillary reflexes, enophthalmos, nystagmus, ptosis, and different-colored irises.
◼ *Pontine hemorrhage.* Bilateral miosis is characteristic of pontine hemorrhage, along with a rapid onset of coma, total paralysis, decerebrate posture, an absent doll's eye sign, and a positive Babinski's sign.
◆ *Uveitis.* Anterior uveitis commonly produces miosis in the affected eye, moderate to severe eye pain, severe conjunctival injection, photophobia, and pus in the anterior chamber. With

posterior uveitis, miosis is accompanied by a gradual onset of eye pain, photophobia, visual floaters, blurred vision and, commonly, a distorted pupil shape.

Mouth lesions

Mouth lesions include ulcers (the most common type), cysts, firm nodules, hemorrhagic lesions, papules, vesicles, bullae, and erythematous lesions. They may occur anywhere on the lips, cheeks, hard and soft palate, salivary glands, tongue, gingivae, or mucous membranes. Many are painful and can be readily detected. Some, however, produce no symptoms; when they occur deep in the mouth, they may be discovered only through a complete oral examination. (See *Common mouth lesions.*)

Assessment

Begin your evaluation with a thorough history. Ask the patient when the lesions appeared and whether he has noticed pain, odor, or drainage. Obtain complete drug and medical histories. Ask about his dental history, including the date of his most recent dental visit.

Next, perform a complete oral examination, noting lesion sites and character. Examine the patient's lips for color and texture. Inspect and palpate the buccal mucosa and tongue for color, texture, and contour; note especially painless ulcers on the sides or base of the tongue. Hold the tongue with a piece of gauze, lift it, and examine its underside and the floor of the mouth. Depress the tongue with a tongue blade, and examine the oropharynx. Inspect the teeth and gums. Palpate the

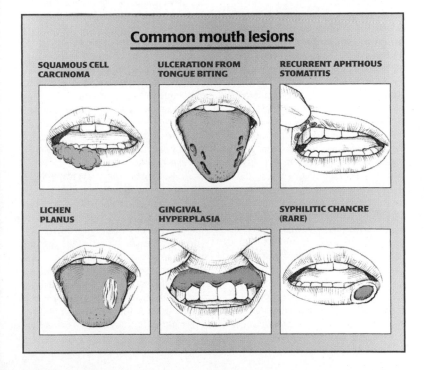

Common mouth lesions

SQUAMOUS CELL CARCINOMA

ULCERATION FROM TONGUE BITING

RECURRENT APHTHOUS STOMATITIS

LICHEN PLANUS

GINGIVAL HYPERPLASIA

SYPHILITIC CHANCRE (RARE)

neck for adenopathy, especially in a patient who smokes tobacco or uses alcohol excessively.

Causes

◆ *Acquired immunodeficiency syndrome (AIDS).* Oral lesions may be an early indication of the immunosuppression that's characteristic of AIDS.

◆ *Actinomycosis (cervicofacial).* Actinomycosis is a chronic fungal infection that typically produces small, firm, flat, and usually painless swellings on the oral mucosa and under the skin of the jaw and neck. They may indurate and abscess, producing fistulas and sinus tracts with a purulent yellow discharge.

◆ *Behçet's syndrome.* Behçet's syndrome is a chronic, progressive syndrome that generally affects young males and produces small, painful ulcers on the lips, gums, buccal mucosa, and tongue.

◆ *Candidiasis.* Candidiasis is a fungal infection that produces soft, elevated plaques on the buccal mucosa, tongue, and sometimes the palate, gingivae, and floor of the mouth. The lesions of acute atrophic candidiasis are red and painful. The lesions of chronic hyperplastic candidiasis are white and firm.

◆ *Discoid lupus erythematosus.* Oral lesions are common, typically appearing on the tongue, buccal mucosa, and palate as erythematous areas with white spots and radiating white striae.

◆ *Erythema multiforme.* Erythema multiforme is an acute inflammatory skin disease that produces a sudden onset of vesicles and bullae on the lips and buccal mucosa.

◆ *Gingivitis (acute necrotizing ulcerative).* Gingivitis is a recurring periodontal condition that causes a sudden onset of gingival ulcers covered with a grayish white pseudomembrane.

◆ *Herpes simplex I.* With primary infection, a brief period of prodromal tingling and itching, fever, and pharyngitis is followed by the eruption of small and irritating vesicles on the tongue, gums, and cheeks.

◆ *Herpes zoster.* Herpes zoster is a viral infection that may produce painful vesicles on the buccal mucosa, tongue, uvula, pharynx, and larynx. Small red nodules typically erupt unilaterally around the thorax or vertically on the arms and legs, and rapidly become vesicles filled with clear fluid or pus.

◆ *Inflammatory fibrous hyperplasia.* Inflammatory fibrous hyperplasia is a painless nodular swelling of the buccal mucosa that results from cheek trauma or irritation. Pink, smooth, pedunculated areas of soft tissue are characteristic.

◆ *Leukoplakia (erythroplakia).* Leukoplakia is a white lesion that can't be removed simply by rubbing the mucosal surface. It may represent dysplasia or early squamous cell carcinoma. Erythroplakia is red and edematous and has a velvety surface. About 90% of all cases of erythroplakia are either dysplasia or cancer.

◆ *Pemphigus.* Pemphigus is a chronic skin disease that's characterized by thin-walled vesicles and bullae that appear in crops on skin or mucous membranes that otherwise appear normal. On the oral mucosa, bullae rupture, leaving painful lesions and raw patches that bleed easily.

◆ *Pyogenic granuloma.* Typically the result of injury, trauma, or irritation, pyogenic granuloma usually appear on the gingivae, but can also erupt on the lips, tongue, or buccal mucosa. The lesions bleed easily because they contain many capillaries.

◆ *Squamous cell carcinoma.* Squamous cell carcinoma is typically a painless ulcer with an elevated, indurated border. It's most common on the lower lip, but it may also occur on the edge of the tongue or floor of the mouth.

◆ *Stomatitis (aphthous)*. Stomatitis is characterized by painful ulcerations of the oral mucosa, usually on the dorsum of the tongue, gingivae, and hard palate.

◆ *Syphilis.* Primary syphilis typically produces a solitary painless, red ulcer on the lip, tongue, palate, tonsil, or gingivae. The ulcer appears as a crater with undulated, raised edges and a shiny center; lip ulcers may develop a crust. During the secondary stage, multiple painless ulcers covered by a grayish white plaque may erupt on the tongue, gingivae, or buccal mucosa. At the tertiary stage, lesions develop on the skin and mucous membranes, especially the tongue and palate.

◆ *Systemic lupus erythematosus.* Oral lesions are common and appear as erythematous areas associated with edema, petechiae, and superficial ulcers with a red halo and a tendency to bleed.

Murmurs

Murmurs are auscultatory sounds heard within the heart chambers or major arteries. Several factors influence a murmur's classification, including timing and duration in the cardiac cycle, auscultatory location, loudness, configuration, pitch, and quality.

Timing can be characterized as systolic (between S_1 and S_2), holosystolic (continuous throughout systole), diastolic (between S_2 and S_1), or continuous throughout systole and diastole; systolic and diastolic murmurs can be further characterized as early, middle, or late. Location refers to the area of maximum loudness, such as the apex, the lower left sternal border, or an intercostal space. Loudness is graded on a scale of 1 to 6. A grade 1 murmur is very faint, only detected after careful auscultation. A grade 2 murmur is a soft, evident murmur. Murmurs considered to be grade 3 are moderately loud. A grade 4 murmur is a loud murmur with a possible intermittent thrill. Grade 5 murmurs are loud and associated with a palpable precordial thrill. Grade 6 murmurs are loud and, like grade 5 murmurs, are associated with a thrill. A grade 6 murmur is audible even when the stethoscope is lifted from the thoracic wall. Configuration, or shape, refers to the nature of loudness—crescendo (grows louder), decrescendo (grows softer), crescendo-decrescendo (first rises, then falls), decrescendo-crescendo (first falls, then rises), plateau (even intensity), or variable (uneven intensity). The murmur's pitch may be high or low. Its quality may be described as harsh, rumbling, blowing, scratching, buzzing, musical, or squeaking.

Murmurs can reflect accelerated blood flow through normal or abnormal valves; forward blood flow through a narrowed or irregular valve or into a dilated vessel; blood backflow through an incompetent valve, septal defect, or patent ductus arteriosus; or decreased blood viscosity. Commonly the result of organic heart disease, murmurs may signal an emergency—for example, a loud holosystolic murmur after an acute myocardial infarction (MI) may signal papillary muscle rupture or a ventricular septal defect. Murmurs may also result from surgical implantation of a prosthetic valve. (See *When murmurs mean emergency,* page 366.)

Some murmurs are innocent, or functional. An innocent systolic murmur is generally soft, medium-pitched, and loudest along the left sternal border at the second or third intercostal space. It's exacerbated by physical activity, excitement, fever, pregnancy,

When murmurs mean emergency

Although not normally a sign of an emergency, murmurs—especially newly developed ones—may signal a serious complication in patients with bacterial endocarditis or a recent acute myocardial infarction (MI).

When caring for a patient with known or suspected bacterial endocarditis, carefully auscultate for new murmurs. Their development, along with crackles, jugular vein distention, orthopnea, and dyspnea, may signal heart failure.

Regular auscultation is also important in a patient who has experienced an acute MI. A loud decrescendo holosystolic murmur at the apex that radiates to the axilla and left sternal border or throughout the chest is significant, particularly in association with a widely split S_2 and an atrial gallop (S_4). This murmur, when accompanied by signs of acute pulmonary edema, usually indicates the development of acute mitral regurgitation due to rupture of the chordae tendineae—a medical emergency.

anemia, or thyrotoxicosis. (See *Detecting congenital murmurs.*)

Assessment

If you discover a murmur, try to determine its type through careful auscultation. (See *Identifying common murmurs,* page 369.) Use the bell of your stethoscope for low-pitched murmurs and the diaphragm for high-pitched murmurs.

Next, obtain a patient history. Ask if the murmur has been known since birth or childhood. Find out if the patient has experienced associated symptoms, particularly palpitations, dizziness, syncope, chest pain, dyspnea, and fatigue. Explore the patient's medical history, noting especially an incidence of rheumatic fever, recent dental work, heart disease, or heart surgery, particularly prosthetic valve replacement.

Perform a systematic physical examination. Note the presence of cardiac arrhythmias, jugular vein distention, and such pulmonary signs and symptoms as dyspnea, orthopnea, and crackles. Does he have peripheral edema?

Causes

◆ *Aortic insufficiency.* Acute aortic insufficiency typically produces a soft, short diastolic murmur over the left sternal border that's best heard when the patient sits and leans forward and at the end of a forced held expiration. S_2 may be soft or absent. Sometimes, a soft, short midsystolic murmur may also be heard over the second right intercostal space. Chronic aortic insufficiency causes a high-pitched, blowing, decrescendo diastolic murmur that's best heard over the second or third right intercostal space or the left sternal border with the patient sitting, leaning forward, and holding his breath after deep expiration. An Austin Flint murmur—a rumbling, mid-to-late diastolic murmur best heard at the apex—may also occur.

◆ *Aortic stenosis.* With aortic stenosis, the murmur is systolic, beginning after S_1 and ending at or before aortic valve closure. It's harsh and grating, medium-pitched, and crescendo-decrescendo. Loudest over the second right intercostal space when the patient is sitting and leaning forward, this murmur may also be heard at the

Detecting congenital murmurs

HEART DEFECT	TYPE OF MURMUR
Aortopulmonary septal defect	*Small defect:* a continuous rough or crackling murmur best heard at the upper left sternal border and below the left clavicle, possibly accompanied by a systolic ejection click. *Large defect:* a harsh systolic murmur heard at the left sternal border.
Atrial septal defect	A mid-systolic, spindle-shaped murmur of grade 2 or 3 intensity heard at the upper left sternal border, with a fixed splitting of S_2. Large shunts may also produce a low- to medium-pitched early diastolic murmur over the lower left sternal border.
Bicuspid aortic valve	An early systolic, loud, high-pitched ejection sound or click that's best heard at the apex and is commonly accompanied by a soft, early or mid-systolic murmur at the upper right sternal border. The aortic component of S_2 is usually accentuated at the apex. This murmur may not be recognized until early childhood.
Coarctation of the aorta	Usually a systolic ejection click at the base of the heart, at the apex, and occasionally over the carotid arteries, usually accompanied by a systolic ejection murmur at the base. This disorder may also produce a blowing diastolic murmur of aortic insufficiency or an apical pansystolic murmur of unknown origin.
Common atrioventricular canal defects (endocardial cushion defect)	*With a competent mitral valve:* a mid-systolic, spindle-shaped murmur of grade 2 or 3 intensity heard at the upper left sternal border, with a fixed splitting of S_2; may be accompanied by a low- to medium-pitched early diastolic murmur over the lower left sternal border. *With an incompetent mitral valve:* an early systolic or holosystolic decrescendo murmur at the apex, along with a widely split S_2 and commonly an S_4.
Ebstein's anomaly	A soft, high-pitched holosystolic blowing murmur that increases with inspiration (Carvallo's sign); best heard over the lower left sternal border and the xiphoid area; possibly accompanied by a low-pitched diastolic rumbling murmur at the apex. Fixed splitting of S_2 and a loud split S_4 also occur.
Left ventricular—right atrial communication	A holosystolic, decrescendo murmur of grades 2 to 4 intensity heard along the lower left sternal border, accompanied by a normal S_2; large shunts also produce a diastolic rumbling murmur over the apex.
Mitral atresia	A nonspecific systolic murmur and a diastolic flow rumble at the lower left sternal border, with one loud S_2.

(continued)

Detecting congenital murmurs *(continued)*

HEART DEFECT	TYPE OF MURMUR
Partial anomalous pulmonary venous connection	A mid-systolic, spindle-shaped grade 2 to 3 murmur at the upper left sternal border, possibly accompanied by a low- to medium-pitched early diastolic murmur over the lower left sternal border.
Patent ductus arteriosus	A continuous rough or crackling murmur best heard at the upper left sternal border and below the left clavicle. The murmur is accentuated late in systole.
Pulmonic insufficiency	An early to mid-diastolic, soft, medium-pitched crescendo-decrescendo murmur best heard at the second or third right intercostal space.
Pulmonic stenosis	An early systolic, harsh, crescendo-decrescendo murmur of grades 4 to 6 intensity heard at the second left intercostal space, possibly radiating along the left sternal border.
Single atrium	A holosystolic regurgitant murmur at the apex, accompanied by a fixed splitting of S_2.
Supravalvular aortic stenosis	A systolic ejection murmur best heard over the second right intercostal space or higher in the episternal notch or over the lower right side of the neck. The aortic closure sound is usually preserved, and no ejection clicks are heard.
Tetralogy of Fallot	A mid-systolic murmur with a systolic thrill palpable at the left mid-sternal border; softer murmurs occurring earlier in systole generally indicate a more severe obstruction.
Tricuspid atresia	Variable, depending on associated defects.
Trilogy of Fallot	A systolic, harsh, crescendo-decrescendo murmur, best heard at the upper left sternal border with radiation toward the left clavicle. The pulmonic component of S_2 becomes progressively softer with increasing degrees of obstruction.
Ventricular septal defect	*Small defect:* usually a holosystolic (but may be limited to early or mid-systole), grades 2 to 4 decrescendo murmur heard along the lower left sternal border, accompanied by a normal S_2. *Large defect:* a holosystolic murmur at the lower left sternal border and a mid-systolic rumbling murmur at the apex, accompanied by an increased S_1 at the lower left sternal border and an increased pulmonic component of S_2.

apex, at the suprasternal notch (Erb's point), and over the carotid arteries. If the patient has advanced disease, S_2 may be heard as a single sound, with inaudible aortic closure. An early systolic ejection click at the apex is typical, but is absent when the valve is severely calcified.

Identifying common murmurs

The timing and configuration of a murmur can help you identify its underlying cause. Learn to recognize the characteristics of these common murmurs shown below.

Aortic insufficiency (chronic)
Thickened valve leaflets fail to close correctly, permitting blood backflow into the left ventricle.

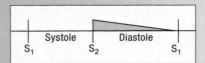

Aortic stenosis
Thickened, scarred, or calcified valve leaflets impede ventricular systolic ejection.

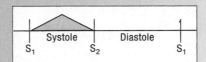

Mitral prolapse
An incompetent mitral valve bulges into the left atrium because of an enlarged posterior leaflet and elongated chordae tendineae.

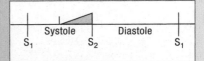

Mitral insufficiency (chronic)
Incomplete mitral valve closure permits blood backflow into the left atrium.

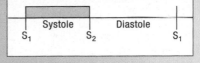

Mitral stenosis
Thickened or scarred valve leaflets cause valve stenosis and restrict blood flow.

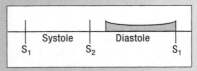

◆ *Cardiomyopathy (hypertrophic).* Hypertrophic cardiomyopathy generates a harsh late systolic murmur, ending at S_2. Best heard over the left sternal border and at the apex, the murmur is commonly accompanied by an audible S_3 or S_4. The murmur decreases with squatting and increases with sitting down.

◆ *Mitral insufficiency.* Acute mitral insufficiency is characterized by a medium-pitched blowing, early systolic or holosystolic decrescendo murmur at the apex, along with a widely split S_2 and commonly an S_4. This murmur doesn't get louder on inspiration as with tricuspid insufficiency. Chronic mitral insufficiency produces a high-pitched, blowing, holosystolic plateau murmur that's loudest at the apex and usually radiates to the axilla or back.

◆ *Mitral prolapse.* Mitral prolapse generates a mid-systolic to late-systolic click with a high-pitched late-systolic crescendo murmur best heard at the apex. Occasionally, multiple clicks may be heard, with or without a systolic murmur.

◆ *Mitral stenosis.* With mitral stenosis, the murmur is soft, low-pitched, rumbling, crescendo-decrescendo, and diastolic, accompanied by a loud S_1 or an opening snap. It's best heard at the apex with the patient in the left lateral position. Mild exercise helps make this murmur audible.

◆ *Myxomas.* A left atrial myxoma (most common) usually produces a mid-diastolic, holosystolic murmur that's loudest at the apex, with an S_4, an early diastolic thudding sound (tumor plop), and a loud, widely split S_1. A right atrial myxoma causes a late diastolic rumbling murmur, a holosystolic crescendo murmur, and tumor plop best heard at the lower left sternal border. A left ventricular myxoma (rare) produces a systolic murmur best heard at the lower left sternal border. A right ventricular myxoma commonly generates a systolic ejection murmur with delayed S_2 and a tumor plop best heard at the left sternal border.

◪ *Papillary muscle rupture.* With papillary muscle rupture—a complication of an acute MI—a loud holosystolic murmur can be auscultated at the apex.

◆ *Rheumatic fever with pericarditis.* A pericardial friction rub along with murmurs and gallops are heard best with the patient leaning forward on his hands and knees during forced expiration. The most common murmurs heard are the systolic murmur of mitral regurgitation, a midsystolic murmur due to swelling of the mitral valve leaflet, and the diastolic murmur of aortic regurgitation.

◆ *Tricuspid insufficiency.* Tricuspid insufficiency is characterized by a soft, high-pitched, holosystolic blowing murmur that increases with inspiration (Carvallo's sign), decreases with exhalation and Valsalva's maneuver, and is

best heard over the lower left sternal border and the xiphoid area.

◆ *Tricuspid stenosis.* Tricuspid stenosis produces a diastolic murmur similar to that of mitral stenosis, but louder with inspiration and decreased with exhalation and Valsalva's maneuver. S_1 may also be louder.

Muscle atrophy

Muscle atrophy results from denervation or prolonged muscle disuse. When deprived of regular exercise, muscle fibers lose bulk and length, producing a visible loss of muscle size and contour and apparent emaciation or deformity in the affected area. Even slight atrophy, which usually results from neuromuscular disease or injury, causes some loss of motion or power. However, atrophy may also stem from metabolic and endocrine disorders and prolonged immobility. Some muscle atrophy also occurs with aging.

Assessment

Ask the patient when and where he first noticed the muscle wasting and how it has progressed. Review the patient's medical history for chronic illnesses; musculoskeletal or neurologic disorders, including trauma; and endocrine and metabolic disorders. Ask about his use of alcohol and drugs, particularly steroids.

Begin the physical examination by determining the location and extent of atrophy. Check all major muscle groups for size, tonicity, and strength. (See *Testing muscle strength*, pages 376 and 377.) Measure the circumference of all limbs, comparing sides. (See *Measuring limb circumference*.) Check for muscle contractures in all limbs by fully extending joints and noting pain or resistance. Complete the examination by palpating peripheral pulses for quality and rate, assessing sensory function, and testing deep tendon reflexes.

Causes

◆ *Amyotrophic lateral sclerosis (ALS).* Initial symptoms of ALS include muscle weakness and atrophy that typically begin in one hand, spread to the arm, and then develop in the other hand and arm. Eventually, weakness and atrophy spread to the trunk, neck, tongue, larynx, pharynx, and legs.

◆ *Hypothyroidism.* Reversible weakness and atrophy of proximal limb muscles may occur in hypothyroidism.

◆ *Meniscal tear.* Quadriceps muscle atrophy, resulting from prolonged knee immobility and muscle weakness, is a classic sign of a meniscal tear.

◆ *Multiple sclerosis (MS).* MS is a degenerative disease that may produce arm and leg atrophy as a result of chronic progressive weakness; spasticity and contractures may also develop.

◆ *Osteoarthritis.* Osteoarthritis is a chronic disorder that eventually causes atrophy proximal to involved joints as a result of progressive weakness and disuse.

◆ *Parkinson's disease.* With Parkinson's disease, muscle rigidity, weakness, and disuse may produce muscle atrophy.

◆ *Peripheral neuropathy.* With peripheral neuropathy, muscle weakness progresses slowly to flaccid paralysis and eventually atrophy. Distal extremity muscles are generally affected first.

◆ *Protein deficiency.* If chronic, protein deficiency may lead to muscle weakness and atrophy. Other findings include chronic fatigue, apathy, anorexia, dry skin, peripheral edema, and dull, sparse, dry hair.

◆ *Rheumatoid arthritis.* Muscle atrophy occurs in the late stages of rheu-

Measuring limb circumference

To ensure accurate and consistent limb circumference measurements, mark and use a consistent reference point each time and measure with the limb in full extension. This illustration shows the correct reference points for arm and leg measurements.

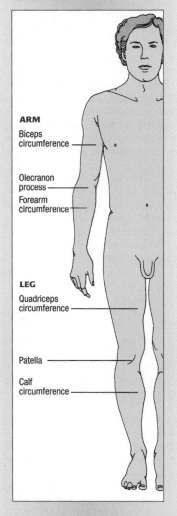

ARM
Biceps circumference

Olecranon process

Forearm circumference

LEG
Quadriceps circumference

Patella

Calf circumference

matoid arthritis as joint pain and stiffness decrease range of motion and discourage muscle use.

◆ *Spinal cord injury.* Trauma to the spinal cord can produce severe muscle weakness and flaccid, then spastic, paralysis, eventually leading to atrophy. Other signs and symptoms depend on the level of injury.

Muscle flaccidity

Flaccid muscles are profoundly weak and soft, with decreased resistance to movement, increased mobility, and a greater than normal range of motion (ROM). The result of disrupted muscle innervation, flaccidity can be localized to a limb or muscle group or generalized over the entire body. Its onset may be acute, such as in trauma, or chronic such as in neurologic disease.

Assessment

Quickly determine the patient's respiratory status, especially noting signs and symptoms of respiratory insufficiency. If the patient isn't in distress, ask about the onset and duration of muscle flaccidity and precipitating factors. Ask about associated symptoms, notably weakness, other muscle changes, and sensory loss or paresthesia.

Examine the affected muscles for atrophy, which indicates a chronic problem. Test muscle strength, and check deep tendon reflexes in all limbs.

Causes

◆ *Amyotrophic lateral sclerosis (ALS).* With ALS, progressive muscle weakness and paralysis are accompanied by generalized flaccidity. Typically, these effects begin in one hand, spread to the arm, and then develop in the other hand and arm. Eventually, they spread to the trunk, neck, tongue, larynx, pharynx, and legs; progressive respiratory muscle weakness leads to respiratory insufficiency.

◆ *Brain lesions.* Frontal and parietal lobe lesions may cause contralateral flaccidity, weakness or paralysis and, eventually, spasticity and possibly contractures.

◆ *Guillain-Barré syndrome.* Guillain-Barré syndrome causes muscle flaccidity. Progression is typically symmetrical and ascending, moving from the feet to the arms and facial nerves within 24 to 72 hours of its onset. Weakness may progress to total motor paralysis and respiratory failure.

◆ *Huntington's disease.* Besides flaccidity caused by Huntington's disease, progressive mental status changes and choreiform movements are major symptoms. Others include poor balance, dysphagia, impaired respirations, and incontinence.

◆ *Muscle disease.* Muscle weakness and flaccidity are features of myopathies and muscular dystrophies.

◆ *Peripheral nerve trauma.* Flaccidity, paralysis, and loss of sensation and reflexes in the innervated area can occur if there has been peripheral nerve trauma.

◆ *Peripheral neuropathy.* With peripheral neuropathy, flaccidity usually occurs in the legs as a result of chronic progressive muscle weakness and paralysis. It may also cause burning pain, glossy red skin, anhidrosis, and a loss of vibration sensation.

◆ *Spinal cord injury.* Spinal shock can result in acute muscle flaccidity or spasticity below the level of injury.

Muscle spasms

Muscle spasms are strong, painful contractions. They can occur in virtually any muscle, but are most common in the calf and foot. Muscle spasms typi-

EMERGENCY INTERVENTIONS

Responding to hypocalcemia

If your patient shows signs of hypocalcemia:
◆ Observe him for laryngospasm.
◆ Provide supplemental oxygen, as necessary.
◆ Prepare for endotracheal intubation and mechanical ventilation, as necessary.

◆ Obtain blood samples for calcium and electrolyte levels and arterial blood gas analysis.
◆ Insert an I.V. catheter for possible administration of a calcium supplement.
◆ Monitor the patient's cardiac status, and prepare to begin resuscitation if necessary.

cally occur from simple muscle fatigue, after exercise, and during pregnancy. However, they may also develop in electrolyte imbalances and neuromuscular disorders or as the result of certain drugs. They're typically precipitated by movement, especially a quick or jerking movement, and can usually be relieved by slow stretching.

Assessment

If the patient complains of frequent or unrelieved spasms in many muscles accompanied by paresthesia in his hands and feet, quickly attempt to elicit Chvostek's and Trousseau's signs. If these signs are present, suspect hypocalcemia. (See *Responding to hypocalcemia.*) If the patient isn't in distress, ask when the spasms began. Is there a particular activity that precipitates them? Did anything worsen or lessen the pain? Ask about other symptoms, such as weakness, sensory loss, or paresthesia.

Evaluate muscle strength and tone and note whether movements precipitate spasms. Test the presence and quality of all peripheral pulses, and examine the limbs for color and temperature changes. Test the capillary refill time, and inspect for edema, especially in the involved area. Observe for signs and symptoms of dehydration. Obtain

a thorough drug and diet history. Ask the patient if he has had recent vomiting or diarrhea. Finally, test reflexes and sensory function in all extremities.

Causes

◆ *Amyotrophic lateral sclerosis (ALS).* With ALS, muscle spasms may accompany progressive muscle weakness and atrophy that typically begin in one hand, spread to the arm, and then spread to the other hand and arm.
◆ *Arterial occlusive disease.* Arterial occlusion typically produces spasms and intermittent claudication in the leg, with residual pain.
◆ *Dehydration.* Sodium loss with dehydration may produce limb and abdominal cramps. Other findings include decreased skin turgor, dry mucous membranes, tachycardia, hypotension, muscle twitching, seizures, and oliguria.
◆ *Drugs.* Common spasm-producing drugs include diuretics, corticosteroids, and estrogens.
◆ *Hypocalcemia.* The classic feature of hypocalcemia is tetany—a syndrome of muscle cramps and twitching, carpopedal and facial muscle spasms, and seizures, possibly with stridor. Chvostek's and Trousseau's signs may be elicited.
◆ *Muscle trauma.* Excessive muscle strain may cause mild to severe

spasms. The injured area may be painful, swollen, reddened, or warm.

◤ *Respiratory alkalosis.* With respiratory alkalosis, the acute onset of muscle spasms may be accompanied by twitching and weakness, carpopedal spasm, and circumoral and peripheral paresthesia.

◆ *Spinal injury or disease.* Muscle spasms can result from spinal injury, such as a cervical extension injury or spinous process fracture, or from spinal disease such as infection.

Muscle spasticity

Spasticity is a state of excessive muscle tone manifested by increased resistance to stretching and heightened reflexes. It's commonly detected by evaluating a muscle's response to passive movement; a spastic muscle offers more resistance when the passive movement is performed quickly. Caused by an upper motor neuron lesion, spasticity usually occurs in the arm and leg muscles. Long-term spasticity results in muscle fibrosis and contractures. (See *How spasticity develops.*)

Assessment

When you detect spasticity, ask the patient about its onset, duration, and progression. What, if any, events precipitate its onset? Has he experienced other muscular changes or related symptoms? Does his medical history reveal an incidence of trauma or a degenerative or vascular disease?

Take the patient's vital signs, and perform a complete neurologic examination. Test the patient's reflexes and evaluate motor and sensory function in all limbs. Evaluate muscles for wasting and contractures. During your examination, keep in mind that generalized spasticity and trismus in a patient with

a recent skin puncture or laceration indicates tetanus. If you suspect this rare disorder, look for signs of respiratory distress. Provide ventilatory support, if necessary, and monitor the patient closely.

Causes

◆ *Amyotrophic lateral sclerosis (ALS).* ALS commonly produces spasticity, spasms, coarse fasciculations, hyperactive deep tendon reflexes (DTRs), and a positive Babinski's sign.

◤ *Epidural hemorrhage.* With epidural hemorrhage, bilateral limb spasticity is a late and ominous sign. Other findings include a momentary loss of consciousness after head trauma, followed by a lucid interval and then a rapid deterioration in the level of consciousness.

◆ *Spinal cord injury.* Spasticity commonly results from cervical and high thoracic spinal cord injury, especially from incomplete lesions. Spastic paralysis in the affected limbs follows initial flaccid paralysis; typically, spasticity and muscle atrophy increase for up to $1\frac{1}{4}$ to 2 years after the injury, and then gradually regress to flaccidity.

◤ *Stroke.* Spastic paralysis may develop on the affected side following the acute stage of a stroke. Associated findings vary with the site and extent of vascular damage.

◤ *Tetanus.* Tetanus is a rare, life-threatening disease that produces varying degrees of spasticity. In generalized tetanus—the most common form—early signs and symptoms include painful jaw and neck stiffness, trismus, headache, irritability, restlessness, a low-grade fever with chills, tachycardia, diaphoresis, and hyperactive DTRs.

How spasticity develops

Motor activity is controlled by pyramidal and extrapyramidal tracts that originate in the motor cortex, basal ganglia, brain stem, and spinal cord. Nerve fibers from the various tracts converge and synapse at the anterior horn in the spinal cord. Together, they maintain segmental muscle tone by modulating the stretch reflex arc. This arc, shown in simplified form below, is basically a negative feedback loop in which muscle stretch (stimulation) causes reflexive contraction (inhibition), thus maintaining muscle length and tone.

Damage to certain tracts results in a loss of inhibition and a disruption of the stretch reflex arc. Uninhibited muscle stretch produces exaggerated, uncontrolled muscle activity, accentuating the reflex arc and eventually resulting in spasticity.

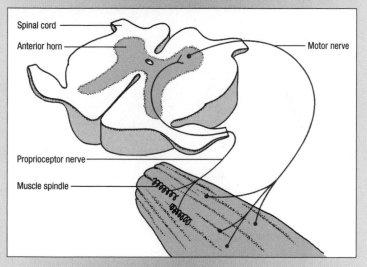

Spinal cord
Anterior horn
Motor nerve
Proprioceptor nerve
Muscle spindle

Muscle weakness

Muscle weakness is detected by observing and measuring the strength of an individual muscle or muscle group. It occurs with certain neurologic, musculoskeletal, metabolic, endocrine, and cardiovascular disorders, as a response to certain drugs, and after prolonged immobilization.

Assessment

Begin by determining the location of the patient's muscle weakness. Ask if he has difficulty with specific movements. Find out when he first noticed the weakness and whether it worsens with exercise or as the day progresses. Also ask about related symptoms, especially muscle or joint pain, altered sensory function, and fatigue. Obtain a medical history, noting chronic disease, such as hyperthyroidism, musculo-

(Text continues on page 378.)

Testing muscle strength

Obtain an overall picture of the patient's motor function by testing strength in 10 selected muscle groups. Ask him to attempt normal range-of-motion movements against your resistance. If the muscle group is weak, vary the amount of resistance as needed to permit accurate assessment. If necessary, position the patient so his limbs don't have to resist gravity, and repeat the test.

Arm muscles

Biceps. With your hand on the patient's hand, have him flex his forearm against your resistance. Watch for biceps contraction.

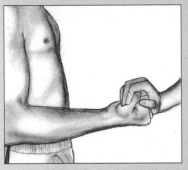

Deltoid. With the patient's arm fully extended, place one hand over his deltoid muscle and the other on his wrist. Ask him to abduct his arm to a horizontal position against your resistance; as he does so, palpate for deltoid contraction.

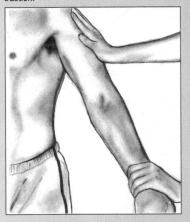

Triceps. Have the patient abduct and hold his arm midway between flexion and extension. Hold and support his arm at the wrist, and ask him to extend it against your resistance. Watch for triceps contraction.

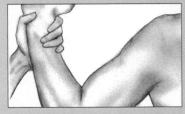

Dorsal interossei. Have the patient extend and spread his fingers, and tell him to try to resist your attempt to squeeze them together.

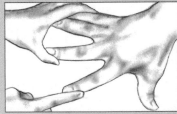

Forearm and hand (grip). Have the patient grasp your middle and index fingers and squeeze as hard as he can. To prevent pain or injury to the examiner, the examiner should cross his fingers.

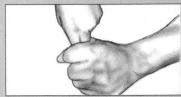

Rate muscle strength on a scale of 0 to 5:
0 = No evidence of muscle contraction
1 = Visible or palpable contraction but no movement
2 = Full muscle movement with force of gravity eliminated
3 = Full muscle movement against gravity but no movement against resistance
4 = Full muscle movement against gravity; partial movement against resistance
5 = Full muscle movement against gravity and resistance—normal strength

Leg muscles

Anterior tibial. With the patient's leg extended, place your hand on his foot and ask him to dorsiflex his ankle against your resistance. Palpate for anterior tibial contraction.

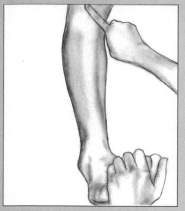

Psoas. While you support his leg, have the patient raise his knee and then flex his hip against your resistance. Watch for psoas contraction.

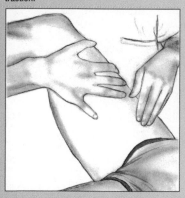

Extensor hallucis longus. With your finger on the patient's great toe, have him dorsiflex the toe against your resistance. Palpate for extensor hallucis contraction.

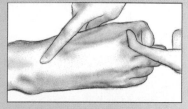

Quadriceps. Have the patient bend his knee slightly while you support his lower leg. Then ask him to extend the knee against your resistance; as he's doing so, palpate for quadriceps contraction.

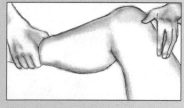

Gastrocnemius. With the patient on his side, support his foot and ask him to plantar flex his ankle against your resistance. Palpate for gastrocnemius contraction.

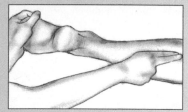

skeletal or neurologic problems, and alcohol and drug use.

Focus your physical examination on evaluating muscle strength bilaterally. (See *Testing muscle strength,* pages 376 and 377.) When testing, make sure that the patient's effort is constant; if it isn't, suspect pain or other reluctance to make the effort. If the patient complains of pain, ease or discontinue testing. Remember that the patient's dominant arm, hand, and leg are somewhat stronger than the nondominant counterparts. Test for range of motion at all major joints, sensory function in the involved areas, and deep tendon reflexes bilaterally.

Causes

◆ *Amyotrophic lateral sclerosis (ALS).* ALS typically begins with muscle weakness and atrophy in one hand that rapidly spread to the arm and then to the other hand and arm.

◆ *Anemia.* With anemia, varying degrees of muscle weakness and fatigue are exacerbated by exertion and temporarily relieved by rest.

◆ *Guillain-Barré syndrome.* With Guillain-Barré syndrome, rapidly progressive, symmetrical weakness and pain ascends from the feet to the arms and facial nerves. It may progress to total motor paralysis and respiratory failure.

◆ *Herniated disk.* Pressure on nerve roots from a herniated disk leads to muscle weakness. Diminished reflexes and sensory changes may also occur.

◆ *Hypercortisolism.* Hypercortisolism may cause limb weakness and eventually atrophy.

◆ *Myasthenia gravis.* Gradually progressive skeletal muscle weakness and fatigue are the cardinal symptoms of myasthenia gravis. Typically, weakness is mild upon awakening, but worsens during the day.

◆ *Osteoarthritis.* Osteoarthritis is a chronic disorder that causes progressive muscle weakness that leads to atrophy.

◆ *Parkinson's disease.* Muscle weakness accompanies rigidity in Parkinson's disease.

◆ *Peripheral nerve trauma.* Prolonged pressure on or injury to a peripheral nerve causes muscle weakness and atrophy. Other findings include paresthesia or sensory loss, pain, and loss of reflexes supplied by the damaged nerve.

◆ *Potassium imbalance.* With hypokalemia, temporary generalized muscle weakness may be accompanied by decreased mentation, leg cramps, polyuria, dizziness, hypotension, and arrhythmias. With hyperkalemia, weakness may progress to flaccid paralysis accompanied by confusion, hyperreflexia, paresthesia, oliguria, and arrhythmias.

◆ *Rhabdomyolysis.* Signs and symptoms of rhabdomyolysis include muscle weakness or pain. Acute renal failure, caused by obstruction and injury from the kidneys' attempt to filter myoglobin from the bloodstream, is common.

◆ *Rheumatoid arthritis.* With rheumatoid arthritis, symmetrical muscle weakness may accompany pain, stiffness, and increased warmth, swelling, and tenderness in involved joints.

◆ *Spinal trauma and disease.* Trauma can cause severe muscle weakness, leading to flaccidity or spasticity and, eventually, paralysis. Infection, tumor, and cervical spondylosis or stenosis can also cause muscle weakness.

◼ *Stroke.* Depending on the site and extent of damage, a stroke may produce contralateral or bilateral weakness of the arms, legs, face, and tongue, possibly progressing to hemiplegia and atrophy.

Mydriasis

Mydriasis—pupillary dilation caused by contraction of the dilator of the iris—is a normal response to decreased light, strong emotional stimuli, and topical administration of mydriatic and cycloplegic drugs. It can also result from ocular and neurologic disorders, eye trauma, and disorders that decrease the patient's level of consciousness (LOC). Mydriasis may be an adverse effect of antihistamines or other drugs.

Assessment

Begin by asking the patient about other eye problems, such as pain, blurring, diplopia, or visual field defects. Obtain a health history, focusing on eye or head trauma, glaucoma and other ocular problems, and neurologic and vascular disorders. In addition, obtain a complete drug history.

Next, perform a thorough eye and pupil examination. Inspect and compare the pupils' size, color, and shape—many people normally have unequal pupils. (See *Grading pupil size*.) Also, test each pupil for light reflex, consensual response, and accommodation. Perform a swinging flashlight test to evaluate a decreased response to direct light coupled with a normal consensual response (Marcus Gunn pupil). Be sure to check the eyes for ptosis, swelling, and ecchymosis. Test visual acuity in both eyes with and without correction. Evaluate extraocular muscle function by checking the six cardinal fields of gaze. (See *Testing extraocular muscles,* page 217.)

Keep in mind that mydriasis appears in two ocular emergencies: acute angle-closure glaucoma and traumatic iridoplegia.

Grading pupil size

To accurately evaluate pupil size, compare the patient's pupils with the scale shown here. Keep in mind that the maximum constriction may be less than 1 mm and the maximum dilation greater than 9 mm.

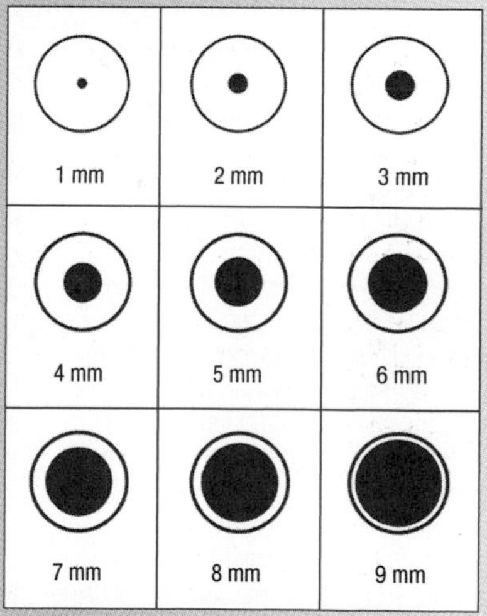

1 mm   2 mm   3 mm
4 mm   5 mm   6 mm
7 mm   8 mm   9 mm

Causes

◆ *Adie's syndrome.* Adie's syndrome is characterized by abrupt unilateral mydriasis, poor or absent pupillary reflexes, blurred vision, and cramplike eye pain.

◆ *Aortic arch syndrome.* Bilateral pupillary mydriasis commonly occurs late in aortic arch syndrome. Other ocular findings include blurred vision, transient vision loss, and diplopia.

◾ *Botulism.* Botulism toxin causes bilateral mydriasis, usually 12 to 36 hours after ingestion. Other early findings are a loss of pupillary reflexes, blurred vision, diplopia, ptosis, strabismus, and extraocular muscle palsies.

◾ *Carotid artery aneurysm.* With carotid artery aneurysm, bitemporal hemianopsia, decreased visual acuity, hemiplegia, a decreased LOC, aphasia, behavioral changes, and hypoesthesia may accompany unilateral mydriasis.

◾ *Glaucoma (acute angle-closure).* Acute angle-closure glaucoma is an ocular emergency that's characterized by moderate mydriasis and the loss of the pupillary reflex in the affected eye, accompanied by an abrupt onset of excruciating pain, redness, decreased visual acuity, blurred vision, halo vision, conjunctival injection, and a cloudy cornea. Without treatment, permanent blindness occurs in 2 to 5 days.

◆ *Oculomotor nerve palsy.* Unilateral mydriasis is commonly the first sign of oculomotor nerve palsy. It's soon followed by ptosis, diplopia, decreased pupillary reflexes, exotropia, and complete loss of accommodation.

◆ *Traumatic iridoplegia.* Eye trauma can paralyze the sphincter of the iris, causing mydriasis and the loss of the pupillary reflex; usually, this is transient. Associated findings include a quivering iris (iridodonesis), ecchymosis, pain, and swelling.

Myoclonus

Myoclonus—sudden, shocklike contractions of a single muscle or muscle group—occurs with various neurologic disorders and may herald the onset of a seizure. These contractions may be isolated or repetitive, rhythmic or arrhythmic, symmetrical or asymmetrical, synchronous or asynchronous, and generalized or focal. They may be precipitated by bright flickering lights, a loud sound, or unexpected physical contact. One type, intention myoclonus, is evoked by intentional muscle movement. Myoclonus occurs normally just before falling asleep and as a part of the natural startle reaction. It also occurs with some poisonings and, rarely, as a complication of hemodialysis.

Assessment

If you observe myoclonus, check for seizure activity. Take the patient's vital signs to rule out arrhythmias or a blocked airway. If the patient is stable, evaluate his level of consciousness (LOC) and mental status. Ask about the frequency, severity, location, and circumstances of myoclonus. Has he ever had a seizure? If so, did myoclonus precede it? Is myoclonus ever precipitated by a sensory stimulus? During the physical examination, check for muscle rigidity and wasting, and test deep tendon reflexes.

Causes

◆ *Alzheimer's disease.* Generalized myoclonus may occur in advanced stages of Alzheimer's disease, a slowly progressive dementia.

◆ *Creutzfeldt-Jakob disease.* Diffuse myoclonic jerks appear early in Creutzfeldt-Jakob disease, a rapidly progressive dementia. Initially random, they gradually become more rhythmic and symmetrical, usually occurring in response to sensory stimuli.

◆ *Encephalitis (viral).* With viral encephalitis, myoclonus is usually intermittent. Associated findings vary, but may include a rapidly decreasing LOC, nuchal rigidity, facial muscle weakness, nystagmus, and ocular palsies.

◆ *Encephalopathy.* Hepatic encephalopathy occasionally produces myoclonic jerks in association with asterixis and focal or generalized seizures. Hypoxic encephalopathy may produce generalized myoclonus or seizures almost immediately after restoration of cardiopulmonary function. The patient may also have a residual intention myoclonus. Uremic encephalopathy commonly produces myoclonic jerks and seizures.

◆ *Epilepsy.* With idiopathic epilepsy, localized myoclonus is usually confined to an arm or leg and occurs singly or in short bursts, usually upon awakening. It's usually more frequent and severe during the prodromal stage of a major generalized seizure, after which it diminishes in frequency and intensity. Myoclonic jerks are usually the first signs of myoclonic epilepsy, the most common cause of progressive myoclonus. At first, myoclonus is infrequent and localized, but over a period of months, it becomes more frequent and involves the entire body, disrupting voluntary movement (intention myoclonus). As the disease progresses, myoclonus is accompanied by generalized seizures and dementia.

N

Nasal flaring

Nasal flaring is the abnormal dilation of the nostrils. Usually occurring during inspiration, nasal flaring may occasionally occur during expiration or throughout the respiratory cycle. It indicates respiratory dysfunction, ranging from mild difficulty to potentially life-threatening respiratory distress.

Assessment

If you note nasal flaring in the patient, quickly evaluate his respiratory status. Absent breath sounds, cyanosis, diaphoresis, and tachycardia point to complete airway obstruction. (See *Responding to nasal flaring.*) When the patient's condition is stabilized, obtain a pertinent history. Ask about cardiac and pulmonary disorders such as asthma. Does the patient have allergies? Has he experienced a recent illness, such as a respiratory tract infection, or trauma? Does the patient smoke or have a history of smoking? Obtain a drug history.

Causes

◄ *Acute respiratory distress syndrome (ARDS).* ARDS causes increased respiratory difficulty and hypoxemia, with nasal flaring, dyspnea, tachypnea, diaphoresis, cyanosis, scattered crackles, and rhonchi.

◄ *Airway obstruction.* Complete obstruction above the tracheal bifurcation causes sudden nasal flaring, absent breath sounds despite intercostal retractions and marked accessory muscle use, tachycardia, diaphoresis, cyanosis and, eventually, respiratory arrest. Partial obstruction causes nasal flaring with inspiratory stridor, gagging, wheezing, a violent cough, marked accessory muscle use, agitation, cyanosis, and hoarseness.

◄ *Anaphylaxis.* Severe reactions can produce respiratory distress with nasal flaring, stridor, wheezing, accessory muscle use, intercostal retractions, and dyspnea.

◆ *Asthma (acute).* An asthma attack can cause nasal flaring, dyspnea, tachypnea, prolonged expiratory wheezing, accessory muscle use, cyanosis, and a dry or productive cough.

◆ *Chronic obstructive pulmonary disease (COPD).* COPD can lead to acute respiratory failure secondary to pulmonary infection or edema. Nasal flaring is accompanied by prolonged pursed-lip expiration, accessory muscle use, and a loose, rattling, productive cough.

◄ *Pneumothorax.* Pneumothorax can result in respiratory distress with nasal

◆

EMERGENCY INTERVENTIONS

Responding to nasal flaring

Nasal flaring can be caused by respiratory difficulties ranging from obstruction to respiratory distress. If the patient shows signs of obstruction, take the following steps:
◆ Deliver back blows or abdominal thrusts, as indicated, to relieve an obstruction.
◆ Prepare for emergency intubation or tracheostomy.
◆ Prepare to begin mechanical ventilation, if indicated.

If the patient displays breathing difficulty, take these steps:

◆ Administer oxygen by nasal cannula or face mask.
◆ Insert an I.V. catheter for the administration of fluids and medications.
◆ Connect the patient to a cardiac monitor.
◆ Obtain a chest X-ray.
◆ Obtain blood samples for arterial blood gas analysis and electrolyte studies.
◆ Prepare for intubation and mechanical ventilation, if necessary.

flaring, dyspnea, tachypnea, sharp chest pain, jugular vein distention, tracheal deviation, and cyanosis. Breath sounds and chest wall motion may be decreased or absent on the affected side. Similar findings can occur with hydrothorax, chylothorax, or hemothorax, depending on the amount of fluid accumulation.

◪ *Pulmonary edema.* Pulmonary edema typically produces nasal flaring, severe dyspnea, wheezing, and a cough that produces frothy, pink sputum. Increased accessory muscle use may occur.

◪ *Pulmonary embolus.* Signs of pulmonary embolus may include nasal flaring, dyspnea, tachypnea, wheezing, cyanosis, a pleural friction rub, and a productive cough (possibly hemoptysis).

Nausea

Nausea is a sensation of profound revulsion to food or of impending vomiting. Typically, it's accompanied by autonomic signs, such as hypersalivation, diaphoresis, tachycardia, pallor, and tachypnea. It's a common symptom of GI disorders, and also occurs with fluid and electrolyte imbalance; infection; metabolic, endocrine, labyrinthine, and cardiac disorders; and as a result of drug therapy, surgery, and radiation. Commonly present during the first trimester of pregnancy, nausea may also arise from severe pain, anxiety, alcohol intoxication, overeating, or ingestion of distasteful food or liquids.

Assessment

Begin by obtaining a complete medical history. Focus on GI, endocrine, and metabolic disorders; recent infections; and cancer and its treatment. If the patient is a female of childbearing age, ask if she is or could be pregnant. Have the patient describe the nausea as well as what causes or relieves it. Ask about related complaints, particularly vomiting (color, amount), abdominal pain, and changes in bowel habits or stool character.

Inspect the skin for jaundice, bruises, and spider angiomas, and assess skin turgor. Next, inspect the abdomen for distention, auscultate for bowel sounds and bruits, palpate for rigidity and tenderness, and test for rebound tenderness. Palpate and percuss the liver for enlargement. Assess other body systems as appropriate.

Causes

◆ *Adrenal insufficiency.* Common GI findings in adrenal insufficiency include nausea, vomiting, anorexia, and diarrhea.

◆ *Appendicitis.* With acute appendicitis, a brief period of nausea may accompany the onset of vague epigastric or periumbilical discomfort, which rapidly progresses to severe stabbing pain localized in the right lower quadrant.

◆ *Cholecystitis (acute).* With acute cholecystitis, nausea commonly follows severe right upper quadrant pain that may radiate to the back or shoulders, usually following meals.

◆ *Cholelithiasis.* With cholelithiasis, nausea accompanies attacks of severe right upper quadrant or epigastric pain after eating fatty foods. Other findings may include epigastric burning, jaundice, and clay-colored stools.

◆ *Diverticulitis.* Besides nausea, diverticulitis causes intermittent crampy abdominal pain, constipation or diarrhea, a low-grade fever and, commonly, a palpable, tender, firm, fixed mass.

◆ *Gastritis.* Nausea is common with gastritis, especially after ingestion of alcohol, aspirin, spicy foods, or caffeine. Vomiting of mucus or blood, epigastric pain, belching, fever, and malaise may also occur.

◆ *Gastroenteritis.* Usually viral, gastroenteritis causes nausea, vomiting, diarrhea, and abdominal cramping.

◆ *Heart failure.* Heart failure may produce nausea and vomiting, particularly with right-sided heart failure.

◆ *Hepatitis.* Nausea is an insidious early symptom of viral hepatitis. Vomiting, fatigue, myalgia and arthralgia, headache, anorexia, photophobia, pharyngitis, cough, and fever also occur early in the preicteric phase.

◆ *Hyperemesis gravidarum.* Unremitting nausea and vomiting that persist beyond the first trimester of pregnancy are characteristic of hyperemesis gravidarum. Vomitus ranges from undigested food, mucus, and bile early in the disorder to a coffee-ground appearance in later stages.

◆ *Intestinal obstruction.* Nausea commonly occurs, especially with high small-intestinal obstruction. Vomiting may be bilious or fecal; abdominal pain is usually episodic and colicky.

◆ *Ménière's disease.* Ménière's disease causes sudden, brief, recurrent attacks of nausea, vomiting, vertigo, tinnitus, diaphoresis, and nystagmus. It also causes hearing loss and ear fullness.

◆ *Mesenteric venous thrombosis.* An insidious or acute onset of nausea, vomiting, and abdominal pain occurs with diarrhea or constipation, abdominal distention, hematemesis, and melena.

◆ *Metabolic acidosis.* Metabolic acidosis is an acid-base imbalance that may produce nausea and vomiting, anorexia, diarrhea, and Kussmaul's respirations.

◆ *Migraine headache.* Nausea and vomiting may occur in the prodromal stage, along with photophobia, light flashes, increased sensitivity to noise, and light-headedness.

◆ *Motion sickness.* With motion sickness, nausea and vomiting are brought on by motion or rhythmic movement. Headache, dizziness, fatigue, diaphoresis, hypersalivation, and dyspnea may also occur.

◼ *Myocardial infarction (MI).* Nausea and vomiting may occur during an MI, but the cardinal symptom is severe substernal chest pain that may radiate to the left arm, jaw, or neck.

◼ *Pancreatitis (acute).* Nausea, usually followed by vomiting, is an early symptom of pancreatitis. Another common finding is steady, severe pain in the epigastrium or left upper quadrant that may radiate to the back.

◆ *Peptic ulcer.* With peptic ulcer, nausea and vomiting may follow attacks of sharp or gnawing, burning epigastric pain. Attacks typically occur when the stomach is empty or after the ingestion of alcohol, caffeine, or aspirin.

◆ *Peritonitis.* Nausea and vomiting usually accompany acute abdominal pain localized to the area of inflammation.

◆ *Preeclampsia.* Nausea and vomiting commonly occur with preeclampsia along with rapid weight gain, oliguria, and a severe frontal headache. The classic diagnostic triad of signs include hypertension, proteinuria, and edema.

Neck pain

Neck pain may originate from any neck structure, ranging from the meninges and cervical vertebrae to its blood vessels, muscles, and lymphatic tissue. This symptom can also be referred from other areas of the body. Its location, onset, and pattern help determine the origin and underlying causes. Neck pain usually results from trauma and degenerative, congenital, inflammatory, metabolic, and neoplastic disorders.

Assessment

If the patient's neck pain is due to trauma, first ensure proper cervical spine immobilization, preferably with a long backboard and a Philadelphia collar. (See *Applying a Philadelphia collar*, page 386.) Then take his vital signs, and perform a quick neurologic examination. Examine the neck for abrasions, swelling, lacerations, erythema, and ecchymoses. If the patient hasn't sustained trauma, find out the severity and onset of his neck pain. Where specifically in the neck does he feel pain? Does anything relieve or worsen the pain? Also, ask about other symptoms such as headaches. Next, focus on the patient's current and past illnesses and injuries, diet, and drug history.

Thoroughly inspect the patient's neck, shoulders, and cervical spine. Assess active range of motion (ROM) in his neck by having him perform flexion, extension, rotation, and lateral side bending. Note the degree of pain produced by these movements. Examine his posture, and test and compare bilateral muscle strength. Check the sensation in his arms, and assess his hand grasp and arm reflexes. Attempt to elicit Brudzinski's and Kernig's signs if there isn't a history of neck trauma, and palpate the cervical lymph nodes for enlargement.

Causes

◆ *Ankylosing spondylitis.* Intermittent, moderate to severe neck pain and stiffness with a severely restricted ROM is characteristic of ankylosing spondylitis.

◆ *Cervical extension injury.* Anterior or posterior neck pain may develop within hours or days following a whiplash or cervical extension injury. Anterior pain usually diminishes with-

Applying a Philadelphia collar

The Philadelphia cervical collar is a lightweight, molded polyethylene collar designed to hold the neck straight with the chin slightly elevated and tucked in. When applied, the collar immobilizes the cervical spine, decreases muscle spasms, and relieves some pain. It also prevents further injury and promotes healing.

When applying the collar, fit it snugly around the patient's neck and attach the Velcro fasteners or buckles at the back. Be sure to check the patient's airway and his neurovascular status to ensure that the collar isn't too tight. Also, make sure that the collar isn't placed too high in front, which can hyperextend the neck. In a patient with a neck sprain, hyperextension may cause the ligaments to heal in a shortened position; in a patient with a cervical spine fracture, it could cause serious neurologic damage.

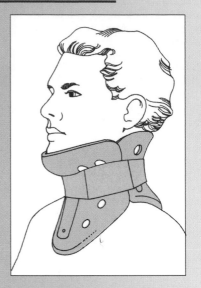

in several days, but posterior pain persists and may even intensify.

◼ *Cervical spine fracture.* Fracture at C1 to C4 can cause sudden death; survivors may experience severe neck pain that restricts all movement, an intense occipital headache, quadriplegia, deformity, and respiratory paralysis.

◆ *Cervical spine tumor.* Metastatic tumors typically produce persistent neck pain that increases with movement and isn't relieved by rest; primary tumors cause mild to severe pain along a specific nerve root.

◆ *Cervical spondylosis.* Cervical spondylosis is a degenerative process that produces posterior neck pain that restricts movement and is aggravated by it. Pain may radiate down either arm and may accompany paresthesia and weakness.

◼ *Esophageal trauma.* An esophageal mucosal tear or a pulsion diverticulum may produce mild neck pain, chest pain, edema, hemoptysis, and dysphagia.

◆ *Herniated cervical disk.* A herniated disk causes variable neck pain that restricts movement and is aggravated by it. It also causes referred pain along a specific dermatome, paresthesia, and arm weakness.

◆ *Laryngeal cancer.* Neck pain that radiates to the ear develops late in laryngeal cancer.

◆ *Lymphadenitis.* With lymphadenitis, enlarged and inflamed cervical lymph nodes cause acute pain and tenderness.

◄ *Meningitis.* With meningitis, neck pain may accompany characteristic nuchal rigidity.

◆ *Neck sprain.* Minor sprains typically produce pain, slight swelling, stiffness, and restricted ROM. Ligament rupture causes pain, marked swelling, ecchymosis, muscle spasms, and nuchal rigidity with head tilt.

◆ *Rheumatoid arthritis.* Rheumatoid arthritis usually affects peripheral joints, but it can also involve the cervical vertebrae. Acute inflammation may cause moderate to severe pain that radiates along a specific nerve root.

◆ *Spinous process fracture.* A fracture near the cervicothoracic junction produces acute pain radiating to the shoulders. Other findings include swelling, exquisite tenderness, restricted ROM, muscle spasms, and deformity.

◄ *Subarachnoid hemorrhage.* Subarachnoid hemorrhage may cause moderate to severe neck pain and rigidity, headache, and a decreased LOC. Kernig's and Brudzinski's signs are present. The patient may describe the headache as, "the worst headache of my life."

◆ *Thyroid trauma.* Besides mild to moderate neck pain, thyroid trauma may cause local swelling and ecchymosis.

◆ *Torticollis.* Torticollis is a neck deformity in which severe neck pain accompanies recurrent unilateral stiffness and muscle spasms that produce a characteristic head tilt.

◄ *Tracheal trauma.* A fracture of the tracheal cartilage produces moderate to severe neck pain and respiratory difficulty. Torn tracheal mucosa produces mild to moderate pain and may result in airway occlusion, hemoptysis, hoarseness, and dysphagia.

Nipple discharge

Nipple discharge can occur spontaneously or can be elicited by nipple stimulation. It's characterized as intermittent or constant, unilateral or bilateral, and by color, consistency, and composition. Its incidence increases with age and parity. This sign rarely occurs (but is more likely to indicate a disorder) in men and in nulligravid, regularly menstruating women. It's relatively common and typically normal in parous women. A thick, grayish discharge—benign epithelial debris from inactive ducts—may occur in middle-age parous women. Colostrum, a thin, yellowish or milky discharge, commonly occurs in the last weeks of pregnancy. Nipple discharge can signal serious underlying disease, particularly when accompanied by other breast changes. Significant causes include endocrine disorders, tumors, certain drugs, and blocked lactiferous ducts.

Assessment

Ask the patient when she first noticed the discharge, and determine its duration, extent, quantity, color, consistency, and smell, if any. Has she had other nipple and breast changes, such as pain, tenderness, itching, warmth, changes in contour, and lumps? Obtain a complete gynecologic and obstetric history, and determine her normal menstrual cycle and the date of her last period. Is the patient taking hormones? Ask if she experiences breast swelling and tenderness, bloating, irritability, headaches, abdominal cramping, nausea, or diarrhea before or during menses. Note the number, date, and outcome of her pregnancies and, if she breast-fed, the approximate time of her

Eliciting nipple discharge

If the patient has a history or evidence of nipple discharge, you can attempt to elicit it during your examination. Help the patient into a supine position, and gently squeeze her nipple between your thumb and index finger (as shown below). Note any discharge through the nipple.

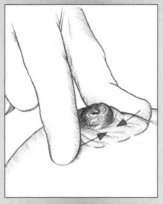

Then place your fingers on the areola, as shown below, and palpate the entire areolar surface, watching for a discharge through areolar ducts.

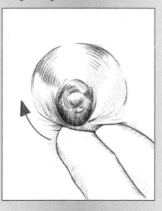

last lactation. Also, check for risk factors of breast cancer.

Start your physical examination by characterizing the discharge. If the discharge isn't spontaneous, try to elicit it. (See *Eliciting nipple discharge.*) Then examine the nipples and breasts with the patient in four different positions: sitting with her arms at her sides, with her arms overhead, with her hands pressing on her hips, and leaning forward so her breasts are suspended. Check for nipple deviation, flattening, retraction, redness, asymmetry, thickening, excoriation, erosion, or cracking. Inspect her breasts for asymmetry, irregular contours, dimpling, erythema, and peau d'orange. With the patient supine, palpate the breasts and axillae for lumps, giving special attention to the areolae. Note the size, location, delineation, consistency, and mobility of any lump you find.

Causes

◆ *Breast abscess.* Breast abscess, most common in breast-feeding women, may produce a thick, purulent discharge from a cracked nipple or infected duct.
◆ *Breast cancer.* Breast cancer may cause bloody, watery, or purulent discharge from a normal-appearing nipple.
◆ *Choriocarcinoma.* Galactorrhea (a white or grayish milky discharge) may result from this highly malignant neoplasm, which can follow pregnancy. Other findings include persistent uterine bleeding and bogginess after delivery or curettage and vaginal masses.
◆ *Drugs.* Galactorrhea can be caused by psychotropic agents, particularly phenothiazines and tricyclic antidepressants; some antihypertensives (reserpine [Serpalan] and methyldopa [Aldomet]); hormonal contraceptives; cimetidine (Tagamet); metoclopramide (Reglan); and verapamil (Calan).

◆ *Intraductal papilloma.* Intraductal papilloma is the primary cause of nipple discharge in the nonpregnant, non–breast-feeding woman. Unilateral serous, serosanguineous, or bloody nipple discharge—usually from only one duct—is its predominant sign.

◆ *Mammary duct ectasia.* A thick, sticky, grayish discharge from multiple ducts may be the first sign of mammary duct ectasia. Other findings include a rubbery, poorly delineated lump beneath the areola, with a blue-green discoloration of the overlying skin, and redness, swelling, tenderness, and burning pain in the areola and nipple.

◆ *Paget's disease.* With Paget's disease, serous or bloody discharge emits from denuded skin on the nipple, which is red, intensely itchy and, possibly, eroded or excoriated. The discharge is usually unilateral.

◆ *Prolactin-secreting pituitary tumor.* Bilateral galactorrhea may occur with a prolactin-secreting pituitary tumor. Other findings include amenorrhea, infertility, decreased libido and vaginal secretions, headaches, and blindness.

◆ *Proliferative (fibrocystic) breast disease.* Proliferative breast disease is a benign disorder that occasionally causes a bilateral clear, milky, or straw-colored discharge, which is rarely purulent or bloody. Multiple round, soft, tender nodules are usually palpable in both breasts, although they may occur singly. Usually, nodules are mobile and are located in the upper outer quadrant.

Nipple retraction

Nipple retraction, the inward displacement of the nipple below the level of surrounding breast tissue, may indicate an inflammatory breast lesion or cancer. It results from scar tissue formation within a lesion or large mammary duct. As the scar tissue shortens, it pulls adjacent tissue inward, causing nipple deviation, flattening and, finally, retraction.

Assessment

Ask the patient when she first noticed the nipple retraction. Has she experienced other nipple changes, such as itching, discoloration, discharge, or excoriation? Has she noticed breast pain, lumps, redness, swelling, or warmth? Obtain a history, noting risk factors of breast cancer, such as a family history or previous malignancy.

Carefully examine both nipples and breasts with the patient sitting upright with her arms at her sides, with her hands pressing on her hips, with her arms overhead, and leaning forward so her breasts are suspended. Look for redness, excoriation, and discharge; nipple flattening and deviation; and breast asymmetry, dimpling, or contour differences. (See *Differentiating nipple retraction from inversion,* page 390.) Try to evert the nipple by gently squeezing the areola. With the patient in a supine position, palpate both breasts for lumps, especially beneath the areola. Mold breast skin over the lump or gently pull it up toward the clavicle, looking for accentuated nipple retraction. Also, palpate axillary lymph nodes.

Causes

◆ *Breast abscess.* Breast abscess, most common in breast-feeding women, occasionally produces unilateral nipple retraction. More common findings include breast pain, erythema, and tenderness; breast induration or a soft mass; and cracked, sore nipples, possibly with a purulent discharge.

Differentiating nipple retraction from inversion

Nipple retraction is sometimes confused with nipple inversion, a common abnormality that's congenital in many patients and doesn't usually signal underlying disease. A *retracted* nipple appears flat and broad, whereas an *inverted* nipple can be pulled out from the sulcus where it hides.

NIPPLE RETRACTION

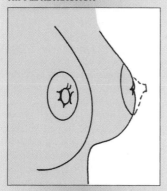

NIPPLE INVERSION

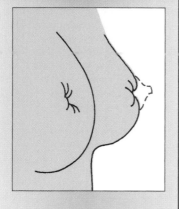

◆ *Breast cancer.* With breast cancer, unilateral nipple retraction is commonly accompanied by a hard, fixed, nontender nodule beneath the areola as well as other breast nodules. Other nipple changes include itching, burning, erosion, and watery or bloody discharge.

◆ *Mammary duct ectasia.* Nipple retraction commonly occurs along with a poorly defined, rubbery nodule beneath the areola, with a blue-green skin discoloration; areolar burning, itching, swelling, tenderness, and erythema; and nipple pain with a thick, sticky, grayish, multiductal discharge.

◆ *Mastitis.* Nipple retraction, deviation, cracking, or flattening may occur in mastitis with a firm and indurated or tender, flocculent, discrete breast nodule; warmth; erythema; tenderness; and edema.

Nocturia

Nocturia—excessive urination at night—may result from disruption of the normal diurnal pattern of urine concentration or from overstimulation of the nerves and muscles that control urination. Normally, more urine is concentrated during the night than during the day. As a result, most people excrete three to four times more urine during the day and can sleep for 6 to 8 hours during the night without being awakened. The patient with nocturia may awaken one or more times during the night to empty his bladder and excrete 700 ml or more of urine.

Although nocturia usually results from renal and lower urinary tract disorders, it may result from certain cardiovascular, endocrine, and metabolic disorders. This common sign may also result from drugs that induce diuresis, particularly when they're taken at night, and from drinking large quantities of fluids, especially caffeinated beverages or alcohol, at bedtime.

Assessment

Begin by exploring the history of the patient's nocturia. When did it begin? How often does it occur? Can the patient identify precipitating factors? Also, note the volume of urine voided. Ask the patient about changes in the color, odor, or consistency of his urine. Has the patient changed his usual pattern or volume of fluid intake? Next, explore associated symptoms. Ask about pain or burning on urination, difficulty initiating a urine stream, costovertebral angle (CVA) tenderness, and flank, upper abdominal, or suprapubic pain.

Determine if the patient or his family has a history of renal or urinary tract disorders or endocrine and metabolic diseases, particularly diabetes. Is the patient taking a drug that increases urine output, such as a diuretic, a cardiac glycoside, or an antihypertensive?

Focus your physical examination on palpating and percussing the kidneys, CVA, and bladder. Carefully inspect the urinary meatus. Inspect a urine specimen for color, odor, and the presence of sediment.

Causes

◆ *Benign prostatic hyperplasia (BPH).* Common in men older than age 50, BPH produces nocturia when significant urethral obstruction develops. Typically, it causes frequency, hesitancy, incontinence, reduced force and caliber of the urine stream and, possibly, hematuria. Oliguria may also occur.

◆ *Cystitis.* All three forms of cystitis— bacterial, chronic interstitial, and viral—may cause nocturia marked by frequent, small voidings and accompanied by dysuria and tenesmus. Hematuria is also common.

◆ *Diabetes insipidus.* The result of antidiuretic hormone deficiency, diabetes insipidus usually produces nocturia early in its course. It's characterized by periodic voiding of moderate to large amounts of urine.

◆ *Diabetes mellitus.* An early sign of diabetes mellitus, nocturia involves frequent, large voidings. Associated findings include daytime polyuria, polydipsia, and polyphagia.

◆ *Hypercalcemic nephropathy.* With hypercalcemic nephropathy, nocturia involves the periodic voiding of moderate to large amounts of urine. Other findings include daytime polyuria and polydipsia.

◆ *Prostate cancer.* The second leading cause of cancer deaths in men, prostate cancer usually produces no symptoms in the early stages. Later, it produces nocturia characterized by frequent voiding of moderate amounts of urine.

◆ *Pyelonephritis (acute).* Nocturia is common with acute pyelonephritis and is usually characterized by frequent voiding of moderate amounts of urine, which may appear cloudy.

◆ *Renal failure (chronic).* Nocturia occurs relatively early in chronic renal failure and is usually characterized by frequent voiding of moderate amounts of urine. As the disorder progresses, oliguria or even anuria develops.

Nuchal rigidity

Commonly an early sign of meningeal irritation, nuchal rigidity refers to neck stiffness that prevents flexion. To elicit this sign, attempt to passively flex the patient's neck and touch his chin to his chest. If nuchal rigidity is present, this maneuver triggers pain and muscle spasms. (Make sure that there's no cervical spinal misalignment, such as a fracture or dislocation, before testing for nuchal rigidity. Severe spinal cord damage could result.) The patient may also notice nuchal rigidity when he attempts to flex his neck during daily activities. This sign isn't reliable in children and infants.

Nuchal rigidity may herald life-threatening subarachnoid hemorrhage or meningitis. It may also be a late sign of cervical arthritis, in which joint mobility is gradually lost.

Assessment

After eliciting nuchal rigidity, attempt to elicit Kernig's and Brudzinski's signs. Quickly evaluate the patient's level of consciousness (LOC). Take his vital signs. Obtain a patient history, relying on family members if an altered LOC prevents the patient from responding. Ask about the onset and duration of neck stiffness. Were there precipitating factors? Also ask about associated signs and symptoms, such as headache, fever, nausea and vomiting, and motor and sensory changes. Check for a history of hypertension, head trauma, cerebral aneurysm or arteriovenous malformation, endocarditis, recent infection (such as sinusitis or pneumonia), or recent dental work. Then, obtain a complete drug history. If the patient has no other signs of meningeal irritation, ask about a history of arthritis or neck trauma. Can the patient recall pulling a muscle in his neck? Inspect the patient's hands for swollen, tender joints, and palpate the neck for pain or tenderness.

Causes

◆ *Cervical arthritis.* With cervical arthritis, nuchal rigidity develops gradually. Initially, the patient may complain of neck stiffness in the early morning or after a period of inactivity. Stiffness then becomes increasingly severe and frequent. Pain on movement, especially with lateral motion or head turning, is common.
◆ *Encephalitis.* Encephalitis may cause nuchal rigidity accompanied by other signs of meningeal irritation, such as positive Kernig's and Brudzinski's signs. Usually, nuchal rigidity appears abruptly and is preceded by headache, vomiting, and fever.
◤ *Meningitis.* Nuchal rigidity is an early sign of meningitis and is accompanied by other signs of meningeal irritation—positive Kernig's and Brudzinski's signs, hyperreflexia and, possibly, opisthotonos. Other early features include a fever with chills, headache, photophobia, and vomiting.
◤ *Subarachnoid hemorrhage.* Nuchal rigidity develops immediately after bleeding into the subarachnoid space. Examination may detect positive Kernig's and Brudzinski's signs. The patient may experience an abrupt onset of a severe headache, photophobia, fever, nausea and vomiting, dizziness, cranial nerve palsies, and focal neurologic signs, such as hemiparesis or hemiplegia.

Nystagmus

Nystagmus refers to the involuntary oscillations of one or, more commonly, both eyeballs. These oscillations are usually rhythmic and may be horizontal, vertical, rotary, or mixed. They may be transient or sustained and may occur spontaneously or on deviation or fixation of the eyes. Minor degrees of nystagmus at the extremes of gaze are normal. Nystagmus when the eyes are stationary and looking straight ahead is always abnormal. Although nystagmus is fairly easy to identify, the patient may be unaware of it unless it affects his vision.

Nystagmus may be classified as pendular or jerk. Pendular nystagmus consists of horizontal (pendular) or vertical (seesaw) oscillations that are equal in rate in both directions and resemble the movements of a clock's pendulum. Jerk nystagmus (convergence-retraction, downbeat, and vestibular), which is more common than pendular nystagmus, has a fast component and then a slow—perhaps unequal—corrective component in the opposite direction. (See *Classifying nystagmus,* page 394.)

Nystagmus results from disease in the visual perceptual area, vestibular system, cerebellum, or brain stem rather than in the extraocular muscles or cranial nerves III, IV, and VI. Occasionally, nystagmus is entirely normal; it's also considered a normal response in the unconscious patient during the doll's eye test (oculocephalic stimulation) or the cold caloric water test (oculovestibular stimulation).

Assessment

Begin by asking the patient how long he's had nystagmus. Does it occur intermittently? Does it affect his vision? Ask about recent infection, especially of the ear or respiratory tract, and about head trauma, stroke, and cancer. Ask about vertigo, dizziness, tinnitus, nausea or vomiting, numbness, weakness, bladder dysfunction, and fever.

Begin the physical examination by assessing the patient's level of consciousness (LOC) and vital signs. Stay alert for signs of increased intracranial pressure. Next, assess nystagmus fully by testing extraocular muscle function: Ask the patient to focus straight ahead and then to follow your finger up, down, and in an "X" across his face. Note when nystagmus occurs as well as its velocity and direction. Finally, test reflexes, motor and sensory function, and the cranial nerves.

Causes

◆ *Brain tumor.* An insidious onset of jerk nystagmus may occur with tumors of the brain stem and cerebellum. Other findings include deafness, dysphagia, nausea and vomiting, vertigo, and ataxia.

◆ *Encephalitis.* With encephalitis, jerk nystagmus is typically accompanied by an altered LOC ranging from lethargy to coma. Usually, it's preceded by the sudden onset of fever, headache, and vomiting.

◤ *Head trauma.* Brain stem injury may cause jerk nystagmus, which is usually horizontal. The patient may also display pupillary changes, an altered respiratory pattern, coma, and decerebrate posture.

◆ *Labyrinthitis (acute).* Acute labyrinthitis is an inner ear inflammation

Classifying nystagmus

Nystagmus may be classified a jerk or pendular.

Jerk nystagmus

Convergence-retraction nystagmus refers to the irregular jerking of the eyes back into the orbi.

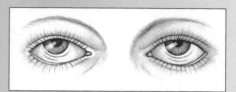

Downbeat nystagmus refers to the irregular downward jerking of the eyes during downward gaze. It can signal lower medullary damage.

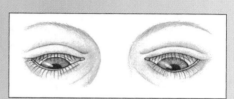

Vestibular nystagmus, the horizontal or rotary movement of the eyes, suggests vestibular disease or cochlear dysfunction.

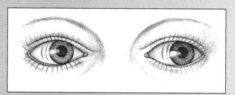

Pendular nystagmus

Horizontal, or pendular, nystagmus refers to oscillations of equal velocity around a center point. It can indicate congenital loss of visual acuity or multiple sclerosis.

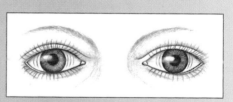

Vertical, or seesaw, nystagmus is the rapid, seesaw movement of the eyes: one eye appears to rise while the other appears to fall. It suggests an optic chiasm lesion.

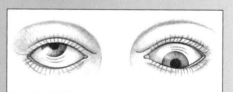

that causes a sudden onset of jerk nystagmus, accompanied by dizziness, vertigo, tinnitus, nausea, and vomiting. The fast component of the nystagmus is toward the unaffected ear. Gradual sensorineural hearing loss may also occur.

◆ *Ménière's disease.* Ménière's disease is characterized by acute attacks of jerk nystagmus, severe nausea and vomiting, dizziness, vertigo, progressive hearing loss, tinnitus, and diaphoresis. Typically, the direction of jerk nystagmus varies from one attack to the next. Attacks may last from 10 minutes to several hours.

◣ *Stroke.* A stroke involving the posterior inferior cerebellar artery may cause sudden horizontal or vertical jerk nystagmus that may be gaze dependent.w

O

Ocular deviation

Ocular deviation refers to abnormal eye movement that may be conjugate (both eyes move together) or disconjugate (one eye moves separately from the other). This common sign may result from ocular, neurologic, endocrine, or systemic disorders that interfere with the muscles, nerves, or brain centers governing eye movement. Occasionally, it signals a life-threatening disorder such as a ruptured cerebral aneurysm. (See *Ocular deviation: Its characteristics and causes in cranial nerve damage.*)

Normally, eye movement is directly controlled by the extraocular muscles innervated by the oculomotor, trochlear, and abducens nerves (cranial nerves III, IV, and VI). Together, these muscles and nerves direct a visual stimulus to fall on corresponding parts of the retina. Disconjugate ocular deviation may result from unequal muscle tone (nonparalytic strabismus) or muscle paralysis associated with cranial nerve damage (paralytic strabismus). Conjugate ocular deviation may result from disorders that affect the centers in the cerebral cortex and brain stem responsible for conjugate eye movement. Typically, such disorders cause gaze

palsy—difficulty moving the eyes in one or more directions.

Assessment

If the patient displays ocular deviation, check his vital signs immediately and assess him for an altered level of consciousness (LOC), pupil changes, motor or sensory dysfunction, and severe headache. If possible, ask the patient's family about behavioral changes. Is there a history of head trauma? If the patient isn't in distress, find out how long he has had the ocular deviation. Is it accompanied by double vision, eye pain, or headache? Also ask if he has noticed associated motor or sensory changes or fever. Check for a history of hypertension, diabetes, allergies, and thyroid, neurologic, or muscular disorders. Then obtain a thorough ocular history. Has the patient ever had extraocular muscle imbalance, eye trauma, or eye surgery?

During the physical examination, observe the patient for partial or complete ptosis. Does he spontaneously tilt his head or turn his face to compensate for ocular deviation? Check for eye redness or periorbital edema. Assess the patient's visual acuity, and then evaluate extraocular muscle function by testing the six cardinal fields of

Ocular deviation: Its characteristics and causes in cranial nerve damage

CHARACTERISTICS	CRANIAL NERVE AND EXTRAOCULAR MUSCLES INVOLVED	PROBABLE CAUSES
Inability to move the eye up-ward, downward, inward, and outward; drooping eyelid; and, except in diabetes, a di-lated pupil in the affected eye	Oculomotor nerve (cranial nerve [CN] III); medial rec-tus, superior rectus, inferior rectus, and inferior oblique muscles	Cerebral aneurysm, diabe-tes, temporal lobe herniation from increased intracranial pressure, brain tumor
Loss of downward and out-ward movement in the affect-ed eye	Trochlear nerve (CN IV); superior oblique muscle	Head trauma
Loss of outward movement in the affected eye	Abducens nerve (CN VI); lateral rectus muscle	Brain tumor

gaze. (See *Testing extraocular muscles,* page 217.)

Causes

◆ *Brain tumor.* The nature of ocular deviation depends on the site and ex-tent of the tumor. Other findings in-clude headache that's most severe in the morning or behavioral changes, dizziness, and vision loss.

◆ *Cavernous sinus thrombosis.* With cavernous sinus thrombosis, ocular de-viation may be accompanied by diplo-pia, photophobia, exophthalmos, orbital and eyelid edema, corneal haziness, and diminished or absent pupillary re-flexes.

◆ *Diabetes mellitus.* A leading cause of isolated third cranial nerve palsy, di-abetes mellitus may cause ocular devi-ation and ptosis. Typically, the patient also complains of the sudden onset of diplopia and pain.

◆ *Encephalitis.* Encephalitis causes oc-ular deviation and diplopia in some cases.

◼ *Head trauma.* The nature of ocular deviation depends on the site and ex-tent of head trauma. The patient may also develop blurred vision, diplopia, nystagmus, headache, and a decreased LOC that may progress to coma.

◆ *Orbital blowout fracture.* In orbital blowout fracture, the inferior rectus muscle may become entrapped, result-ing in limited extraocular movement and ocular deviation. Typically, the pa-tient's upward gaze is absent. Other di-rections of gaze may be affected if ede-ma is dramatic. The globe may also be displaced downward and inward.

◆ *Orbital tumor.* Ocular deviation oc-curs as the tumor gradually enlarges. Associated findings include proptosis, diplopia and, possibly, blurred vision.

◼ *Stroke.* Stroke may cause ocular de-viation, depending on the site and extent of the stroke. Other findings are variable and include homonymous hemianopsia, blurred vision, and diplopia.

◆ *Thyrotoxicosis.* Thyrotoxicosis may produce exophthalmos which, in turn, causes limited extraocular movement and ocular deviation. Usually, the patient's upward gaze weakens first, followed by diplopia. Other findings include lid retraction, a wide-eyed staring gaze, excessive tearing, and edematous eyelids.

Oligomenorrhea

In most women, menstrual bleeding occurs every 28 days, plus or minus 4 days. Although some variation is normal, menstrual bleeding at intervals of greater than 36 days may indicate oligomenorrhea—abnormally infrequent menstrual bleeding characterized by three to six menstrual cycles per year. When menstrual bleeding does occur, it's usually profuse, prolonged (up to 10 days), and laden with clots and tissue. Occasionally, scant bleeding or spotting occurs between these heavy menses.

Oligomenorrhea may develop suddenly or follow a period of gradually lengthening cycles. Although it may alternate with normal menstrual bleeding, it can progress to secondary amenorrhea. Because it's commonly associated with anovulation, it's common in infertile, early postmenarchal, and perimenopausal women. This sign usually reflects abnormalities of the hormones that govern normal endometrial function. It may result from ovarian, hypothalamic, pituitary, thyroid, and other metabolic disorders or from the effects of certain drugs. It may also result from emotional or physical stress, such

as sudden weight change, a debilitating illness, or rigorous physical training.

Assessment

After asking the patient's age, find out when menarche occurred. Has the patient ever experienced normal menstrual cycles? When did she begin having abnormal cycles? Ask her to describe the pattern of bleeding. How many days does the bleeding last? How frequently does it occur? Are there clots and tissue fragments in her menstrual flow? Note when she last had menstrual bleeding. Next, determine if she's having symptoms of ovulatory bleeding. Does she experience any mild, cramping abdominal pain 14 days before she bleeds? Is the bleeding accompanied by premenstrual symptoms, such as breast tenderness, irritability, bloating, weight gain, nausea, or diarrhea? Does she have cramping or pain with bleeding? Also, check for a history of infertility. Ask if she's currently using hormonal contraceptives or if she has ever used them in the past. If she has, find out when she stopped taking them.

Then ask about previous gynecologic disorders such as ovarian cysts. If the patient is breast-feeding, has she experienced problems with milk production? If she hasn't been breast-feeding recently, has she noticed milk leaking from her breasts? Ask about recent weight gain or loss. Ask if she's exercising more vigorously than usual.

Screen for metabolic disorders by asking about excessive thirst, frequent urination, or fatigue. Has the patient been jittery or had palpitations? Ask about headaches, dizziness, and impaired peripheral vision. Complete the history by finding out what drugs the patient is taking.

Begin the physical examination by taking the patient's vital signs and weighing her. Inspect for increased facial hair growth, sparse body hair, male distribution of fat and muscle, acne, and clitoral enlargement. Note if the skin is abnormally dry or moist, and check hair texture. Also, be alert for signs of psychological or physical stress. Rule out pregnancy with a blood or urine pregnancy test.

Causes

◆ *Adrenal hyperplasia.* In adrenal hyperplasia, oligomenorrhea may occur with signs of androgen excess, such as clitoral enlargement and male distribution of hair, fat, and muscle mass.
◆ *Anorexia nervosa.* Anorexia nervosa may cause sporadic oligomenorrhea or amenorrhea. Its cardinal symptom, however, is a morbid fear of being fat associated with weight loss of more than 20% of ideal body weight.
◆ *Diabetes mellitus.* Oligomenorrhea may be an early sign in diabetes mellitus. In type 1 diabetes, the patient may have never had normal menses.
◆ *Drugs.* Drugs that increase androgen levels—such as corticosteroids, corticotropin, danazol (Danocrine), and injectable and implanted hormonal contraceptives—may cause oligomenorrhea. Other drugs that may cause oligomenorrhea include phenothiazine derivatives, amphetamines, and antihypertensive drugs, which increase prolactin levels.
◆ *Hypothyroidism.* Besides oligomenorrhea, hypothyroidism may result in dry, flaky, inelastic skin; fatigue; forgetfulness; cold intolerance; unexplained weight gain; ptosis; dry, sparse hair; and thick, brittle nails.
◆ *Prolactin-secreting pituitary tumor.* The first sign of a prolactin-secreting pituitary tumor may be oligomenorrhea or amenorrhea, accompanied by unilateral or bilateral galactorrhea.
◆ *Thyrotoxicosis.* Thyrotoxicosis may produce oligomenorrhea along with reduced fertility. Cardinal findings include weight loss despite increased appetite, tachycardia, palpitations, diarrhea, tremors, diaphoresis, and heat intolerance.

Oliguria

Oliguria is a cardinal sign of renal and urinary tract disorders. It's clinically defined as urine output of less than 400 ml/24 hours. Typically, oliguria occurs abruptly and may herald serious—possibly life-threatening—hemodynamic instability. Its causes can be classified as prerenal (decreased renal blood flow), intrarenal (intrinsic renal damage), or postrenal (urinary tract obstruction); the pathophysiology differs for each classification. (See *How oliguria develops,* pages 400 and 401.) Oliguria associated with a prerenal or postrenal cause is usually promptly reversible with treatment; however, it may lead to intrarenal damage if untreated. Oliguria associated with an intrarenal cause is usually more persistent and may be irreversible.

Assessment

Begin by asking the patient about his usual daily voiding pattern, including frequency and amount. When did he first notice changes in this pattern? Has he noticed changes in the color, odor, or consistency of his urine? Ask about pain or burning on urination. Has the patient had a fever? Note his normal daily fluid intake. Has he recently been drinking more or less than usual? Has he had recent episodes of diarrhea or vomiting that might cause fluid loss?
(Text continues on page 402.)

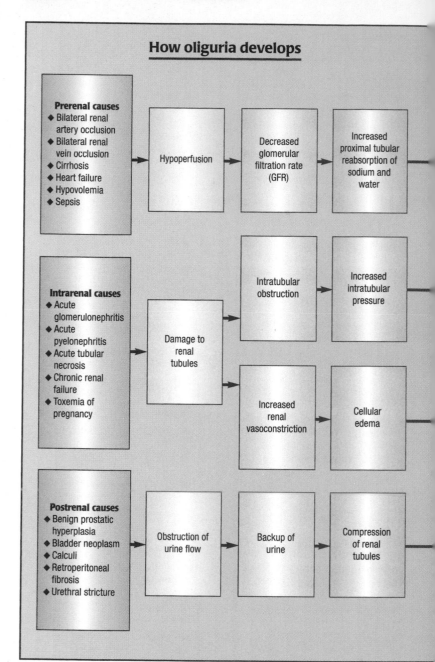

How oliguria develops

Prerenal causes
- Bilateral renal artery occlusion
- Bilateral renal vein occlusion
- Cirrhosis
- Heart failure
- Hypovolemia
- Sepsis

→ Hypoperfusion → Decreased glomerular filtration rate (GFR) → Increased proximal tubular reabsorption of sodium and water →

Intrarenal causes
- Acute glomerulonephritis
- Acute pyelonephritis
- Acute tubular necrosis
- Chronic renal failure
- Toxemia of pregnancy

→ Damage to renal tubules → Intratubular obstruction → Increased intratubular pressure →

→ Increased renal vasoconstriction → Cellular edema →

Postrenal causes
- Benign prostatic hyperplasia
- Bladder neoplasm
- Calculi
- Retroperitoneal fibrosis
- Urethral stricture

→ Obstruction of urine flow → Backup of urine → Compression of renal tubules →

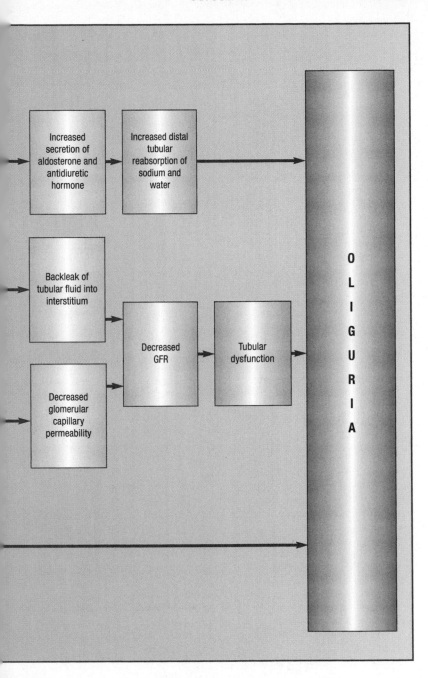

Next, explore associated complaints, especially fatigue, loss of appetite, thirst, dyspnea, chest pain, or recent weight gain or loss. Check for a history of renal, urinary tract, or cardiovascular disorders. Was the patient exposed to nephrotoxic agents, such as heavy metals, organic solvents, anesthetics, or radiographic contrast media? Next, obtain a drug history.

Begin the physical examination by checking the patient's vital signs and weighing him. Assess his overall appearance for edema. Palpate both kidneys for tenderness and enlargement, and percuss for costovertebral angle (CVA) tenderness. Also, inspect the flank area for edema or erythema. Auscultate the heart and lungs for abnormal sounds and the flank area for renal artery bruits. Assess the patient for edema or signs of dehydration such as dry mucous membranes.

Obtain a urine sample, and inspect it for abnormal color, odor, or sediment. Use reagent strips to test for glucose, protein, and blood. Also use a urinometer to measure specific gravity.

Causes

◆ *Acute tubular necrosis (ATN).* Oliguria is an early sign of ATN and may occur abruptly (in shock) or gradually (in nephrotoxicity). Usually, it persists for about 2 weeks, followed by polyuria. Related findings include signs of hyperkalemia, uremia, and heart failure.

◆ *Calculi.* Oliguria or anuria may result from calculi lodging in the kidneys, ureters, bladder outlet, or urethra. Other findings include urinary frequency and urgency, dysuria, hematuria, or pyuria and renal colic.

◆ *Drugs.* Oliguria may result from such drugs as diuretics, aminoglycosides, chemotherapeutic agents, adrenergics, anticholinergics, sulfonamides, and acyclovir (Zovirax).

◆ *Glomerulonephritis (acute).* Acute glomerulonephritis produces oliguria or anuria. Other findings include mild fever, fatigue, gross hematuria, proteinuria, generalized edema, and elevated blood pressure.

◆ *Heart failure.* Oliguria may occur in left-sided heart failure as a result of low cardiac output and decreased renal perfusion. In advanced or chronic heart failure, the patient may develop orthopnea, cyanosis, clubbing, a ventricular gallop, diastolic hypertension, cardiomegaly, and hemoptysis.

◆ *Hypovolemia.* Any disorder that decreases circulating fluid volume can produce oliguria. Other findings include orthostatic hypotension, fatigue, profound thirst, sunken eyeballs, poor skin turgor, and dry mucous membranes.

◆ *Pyelonephritis (acute).* The sudden onset of oliguria in acute pyelonephritis is accompanied by high fever with chills, fatigue, CVA tenderness, weakness, nocturia, hematuria, urinary frequency and urgency, and tenesmus.

◆ *Renal failure (chronic).* Oliguria is a major sign of end-stage chronic renal failure. Other findings reflect progressive uremia.

◆ *Toxemia of pregnancy.* In severe preeclampsia, oliguria may be accompanied by elevated blood pressure, dizziness, diplopia, blurred vision, epigastric pain, nausea and vomiting, irritability, and a severe frontal headache. Typically, preeclampsia is preceded by generalized edema and sudden weight gain.

◆ *Urethral stricture.* Urethral stricture produces oliguria accompanied by chronic urethral discharge, urinary frequency and urgency, dysuria, pyuria, and a diminished urine stream.

Opisthotonos

Opisthotonos is a sign of severe meningeal irritation. It's a severe, prolonged spasm characterized by a hyperextended neck, heels bent back, arms and hands flexed at the joints, and a strongly arched, rigid back. Usually, this posture occurs spontaneously and continuously; however, it may be aggravated by movement. Opisthotonos represents a protective reflex because it immobilizes the spine, alleviating the pain associated with meningeal irritation.

Although opisthotonos is usually caused by meningitis, it may also result from subarachnoid hemorrhage, Arnold-Chiari syndrome, or tetanus. Occasionally, it occurs in achondroplastic dwarfism, although not necessarily as an indicator of meningeal irritation. Opisthotonos is far more common in children—especially infants—than in adults. It's also more exaggerated in children because of nervous system immaturity. (See *Opisthotonos: Sign of meningeal irritation*.)

Assessment

If the patient is stuporous or comatose, immediately evaluate his vital signs. If his condition permits, obtain a history. If the patient is a young child or an in-

---

Opisthotonos: Sign of meningeal irritation

In opisthotonos, the back is severely arched with the neck hyperextended. The heels bend back on the legs, and the arms and hands flex rigidly at the joints, as shown.

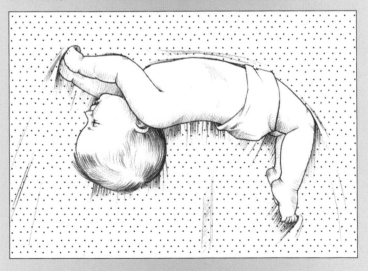

fant, consult with a relative. Ask about a history of cerebral aneurysm, arteriovenous malformation, and hypertension. Note a recent infection that may have spread to the nervous system. Explore associated findings, such as headaches, chills, and vomiting. Obtain a drug history.

Focus the physical examination on the patient's neurologic status. Evaluate his level of consciousness, and test sensorimotor and cranial nerve function. Then check for Brudzinski's and Kernig's signs and for nuchal rigidity.

Causes

◆ *Antipsychotics.* Phenothiazines and other antipsychotic drugs may cause opisthotonos, usually as part of an acute dystonic reaction.

◼ *Arnold-Chiari syndrome.* With Arnold-Chiari syndrome, opisthotonos typically occurs with hydrocephalus and its characteristic enlarged head; thin, shiny scalp with distended veins; and underdeveloped neck muscles.

◼ *Meningitis.* In meningitis, opisthotonos accompanies other signs of meningeal irritation, including nuchal rigidity, positive Brudzinski's and Kernig's signs, and hyperreflexia. Meningitis also causes signs of infection and increased intracranial pressure.

◼ *Subarachnoid hemorrhage.* Subarachnoid hemorrhage may produce opisthotonos along with other signs of meningeal irritation, such as nuchal rigidity and positive Kernig's and Brudzinski's signs.

◼ *Tetanus.* Tetanus is an infection that can cause opisthotonos. Initially, trismus (lockjaw) occurs. Eventually, muscle spasms may affect the abdomen, the back, or the face. Spasms may affect the respiratory muscles, causing distress.

Orthopnea

Orthopnea—difficulty breathing in the supine position—is a common symptom of cardiopulmonary disorders that produce dyspnea. It's usually a subtle symptom; the patient may complain that he can't catch his breath when lying down, or he may mention that he sleeps most comfortably in a reclining chair or propped up by pillows. The common classification of two- or three-pillow orthopnea is derived from this complaint.

Orthopnea results from increased hydrostatic pressure in the pulmonary vasculature related to gravitational effects in the supine position. Orthopnea may be aggravated by obesity or pregnancy, which restricts diaphragmatic excursion. Sitting in an upright position relieves orthopnea by placing much of the pulmonary vasculature above the left atrium, thereby reducing mean hydrostatic pressure, and by enhancing diaphragmatic excursion, which increases inspiratory volume.

Assessment

Begin by asking about a history of cardiopulmonary disorders, such as myocardial infarction, rheumatic heart disease, valvular disease, asthma, emphysema, or chronic bronchitis. Does the patient smoke? If so, how much? Explore associated symptoms, especially noting complaints of coughing, nocturnal or exertional dyspnea, fatigue, weakness, loss of appetite, or chest pain. Does the patient use alcohol or have a history of heavy alcohol use?

When examining the patient, check for other signs of increased respiratory effort, such as accessory muscle use, shallow respirations, and tachypnea. Also note barrel chest. Inspect the patient's skin for pallor or cyanosis and the fingers for clubbing. Observe and palpate for edema. Check for jugular vein distention. Auscultate the lungs for crackles, rhonchi, or wheezing. Also auscultate the heart. Monitor the patient's oxygen saturation.

Causes

◆ *Chronic obstructive pulmonary disease (COPD).* COPD typically produces orthopnea and other dyspneic complaints, accompanied by accessory muscle use, tachypnea, tachycardia, and paradoxical pulse. Auscultation may reveal diminished breath sounds, rhonchi, crackles, and wheezing.
◆ *Left-sided heart failure.* Orthopnea occurs late in left-sided heart failure. If heart failure is acute, orthopnea may begin suddenly; if chronic, it may become constant. The earliest symptom of this disorder is progressively severe dyspnea. Other common early symptoms include Cheyne-Stokes respirations, paroxysmal nocturnal dyspnea, fatigue, weakness, and cough that may occasionally produce clear or blood-tinged sputum.
◪ *Mediastinal tumor.* Orthopnea is an early sign of a mediastinal tumor, resulting from pressure of the tumor against the trachea, bronchus, or lung when the patient lies down. When the tumor enlarges, it produces retrosternal chest pain, a dry cough, hoarseness, dysphagia, stertorous respirations, palpitations, and cyanosis.

Orthostatic hypotension

In orthostatic hypotension, the patient's blood pressure drops 15 to 20 mm Hg or more—possibly with an increase in the heart rate of 20 beats/ minute—when he rises from a supine to a sitting or standing position. (Blood pressure should be measured 5 minutes after the patient has changed his position.) This common sign indicates failure of compensatory vasomotor responses to adjust to position changes. It's typically associated with light-headedness, syncope, or blurred vision and may occur in a hypotensive, normotensive, or hypertensive patient. Although commonly a nonpathologic sign in an elderly person, orthostatic hypotension may result from prolonged bed rest, fluid and electrolyte imbalance, endocrine or systemic disorders, and the effects of drugs.

Assessment

To detect orthostatic hypotension, take and compare blood pressure readings with the patient supine, sitting, and standing. If you obtain a positive finding, quickly check for tachycardia, an altered level of consciousness, and pale, clammy skin. Suspect hypovolemic shock if these signs are present. If the patient is in no danger, obtain a history. Ask the patient if he frequently experiences dizziness, weakness, or fainting when he stands. Also ask about associated symptoms, particularly fatigue, orthopnea, impotence, nausea, headaches, abdominal or chest discomfort, and GI bleeding. Then obtain a complete drug history.

Begin the physical examination by checking the patient's skin turgor. Palpate peripheral pulses, and auscultate the heart and lungs. Finally, test muscle strength and observe the patient's gait for unsteadiness.

Causes

◆ *Adrenal insufficiency.* Adrenal insufficiency typically begins insidiously and progresses to more severe signs and symptoms. Orthostatic hypotension may be accompanied by fatigue, muscle weakness, poor coordination, anorexia, nausea and vomiting, fasting hypoglycemia, weight loss, abdominal pain, irritability, and a weak, irregular pulse. Another common feature is hyperpigmentation—bronze coloring of the skin—that's especially prominent on the face, lips, gums, tongue, buccal mucosa, elbows, palms, knuckles, waist, and knees.

◆ *Alcoholism.* Chronic alcoholism can lead to the development of peripheral neuropathy, which can present as orthostatic hypotension. Impotence is also a major issue in these patients.

◆ *Amyloidosis.* Orthostatic hypotension is commonly associated with amyloid infiltration of the autonomic nerves. Other signs and symptoms vary widely and include angina, tachycardia, dyspnea, orthopnea, fatigue, and cough.

◆ *Drugs.* Certain drugs may cause orthostatic hypotension by reducing circulating blood volume, causing blood vessel dilation, or depressing the sympathetic nervous system. These drugs include antihypertensives, tricyclic antidepressants, phenothiazines, levodopa (Dopar), nitrates, monoamine oxidase inhibitors, spinal anesthesia, and large doses of diuretics.

◆ *Hyperaldosteronism.* Hyperaldosteronism typically produces orthostatic hypotension with sustained elevated blood pressure. Most other clinical effects of hyperaldosteronism result from hypokalemia, which increases neuromuscular irritability.

◆ *Hyponatremia.* With hyponatremia, orthostatic hypotension is typically accompanied by profound thirst, tachycardia, abdominal cramps, muscle twitching and weakness, oliguria or anuria, cold clammy skin, and poor skin turgor.

◆ *Hypovolemia.* Mild to moderate hypovolemia may cause orthostatic hypotension associated with fatigue, muscle weakness, nausea, and profound thirst.

Ortolani's sign

Ortolani's sign—a click, clunk, or popping sensation that's felt and commonly heard when a neonate's hip is flexed 90 degrees and abducted—is an indication of developmental dysplasia of the hip (DDH). Ortolani's sign results when the femoral head enters or exits the acetabulum. Screening for this sign is an important part of neonatal care because early detection and treatment of DDH improves the neonate's chances of growing with a correctly formed, functional joint.

Assessment

During assessment for Ortolani's sign, the neonate should be relaxed and lying supine. (See *Detecting developmental dysplasia of the hip.*) After eliciting Ortolani's sign, evaluate the neonate for asymmetrical gluteal folds, limited hip abduction, and unequal leg length.

Causes

◆ *DDH.* With complete dysplasia, the affected leg may appear shorter or the affected hip may appear more prominent.

Detecting developmental dysplasia of the hip

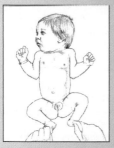

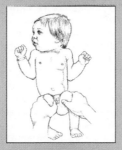

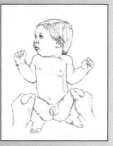

When assessing the neonate, attempt to elicit Ortolani's sign to detect developmental dysplasia of the hip (DDH). Begin by placing the neonate in a supine position with his knees and hips flexed. Observe for symmetry.

Place your hands on the neonate's knees, with your index fingers along his lateral thighs on the greater trochanter. Then raise his knees to a 90-degree angle with his back.

Abduct the neonate's thighs so that the lateral aspect of his knees lies almost flat on the table. If the neonate has a dislocated hip, you'll feel and usually hear a click, clunk, or popping sensation (Ortolani's sign) as the head of the femur moves out of the acetabulum. The neonate may also give a sudden cry of pain. Make sure to distinguish a positive Ortolani's sign from the normal clicks caused by hip rotation, from signs that don't elicit the sensation of instability, or from simultaneous movement of the knee.

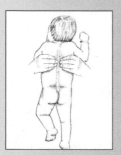

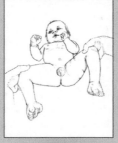

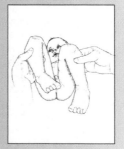

If you elicit a positive Ortolani's sign, look for other signs of DDH.

Flex the neonate's hips to detect limited abduction.

Flex the neonate's knees, and observe for apparent shortening of the femur.

Otorrhea

Otorrhea—drainage from the ear—may be bloody (otorrhagia), purulent, clear, or serosanguineous. Its onset, duration, and severity provide clues to the underlying cause. This sign may result from disorders that affect the external ear canal or the middle ear, including allergy, infection, neoplasms, trauma, and collagen diseases. Otorrhea may occur alone or with other symptoms such as ear pain.

Assessment

Begin your evaluation by asking the patient when otorrhea began, noting how he recognized it. Did he clean the drainage from deep within the ear canal, or did he wipe it from the auricle? Have him describe the color, consistency, and odor of the drainage. Is it clear, purulent, or bloody? Does it occur in one or both ears? Is it continuous or intermittent? If the patient wears cotton in his ear to absorb the drainage, ask how often he changes it.

Then explore associated otologic symptoms, especially pain. Is there tenderness on movement of the pinna or tragus? Ask about vertigo, which is absent in disorders of the external ear canal. Also ask about tinnitus.

Next, check the patient's medical history for recent upper respiratory infection or head trauma. Ask how he cleans his ears. Is he an avid swimmer? Note a history of cancer, dermatitis, or immunosuppressant therapy.

Focus the physical examination on the patient's external ear, middle ear, and tympanic membrane. (If his symptoms are unilateral, examine the uninvolved ear first so as not to cross-contaminate.) Inspect the external ear, and apply pressure on the tragus and mastoid area to elicit tenderness. Then insert an otoscope, using the largest speculum that will comfortably fit into the ear canal. If necessary, clean cerumen, pus, or other debris from the canal. Observe for edema, erythema, crusts, or polyps. Inspect the tympanic membrane, which should look like a shiny, pearl-gray cone. Note color changes, perforation, absence of the normal light reflex (a cone of light appearing toward the bottom of the drum), or a bulging membrane.

Next, test hearing acuity. Have the patient occlude one ear while you whisper some common two-syllable words toward the unoccluded ear. Stand behind him so he doesn't read your lips, and ask him to repeat what he heard. Perform the test on the other ear using different words. Then use a tuning fork to perform Weber's test and the Rinne test. (See *Differentiating conductive from sensorineural hearing loss,* page 294.) Complete your assessment by palpating the patient's neck and his preauricular, parotid, and post-auricular (mastoid) areas for lymphadenopathy. Also, test the function of cranial nerves VII, IX, X, and XI.

Causes

◆ *Aural polyps.* Aural polyps may produce foul, purulent and, perhaps, blood-streaked discharge. If they occlude the external ear canal, the polyps may cause partial hearing loss.

◆ *Basilar skull fracture.* With a basilar skull fracture, otorrhea may be clear and watery and positive for glucose (representing cerebrospinal fluid leakage) or bloody (representing hemorrhage). Basilar skull fracture may be accompanied by hearing loss, rhinorrhea, periorbital ecchymosis, and mastoid ecchymosis.

◆ *Epidural abscess.* In epidural abscess, profuse, creamy otorrhea is accompanied by steady, throbbing ear pain; fever; and a temporal or temporoparietal headache on the ipsilateral side.

◆ *Myringitis (infectious).* With acute infectious myringitis, small, reddened, blood-filled blebs erupt in the external ear canal, the tympanic membrane and, occasionally, the middle ear. Spontaneous rupture of these blebs causes serosanguineous otorrhea. Other findings include severe ear pain and tenderness over the mastoid process.

◆ *Otitis externa.* Otitis externa may be acute, chronic, or malignant.

Acute otitis externa, commonly known as swimmer's ear, usually causes purulent, yellow, sticky, foul-smelling otorrhea. Inspection may reveal white-green debris in the external ear canal. Other findings include partial conductive hearing loss and severe tenderness with movement of the mastoid, tragus, mouth, or jaw.

Chronic otitis externa usually causes scanty, intermittent otorrhea that may be serous or purulent and possibly foul-smelling. Its primary symptom, however, is itching.

◪ Malignant otitis externa produces debris in the ear canal that may build up against the tympanic membrane, causing severe pain that's especially acute during manipulation of the tragus or auricle. Malignant otitis externa is a fulminant bacterial infection and is most common in patients with diabetes and in immunosuppressed patients.

◆ *Otitis media.* With acute otitis media, rupture of the tympanic membrane produces bloody, purulent otorrhea and relieves continuous or intermittent ear pain. With acute suppurative otitis

media, the patient may also exhibit signs and symptoms of an upper respiratory infection. Chronic otitis media causes intermittent, purulent, foul-smelling otorrhea commonly associated with tympanic membrane perforation.

◆ *Trauma.* Bloody otorrhea may result from trauma (such as a blow to the external ear), a foreign body in the ear, or barotrauma. Usually, bleeding is minimal or moderate; it may be accompanied by partial hearing loss.

◆ *Tumor (malignant).* Squamous cell carcinoma of the external ear causes hearing loss, purulent otorrhea with itching, and deep, boring ear pain. In late stages, facial paralysis may result. In squamous cell carcinoma of the middle ear, blood-tinged otorrhea occurs early, typically accompanied by hearing loss on the affected side.

PQ

Pallor

Pallor is abnormal paleness or loss of skin color that may develop suddenly or gradually. Although generalized pallor affects the entire body, it's most apparent on the face, conjunctiva, oral mucosa, and nail beds. Localized pallor commonly affects a single limb.

How easily pallor is detected varies with skin color and the thickness and vascularity of underlying subcutaneous tissue. At times, it's merely a subtle lightening of skin color that may be difficult to detect, especially in dark-skinned persons; sometimes it's evident only on the conjunctiva and oral mucosa.

Pallor may result from decreased peripheral oxyhemoglobin (diminished peripheral blood flow associated with peripheral vasoconstriction or arterial occlusion or with low cardiac output) or decreased total oxyhemoglobin (usually results from anemia, the chief cause of pallor). Transient peripheral vasoconstriction may occur with exposure to cold, causing nonpathologic pallor. (See *How pallor develops*.)

Assessment

If generalized pallor develops suddenly, quickly look for signs of shock. If the patient's condition permits, take a complete history. Does the patient have a history of anemia or a chronic disorder that might lead to pallor, such as renal failure, heart failure, or diabetes? Ask about the patient's diet, particularly his intake of red meat and leafy, green vegetables. Then explore the pallor more fully. Find out when the patient first noticed it. Is it constant or intermittent? Does it occur when he's exposed to cold? Does it occur when he's under emotional stress? Explore associated signs and symptoms. If pallor is confined to one or both legs, ask the patient if walking is painful. Do his legs feel cold or numb? If pallor is confined to his fingers, ask about tingling and numbness.

Start the physical examination by checking the patient's vital signs. Make sure to check for orthostatic hypotension. Auscultate the heart for gallops and murmurs and the lungs for crackles. Check the patient's skin temperature—cold extremities commonly occur with vasoconstriction or arterial occlusion. Also note skin ulceration. Examine the abdomen for splenomegaly. Finally, palpate peripheral pulses. An ab-

How pallor develops

Pallor may result from decreased peripheral oxyhemoglobin or decreased total oxyhemoglobin. This chart illustrates the progression to pallor.

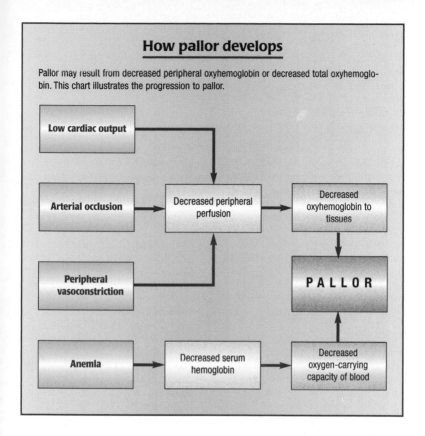

sent pulse in a pale extremity may indicate arterial occlusion; a weak pulse may indicate low cardiac output.

Causes

◆ *Anemia.* With anemia, pallor typically develops gradually. The patient's skin may also appear sallow or grayish.
◆ *Arterial occlusion (acute).* In arterial occlusion, which usually results from an embolus, pallor develops abruptly. In the affected extremity, a line of demarcation develops, separating the cool, pale, cyanotic, and mottled skin below the occlusion from the normal skin above it.
◆ *Arterial occlusive disease (chronic).* With arterial occlusive disease, pallor is specific to an extremity—usually one leg but occasionally both legs or an arm. It develops gradually from obstructive arteriosclerosis or a thrombus and is aggravated by elevating the extremity.
◆ *Frostbite.* Pallor is localized to the frostbitten area, such as the feet, hands, nose, or ears. Typically, the area feels cold, waxy and, perhaps, hard in deep frostbite. The skin doesn't blanch, and sensation may be absent. As the

area thaws, the skin turns purplish blue.

◆ *Orthostatic hypotension.* With orthostatic hypotension, pallor occurs abruptly on rising from a recumbent position to a sitting or standing position.

◆ *Raynaud's disease.* Pallor of the fingers upon exposure to cold or stress is a hallmark of Raynaud's disease. Typically, the fingers abruptly turn pale, then cyanotic; with rewarming, they become red and paresthetic.

◼ *Shock.* Two forms of shock—hypovolemic and cardiogenic—initially cause an acute onset of pallor and cool, clammy skin. Other early signs and symptoms include restlessness, thirst, slight tachycardia, hypotension, and tachypnea.

Palpitations

Defined as a conscious awareness of one's heartbeat, palpitations are usually felt over the precordium or in the throat or neck. The patient may describe them as pounding, jumping, turning, fluttering, or flopping or as missing or skipping beats. Palpitations may be regular or irregular, fast or slow, paroxysmal or sustained.

Although usually insignificant, palpitations may result from a cardiac or metabolic disorder or from the effects of certain drugs. Nonpathologic palpitations may occur with a newly implanted prosthetic valve because the valve's clicking sound heightens the patient's awareness of his heartbeat. Transient palpitations may accompany emotional or physical stress. They can also accompany the use of stimulants, such as tobacco and caffeine.

To help characterize the palpitations, ask the patient to simulate their rhythm by tapping his finger on a hard surface. An irregular "skipped beat" rhythm points to premature ventricular contractions, whereas an episodic racing rhythm that ends abruptly suggests paroxysmal atrial tachycardia.

Assessment

If the patient complains of palpitations, ask him about dizziness and shortness of breath. Then inspect for pale, cool, clammy skin. Check his vital signs, noting hypotension and an irregular or abnormal pulse. If these signs are present, suspect cardiac arrhythmia. If the patient isn't in distress, perform a complete cardiac assessment. Ask if he has a cardiovascular or pulmonary disorder, which may produce arrhythmias. Does the patient have a history of hypertension or hypoglycemia? Make sure to obtain a drug history. Has the patient recently started cardiac glycoside therapy? Also ask about caffeine, tobacco, and alcohol consumption.

Then explore associated symptoms, such as weakness, fatigue, and angina. Finally, auscultate for gallops, murmurs, and abnormal breath sounds.

Causes

◆ *Anxiety attack (acute).* Anxiety is the most common cause of palpitations in children and adults. With anxiety, palpitations may be accompanied by diaphoresis, facial flushing, trembling, and hyperventilation (that may lead to dizziness, weakness, and syncope).

◼ *Cardiac arrhythmias.* With a cardiac arrhythmia, paroxysmal or sustained palpitations may be accompanied by dizziness, weakness, and fatigue. The patient may also experience an irregular, rapid, or slow pulse rate.

◆ *Drugs.* Palpitations may result from drugs that precipitate cardiac arrhythmias or increase cardiac output. These include such drugs as cardiac glycosides, thyroid supplements, ganglionic blockers, beta-adrenergic blockers, calcium channel blockers, atropine, minoxidil (Rogaine), and sympathomimetics such as cocaine.

◆ *Hypertension.* With hypertension, the patient may be asymptomatic or may complain of sustained palpitations alone or with a headache, dizziness, tinnitus, and fatigue.

◆ *Hypocalcemia.* Typically, hypocalcemia produces palpitations, weakness, and fatigue. It progresses from paresthesia to muscle tension and carpopedal spasms. The patient may also exhibit muscle twitching.

◆ *Mitral prolapse.* Mitral prolapse is a valvular disorder that may cause paroxysmal palpitations accompanied by sharp, stabbing, or aching precordial pain. The hallmark of this disorder is a midsystolic click followed by an apical systolic murmur.

◆ *Mitral stenosis.* Early findings of mitral stenosis typically include sustained palpitations accompanied by exertional dyspnea and fatigue. Auscultation reveals a loud first heart sound or opening snap and a rumbling diastolic murmur at the apex.

◆ *Thyrotoxicosis.* Sustained palpitations are a characteristic symptom of thyrotoxicosis. They may be accompanied by tachycardia, dyspnea, weight loss despite increased appetite, tremors, diaphoresis, and heat intolerance.

Papular rash

A papular rash consists of small, raised, circumscribed and, perhaps, discolored (red to purple) lesions known as *papules.* The rash may erupt anywhere on the body in various configurations and may be acute or chronic. Papular rashes characterize many cutaneous disorders; they may also result from an allergy and from infectious, neoplastic, and systemic disorders. (To compare papules with other skin lesions, see *Recognizing common skin lesions,* page 414.)

Assessment

Begin your assessment by fully evaluating the papular rash. Note its color, configuration, and location on the patient's body. Find out when it erupted. Has the patient noticed changes in the rash since then? Is it itchy or burning, or painful or tender? Has there ever been discharge or drainage from the rash? If so, have the patient describe it. Also have him describe associated signs and symptoms, such as fevers, headaches, and GI distress.

Next, obtain a medical history, including allergies, previous rashes or skin disorders, infections, childhood diseases, sexual history (including sexually transmitted diseases), and cancers. Has the patient recently been bitten by an insect or rodent or been exposed to anyone with an infectious disease? Finally, obtain a complete drug history.

Causes

◆ *Acne vulgaris.* With acne vulgaris, rupture of enlarged comedones pro-

Recognizing common skin lesions

Macule

A small (usually less than 1 cm in diameter), flat blemish or discoloration that can be brown, tan, red, or white and has the same texture as surrounding skin

Bulla

A raised, thin-walled blister greater than 0.5 cm in diameter, containing clear or serous fluid

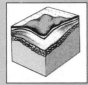

Vesicle

A small (less than 0.5 cm in diameter), thin-walled, raised blister containing clear, serous, purulent, or bloody fluid

Pustule

A circumscribed, pus- or lymph-filled elevated lesion that varies in diameter and may be firm or soft and white or yellow

Wheal

A slightly raised, firm lesion of variable size and shape, surrounded by edema; skin appearing red or pale

Nodule

A small, firm, circumscribed elevated lesion 1 to 2 cm in diameter with possible skin discoloration

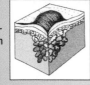

Papule

A small, solid, raised lesion less than 1 cm in diameter, with red, brown, or purple skin discoloration

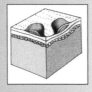

Tumor

A solid, raised mass usually larger than 2 cm in diameter with possible skin discoloration

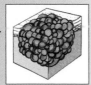

duces inflamed—and, perhaps painful and pruritic—papules, pustules, nodules, or cysts on the face and sometimes the shoulders, chest, and back.

◆ *Dermatomyositis.* Gottron's papules—flat, violet-colored lesions on the dorsa of the finger joints and the nape of the neck and shoulders—are characteristic of dermatomyositis, as is the dusky lilac discoloration of periorbital tissue and lid margins. They may be accompanied by a transient, erythematous, macular rash in a malar distribution on the face.

◆ *Follicular mucinosis.* With follicular mucinosis, perifollicular papules or plaques are accompanied by prominent alopecia.

◆ *Fox-Fordyce disease.* Fox-Fordyce disease is a chronic disorder that's marked by pruritic papules on the axillae, pubic area, and areolae associated with apocrine sweat gland inflammation. Sparse hair growth in these areas is also common.

◆ *Granuloma annulare.* Granuloma annulare is a benign, chronic disorder that produces papules that usually coalesce to form plaques. The papules spread peripherally to form a ring with a normal or slightly depressed center. They usually appear on the feet, legs, hands, or fingers and may be pruritic.

◆ *Human immunodeficiency virus (HIV) infection.* Acute infection with HIV typically causes a generalized maculopapular rash. Other signs and symptoms include fever, malaise, sore throat, and headache. Most patients don't recall these symptoms of acute infection.

◆ *Kaposi's sarcoma.* Kaposi's sarcoma is characterized by purple or blue papules or macules of vascular origin on the skin, mucous membranes, and viscera. These lesions decrease in size with firm pressure and then return to their original size within 10 to 15 seconds. They may become scaly and ulcerate with bleeding.

◆ *Lichen planus.* Discrete, flat, angular or polygonal, violet papules, commonly marked with white lines or spots, are characteristic of lichen planus. The papules may be linear or coalesce into plaques and usually appear on the lumbar region, genitalia, ankles, anterior tibiae, and wrists.

◆ *Necrotizing vasculitis.* With necrotizing vasculitis, crops of purpuric papules are typical. Some patients also develop low-grade fever, headache, myalgia, arthralgia, and abdominal pain.

◆ *Pityriasis rosea.* Pityriasis rosea begins with an erythematous "herald patch"—a slightly raised, oval lesion about ¾″ to 2½″ (2 to 6.5 cm) in diameter that may appear anywhere on the body. A few days to weeks later, yellow to tan or erythematous patches with scaly edges appear on the trunk, arms, and legs in a characteristic "pine tree" pattern.

◆ *Polymorphic light eruption.* Abnormal reactions to light may produce papular, vesicular, or nodular rashes on sun-exposed areas. Other symptoms include pruritus, headache, and malaise.

◆ *Psoriasis.* Psoriasis is a common chronic disorder that begins with small, erythematous papules on the scalp, chest, elbows, knees, back, buttocks, and genitalia. These papules are sometimes pruritic and painful. Eventually they enlarge and coalesce, forming elevated, red, scaly plaques covered by characteristic silver scales, except in moist areas such as the genitalia.

◆ *Rosacea.* Rosacea is a hyperemic disorder characterized by persistent erythema, telangiectasia, and recurrent eruption of papules and pustules on the forehead, malar areas, nasal creases, and chin.

◆ *Seborrheic keratosis.* With seborrheic keratosis, a cutaneous disorder, benign skin tumors begin as small, yellow-brown papules on the chest, back, or abdomen, eventually enlarging and becoming deeply pigmented. However, in blacks, these papules may remain small and affect only the malar part of the face (dermatosis papulosa nigra).

◆ *Syringoma.* With syringoma, adenoma of the sweat glands produces a yellowish or erythematous papular rash on the face (especially the eyelids), neck, and upper chest.

◆ *Systemic lupus erythematosus (SLE).* SLE is characterized by a "butterfly rash" of erythematous maculopapules or discoid plaques that appears in a malar distribution across the nose and cheeks.

Paralysis

Paralysis is the total loss of voluntary motor function and results from severe cortical or pyramidal tract damage. It can occur with a cerebrovascular disorder, degenerative neuromuscular disease, trauma, tumor, or central nervous system infection. Acute paralysis may be an early indicator of a life-threatening disorder such as Guillain-Barré syndrome.

Paralysis can be local or widespread, symmetrical or asymmetrical, transient or permanent, and spastic or flaccid. It's commonly classified according to location and severity as paraplegia, quadriplegia, or hemiplegia. Incomplete paralysis with profound weakness may precede total paralysis in some patients.

Assessment

If paralysis has developed suddenly, suspect trauma or an acute vascular insult. Quickly determine the patient's level of consciousness (LOC) and respiratory function, and check his vital signs. Elevated systolic blood pressure, widening pulse pressure, and bradycardia may signal increasing intracranial pressure (ICP). (See *Responding to paralysis.*)

If the patient is in no immediate danger, perform a complete neurologic assessment. Start with the history, relying on family members for information, if necessary. Ask about the onset, duration, intensity, and progression of paralysis and about the events preceding its development. Focus medical history questions on the incidence of degenerative neurologic or neuromuscular disease, recent infectious illness, sexually transmitted disease, cancer, or recent injury. Explore related signs and symptoms, noting fevers, headaches, vision disturbances, dysphagia, nausea and vomiting, bowel or bladder dysfunction, muscle pain or weakness, and fatigue.

Next, perform a complete neurologic examination, testing cranial nerve (CN), motor, and sensory function and deep tendon reflexes. Assess strength in all major muscle groups, and note muscle atrophy. (See *Testing muscle strength,* pages 376 and 377.) Document all findings to serve as a baseline.

Causes

◆ *Amyotrophic lateral sclerosis (ALS).* ALS is an invariably fatal disorder that produces spastic or flaccid paralysis, which eventually progresses to total paralysis in the body's major muscle groups. Earlier findings include pro-

EMERGENCY INTERVENTIONS

Responding to paralysis

If you suspect trauma or an acute vascular insult in a patient with paralysis:
◆ Make sure that his spine is properly immobilized.
◆ Elevate his head 30 degrees, if possible, to decrease intracranial pressure.

◆ Be prepared to administer oxygen, insert an artificial airway, or assist with intubation and mechanical ventilation, as needed.

gressive muscle weakness, fasciculations, and muscle atrophy, usually beginning in the arms and hands.
◆ *Bell's palsy.* Bell's palsy, a disease of CN VII, causes transient, unilateral facial muscle paralysis. The affected muscles sag, and eyelid closure is impossible. Other signs include increased tearing, drooling, and a diminished or absent corneal reflex.

⌑ *Botulism.* Botulism is a bacterial toxin infection that can cause rapidly descending muscle weakness that progresses to paralysis within 2 to 4 days after the ingestion of contaminated food. Respiratory muscle paralysis leads to dyspnea and respiratory arrest.

⌑ *Brain abscess.* Advanced abscess in the frontal or temporal lobe can cause hemiplegia accompanied by other late findings, such as ocular disturbances, unequal pupils, a decreased LOC, ataxia, tremors, and signs of infection.
◆ *Brain tumor.* A tumor affecting the motor cortex of the frontal lobe may cause contralateral hemiparesis that progresses to hemiplegia. Onset is gradual, but paralysis is permanent without treatment.
◆ *Conversion disorder.* Hysterical paralysis, a classic symptom of conversion disorder, is characterized by the loss of voluntary movement with no obvious physical cause.

◆ *Drugs.* The therapeutic use of neuromuscular blockers, such as pancuronium or curare, produces paralysis.

⌑ *Encephalitis.* Variable paralysis develops in the late stages of encephalitis. Earlier signs and symptoms include a rapidly decreasing LOC, fever, headache, photophobia, vomiting, and signs of meningeal irritation.

⌑ *Guillain-Barré syndrome.* Guillain-Barré syndrome is characterized by a rapidly developing, but reversible, ascending paralysis. It commonly begins as leg muscle weakness and progresses symmetrically. Respiratory muscle paralysis may be life-threatening.

⌑ *Head trauma.* Cerebral injury can cause paralysis due to cerebral edema and increased ICP. The onset is usually sudden. The location and extent vary, depending on the injury.
◆ *Multiple sclerosis (MS).* With MS, paralysis commonly waxes and wanes until the later stages, when it may become permanent. Its extent can range from monoplegia to quadriplegia. In most patients, vision and sensory disturbances (paresthesia) are the earliest symptoms.
◆ *Myasthenia gravis.* With myasthenia gravis, profound muscle weakness and abnormal fatigability may produce paralysis of certain muscle groups. Paralysis is usually transient in early stages,

Understanding spinal cord syndromes

When a patient's spinal cord is incompletely severed, he experiences partial motor and sensory loss. Most incomplete cord lesions fit into one of the syndromes described below.

Anterior cord syndrome, usually resulting from a flexion injury, causes motor paralysis and loss of pain and temperature sensation below the level of injury. Touch, proprioception, and vibration sensation are usually preserved.

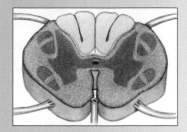

Brown-Séquard syndrome can result from flexion, rotation, or penetration injury. It's characterized by unilateral motor paralysis ipsilateral to the injury and a loss of pain and temperature sensation contralateral to the injury.

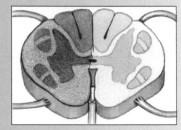

Central cord syndrome is caused by hyperextension or flexion injury. Motor loss is variable and greater in the arms than in the legs; sensory loss is usually slight.

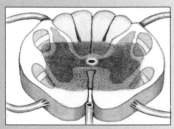

Posterior cord syndrome, produced by a cervical hyperextension injury, causes only a loss of proprioception and light touch sensation. Motor function remains intact.

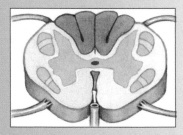

but becomes more persistent as the disease progresses.

◆ *Parkinson's disease.* Tremors, bradykinesia, and lead-pipe or cogwheel rigidity are the classic signs of Parkinson's disease. Extreme rigidity can progress to paralysis, particularly in the extremities. In most cases, paralysis resolves with prompt treatment of the disease.

◆ *Peripheral neuropathy.* Typically, peripheral neuropathy produces muscle weakness that may lead to flaccid paralysis and atrophy.

🔾 *Rabies.* Rabies is an acute disorder that produces progressive flaccid paralysis, vascular collapse, coma, and death within 2 weeks of contact with an infected animal.

◆ *Seizure disorders.* Seizures, particularly focal seizures, can cause transient local paralysis. Any part of the body may be affected, although paralysis tends to occur contralateral to the side of the irritable focus.

◆ *Spinal cord injury.* Complete spinal cord transection results in permanent spastic paralysis below the level of injury. Reflexes may return after spinal shock resolves. Partial transection causes variable paralysis and paresthesia, depending on the location and extent of injury. (See *Understanding spinal cord syndromes.*)

◆ *Spinal cord tumors.* Paresis, pain, paresthesia, and variable sensory loss may occur along the nerve distribution pathway served by the affected cord segment. Eventually, these symptoms may progress to spastic paralysis.

🔾 *Stroke.* Stroke involving the motor cortex can produce contralateral paresis or paralysis. Onset may be sudden or gradual, and paralysis may be transient or permanent. Associated signs and symptoms vary widely.

🔾 *Subarachnoid hemorrhage.* Subarachnoid hemorrhage can produce sudden paralysis. The condition may be temporary, resolving with decreasing edema, or permanent, if tissue destruction has occurred.

◆ *Syringomyelia.* Syringomyelia is a degenerative spinal cord disease that produces segmental paresis, leading to flaccid paralysis of the hands and arms. Reflexes are absent, and loss of pain and temperature sensation is distributed over the neck, shoulders, and arms in a capelike pattern.

◆ *Transient ischemic attack (TIA).* Episodic TIAs may cause transient unilateral paralysis accompanied by blurred or double vision, paresthesia, dizziness, aphasia, dysarthria, a decreased LOC, and other site-dependent findings.

Paresthesia

Paresthesia is an abnormal sensation or combination of sensations—commonly described as numbness, prickling, or tingling—felt along peripheral nerve pathways; these sensations generally aren't painful. Unpleasant or painful sensations, on the other hand, are termed *dysesthesias.* Paresthesia may develop suddenly or gradually and may be transient or permanent.

Paresthesia is a common symptom of many neurologic disorders and may also result from a systemic disorder or particular drug. It may reflect damage or irritation of the parietal lobe, thalamus, spinothalamic tract, or spinal or peripheral nerves—the neural circuit that transmits and interprets sensory stimuli.

Assessment

Begin your assessment by exploring the paresthesia. When did abnormal sensations begin? Have the patient describe their characteristics and distribution. Also, ask about associated signs and symptoms, such as sensory loss and paresis or paralysis. Next, take a medical history, including neurologic, cardiovascular, metabolic, renal, and chronic inflammatory disorders, such as arthritis or lupus. Has the patient recently sustained a traumatic injury or had surgery or an invasive procedure that may have damaged peripheral nerves?

Focus the physical examination on the patient's neurologic status. Assess his level of consciousness (LOC) and cranial nerve function. Test muscle strength and deep tendon reflexes (DTRs) in limbs affected by paresthesia. Systematically evaluate light touch, pain, temperature, vibration, and position sensation. (See *Testing for analgesia*, page 90.) Also, note skin color and temperature and palpate pulses.

Causes

◆ *Arterial occlusion (acute).* With acute arterial occlusion, sudden paresthesia and coldness may develop in one or both legs with a saddle embolus. Paresis, intermittent claudication, and aching pain at rest are also characteristic. The extremity becomes mottled with a line of temperature and color demarcation at the level of occlusion. Pulses are absent below the occlusion, and the capillary refill time is increased.

◆ *Arteriosclerosis obliterans.* Arteriosclerosis obliterans produces paresthesia, intermittent claudication (most common symptom), diminished or absent popliteal and pedal pulses, pallor, paresis, and coldness in the affected leg.

◆ *Arthritis.* Rheumatoid or osteoarthritic changes in the cervical spine may cause paresthesia in the neck, shoulders, and arms. Occasionally, the lumbar spine is affected, causing paresthesia in one or both legs and feet.

◆ *Brain tumor.* Tumors affecting the sensory cortex in the parietal lobe may cause progressive contralateral paresthesia accompanied by agnosia, apraxia, agraphia, homonymous hemianopsia, and a loss of proprioception.

◆ *Buerger's disease.* With Buerger's disease, a smoking-related inflammatory occlusive disorder, exposure to cold makes the feet cold, cyanotic, and numb; later, they redden, become hot, and tingle. Intermittent claudication, which is aggravated by exercise and relieved by rest, is also common.

◆ *Diabetes mellitus.* Diabetic neuropathy can cause paresthesia with a burning sensation in the hands and feet. Other findings include fatigue, polyuria, polydipsia, weight loss, polyphagia, and insidious, permanent anosmia.

▧ *Guillain-Barré syndrome.* With Guillain-Barré syndrome, transient paresthesia may precede muscle weakness, which usually begins in the legs and ascends to the arms and facial nerves. Weakness may progress to total paralysis.

◆ *Head trauma.* Unilateral or bilateral paresthesia may occur when head trauma causes a concussion or contusion; however, sensory loss is more common.

◆ *Herniated disk.* Herniation of a thoracic, lumbar, or cervical disk may cause acute or gradual onset of paresthesia along the distribution pathways of affected spinal nerves.

◆ *Herpes zoster.* Paresthesia is an early symptom of herpes zoster and occurs in the dermatome supplied by the affected spinal nerve. Within several days, this dermatome is marked by a pruritic, erythematous, vesicular rash associated with sharp, shooting, or burning pain.

◆ *Hyperventilation syndrome.* Usually triggered by acute anxiety, hyperventilation syndrome may produce transient paresthesia in the hands, feet, and perioral area.

◆ *Migraine headache.* Paresthesia in the hands, face, and perioral area may herald an impending migraine headache. Other prodromal symptoms include scotomas, hemiparesis, confusion, dizziness, and photophobia.

◆ *Multiple sclerosis (MS).* With MS, demyelination of the sensory cortex or spinothalamic tract may produce paresthesia—typically one of the earliest symptoms. Like other findings of MS, paresthesia commonly waxes and wanes until the later stages, when it may become permanent.

◆ *Peripheral nerve trauma.* Injury to a major peripheral nerve can cause paresthesia—commonly dysesthesia—in the area supplied by that nerve. Paresthesia begins shortly after trauma and may be permanent.

◆ *Peripheral neuropathy.* Peripheral neuropathy can cause progressive paresthesia in all extremities. The patient also commonly displays muscle weakness, which may lead to flaccid paralysis and atrophy.

◆ *Rabies.* Paresthesia, coldness, and itching at the site of an animal bite herald the prodromal stage of rabies.

◆ *Raynaud's disease.* Exposure to cold or stress makes the fingers turn pale, cold, and cyanotic; with rewarming, they become red and paresthetic.

◆ *Seizure disorders.* Seizures originating in the parietal lobe usually cause paresthesia of the lips, fingers, and toes. The paresthesia may act as auras that precede tonic-clonic seizures.

◆ *Spinal cord injury.* Paresthesia may occur in partial spinal cord transection, after spinal shock resolves. It may be unilateral or bilateral, occurring at or below the level of the lesion. Associated sensory and motor loss is variable. (See *Understanding spinal cord syndromes,* page 418.)

◆ *Spinal cord tumors.* Paresthesia, paresis, pain, and sensory loss along nerve pathways served by the affected cord segment result from such tumors.

◆ *Stroke.* Although contralateral paresthesia may occur with stroke, sensory loss is more common. Associated findings vary with the artery affected and may include contralateral hemiplegia, a decreased LOC, and homonymous hemianopsia.

◆ *Tabes dorsalis.* With tabes dorsalis, paresthesia—especially of the legs—is a common, but late, symptom. Other findings include ataxia, loss of proprioception and pain and temperature sensation, absent DTRs, Charcot's joints, Argyll Robertson pupils (characterized by miosis, irregular shape, and a loss of direct and consensual pupillary reflex to light, with normal pupillary constriction when looking at something near), incontinence, and impotence.

◆ *Transient ischemic attack (TIA).* Paresthesia typically occurs abruptly with a TIA and is limited to one arm or another isolated part of the body. It usually lasts about 10 minutes and is accompanied by paralysis or paresis.

Paroxysmal nocturnal dyspnea

Typically dramatic and terrifying to the patient, this sign refers to an attack of dyspnea that abruptly awakens the patient. Common findings include diaphoresis, coughing, wheezing, and chest discomfort. The attack abates after the patient sits up or stands for several minutes but may recur every 2 to 3 hours.

Paroxysmal nocturnal dyspnea is a sign of left-sided heart failure. It may result from decreased respiratory drive, impaired left ventricular function, enhanced reabsorption of interstitial fluid, or increased thoracic blood volume. All of these pathophysiologic mechanisms cause dyspnea to worsen when the patient lies down.

Assessment

Begin by exploring the patient's complaint of dyspnea. Does he have dyspneic attacks only at night or at other times as well, such as after exertion or while sitting down? If so, what type of activity triggers the attack? Does he experience coughing, wheezing, fatigue, or weakness during an attack? Find out if he has a history of lower extremity edema or jugular vein distention. Ask if he sleeps with his head elevated. If so, how many pillows does he use? Or, does he sleep in a reclining chair? Obtain a cardiopulmonary history. Does the patient have a history of a myocardial infarction, coronary artery disease, or hypertension? Has he had chronic bronchitis, emphysema, or asthma? Has he had cardiac surgery?

Next, perform a physical examination. Begin by checking the patient's vital signs and forming an overall impression of his appearance. Is he noticeably cyanotic or edematous? Auscultate the lungs for crackles and wheezing and the heart for gallops and arrhythmias.

Causes

◆ *Left-sided heart failure.* Dyspnea—on exertion, during sleep, and eventually even at rest—is an early sign of left-sided heart failure. This sign is characteristically accompanied by Cheyne-Stokes respirations, diaphoresis, weakness, wheezing, and persistent, nonproductive cough or cough that produces clear or blood-tinged sputum. As the patient's condition worsens, he develops tachycardia, tachypnea, alternating pulse (commonly initiated by a premature beat), a ventricular gallop, crackles, and peripheral edema. With advanced left-sided heart failure, the patient may also exhibit severe orthopnea, cyanosis, clubbing, hemoptysis, and cardiac arrhythmias as well as signs and symptoms of shock, such as hypotension, a weak pulse, and cold, clammy skin.

Peau d'orange

Usually a late sign of breast cancer, peau d'orange (orange peel skin) is the edematous thickening and pitting of breast skin. This slowly developing sign can also occur with breast or axillary lymph node infection, erysipelas, or Graves' disease. Its striking orange peel appearance stems from lymphatic edema around deepened hair follicles. (See *Recognizing peau d'orange*.)

Assessment

Ask the patient when she first detected peau d'orange. Has she noticed lumps, pain, or other breast changes? Does she have related signs and symptoms, such as malaise, achiness, or weight loss? Is she lactating, or has she recently weaned her infant? Has she had previous axillary surgery that may have impaired lymphatic drainage of the breast?

In a well-lit examining room, observe the patient's breasts. Estimate the extent of the peau d'orange, and check for erythema. Assess the nipples for discharge, deviation, retraction, dimpling, and cracking. Gently palpate the area of peau d'orange, noting warmth or induration. Then palpate the entire breast, noting fixed or mobile lumps, and the axillary lymph nodes, noting enlargement. Finally, take the patient's temperature.

Causes

◆ *Breast abscess.* Breast abscess, which usually affects lactating women with milk stasis, causes peau d'orange, malaise, breast tenderness and erythema, and sudden fever that may be accompanied by shaking chills. A cracked nipple may produce a purulent discharge, and an indurated or palpable soft mass may be present.
◆ *Breast cancer.* Advanced breast cancer is the most likely cause of peau d'orange, which usually begins in the dependent part of the breast or the areola. Palpation typically reveals a firm, immobile mass that adheres to the skin

Recognizing peau d'orange

In peau d'orange, the skin appears to be pitted (as shown here). This condition usually indicates late-stage breast cancer.

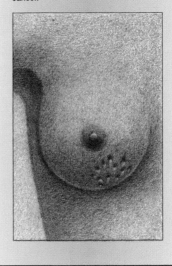

above the area of peau d'orange. Inspection of the breasts may reveal changes in contour, size, or symmetry. Inspection of the nipples may reveal deviation, erosion, retraction, and a thin and watery, bloody, or purulent discharge. The patient may report a burning and itching sensation in the nipples as well as a sensation of warmth or heat in the breast.

Pericardial friction rub

Commonly transient, a pericardial friction rub is a scratching, grating, or

Pericardial friction rub or murmur?

Is the sound you hear a pericardial friction rub or a murmur? Here's how to tell. The classic pericardial friction rub has three sound components, which are related to the phases of the cardiac cycle. In some patients, however, the rub's presystolic and early diastolic sounds may be inaudible, causing the rub to resemble the murmur of mitral insufficiency or aortic stenosis and insufficiency.

If you don't detect the classic three-component sound, you can distinguish a pericardial friction rub from a murmur by auscultating again and asking yourself these questions:

How deep is the sound?
A pericardial friction rub usually sounds superficial; a murmur sounds deeper in the chest.

Does the sound radiate?
A pericardial friction rub usually doesn't radiate; a murmur may radiate widely.

Does the sound vary with inspiration or changes in patient position?
A pericardial friction rub is usually loudest during inspiration and is best heard when the patient leans forward. A murmur varies in timing and duration with both factors.

best heard along the lower left sternal border during deep inspiration. It indicates pericarditis, which can result from an acute infection, a cardiac or renal disorder, postpericardiotomy syndrome, or the use of certain drugs.

Occasionally, a pericardial friction rub can resemble a murmur or a pleural friction rub. (See *Pericardial friction rub or murmur?*) However, the classic pericardial friction rub has three components. (See *Understanding pericardial friction rubs.*)

Assessment

Obtain a complete medical history, especially noting cardiac dysfunction. Has the patient recently had a myocardial infarction or cardiac surgery? Has he ever had pericarditis or a rheumatic disorder, such as rheumatoid arthritis or systemic lupus erythematosus? Does he have chronic renal failure or an infection? If the patient complains of chest pain, ask him to describe its character and location. What relieves the pain? What worsens it?

Check the patient's vital signs, particularly noting hypotension, tachycardia, an irregular pulse, tachypnea, and fever. Inspect for jugular vein distention, edema, ascites, and hepatomegaly. Auscultate the lungs for crackles. (See *Comparing auscultation findings*, pages 426 and 427.)

Causes

◆ *Pericarditis (acute).* A pericardial friction rub is the hallmark of acute pericarditis. This disorder also causes sharp precordial or retrosternal pain that usually radiates to the left shoulder, neck, and back. The pain worsens when the patient breathes deeply,

crunching sound that occurs when two inflamed layers of the pericardium slide over each other. Ranging from faint to loud, this abnormal sound is

Understanding pericardial friction rubs

The complete, or classic, pericardial friction rub is triphasic. Its three sound components are linked to phases of the cardiac cycle. The presystolic component (A) reflects atrial systole and precedes the first heart sound (S$_1$). The systolic component (B)—usually the loudest—reflects ventricular systole and occurs between the S$_1$ and second heart sound (S$_2$). The early diastolic component (C) reflects ventricular diastole and follows the S$_2$.

Sometimes, the early diastolic component merges with the presystolic component, producing a diphasic to-and-fro sound on auscultation. In other patients, auscultation may detect only one component—a monophasic rub, typically during ventricular systole.

TRIPHASIC RUB

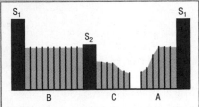

DIPHASIC RUB

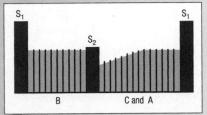

MONOPHASIC RUB

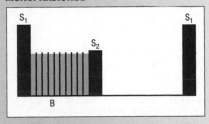

coughs, or lies flat and, possibly, when he swallows. It abates when he sits up and leans forward. The patient may also develop a fever, dyspnea, tachycardia, and arrhythmias.

◆ *Pericarditis (chronic constrictive).* With chronic constrictive pericarditis, a pericardial friction rub develops gradually and is accompanied by signs of decreased cardiac filling and output, such as peripheral edema, ascites, jugular vein distention on inspiration, and hepatomegaly. Dyspnea, orthopnea, paradoxical pulse, and chest pain may also occur.

(Text continues on page 428.)

Comparing auscultation findings

During auscultation, you may detect a pleural friction rub, a pericardial friction rub, or crackles—three abnormal sounds that are commonly confused. Use these illustrations to help clarify auscultation findings.

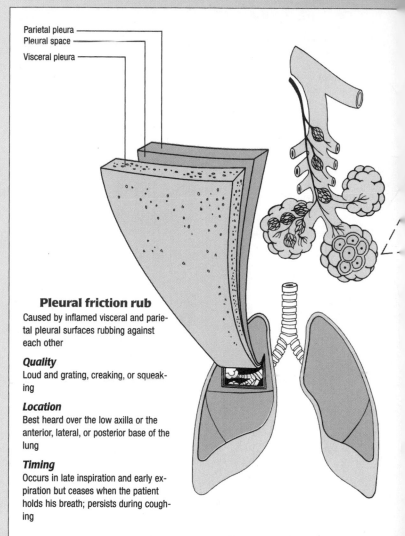

Parietal pleura
Pleural space
Visceral pleura

Pleural friction rub

Caused by inflamed visceral and parietal pleural surfaces rubbing against each other

Quality
Loud and grating, creaking, or squeaking

Location
Best heard over the low axilla or the anterior, lateral, or posterior base of the lung

Timing
Occurs in late inspiration and early expiration but ceases when the patient holds his breath; persists during coughing

Crackles

Caused by air suddenly entering fluid-filled airways

Quality

Popping or rattling

Location

Best heard at less distended and more dependent areas of the lungs, usually at the bases

Timing

Occurs during inspiration or expiration; doesn't clear with cough; stops when the patient holds his breath

Pericardial friction rub

Caused by inflamed layers of the pericardium rubbing against each other

Quality

Hard and grating, scratching, or crunching

Location

Best heard along the lower left sternal border

Timing

Occurs in relation to heartbeat; most noticeable during deep inspiration and continues even when the patient holds his breath

Peristaltic waves, visible

With intestinal obstruction, peristalsis temporarily increases in strength and frequency as the intestine contracts to force its contents past the obstruction. As a result, visible peristaltic waves may roll across the abdomen. Typically, these waves appear suddenly and vanish quickly because increased peristalsis overcomes the obstruction or the GI tract becomes atonic. Peristaltic waves are best detected by stooping at the patient's side and inspecting his abdominal contour while he's in a supine position. Visible peristaltic waves may also reflect normal stomach and intestinal contractions in thin patients or in malnourished patients with abdominal muscle atrophy.

Assessment

After observing peristaltic waves, collect pertinent history data. Ask about a history of pyloric ulcer, stomach cancer, or chronic gastritis, which can lead to pyloric obstruction. Also ask about conditions leading to intestinal obstruction, such as intestinal tumors or polyps, gallstones, chronic constipation, and hernia. Has the patient had recent abdominal surgery? Be sure to obtain a drug history.

Determine if the patient has related symptoms. Spasmodic abdominal pain, for example, accompanies small-bowel obstruction, whereas colicky pain accompanies pyloric obstruction. Is the patient experiencing nausea and vomiting? If he has vomited, ask about the consistency, amount, and color of the vomitus. Lumpy vomitus may contain undigested food particles; green or brown vomitus may contain bile or fecal matter.

Next, with the patient in a supine position, inspect the abdomen for distention, surgical scars and adhesions, or visible loops of bowel. Auscultate for bowel sounds, noting high-pitched, tinkling sounds. Then jar the patient's bed (or roll the patient from side to side), and auscultate for a succussion splash—a splashing sound in the stomach from retained secretions due to pyloric obstruction. Palpate the abdomen for rigidity and tenderness, and percuss for tympany. Check the skin and mucous membranes for dryness and poor skin turgor, indicating dehydration. Check the patient's vital signs, noting tachycardia and hypotension, which indicate hypovolemia.

Causes

◆ *Large-bowel obstruction.* Visible peristaltic waves in the upper abdomen are an early sign of large-bowel obstruction. Obstipation, however, may be the earliest finding.
◆ *Pyloric obstruction.* Peristaltic waves may be detected in a swollen epigastrium or in the left upper quadrant, usually beginning near the left rib margin and rolling from left to right. Related findings include vague epigastric discomfort or colicky pain after eating, nausea, vomiting, anorexia, and weight loss. Auscultation reveals a loud succussion splash.
◆ *Small-bowel obstruction.* Early signs of mechanical obstruction of the small bowel include peristaltic waves rolling across the upper abdomen and intermittent, cramping periumbilical pain. Associated signs and symptoms include nausea; vomiting of bilious or, later, fecal matter; and constipation. In partial

obstruction, diarrhea may occur. Hyperactive bowel sounds and slight abdominal distention also occur early.

Photophobia

A common symptom, photophobia is an abnormal sensitivity to light. In many patients, photophobia simply indicates increased eye sensitivity without underlying disease. For example, it can stem from wearing contact lenses excessively or using poorly fitted lenses. However, in others, this symptom can result from a systemic disorder, an ocular disorder or trauma, or the use of certain drugs.

Assessment

If the patient reports photophobia, find out when it began and how severe it is. Did it follow eye trauma, a chemical splash, or exposure to the rays of a sun lamp? If photophobia results from trauma, avoid manipulating the eyes. Ask the patient about eye pain, and have him describe its location, duration, and intensity. Does he have a sensation of a foreign body in his eye? Does he have other signs and symptoms, such as increased tearing, vision changes, nuchal rigidity, or severe headache?

Next, check the patient's vital signs and assess his neurologic status. Assess visual acuity, unless the cause is a chemical burn. Then perform a careful eye examination, inspecting the eyes' external structures for abnormalities. Examine the conjunctiva and sclera, noting their color. Characterize the amount and consistency of any discharge. Check pupillary reaction to light. Evaluate extraocular muscle function by testing the six cardinal fields of gaze, and test visual acuity in both eyes.

Causes

◆ *Burns.* With a chemical burn, photophobia and eye pain may be accompanied by erythema and blistering on the face and lids, miosis, diffuse conjunctival injection, and corneal changes. The patient experiences blurred vision and may be unable to keep his eyes open. With an ultraviolet radiation burn, photophobia occurs with moderate to severe eye pain. These symptoms develop about 12 hours after exposure to the rays of a welding arc or sun lamp.

◆ *Conjunctivitis.* When conjunctivitis affects the cornea, it causes photophobia. Other common findings include conjunctival injection, increased tearing, and a foreign-body sensation. Allergic conjunctivitis is distinguished by a stringy eye discharge and milky red injection. Bacterial conjunctivitis tends to cause a copious, mucopurulent, flaky eye discharge that may make the eyelids stick together in addition to brilliant red conjunctiva. Fungal conjunctivitis produces a thick, purulent discharge, extreme redness, and crusting, sticky eyelids. Viral conjunctivitis causes copious tearing with little discharge as well as enlargement of the preauricular lymph nodes.

◆ *Corneal abrasion.* A common finding with corneal abrasion, photophobia is usually accompanied by excessive tearing, conjunctival injection, visible corneal damage, and a foreign-body sensation in the eye.

◆ *Corneal ulcer.* A corneal ulcer is a vision-threatening disorder that causes severe photophobia and eye pain aggravated by blinking. Impaired visual acuity may accompany blurring, eye discharge, and sticky eyelids.

◆ *Iritis (acute).* Severe photophobia may result from acute iritis, along with marked conjunctival injection, moderate to severe eye pain, and blurred vision. The pupil may be constricted and may respond poorly to light.

◆ *Keratitis (interstitial).* Keratitis is a corneal inflammation that causes photophobia, eye pain, blurred vision, dramatic conjunctival injection, and grayish pink corneas.

▧ *Meningitis (acute bacterial).* A common symptom of meningitis, photophobia may occur with other signs of meningeal irritation, such as nuchal rigidity, hyperreflexia, severe headache, and opisthotonos.

◆ *Migraine headache.* Photophobia and noise sensitivity are prominent findings of a common migraine. Typically severe, this aching or throbbing headache may also cause fatigue, blurred vision, nausea, and vomiting.

◆ *Uveitis.* Anterior and posterior uveitis can cause photophobia. Typically, anterior uveitis also produces moderate to severe eye pain, severe conjunctival injection, and a small, nonreactive pupil. Posterior uveitis develops slowly, causing visual floaters, eye pain, pupil distortion, conjunctival injection, and blurred vision.

Pleural friction rub

Commonly resulting from a pulmonary disorder or trauma, this loud, coarse, grating, creaking, or squeaking sound may be auscultated over one or both lungs during late inspiration or early expiration. It's heard best over the low axilla or the anterior, lateral, or posterior bases of the lung fields with the pa-

tient upright. Sometimes intermittent, it may resemble crackles or a pericardial friction rub. (See *Comparing auscultation findings,* pages 426 and 427.)

A pleural friction rub indicates inflammation of the visceral and parietal pleural lining, which causes congestion and edema. The resultant fibrinous exudate covers both pleural surfaces, displacing the fluid that's normally between them and causing the surfaces to rub together.

Assessment

When you detect a pleural friction rub, quickly look for signs of respiratory distress, including shallow or decreased respirations, wheezing or stridor, dyspnea, increased accessory muscle use, intercostal or suprasternal retractions, cyanosis, and nasal flaring. Check for hypotension, tachycardia, and a decreased level of consciousness. (See *Responding to respiratory distress.*) If the patient isn't in severe distress, explore related symptoms. Find out if he has had chest pain. If so, ask him to describe its location and severity. How long does his chest pain last? Does the pain radiate to his shoulder, neck, or upper abdomen? Does the pain worsen with breathing, movement, coughing, or sneezing? Does the pain abate if he splints his chest, holds his breath, or exerts pressure or lies on the affected side?

Ask the patient about a history of rheumatoid arthritis, a respiratory or cardiovascular disorder, recent trauma, asbestos exposure, or radiation therapy. If he smokes, obtain a history in pack-years.

Characterize the pleural friction rub by auscultating the lungs with the patient sitting upright and breathing

EMERGENCY INTERVENTIONS

Responding to respiratory distress

If you detect signs of respiratory distress in a patient:
◆ Open and maintain an airway.
◆ Administer supplemental oxygen.
◆ Prepare for endotracheal intubation and mechanical ventilation, if needed.

◆ Insert a large-bore I.V. catheter to deliver drugs and I.V. fluids.
◆ Elevate the patient's head 30 degrees.
◆ Monitor cardiac and respiratory status constantly.
◆ Check vital signs frequently.

deeply and slowly through his mouth. Is the friction rub unilateral or bilateral? Also, listen for absent or diminished breath sounds, noting their location and timing in the respiratory cycle. Do abnormal breath sounds clear with coughing? Observe the patient for clubbing and pedal edema, which may indicate a chronic disorder. Then palpate for decreased chest motion and percuss for flatness or dullness.

Causes

◆ *Asbestosis.* Besides a pleural friction rub, asbestosis may cause exertional dyspnea, cough, chest pain, and crackles. Clubbing is a late sign.
◆ *Lung cancer.* A pleural friction rub may be heard in the affected area of the lung. Other findings include a cough (with possible hemoptysis), dyspnea, chest pain, weight loss, anorexia, fatigue, clubbing, fever, and wheezing.
◆ *Pleurisy.* A pleural friction rub occurs early in pleurisy. However, the cardinal symptom is sudden, intense chest pain that's usually unilateral and located in the lower and lateral parts of the chest. Deep breathing, coughing, or thoracic movement aggravates the

pain. Decreased breath sounds and inspiratory crackles may be heard over the painful area.
◆ *Pneumonia (bacterial).* A pleural friction rub occurs with bacterial pneumonia, which usually starts with a dry, painful, hacking cough that rapidly becomes productive. Other signs and symptoms develop suddenly. Auscultation reveals decreased breath sounds and fine crackles.
◆ *Pulmonary embolism.* An embolism can cause a pleural friction rub over the affected area of the lung. Usually, the first symptom is sudden dyspnea, which may be accompanied by angina or unilateral pleuritic chest pain.
◆ *Systemic lupus erythematosus (SLE).* Pulmonary involvement with SLE can cause a pleural friction rub, hemoptysis, dyspnea, pleuritic chest pain, and crackles.
◆ *Tuberculosis (TB; pulmonary).* With pulmonary TB, a pleural friction rub may occur over the affected part of the lung. Early signs and symptoms include weight loss, night sweats, low-grade fever in the afternoon, malaise, dyspnea, anorexia, and easy fatigability.

Polydipsia

Polydipsia refers to excessive thirst, a common symptom associated with endocrine disorders and certain drugs. It may reflect decreased fluid intake, increased urine output, or excessive loss of water and salt.

Assessment

Obtain a history. Find out how much fluid the patient drinks each day. How often and how much does he typically urinate? Does the need to urinate awaken him at night? Determine if he or anyone in his family has diabetes or kidney disease. What medications does he use?

Begin your physical assessment by taking his blood pressure and pulse when he's in supine and standing positions. A decrease of 10 mm Hg in systolic pressure and a pulse rate increase of 10 beats/minute from the supine to the sitting or standing position may indicate hypovolemia. If you detect these changes, ask the patient about recent weight loss. Check for signs of dehydration, such as dry mucous membranes and decreased skin turgor. Infuse I.V. replacement fluids as ordered.

Causes

◆ *Diabetes insipidus.* Diabetes insipidus characteristically produces polydipsia and may also cause excessive voiding of dilute urine and mild to moderate nocturia. Fatigue and signs of dehydration occur in severe cases.

◆ *Diabetes mellitus.* Polydipsia is a classic finding with diabetes mellitus—a consequence of the hyperosmolar state. Other characteristic findings include polyuria, polyphagia, nocturia, weakness, fatigue, and weight loss.

◆ *Drugs.* Diuretics and demeclocycline (Declomycin) may produce polydipsia. Phenothiazines and anticholinergics can cause dry mouth, making the patient so thirsty that he drinks compulsively.

◆ *Hypercalcemia.* As hypercalcemia progresses, the patient develops polydipsia, polyuria, nocturia, constipation, paresthesia and, occasionally, hematuria and pyuria. Severe hypercalcemia can progress quickly to vomiting, a decreased level of consciousness, and renal failure.

◆ *Hypokalemia.* Hypokalemia is an electrolyte imbalance that can cause nephropathy, resulting in polydipsia, polyuria, and nocturia.

◆ *Psychogenic polydipsia.* Psychogenic polydipsia is an uncommon disorder that causes polydipsia and polyuria. It may occur with any psychiatric disorder, but it's more common with schizophrenia.

◆ *Renal disorders (chronic).* Chronic renal disorders, such as glomerulonephritis and pyelonephritis, damage the kidneys, causing polydipsia and polyuria. Other findings include nocturia, elevated blood pressure, and pallor.

◆ *Sheehan's syndrome.* Polydipsia, polyuria, and nocturia occur with Sheehan's syndrome, a disorder of postpartum pituitary necrosis. Other findings include failure to lactate, amenorrhea, and decreased pubic and axillary hair growth.

◆ *Sickle cell anemia.* As nephropathy develops with sickle cell anemia, polydipsia and polyuria occur.

Polyphagia

Polyphagia refers to voracious or excessive eating. This common symptom can be persistent or intermittent, resulting primarily from endocrine and psychological disorders as well as the use of certain drugs. Depending on the underlying cause, polyphagia may cause weight gain.

Assessment

Begin your evaluation by asking the patient what he has had to eat and drink within the past 24 hours. (If he easily recalls this information, ask about his intake for the previous 2 days for a broader view of his dietary habits.) Note the frequency of meals and the amount and types of food eaten. Find out if the patient's eating habits have changed recently. Has he always had a large appetite? Does his overeating alternate with periods of anorexia? Ask about conditions that may trigger overeating, such as stress and depression. If the patient is female, also ask about menstruation. Does the patient actually feel hungry, or does he eat simply because food is available? Does he ever vomit or have a headache after overeating?

Explore related signs and symptoms. Has the patient recently gained or lost weight? Does he feel tired, nervous, or excitable? Has he experienced heat intolerance, dizziness, palpitations, diarrhea, or increased thirst or urination? Obtain a complete drug history, including the use of laxatives or enemas.

During the physical examination, weigh the patient. Tell him his current weight, and watch for an expression of disbelief or anger. Inspect the skin to detect dryness or poor turgor. Palpate the thyroid for enlargement.

Causes

◆ *Anxiety.* Polyphagia may result from mild to moderate anxiety or emotional stress.
◆ *Bulimia.* Most common in women ages 18 to 29, bulimia causes polyphagia that alternates with self-induced vomiting, fasting, or diarrhea. The patient typically weighs less than normal but has a morbid fear of obesity.
◆ *Diabetes mellitus.* With diabetes mellitus, polyphagia occurs with weight loss, polydipsia, and polyuria. It's accompanied by nocturia, fatigue, and signs of dehydration, such as dry mucous membranes and poor skin turgor.
◆ *Premenstrual syndrome (PMS).* Appetite changes, typified by food cravings and binges, are common with PMS. Abdominal bloating, the most common associated finding, may occur with behavioral changes.

Polyuria

A relatively common sign, polyuria is the daily production and excretion of more than 3 L of urine. It's usually reported by the patient as increased urination, especially when it occurs at night. Overhydration, consumption of caffeine or alcohol, and excessive ingestion of salt, glucose, or other hyperosmolar substances are aggravating factors.

Polyuria also results from the use of certain drugs or from a psychological, neurologic, or renal disorder. It can reflect central nervous system dysfunction that diminishes or suppresses antidiuretic hormone (ADH) secretion, which regulates fluid balance. Or, when ADH levels are normal, it can reflect renal impairment. In both of these pathophysiologic mechanisms, the renal tubules fail to reabsorb sufficient water, causing polyuria.

Assessment

Because the patient with polyuria is at risk for developing hypovolemia, evaluate his fluid status first. Check his vital signs, noting increased body temperature, tachycardia, and orthostatic hypotension (greater than or equal to a decrease of 10 mm Hg in systolic blood pressure and an increase of 10 beats/ minute in heart rate upon standing). Inspect for dry skin and mucous membranes, decreased skin turgor and elasticity, and reduced perspiration. Is the patient unusually tired or thirsty? Has he recently lost more than 5% of his body weight?

If the patient doesn't display signs of hypovolemia, explore the frequency and pattern of the polyuria. When did it begin? How long has it lasted? Was it precipitated by a certain event? Ask him to describe the pattern and amount of his daily fluid intake. Check for a history of visual deficits, headaches, or head trauma, which may precede diabetes insipidus. Also check for a history of urinary tract obstruction, diabetes mellitus, renal disorders, chronic hypokalemia or hypercalcemia, or psychiatric disorders. Ask if the patient is taking any drugs.

Perform a neurologic examination, noting any change in the patient's level of consciousness. Then palpate the bladder and inspect the urethral mea-tus. Obtain a urine specimen, and check its specific gravity.

Causes

◆ *Acute tubular necrosis.* During the diuretic phase of acute tubular necrosis, polyuria of less than 8 L/day gradually subsides after 8 to 10 days. Urine specific gravity (1.010 or less) increases as polyuria subsides.
◆ *Diabetes insipidus.* Polyuria of about 5 L/day with a specific gravity of 1.005 or less is common with diabetes insipidus, although extreme polyuria— up to 30 L/day—occasionally occurs, commonly accompanied by polydipsia and signs of dehydration.
◆ *Diabetes mellitus.* With diabetes mellitus, polyuria seldom exceeds 5 L/ day; however, urine specific gravity typically exceeds 1.020. The patient usually reports polydipsia, polyphagia, weight loss, and fatigue.
◆ *Drugs.* Diuretics characteristically produce polyuria. Cardiotonics, vitamin D, demeclocycline (Declomycin), phenytoin (Dilantin), lithium (Eskalith), and propoxyphene (Darvon) can also produce polyuria.
◆ *Glomerulonephritis (chronic).* Polyuria gradually progresses to oliguria with chronic glomerulonephritis. Urine output is usually less than 4 L/day; specific gravity is about 1.010. Nocturia, hematuria, frothy or malodorous urine, and mild to severe proteinuria may occur.
◆ *Postobstructive uropathy.* After resolution of a urinary tract obstruction, polyuria—usually more than 5 L/day with a specific gravity of less than 1.010—occurs for several days before gradually subsiding. Bladder distention and edema may occur with nocturia and weight loss.

◆ *Psychogenic polydipsia.* Most common in people older than age 30, psychogenic polydipsia usually produces dilute polyuria of 3 to 15 L/day, depending on fluid intake. The patient may appear depressed and experience headache and blurred vision.

Priapism

A urologic emergency, priapism is a persistent, painful erection that's unrelated to sexual excitation. This relatively rare sign may begin during sleep and appear to be a normal erection, but it may last for several hours or days. It's usually accompanied by a severe, constant, dull aching in the penis. Despite the pain, the patient may be too embarrassed to seek medical help and may try to relieve the condition through continued sexual activity.

Priapism occurs when the veins of the corpora cavernosa fail to drain correctly, resulting in persistent engorgement of the tissues. Without prompt treatment, penile ischemia and thrombosis occur. (See *Responding to priapism.*) In about one-half of all cases, priapism is idiopathic and develops without apparent predisposing factors. Secondary priapism can result from a blood disorder, neoplasm, trauma, or the use of certain drugs.

Assessment

If the patient's condition permits, ask him when the priapism began. Is it continuous or intermittent? Has he ever experienced a prolonged erection before? If so, what did he do to relieve it? How long did he remain without swelling? Does he have pain or tenderness when he urinates? Has he noticed changes in sexual function?

Explore the patient's medical history. If he reports sickle cell anemia, find out about factors that could precipitate a crisis, such as dehydration and infection. Ask if he has recently suffered genital trauma. Obtain a thorough drug history, and ask if he has had drugs injected or objects inserted into his penis.

Examine the patient's penis, noting its color and temperature. Check for loss of sensation and signs of infection, such as redness or drainage. Finally, check his vital signs, particularly noting any fever.

Causes

◆ *Drugs.* Priapism can result from the use of a phenothiazine, thioridazine

---

EMERGENCY INTERVENTIONS

Responding to priapism

If the patient has priapism:
◆ Apply an ice pack to the penis.
◆ Administer an analgesic as ordered.

◆ Prepare to insert an indwelling urinary catheter to relieve urine retention.
◆ Keep in mind that irrigation and surgery may be required.

(Mellaril), trazodone (Desyrel), an androgenic steroid, an anticoagulant, or an antihypertensive. It may also occur with medications used in treating erectile dysfunction.

◆ *Penile cancer.* Cancer that exerts pressure on the corpora cavernosa can cause priapism. Usually, the first sign is a painless ulcerative lesion or an enlarging warty growth on the glans or foreskin, which may be accompanied by localized pain, a foul-smelling discharge from the prepuce, a firm lump near the glans, and lymphadenopathy.

◆ *Sickle cell anemia.* With sickle cell anemia, painful priapism can occur without warning, usually on awakening. The patient may have a history of priapism, impaired growth and development, and an increased susceptibility to infection.

◆ *Spinal cord injury.* With spinal cord injury, the patient may be unaware of the onset of priapism. Related findings depend on the extent and level of injury and may include autonomic signs such as bradycardia.

◼ *Stroke.* A stroke may cause priapism, but sensory loss and aphasia may prevent the patient from noticing or describing it. Other findings depend on the stroke's location and extent.

Pruritus

Pruritus is an unpleasant itching sensation that affects the skin, certain mucous membranes, and the eyes. Commonly provoking scratching to gain relief, it's most severe at night and may be exacerbated by increased skin temperature, poor skin turgor, local vasodilation, dermatoses, and stress.

The most common symptom of dermatologic disorders, pruritus may also result from a local or systemic disorder or from drug use. Physiologic pruritus, such as pruritic urticarial papules and plaques of pregnancy, may occur in primigravidas late in the third trimester. Pruritus can also stem from emotional upset or contact with skin irritants.

Assessment

If the patient reports pruritus, have him describe its onset, frequency, and intensity. If pruritus occurs at night, ask whether it prevents him from falling asleep or awakens him after he falls asleep. (Generally, pruritus related to dermatoses prevents—but doesn't disturb—sleep.) Is the itching localized or generalized? When is it most severe? How long does it last? Is there a relationship to activities (physical exertion, bathing, applying makeup, or the use of perfumes)?

Ask the patient how he cleans his skin. In particular, look for excessive bathing, harsh soaps, contact allergy, and excessively hot water. Ask about the patient's general health and the medications he takes. Has he recently traveled abroad? Does he have pets? Does anyone else in the house report itching? Does stress, fear, depression, or illness seem to aggravate the itching? Does he have occupational exposure to known skin irritants, such as glass fiber insulation or chemicals, or other skin irritants? Ask about previous skin disorders and related symptoms. Then obtain a complete drug history.

Examine the patient for signs of scratching, such as excoriation, purpura, scabs, scars, or lichenification. Look for primary lesions to help confirm dermatoses.

Causes

◆ *Anemia (iron deficiency).* Iron deficiency anemia occasionally produces pruritus.

◆ *Conjunctivitis.* All forms of conjunctivitis cause eye itching, burning, and pain along with photophobia, conjunctival injection, a foreign-body sensation, excessive tearing, and a feeling of fullness around the eye.

◆ *Dermatitis.* Several types of dermatitis can cause pruritus accompanied by a skin lesion. Atopic dermatitis begins with intense, severe pruritus and an erythematous rash on dry skin at flexion points (antecubital fossa, popliteal area, and neck). During a flare-up, scratching may produce edema, scaling, and pustules. With chronic atopic dermatitis, lesions may progress to dry, scaly skin with white dermatographia, blanching, and lichenification.

Mild irritants and allergies can cause contact dermatitis, with itchy small vesicles that may ooze and scale and are surrounded by redness. A severe reaction can produce marked localized edema.

Dermatitis herpetiformis, most common in men between ages 20 and 50, initially causes intense pruritus and stinging. Between 8 and 12 hours later, symmetrically distributed lesions form on the buttocks, shoulders, elbows, and knees. These lesions are erythematous and papular, bullous, or pustular.

◆ *Hepatobiliary disease.* An important diagnostic clue to liver and gallbladder disease, pruritus is commonly accompanied by jaundice and may be generalized or localized to the palms and soles. Other characteristics include right upper quadrant pain, clay-colored stools, epigastric burning, and bitter fluid regurgitation.

◆ *Herpes zoster.* Within 2 to 4 days of a fever and malaise, pruritus, paresthesia or hyperesthesia, and severe, deep pain from cutaneous nerve involvement develop on the trunk or the arms and legs in a dermatome distribution.

◆ *Lichen simplex chronicus.* With lichen simplex chronicus, persistent rubbing and scratching cause localized pruritus and a circumscribed scaling patch with sharp margins. Later, the skin thickens and papules form.

◆ *Myringitis (chronic).* Myringitis produces pruritus in the affected ear, along with a purulent discharge and gradual hearing loss.

◆ *Pediculosis.* A prominent symptom, pruritus occurs in the area of infestation. Pediculosis capitis (head lice) may also cause scalp excoriation from scratching, along with matted, foul-smelling, lusterless hair; occipital and cervical lymphadenopathy; and oval, gray-white nits on hair shafts. Pediculosis corporis (body lice) initially causes small red papules (usually on the shoulders, trunk, or buttocks) that become urticarial from scratching. With pediculosis pubis (pubic lice), scratching commonly produces skin irritation. Nits or adult lice and erythematous, itching papules may appear in pubic hair or in hair around the anus, abdomen, or thighs.

◆ *Psoriasis.* Pruritus and pain are common in psoriasis. This skin disorder typically begins with small erythematous papules that enlarge or coalesce to form red elevated plaques with silver scales on the scalp, chest, elbows, knees, back, buttocks, and genitals. Nail pitting may occur.

◆ *Scabies.* Typically, scabies causes localized pruritus that awakens the patient. It may become generalized and persist for up to 2 weeks after treatment. Threadlike lesions several millimeters long appear with a swollen nodule or red papule.

◆ *Tinea pedis.* Tinea pedis is a fungal infection that causes severe foot pruritus, pain with walking, scales and blisters between the toes, and a dry, scaly squamous inflammation on the entire sole.

◆ *Urticaria.* Extreme pruritus and stinging occur as transient, erythematous or whitish wheals form on the skin or mucous membranes. Prickly sensations typically precede the wheals, which may affect any part of the body and may range from pinpoint to palm-sized or larger.

◆ *Vaginitis.* Vaginitis commonly causes localized pruritus and a foul-smelling vaginal discharge that may be purulent, white or gray, and curdlike. Perineal pain and urinary dysfunction may also occur.

Psoas sign

A positive psoas sign—increased abdominal pain when the patient moves his leg against resistance—indicates direct or reflexive irritation of the psoas muscles. This sign, which can be elicited on the right or left side, usually indicates appendicitis but may also occur with localized abscesses. It's elicited in

Eliciting a psoas sign

You can use two techniques to elicit a psoas sign in an adult with abdominal pain. With either technique, increased abdominal pain is a positive result, indicating psoas muscle irritation from an inflamed appendix or a localized abscess.

With the patient in a supine position, instruct her to move her flexed left leg against your hand to test for a left psoas sign. Then perform this maneuver on the right leg to test for a right psoas sign.

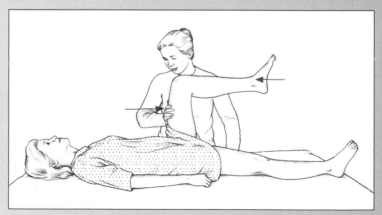

a patient with abdominal or lower back pain *after* completion of an abdominal examination to prevent spurious assessment findings. (See *Eliciting a psoas sign.*)

Assessment

If you elicit a positive psoas sign in a patient with abdominal pain, suspect appendicitis. (See *Responding to a positive psoas sign,* page 440.) Quickly check the patient's vital signs. Also check for the Rovsing sign by deeply palpating the patient's left lower quadrant. If he reports pain in the right lower quadrant, the sign is positive, indicating peritoneal irritation.

Causes

◆ *Appendicitis.* An inflamed retrocecal appendix can cause a positive right psoas sign. Early epigastric and periumbilical pain disappears, only to worsen and localize in the right lower quadrant. This pain also worsens with walking or coughing. A positive obturator sign may also be evident.

◆ *Retroperitoneal abscess.* After a lower retroperitoneal infection, an iliac or lumbar abscess can produce a positive right or left psoas sign and fever. An iliac abscess causes iliac or inguinal pain that may radiate to the hip, thigh, flank, or knee. A lumbar abscess usually produces back tenderness and

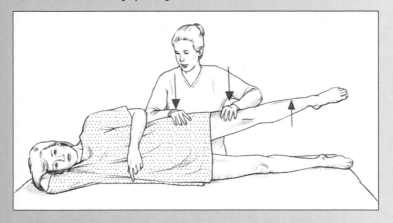

To test for a left psoas sign, turn the patient onto her right side. Then instruct her to push her left leg upward from the hip against your hand. Next, turn the patient onto her left side and repeat this maneuver to test for a right psoas sign.

EMERGENCY INTERVENTIONS

Responding to a positive psoas sign

If you elicit a positive psoas sign in a patient with abdominal pain, prepare him for surgery:
◆ Explain the procedure.
◆ Restrict food and fluids.

◆ Withhold analgesics (which can mask symptoms).
◆ Insert an I.V. catheter and administer I.V. fluids as ordered.
◆ Don't give a cathartic or an enema.

spasms on the affected side with a palpable lumbar mass.

Psychotic behavior

Psychotic behavior reflects an inability or unwillingness to recognize and acknowledge reality and to relate with others. It may begin suddenly or insidiously, progressing from vague complaints of fatigue, insomnia, or headaches to withdrawal, social isolation, and preoccupation with certain issues, resulting in gross impairment in functioning.

Various behaviors together or separately can constitute psychotic behavior, including delusions, illusions, hallucinations, bizarre language, and perseveration. Delusions are persistent beliefs that have no basis in reality or in the patient's knowledge or experience, such as delusions of grandeur. Illusions are misinterpretations of external sensory stimuli such as a mirage in the desert. In contrast, hallucinations are sensory perceptions that don't result from external stimuli. Bizarre language reflects a communication disruption. It can range from echolalia (purposeless repetition of a word or phrase) and clang association (repeti-

tion of words or phrases that sound similar) to neologisms (creation and use of words whose meaning only the patient knows). Perseveration, a persistent verbal or motor response, may indicate organic brain disease. Motor changes include inactivity, excessive activity, and repetitive movements.

Assessment

Because the patient's behavior can make it difficult—or potentially dangerous—to obtain pertinent information, conduct the interview in a calm, safe, and well-lit room. Provide enough personal space to avoid threatening or agitating the patient. Ask him to describe his problem and the circumstances that may have precipitated it. Obtain a drug history, noting especially the use of an antipsychotic, and explore his use of alcohol and other drugs. Ask about recent illnesses or accidents.

As the patient talks, watch for cognitive, linguistic, or perceptual abnormalities such as delusions. Do thoughts and actions seem to match? Look for unusual gestures, posture, gait, tone of voice, and mannerisms. Does the patient appear to be responding to stimuli?

Controlling psychotic behavior

A patient who displays psychotic behavior may be terrified and unable to differentiate between himself and his environment. To control his behavior and prevent injury to the patient, staff, and others, follow these guidelines:

◆ Remove potentially dangerous objects, such as belts or metal utensils, from the patient's environment.

◆ Help the patient discern what's real and unreal in an honest and genuine way.

◆ Be straightforward, concise, and nonthreatening when speaking to the patient. Discuss simple, concrete subjects, and avoid theories or philosophical issues.

◆ Positively reinforce the patient's perceptions of reality, and correct his misperceptions in a matter-of-fact way.

◆ *Never* argue with the patient, but also don't support his misperceptions.

◆ If the patient is frightened, stay with him.

◆ Touch the patient to provide reassurance *only* if you've done this before and know that it's safe.

◆ Move the patient to a safer, less-stimulating environment.

◆ Provide one-on-one care if the patient's behavior is extremely bizarre, disturbing to other patients, or dangerous to himself.

◆ Medicate the patient appropriately as prescribed.

Interview the patient's family. Which family members does he seem closest to? How does the family describe the patient's relationships, communication patterns, and role? Has a family member ever been hospitalized for psychiatric or emotional illness? Ask about the patient's compliance with his drug regimen.

Finally, evaluate the patient's environment, educational and employment history, and socioeconomic status. How does the patient spend his leisure time? Does he have friends? Has he ever had a close emotional relationship? Help him develop a conception of reality by calling him by his preferred name, telling him your name, describing where he is, and using clocks and calendars. (See *Controlling psychotic behavior*.)

Causes

◆ *Drugs.* Certain drugs can cause psychotic behavior. (See *Psychotic behavior: An adverse drug effect,* page 442.) However, almost any drug can provoke psychotic behavior as a rare, severe adverse or idiosyncratic reaction.

◆ *Organic disorders.* Various organic disorders, such as alcohol withdrawal syndrome, cocaine or amphetamine intoxication, cerebral hypoxia, and nutritional disorders, can produce psychotic behavior. Endocrine disorders, such as adrenal dysfunction, and severe infections, such as encephalitis, can also cause psychotic behavior. Neurologic causes include Alzheimer's disease and other dementias.

◆ *Psychiatric disorders.* Psychotic behavior usually occurs with bipolar disorder, personality disorder, schizophrenia, and some pervasive developmental disorders.

Psychotic behavior:
An adverse drug effect

Certain drugs can cause psychotic behavior and other psychiatric signs and symptoms, ranging from depression to violent behavior. Usually, these effects occur during therapy and resolve when the drug is discontinued. If the patient is receiving one of these common drugs and exhibits the behavior described, the dosage may have to be changed or another drug may have to be substituted.

DRUG	PSYCHIATRIC SIGNS AND SYMPTOMS
Albuterol (Proventil)	Hallucinations, paranoia
Alprazolam (Xanax)	Anger, hostility
Amantadine (Symmetrel)	Visual hallucinations, nightmares
Asparaginase (Elspar)	Confusion, depression, paranoia
Atropine and anticholinergics	Auditory, visual, and tactile hallucinations; memory loss; delirium; fear; paranoia
Bromocriptine (Parlodel)	Mania, delusions, sudden relapse of schizophrenia, paranoia, aggressive behavior
Cimetidine (Tagamet)	Hallucinations, paranoia, confusion, depression, delirium
Clonidine (Catapres)	Delirium, hallucinations, depression
Corticosteroids (prednisone [Deltasone], corticotrophin [ACTH], cortisone [Cortone])	Mania, catatonia, depression, confusion, paranoia, hallucinations
Cycloserine (Seromycin)	Anxiety, depression, confusion, paranoia, hallucinations
Dapsone	Insomnia, agitation, hallucinations
Diazepam (Valium)	Suicidal thoughts, rage, hallucinations, depression
Digoxin (Lanoxin)	Agitation, paranoia, auditory and visual hallucinations, panic
Disopyramide (Norpace)	Delirium, auditory hallucinations, paranoia, depression
Disulfiram (Antabuse)	Hostility, depression, paranoia, hallucinations
Indomethacin (Indocin)	Paranoia, euphoria, amnesia, visual hallucinations
Lidocaine (Anestacon)	Disorientation, hallucinations, paranoia
Methyldopa	Severe depression, amnesia, paranoia, hallucinations
Propranolol (Inderal)	Severe depression, hallucinations, paranoia, confusion
Thyroid hormones	Mania, hallucinations, paranoia
Vincristine (Oncovin)	Hallucinations

Ptosis

Ptosis is the excessive drooping of one or both upper eyelids. This sign can be constant, progressive, or intermittent and unilateral or bilateral. When it's unilateral, it's easy to detect by comparing the eyelids' relative positions. When it's bilateral or mild, it's difficult to detect—the eyelids may be abnormally low, covering the upper part of the iris or even part of the pupil instead of overlapping the iris slightly. Other clues include a furrowed forehead or a tipped-back head—both of these help the patient see under his drooping lids. With severe ptosis, the patient may not be able to raise his eyelids voluntarily. Because ptosis can resemble enophthalmos, exophthalmometry may be required.

Ptosis can be classified as congenital or acquired. Classification is important for proper treatment. Congenital ptosis results from levator muscle underdevelopment or disorders of the third cranial (oculomotor) nerve. Acquired ptosis may result from trauma to or inflammation of these muscles and nerves or from certain drugs, a systemic disease, an intracranial lesion, or a life-threatening aneurysm. However, the most common cause is advanced age, which reduces muscle elasticity and produces senile ptosis.

Assessment

Ask the patient when he first noticed his drooping eyelid. Also, ask him if it has worsened or improved since he first noticed it. Find out if he has recently suffered a traumatic eye injury. (If he has, avoid manipulating the eye to prevent further damage.) Ask about eye pain or headaches, and determine its location and severity. Has the patient experienced vision changes? Obtain a drug history, noting especially the use of a chemotherapeutic drug.

Assess the degree of ptosis, and check for eyelid edema, exophthalmos, deviation, and conjunctival injection. Evaluate extraocular muscle function by testing the six cardinal fields of gaze. (See *Testing extraocular muscles*, page 217.) Carefully examine the pupils' size, color, shape, and reaction to light, and test visual acuity.

Causes

◆ *Botulism.* Acute cranial nerve dysfunction as a result of botulism causes hallmark signs of ptosis, dysarthria, dysphagia, and diplopia.

◼ *Cerebral aneurysm.* An aneurysm that compresses the oculomotor nerve can cause sudden ptosis, along with diplopia, a dilated pupil, and an inability to rotate the eye.

◆ *Lacrimal gland tumor.* A lacrimal gland tumor commonly produces mild to severe ptosis, depending on the tumor's size and location. It may also cause brow elevation, exophthalmos, eye deviation and, possibly, eye pain.

◆ *Myasthenia gravis.* Commonly the first sign of myasthenia gravis, gradual bilateral ptosis may be mild to severe and is accompanied by weak eye closure and diplopia.

◆ *Ocular muscle dystrophy.* With ocular muscle dystrophy, bilateral ptosis progresses slowly to complete eyelid closure. Other findings include progressive external ophthalmoplegia and muscle weakness and atrophy of the upper face, neck, trunk, and limbs.

◆ *Ocular trauma.* Trauma to the nerve or muscles that control the eyelids can cause mild to severe ptosis. Depending on the damage, eye pain, lid swelling, ecchymosis, and decreased visual acuity may also occur.

◆ *Parry-Romberg syndrome.* Unilateral ptosis and facial hemiatrophy occur with Parry-Romberg syndrome. Other signs include miosis, sluggish pupil reaction to light, enophthalmos, different-colored irises, ocular muscle paralysis, nystagmus, and neck, shoulder, trunk, and extremity atrophy.

Pulse, absent or weak

An absent or weak pulse may be generalized or affect only one extremity. When generalized, this sign is an important indicator of such life-threatening conditions as shock and arrhythmia. Localized loss or weakness of a pulse that's normally present and strong may indicate acute arterial occlusion, which could require emergency surgery. However, the pressure of palpation may temporarily diminish or obliterate superficial pulses, such as the posterior tibial or the dorsal pedal. Thus, bilateral weakness or absence of these pulses doesn't necessarily indicate underlying disease. (See *Evaluating peripheral pulses.*)

Assessment

If you detect an absent or a weak pulse, quickly palpate the remaining arterial pulses to distinguish between localized or generalized loss or weakness. Then quickly check the patient's other vital signs, evaluate his cardiopulmonary status, and obtain a brief history. Based on your findings, proceed with emergency interventions. (See *Managing an absent or a weak pulse,* pages 446 and 447.)

Causes

◙ *Aortic aneurysm (dissecting).* When a dissecting aneurysm affects circulation to the innominate, left common carotid, subclavian, or femoral artery, it causes weak or absent arterial pulses distal to the affected area. Tearing pain usually develops suddenly in the chest and neck and may radiate to the upper and lower back and abdomen.

◆ *Aortic arch syndrome (Takayasu's arteritis).* Aortic arch syndrome produces weak or abruptly absent carotid pulses and unequal or absent radial pulses. These signs are usually preceded by malaise, night sweats, pallor, nausea, anorexia, weight loss, arthralgia, and Raynaud's phenomenon.

◆ *Aortic bifurcation occlusion (acute).* Aortic bifurcation occlusion produces abrupt absence of all leg pulses. The patient reports moderate to severe pain in the legs, which are cold, pale, numb, and flaccid.

◆ *Aortic stenosis.* With aortic stenosis, the carotid pulse is sustained but weak. Dyspnea (especially on exertion or paroxysmal nocturnal), chest pain, and syncope dominate the clinical picture.

◙ *Arrhythmias.* Cardiac arrhythmias may produce generalized weak pulses accompanied by cool, clammy skin. Other findings reflect the arrhythmia's severity and may include hypotension, chest pain, dyspnea, and dizziness.

◆ *Arterial occlusion.* With acute occlusion, arterial pulses distal to the obstruction are unilaterally weak and then absent. The affected limb is cool, pale, and cyanotic, with an increased capillary refill time. The patient complains of moderate to severe pain and paresthesia. A line of color and temperature demarcation develops at the level of obstruction.

◙ *Cardiac tamponade.* Cardiac tamponade causes a weak, rapid pulse accompanied by these classic findings: paradoxical pulse, jugular vein distention, hypotension, and muffled heart sounds.

◆ *Coarctation of the aorta.* Findings of coarctation of the aorta include bounding pulses in the arms and neck, with decreased pulsations and systolic pulse pressure in the lower extremities.

◆ *Peripheral vascular disease.* Peripheral vascular disease causes a weakening and loss of peripheral pulses. The patient complains of aching pain distal to the occlusion that worsens with exercise and abates with rest. The skin feels cool and shows decreased hair growth.

◼ *Pulmonary embolism.* Pulmonary embolism causes a generalized weak, rapid pulse. It may also cause an abrupt onset of chest pain, tachycardia, dyspnea, apprehension, syncope, diaphoresis, and cyanosis.

◼ *Shock (anaphylactic).* With anaphylactic shock, pulses become rapid and weak and then uniformly absent within seconds or minutes after exposure to an allergen. This is preceded by hypotension, a pounding headache and, possibly, urticaria.

◼ *Shock (cardiogenic).* With cardiogenic shock, peripheral pulses are absent and central pulses are weak, depending on the degree of vascular collapse. Pulse pressure is narrow. A drop in systolic blood pressure to 30 mm Hg below baseline or a sustained reading below 80 mm Hg produces poor tissue perfusion.

◼ *Shock (hypovolemic).* With hypovolemic shock, all pulses in the extremities become weak and then uniformly absent, depending on the severity of hypovolemia. As shock progresses, remaining pulses become thready and more rapid.

◼ *Shock (septic).* With septic shock, all pulses in the extremities first become weak. Depending on the degree of vascular collapse, pulses may then become uniformly absent.

◆ *Thoracic outlet syndrome.* A patient with thoracic outlet syndrome may de-

---

Evaluating peripheral pulses

The rate, amplitude, and symmetry of peripheral pulses provide important clues to cardiac function and the quality of peripheral perfusion. To gather these clues, palpate peripheral pulses lightly with the pads of your index, middle, and ring fingers, as space permits.

Rate

Count all pulses for at least 30 seconds (60 seconds when recording vital signs). The normal rate is between 60 and 100 beats/minute.

Amplitude

Palpate the blood vessel during ventricular systole. Describe pulse amplitude by using a scale such as the one below:
  4+ = bounding
  3+ = increased
  2+ = normal
  1+ = weak, thready
  0 = absent.
  Use a stick figure to easily document the location and amplitude of all pulses.

Symmetry

Simultaneously palpate pulses (except for the carotid pulse) on both sides of the patient's body, and note inequality. Always assess peripheral pulses methodically, moving from the arms to the legs.

---

velop gradual or abrupt weakness or loss of the pulses in the arms, depending on how quickly vessels in the neck compress. These pulse changes commonly occur after the patient works with his hands above his shoulders, lifts a weight, or abducts his arm.

(Text continues on page 448.)

EMERGENCY INTERVENTIONS

Managing an absent or a weak pulse

An absent or a weak pulse can result from any one of several life-threatening disorders. Your evaluation and interventions will vary, depending on whether the weak or absent pulse is generalized or localized to one extremity. They'll also depend on associated signs and symptoms. Use the flowchart below to help you establish priorities for successfully managing this emergency.

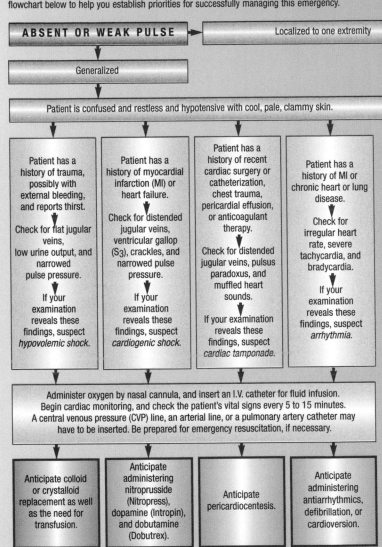

ABSENT OR WEAK PULSE → Localized to one extremity

Generalized

Patient is confused and restless and hypotensive with cool, pale, clammy skin.

Patient has a history of trauma, possibly with external bleeding, and reports thirst.	Patient has a history of myocardial infarction (MI) or heart failure.	Patient has a history of recent cardiac surgery or catheterization, chest trauma, pericardial effusion, or anticoagulant therapy.	Patient has a history of MI or chronic heart or lung disease.
Check for flat jugular veins, low urine output, and narrowed pulse pressure.	Check for distended jugular veins, ventricular gallop (S3), crackles, and narrowed pulse pressure.	Check for distended jugular veins, pulsus paradoxus, and muffled heart sounds.	Check for irregular heart rate, severe tachycardia, and bradycardia.
If your examination reveals these findings, suspect *hypovolemic shock.*	If your examination reveals these findings, suspect *cardiogenic shock.*	If your examination reveals these findings, suspect *cardiac tamponade.*	If your examination reveals these findings, suspect *arrhythmia.*

Administer oxygen by nasal cannula, and insert an I.V. catheter for fluid infusion. Begin cardiac monitoring, and check the patient's vital signs every 5 to 15 minutes. A central venous pressure (CVP) line, an arterial line, or a pulmonary artery catheter may have to be inserted. Be prepared for emergency resuscitation, if necessary.

Anticipate colloid or crystalloid replacement as well as the need for transfusion.	Anticipate administering nitroprusside (Nitropress), dopamine (Intropin), and dobutamine (Dobutrex).	Anticipate pericardiocentesis.	Anticipate administering antiarrhythmics, defibrillation, or cardioversion.

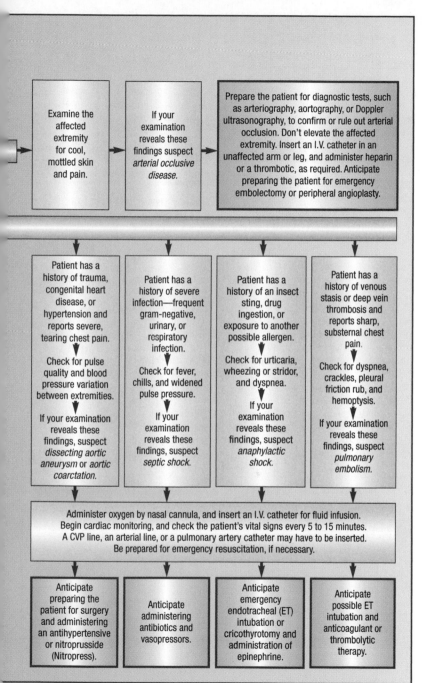

Examine the affected extremity for cool, mottled skin and pain.

If your examination reveals these findings suspect *arterial occlusive disease*.

Prepare the patient for diagnostic tests, such as arteriography, aortography, or Doppler ultrasonography, to confirm or rule out arterial occlusion. Don't elevate the affected extremity. Insert an I.V. catheter in an unaffected arm or leg, and administer heparin or a thrombotic, as required. Anticipate preparing the patient for emergency embolectomy or peripheral angioplasty.

Patient has a history of trauma, congenital heart disease, or hypertension and reports severe, tearing chest pain.

Check for pulse quality and blood pressure variation between extremities.

If your examination reveals these findings, suspect *dissecting aortic aneurysm* or *aortic coarctation*.

Patient has a history of severe infection—frequent gram-negative, urinary, or respiratory infection.

Check for fever, chills, and widened pulse pressure.

If your examination reveals these findings, suspect *septic shock*.

Patient has a history of an insect sting, drug ingestion, or exposure to another possible allergen.

Check for urticaria, wheezing or stridor, and dyspnea.

If your examination reveals these findings, suspect *anaphylactic shock*.

Patient has a history of venous stasis or deep vein thrombosis and reports sharp, substernal chest pain.

Check for dyspnea, crackles, pleural friction rub, and hemoptysis.

If your examination reveals these findings, suspect *pulmonary embolism*.

Administer oxygen by nasal cannula, and insert an I.V. catheter for fluid infusion. Begin cardiac monitoring, and check the patient's vital signs every 5 to 15 minutes. A CVP line, an arterial line, or a pulmonary artery catheter may have to be inserted. Be prepared for emergency resuscitation, if necessary.

Anticipate preparing the patient for surgery and administering an antihypertensive or nitroprusside (Nitropress).

Anticipate administering antibiotics and vasopressors.

Anticipate emergency endotracheal (ET) intubation or cricothyrotomy and administration of epinephrine.

Anticipate possible ET intubation and anticoagulant or thrombolytic therapy.

Pulse, bounding

Produced by large waves of pressure as blood ejects from the left ventricle with each contraction, a bounding pulse is strong and easily palpable and may be visible over superficial peripheral arteries. It's characterized by regular, recurrent expansion and contraction of the arterial walls and isn't obliterated by the pressure of palpation. A healthy person develops a bounding pulse during exercise, pregnancy, and periods of anxiety. However, this sign also results from fever and certain endocrine, hematologic, and cardiovascular disorders that increase the basal metabolic rate.

Assessment

After you detect a bounding pulse, check the patient's other vital signs and then auscultate the heart and lungs for abnormal sounds, rates, or rhythms. Ask the patient if he has noticed weakness, fatigue, shortness of breath, or other health changes. Review his medical history for hyperthyroidism, anemia, or a cardiovascular disorder, and ask about his use of alcohol.

Causes

◆ *Alcoholism (acute)*. Vasodilation produces a rapid, bounding pulse and flushed face. An odor of alcohol on the breath and an ataxic gait are common.
◆ *Aortic insufficiency*. Sometimes called a *water-hammer pulse,* the bounding pulse associated with aortic insufficiency is characterized by rapid, forceful expansion of the arterial pulse followed by rapid contraction. Widened pulse pressure also occurs. This disorder may produce findings associated with left-sided heart failure and cardiovascular collapse.
◆ *Febrile disorder*. Fever can cause a bounding pulse. Accompanying findings reflect the specific disorder.
◆ *Thyrotoxicosis*. Thyrotoxicosis produces a rapid, full, bounding pulse. Associated findings include tachycardia, palpitations, a third or fourth heart sound gallop, weight loss despite increased appetite, and heat intolerance.

Pulse pressure, narrowed

Pulse pressure, the difference between systolic and diastolic blood pressures, is measured by sphygmomanometry or intra-arterial monitoring. Normally, systolic pressure exceeds diastolic by about 40 mm Hg. Narrowed pressure—a difference of less than 30 mm Hg—occurs when peripheral vascular resistance increases, cardiac output declines, or intravascular volume markedly decreases.

With conditions that cause mechanical obstruction, such as aortic stenosis, pulse pressure is directly related to the severity of the underlying condition. Usually a late sign, narrowed pulse pressure alone doesn't signal an emergency, even though it commonly occurs with shock and other life-threatening disorders.

Assessment

After you detect a narrowed pulse pressure, check for other signs of heart failure, such as hypotension, tachycardia, dyspnea, jugular vein distention, pulmonary crackles, and decreased urine output. Also check for changes in skin temperature or color, the strength of peripheral pulses, and the patient's level of consciousness (LOC). Auscultate the heart for murmurs. Ask about a history of chest pain, dizziness, or syncope.

Causes

◼ *Cardiac tamponade.* With cardiac tamponade, pulse pressure narrows by 10 to 20 mm Hg. Paradoxical pulse, jugular vein distention, hypotension, and muffled heart sounds are classic. The patient may exhibit dyspnea, tachypnea, a decreased LOC, and a weak, rapid pulse.
◆ *Heart failure.* Narrowed pulse pressure occurs relatively late with heart failure and may accompany tachypnea, palpitations, dependent edema, chest tightness, hypotension, diaphoresis, pallor, and oliguria.
◼ *Shock.* With all forms of shock, narrowed pulse pressure occurs late.

Pulse pressure, widened

Pulse pressure is the difference between systolic and diastolic blood pressures. Normally, systolic pressure is about 40 mm Hg higher than diastolic pressure. Widened pulse pressure—a difference of more than 50 mm Hg—commonly occurs as a physiologic response to fever, hot weather, exercise, anxiety, anemia, or pregnancy. However, it can also result from certain neurologic disorders—especially life-threatening increased intracranial pressure (ICP)—or from cardiovascular disorders, such as aortic insufficiency, that cause blood backflow into the heart with each contraction. Widened pulse pressure can easily be identified by monitoring arterial blood pressure.

It's commonly detected during routine sphygmomanometry recordings.

Assessment

If the patient's level of consciousness (LOC) is decreased and you suspect that his widened pulse pressure results from increased ICP, check his vital signs. Perform a thorough neurologic examination to serve as a baseline for assessing subsequent changes. Use the Glasgow Coma Scale to evaluate the patient's LOC. (See *Glasgow Coma Scale,* page 342.) Also, check cranial nerve function—especially in cranial nerves III, IV, and VI—and assess pupillary reactions, reflexes, and muscle tone. If you don't suspect increased ICP, ask about associated symptoms, such as chest pain, shortness of breath, weakness, fatigue, or syncope. Check for edema, and auscultate for murmurs.

Causes

◼ *Aortic insufficiency.* With acute aortic insufficiency, pulse pressure widens progressively as the valve deteriorates and a bounding pulse and an atrial or a ventricular gallop develop. These signs may be accompanied by chest pain, palpitations, pallor, pulsus bisferiens, signs of heart failure, and strong, abrupt carotid pulsations.
◆ *Arteriosclerosis.* With arteriosclerosis, reduced arterial compliance causes progressive widening of pulse pressure, which becomes permanent without treatment of the underlying disorder.
◆ *Febrile disorder.* Fever can cause widened pulse pressure. Accompanying symptoms vary depending on the specific disorder.
◼ *Increased ICP.* Widening pulse pressure is an intermediate to late sign of increased ICP. Although a decreased

LOC is the earliest and most sensitive indicator, the onset and progression of widening pulse pressure also parallel rising ICP. (A gap of 50 mm Hg can signal a rapid deterioration in the patient's condition.) Assessment reveals Cushing's triad: bradycardia, hypertension, and widening pulse pressure.

Pulse rhythm abnormality

An abnormal pulse rhythm is an irregular expansion and contraction of the peripheral arterial walls. It may be persistent or sporadic and rhythmic or ar-

Abnormal pulse rhythm: A clue to cardiac arrhythmias

An abnormal pulse rhythm may be your only clue that the patient has a cardiac arrhythmia, but this sign doesn't help you pinpoint the specific type of arrhythmia. For that, you need a cardiac monitor or an electrocardiogram (ECG) machine. These devices record the electrical current generated by the heart's conduction system and display this information on an oscilloscope screen or a strip-chart recorder. Besides rhythm disturbances, they can identify conduction defects and electrolyte imbalances.

The ECG strips below show some common cardiac arrhythmias that can cause abnormal pulse rhythms.

ARRHYTHMIA

Sinus arrhythmia

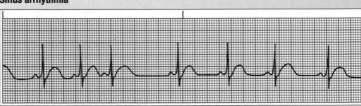

Premature atrial contractions (PACs)

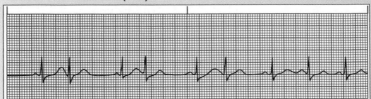

rhythmic. Detected by palpating the radial or carotid pulse, an abnormal rhythm is typically reported first by the patient, who complains of palpitations. This important finding reflects an underlying cardiac arrhythmia, which may range from benign to life-threatening. Arrhythmias are commonly associated with cardiovascular, renal, respiratory, metabolic, and neurologic disorders as well as the findings of drugs, diagnostic tests, and treatments. (See *Abnormal pulse rhythm: A clue to cardiac arrhythmias.*)

(*Text continues on page 454.*)

ULSE RHYTHM AND RATE	CLINICAL IMPLICATIONS
Irregular rhythm; fast, slow, or normal rate	◆ Reflex vagal tone inhibition (heart rate increases with inspiration and decreases with expiration) related to normal respiratory cycle ◆ May result from drugs, as in digoxin toxicity ◆ Occurs most commonly in children and young adults
Irregular rhythm during PACs; fast, slow, or normal rate	◆ Occasional PAC possibly normal ◆ Isolated PACs indicative of atrial irritation—for example, from anxiety or excessive caffeine intake (increasing PACs may herald other atrial arrhythmias). ◆ May result from heart failure, chronic obstructive pulmonary disease (COPD), or use of a cardiac glycoside, aminophylline, or medications that prolong the absolute refractory period of the sinoatrial node

(continued)

Abnormal pulse rhythm:
A clue to cardiac arrhythmias *(continued)*

ARRHYTHMIA

Paroxysmal atrial tachycardia

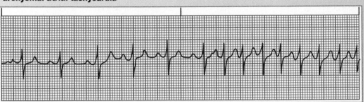

Atrial fibrillation

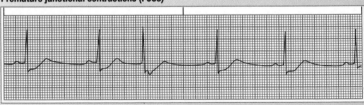

Premature junctional contractions (PJCs)

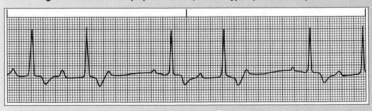

Second-degree atrioventricular (AV) heart block, Mobitz Type I (Wenckebach)

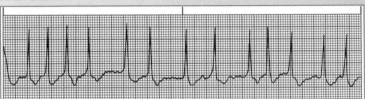

PULSE RHYTHM AND RATE	CLINICAL IMPLICATIONS
Regular rhythm with abrupt onset and termination of arrhythmia; heart rate exceeding 160 beats/minute	◆ May occur in otherwise healthy persons who are suffering from physical or psychological stress, hypoxia, or digoxin toxicity; who use marijuana; or who consume excessive amounts of caffeine or other stimulants ◆ May precipitate angina or heart failure
Irregular rhythm; atrial rate exceeding 400 beats/minute; ventricular rate variable	◆ May result from heart failure, COPD, hypertension, sepsis, pulmonary embolus, mitral valve disease, digoxin toxicity (rarely), atrial irritation, postcoronary bypass, or valve replacement surgery ◆ Because atria don't contract, preload isn't consistent, so cardiac output changes with each beat. Emboli may also result.
Irregular rhythm during PJCs; fast, slow, or normal rate	◆ May result from myocardial infarction (MI) or ischemia, excessive caffeine intake and, most commonly, digoxin toxicity (from enhanced automaticity)
Irregular ventricular rhythm; fast, slow, or normal rate	◆ Usually transient; may progress to complete heart block ◆ May result from inferior-wall MI, digoxin or quinidine toxicity, vagal stimulation, electrolyte imbalance, or arteriosclerotic heart disease

(continued)

Abnormal pulse rhythm:
A clue to cardiac arrhythmias *(continued)*

ARRHYTHMIA

Second-degree AV heart block, Mobitz Type II

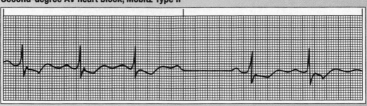

Premature ventricular contractions (multifocal)

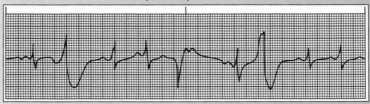

Assessment

Quickly look for signs of reduced cardiac output, such as a decreased level of consciousness, hypotension, or dizziness. Promptly obtain an electrocardiogram and possibly a chest X-ray, and begin cardiac monitoring. Closely monitor the patient's vital signs, pulse quality, and cardiac rhythm because accompanying bradycardia or tachycardia may cause further deterioration of cardiac output. If the patient's condition permits, ask if he's experiencing pain. If so, find out about its onset and location. Does the pain radiate? Ask about a history of heart disease and treatment for arrhythmias. Obtain a drug history, and check the patient's compliance. Also, ask about caffeine or alcohol intake. Digoxin (Lanoxin) toxicity, cessation of an antiarrhythmic, and the use of quinidine, a sympathomimetic (such as epinephrine), caffeine, or alcohol may cause arrhythmias.

Next, check the patient's apical and peripheral arterial pulses. An apical rate exceeding a peripheral arterial rate indicates a pulse deficit, which may also cause associated signs and symptoms of low cardiac output. Evaluate heart sounds: A long pause between S_1, the first heart sound (*lub*), and S_2, the second heart sound (*dub*), may indicate a conduction defect. A faint or absent S_1 and an easily audible S_2 may indicate atrial fibrillation or flutter. You

PULSE RHYTHM AND RATE	CLINICAL IMPLICATIONS
Irregular ventricular rhythm; slow or normal rate	◆ May progress to complete heart block ◆ May result from degenerative disease of conduction system, ischemia of AV node in an anterior-wall MI, anteroseptal infarction, electrolyte imbalance, or digoxin or quinidine toxicity
Usually irregular rhythm with a long pause after the premature beat; fast, slow, or normal rate	◆ Arise from different ventricular sites or from the same site with changing patterns of conduction ◆ May result from caffeine or stress, alcohol ingestion, myocardial ischemia or infarction, myocardial irritation by pacemaker electrodes, hypocalcemia, hypercalcemia, digoxin toxicity, or exercise

may hear the two heart sounds close together on certain beats—possibly indicating premature atrial contractions—or other variations in heart rate or rhythm. Take the patient's apical and radial pulses while you listen for heart sounds. With some arrhythmias, such as premature ventricular contractions, you may hear the beat with your stethoscope but not feel it over the radial artery. This indicates an ineffective contraction that failed to produce a peripheral pulse. Count the apical pulse for 60 seconds, noting the frequency of skipped peripheral beats. Report your findings to the practitioner.

Causes

🔹 *Cardiac arrhythmias.* An abnormal pulse rhythm may be the only sign of a cardiac arrhythmia. The patient may complain of palpitations, a fluttering heartbeat, or weak and skipped beats. Pulses may be weak and rapid or slow. Depending on the specific arrhythmia, dull chest pain or discomfort and hypotension may occur. Associated findings, if any, reflect decreased cardiac output.

Pulsus alternans

A sign of severe left-sided heart failure, pulsus alternans (alternating pulse) is a

Comparing arterial pressure waves

The waveforms shown here help differentiate a normal arterial pulse from pulsus alternans and pulsus paradoxus.

Normal arterial pulse

The percussion wave in a *normal arterial pulse* reflects ejection of blood into the aorta (early systole). The tidal wave is the peak of the pulse wave (later systole), and the dicrotic notch marks the beginning of diastole.

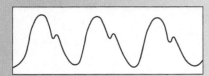

Pulsus alternans

Pulsus alternans is a beat-to-beat alteration in pulse size and intensity. Although the rhythm of pulsus alternans is regular, the volume varies. If you take the blood pressure of a patient with this abnormality, you'll first hear a loud Korotkoff sound and then a soft sound, continually alternating. Pulsus alternans commonly accompanies states of poor contractility that occur with left-sided heart failure.

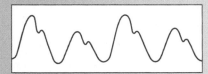

Pulsus bisferiens

Pulsus bisferiens is a double-beating pulse with two systolic peaks. The first beat reflects pulse pressure; the second, reverberation from the periphery. Pulsus bisferiens commonly occurs with aortic insufficiency (aortic stenosis, aortic regurgitation), hypertrophic cardiomyopathy, or high cardiac output states.

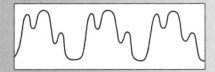

Pulsus paradoxus

Pulsus paradoxus is an exaggerated decline in blood pressure during inspiration, resulting from an increase in negative intrathoracic pressure. Pulsus paradoxus that exceeds 10 mm Hg is considered abnormal and may result from cardiac tamponade, constrictive pericarditis, or severe lung disease.

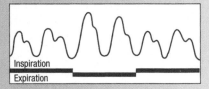

Inspiration
Expiration

beat-to-beat change in the size and intensity of a peripheral pulse. Although pulse rhythm remains regular, strong and weak contractions alternate. (See *Comparing arterial pressure waves*.) An alteration in the intensity of heart sounds and of existing heart murmurs may accompany this sign.

Pulsus alternans is thought to result from the change in stroke volume that occurs with beat-to-beat alteration in the left ventricle's contractility. Recumbency or exercise increases venous return and reduces the abnormal pulse, which typically disappears with treatment for heart failure. Rarely, a patient with normal left ventricular function has pulsus alternans, but the abnormal pulse seldom persists for more than 10 to 12 beats.

Assessment

Pulsus alternans indicates a critical change in the patient's status. When you detect it, be sure to quickly check his other vital signs. Closely evaluate the patient's heart rate, respiratory pattern, and blood pressure. Also, auscultate for a ventricular gallop and increased crackles. Although most easily detected by sphygmomanometry, you can detect pulsus alternans by palpating the brachial, radial, or femoral artery when systolic pressure varies from beat to beat by more than 20 mm Hg. Because the small changes in arterial pressure that occur during normal respirations may obscure this abnormal pulse, you'll need to have the patient hold his breath during palpation. Apply light pressure to avoid obliterating the weaker pulse.

When using a sphygmomanometer to detect pulsus alternans, inflate the cuff 10 to 20 mm Hg above the systolic pressure as determined by palpation and then slowly deflate it. At first, you'll hear only the strong beats. With further deflation, all beats will become audible and palpable and then equally intense. (The difference between this point and the peak systolic level is commonly used to determine the degree of pulsus alternans.) When the cuff is removed, pulsus alternans returns. Occasionally, the weak beat is so small that no palpable pulse is detected at the periphery. This produces total pulsus alternans, an apparent halving of the pulse rate.

Causes

◆ *Left-sided heart failure.* With left-sided heart failure, pulsus alternans is commonly initiated by a premature beat and is almost always associated with a ventricular gallop. Other findings include hypotension, cyanosis, fatigue, and weakness.

Pulsus bisferiens

A bisferious pulse is a hyperdynamic, double-beating pulse characterized by two systolic peaks separated by a midsystolic dip. Both peaks may be equal or either may be larger; however, the first peak is usually taller or more forceful than the second. The first peak (percussion wave) is believed to be the pulse pressure; the second (tidal wave), reverberation from the periphery. Pulsus bisferiens occurs in conditions in which a large blood volume is rapidly ejected from the left ventricle, as in aortic insufficiency. The pulse can be palpated in peripheral arteries or observed on an arterial pressure wave recording.

To detect pulsus bisferiens, lightly palpate the carotid, brachial, radial, or femoral artery. (The pulse is easiest to palpate in the carotid artery.) At the same time, listen to the patient's heart sounds to determine if the two palpable peaks occur during systole. If they do, you'll feel the double pulse between the first and second heart sounds. (See *Comparing arterial pressure waves,* page 456.)

Assessment

After you detect a bisferious pulse, review the patient's history for cardiac disorders. Next, find out what medication he's taking, if any, and ask if he has other illnesses. Also ask about associated signs and symptoms, such as dyspnea, chest pain, or fatigue. Find out how long he has had these symptoms and if they change with activity or rest. Then check his vital signs and auscultate for abnormal heart or breath sounds.

Causes

◆ *Aortic insufficiency.* Aortic insufficiency is the most common organic cause of a bisferious pulse. Most patients with chronic aortic insufficiency are asymptomatic until ages 40 to 50. However, exertional dyspnea, worsening fatigue, orthopnea and, eventually, paroxysmal nocturnal dyspnea may develop. Aortic insufficiency may produce signs and symptoms of left-sided heart failure and cardiovascular collapse. The patient may also exhibit widened pulse pressure and one or more murmurs, especially an apical diastolic rumble (Austin Flint murmur).
◆ *High cardiac output states.* Pulsus bisferiens commonly occurs with high output states, such as anemia, thyro-

toxicosis, fever, and exercise. Associated findings vary with the underlying cause and may include moderate tachycardia, a cervical venous hum, and widened pulse pressure.
◆ *Hypertrophic obstructive cardiomyopathy.* About 40% of patients with hypertrophic obstructive cardiomyopathy have pulsus bisferiens because of a pressure gradient in the left ventricular outflow tract. Recorded more often than it's palpated, the pulse rises rapidly. The first wave is the more forceful one.

Pulsus paradoxus

Pulsus paradoxus, or paradoxical pulse, is an exaggerated decline in blood pressure during inspiration. Normally, systolic pressure falls less than 10 mm Hg during inspiration. In pulsus paradoxus, it falls more than 10 mm Hg. (See *Comparing arterial pressure waves,* page 456.) When systolic pressure falls more than 20 mm Hg, the peripheral pulses may be barely palpable or may disappear during inspiration.

Pulsus paradoxus is thought to result from an exaggerated inspirational increase in negative intrathoracic pressure. Normally, systolic pressure drops during inspiration because of blood pooling in the pulmonary system. This, in turn, reduces left ventricular filling and stroke volume and transmits negative intrathoracic pressure to the aorta. Conditions associated with large intrapleural pressure swings, such as asthma, or those that reduce left-sided heart filling, such as pericardial tamponade, produce pulsus paradoxus.

Assessment

To accurately detect and measure pulsus paradoxus, use a sphygmomanometer or an intra-arterial monitoring device. Inflate the blood pressure cuff 10 to 20 mm Hg beyond the peak systolic pressure. Then deflate the cuff at a rate of 2 mm Hg/second until you hear the first Korotkoff sound during expiration. Note the systolic pressure. As you continue to slowly deflate the cuff, observe the patient's respiratory pattern. If pulsus paradoxus is present, the Korotkoff sounds disappear with inspiration and return with expiration. Continue to deflate the cuff until you hear Korotkoff sounds during inspiration and expiration, and again note the systolic pressure. Subtract this reading from the first one to determine the degree of pulsus paradoxus. A difference of more than 10 mm Hg is abnormal.

You can also detect pulsus paradoxus by palpating the radial pulse over several cycles of slow inspiration and expiration. Marked pulse diminution during inspiration indicates pulsus paradoxus. When you check for pulsus paradoxus, remember that irregular heart rhythms and tachycardia cause variations in pulse amplitude and must be ruled out before true pulsus paradoxus can be identified.

Pulsus paradoxus may signal cardiac tamponade—a life-threatening complication of pericardial effusion that occurs when sufficient blood or fluid accumulates to compress the heart. When you detect pulsus paradoxus, quickly check the patient's other vital signs. Check for additional signs and symptoms of cardiac tamponade, such as dyspnea, tachypnea, diaphoresis, jugular vein distention, tachycardia, narrowed pulse pressure, and hypotension. If the patient doesn't have cardiac tamponade, find out if he has a history of chronic cardiac or pulmonary disease. Ask about the development of associated signs and symptoms, such as cough or chest pain. Then auscultate for abnormal breath sounds.

Causes

◼ *Cardiac tamponade.* Pulsus paradoxus commonly occurs with cardiac tamponade, but it may be difficult to detect if intrapericardial pressure rises abruptly and profound hypotension occurs. With severe tamponade, assessment also reveals these classic findings: hypotension, diminished or muffled heart sounds, and jugular vein distention.

◆ *Chronic obstructive pulmonary disease (COPD).* The wide fluctuations in intrathoracic pressure that characterize COPD produce pulsus paradoxus and possibly tachycardia. Other findings vary but may include dyspnea, tachypnea, wheezing, a productive or nonproductive cough, accessory muscle use, barrel chest, and clubbing. The patient may show labored, pursed-lip breathing after exertion or even at rest.

◆ *Pericarditis (chronic constrictive).* Pulsus paradoxus can occur in up to 50% of patients with pericarditis. Other findings include a pericardial friction rub, chest pain, exertional dyspnea, orthopnea, hepatomegaly, and ascites. Patients also exhibit peripheral edema and Kussmaul's sign—jugular vein distention that becomes more prominent on inspiration.

◼ *Pulmonary embolism (massive).* Decreased left ventricular filling and stroke volume in massive pulmonary embolism produce pulsus paradoxus as well as syncope and severe dyspnea, tachypnea, and pleuritic chest pain.

The patient appears cyanotic, with jugular vein distention.

Pupils, nonreactive

Nonreactive (fixed) pupils fail to constrict in response to light or to dilate when the light is removed. The development of a unilateral or bilateral nonreactive response indicates an important change in the patient's condition and may signal a life-threatening emergency and possibly brain death. It also occurs with the use of certain optic drugs.

Assessment

If the patient is unconscious and develops unilateral or bilateral nonreactive pupils, quickly check his vital signs. Be alert for the development of untoward changes in the patient's condition. Remember that a unilateral dilated, nonreactive pupil may be an early sign of uncal brain herniation. If the patient is conscious, obtain a brief history. Ask if he's using eye drops. If he is, find out when they were last instilled. Also ask if he's experiencing pain. Check the patient's visual acuity in both eyes. Then test the pupillary reaction to accommodation: Normally, both pupils constrict equally as the patient shifts his glance from a distant to a near object.

To evaluate pupillary reaction to light, first test the patient's direct light reflex. Darken the room, and cover one of the patient's eyes while you hold open the opposite eyelid. Using a bright penlight, bring the light toward the patient from the side and shine it directly into his opened eye. If normal, the pupil will promptly constrict. Next, test the consensual light reflex. Hold the patient's eyelids open, and shine

the light into one eye while watching the pupil of the opposite eye. If normal, both pupils will promptly constrict. Repeat both procedures in the opposite eye. A unilateral or bilateral nonreactive response indicates dysfunction of cranial nerves (CNs) II and III, which mediate the pupillary light reflex. (See *Innervation of direct and consensual light reflexes*.)

Next, hold a penlight at the side of each eye and examine the cornea and iris for abnormalities. Measure intraocular pressure (IOP) with a tonometer, or estimate IOP by placing your second and third fingers over the patient's closed eyelid. If the eyeball feels rock-hard, suspect elevated IOP. Ophthalmoscopic and slit-lamp examinations of the eye will need to be performed. If the patient has experienced ocular trauma, don't manipulate the affected eye. After the examination, cover the affected eye with a protective metal shield but don't let the shield rest on the globe.

Causes

◆ *Drugs.* Instillation of a topical mydriatic and a cycloplegic may induce a temporarily nonreactive pupil in the affected eye. Opiates, such as heroin and morphine, cause pinpoint pupils with a minimal light response that can be seen only with a magnifying glass. Atropine poisoning produces widely dilated, nonreactive pupils.

◪ *Encephalitis.* As encephalitis progresses, initially sluggish pupils become dilated and nonreactive. Decreased accommodation and other symptoms of cranial nerve palsies, such as dysphagia, develop.

◆ *Glaucoma (acute angle-closure).* With acute angle-closure glaucoma, an ophthalmic emergency, examination reveals a moderately dilated, nonreactive

Innervation of direct and consensual light reflexes

Two reactions—direct and consensual—constitute the pupillary light reflex. Normally, when a light is shined directly onto the retina of one eye, the parasympathetic nerves are stimulated to cause brisk constriction of that pupil—the *direct light reflex*. The pupil of the opposite eye also constricts—the *consensual light reflex*.

The optic nerve (cranial nerve [CN] II) mediates the afferent arc of this reflex from each eye, whereas the oculomotor nerve (CN III) mediates the efferent arc to both eyes. A nonreactive or sluggish response in one or both pupils indicates dysfunction of these cranial nerves, usually due to degenerative disease of the central nervous system.

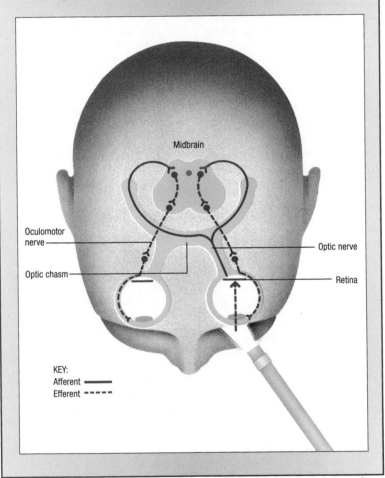

Midbrain

Oculomotor nerve

Optic chasm

Optic nerve

Retina

KEY:
Afferent ━━━━━
Efferent ─────

pupil in the affected eye. Conjunctival injection, corneal clouding, and decreased visual acuity also occur. The patient experiences a sudden onset of blurred vision, followed by excruciating pain in and around the affected eye, and commonly reports seeing halos around white lights at night.

◧ *Oculomotor nerve palsy.* Commonly, the first signs of oculomotor nerve palsy are a dilated, nonreactive pupil and loss of the accommodation reaction. These findings may occur in one or both eyes, depending on whether the palsy is unilateral or bilateral. Among the causes of total CN III palsy is life-threatening brain herniation. Central herniation causes bilateral midposition nonreactive pupils, whereas uncal herniation initially causes a unilateral dilated, nonreactive pupil.

◆ *Uveitis.* A small, nonreactive pupil that appears suddenly with severe eye pain, conjunctival injection, and photophobia typifies anterior uveitis. With posterior uveitis, similar findings develop insidiously, along with blurred vision and a distorted pupil shape.

Pupils, sluggish

A sluggish pupillary reaction is an abnormally slow pupillary response to light. It can occur in one pupil or both, unlike the normal reaction, which is always bilateral. A sluggish reaction accompanies degenerative disease of the central nervous system and diabetic neuropathy. It can occur normally in elderly people, whose pupils become smaller and less responsive with age.

Assessment

To assess pupillary reaction to light, first test the patient's direct light reflex. Darken the room, and cover one of the patient's eyes while you hold open the opposite eyelid. Using a bright penlight, bring the light toward the patient from the side and shine it directly into his opened eye. If normal, the pupil will promptly constrict. Next, test the consensual light reflex. Hold both of the patient's eyelids open, and shine the light into one eye while watching the pupil of the opposite eye. If normal, both pupils will promptly constrict. Repeat both procedures to test light reflexes in the opposite eye. A sluggish reaction in one or both pupils indicates dysfunction of cranial nerves II and III, which mediate the pupillary light reflex. (See *Innervation of direct and consensual light reflexes,* page 461.)

If you detect a sluggish pupillary reaction, determine the patient's visual function. Start by testing visual acuity in both eyes. Then test the pupillary reaction to accommodation; the pupils should constrict equally as the patient shifts his glance from a distant to a near object. Next, hold a penlight at the side of each eye and examine the cornea and iris for irregularities, scars, and foreign bodies. Measure intraocular pressure (IOP) with a tonometer, or estimate IOP by placing your fingers over the patient's closed eyelid. If the eyeball feels rock-hard, suspect elevated IOP. Also, ophthalmoscopic and slit-lamp examinations of the eye will need to be performed.

Causes

◆ *Adie's syndrome.* Adie's syndrome produces an abrupt onset of unilateral mydriasis and a sluggish pupillary response that may progress to a nonreactive response. The patient may complain of blurred vision and cramplike eye pain. Eventually, both eyes may be affected.

◾ *Encephalitis.* Encephalitis initially produces a bilateral sluggish pupillary response. Later, pupils become dilated and nonreactive and decreased accommodation may occur, along with other cranial nerve palsies, such as dysphagia and facial weakness.

◆ *Herpes zoster.* The patient with herpes zoster affecting the nasociliary nerve may have a sluggish pupillary response. Examination of the conjunctiva reveals follicles. Additional ocular findings include a serous discharge, absence of tears, ptosis, and extraocular muscle palsy.

◆ *Iritis (acute).* With iritis, the affected eye exhibits a sluggish pupillary response and conjunctival injection. The pupil may remain constricted; if posterior synechiae have formed, the pupil will also be irregularly shaped. The patient reports a sudden onset of eye pain and photophobia and may also have blurred vision.

◆ *Myotonic dystrophy.* With myotonic dystrophy, sluggish pupillary reaction may be accompanied by lid lag, ptosis, miosis and, possibly, diplopia. The patient may develop decreased visual acuity from cataract formation.

◆ *Tertiary syphilis.* A sluggish pupillary reaction (especially in Argyll Robertson pupils) occurs in the late stage of neurosyphilis, along with marked weakness of the extraocular muscles, visual field defects and, possibly, cataractous changes in the lens. The patient may complain of orbital rim pain, which worsens at night. He may also exhibit lid edema, decreased visual acuity, and exophthalmos.

◆ *Wernicke's disease.* Initially, Wernicke's disease produces an intention tremor accompanied by a sluggish pupillary reaction. Later, pupils may become nonreactive. Additional ocular findings include diplopia, gaze paralysis, nystagmus, ptosis, decreased visual acuity, and conjunctival injection.

Purpura

Purpura is the extravasation of red blood cells from the blood vessels into the skin, subcutaneous tissue, or mucous membranes. It's characterized by discoloration that's easily visible through the epidermis, usually purplish or brownish red. Purpuric lesions include petechiae, ecchymoses, and hematomas. (See *Identifying purpuric lesions,* page 464.) Purpura differs from erythema in that it doesn't blanch with pressure because it involves blood in the tissues, not just dilated vessels.

Purpura results from damage to the endothelium of small blood vessels, a coagulation defect, ineffective perivascular support, capillary fragility and permeability, or a combination of these factors. These faulty hemostatic factors, in turn, can result from thrombocytopenia or another hematologic disorder, an invasive procedure, or the use of an anticoagulant.

Additional causes are nonpathologic. Purpura can be a consequence of aging, when loss of collagen decreases connective tissue support of upper skin blood vessels. In an elderly or cachectic person, skin atrophy and inelasticity and loss of subcutaneous fat increase susceptibility to minor trauma, causing purpura to appear along the veins of the forearms, hands, legs, and feet. Prolonged coughing or vomiting can produce crops of petechiae in loose face and neck tissue. Violent muscle contraction, as occurs in seizures or weight lifting, sometimes results in localized ecchymoses from increased intraluminal pressure and rupture. A high fever, which increases capillary fragility, can also produce purpura.

Identifying purpuric lesions

Purpuric lesions fall into three categories: petechiae, ecchymoses, and hematomas.

Petechiae

Petechiae are painless, round, pinpoint lesions, 1 to 3 mm in diameter. Caused by extravasation of red blood cells into cutaneous tissue, these red or purple lesions usually arise on dependent portions of the body. They appear and fade in crops and can group to form ecchymoses.

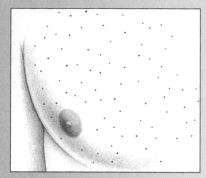

Ecchymoses

Ecchymoses, another form of blood extravasation, are larger than petechiae. These purple, blue, or yellow-green bruises vary in size and shape and can arise anywhere on the body as a result of trauma. Ecchymoses usually appear on the arms and legs of patients with bleeding disorders.

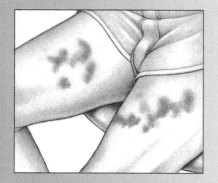

Hematomas

Hematomas are palpable ecchymoses that are painful and swollen. Usually the result of trauma, superficial hematomas are red, whereas deep hematomas are blue. Hematomas commonly exceed 1 cm in diameter, but their size varies widely.

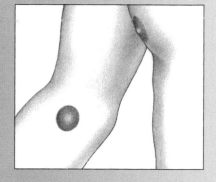

Assessment

Ask the patient when he first noticed the lesion and whether he has noticed other lesions on his body. Does he or his family have a history of bleeding disorders or easy bruising? Find out what medications he's taking, and ask him to describe his diet. Ask about recent trauma or transfusions and the development of associated signs, such as epistaxis, bleeding gums, hematuria, and hematochezia. Also ask about systemic complaints that may suggest infection, such as fever. If the patient is female, ask about heavy menstrual flow.

Inspect the patient's entire skin surface to determine the type, size, location, distribution, and severity of purpuric lesions. Also inspect the mucous membranes. Remember that the same mechanisms that cause purpura can also cause internal hemorrhage, although purpura isn't a cardinal indicator of this condition.

Causes

◆ *Autoerythrocyte sensitivity.* With autoerythrocyte sensitivity, painful ecchymoses appear either singly or in groups, usually preceded by local itching, burning, or pain.

▨ *Disseminated intravascular coagulation (DIC).* DIC can cause varying degrees of purpura, depending on its severity and underlying cause. Rarely, the patient develops purpura fulminans, with symmetrical cutaneous and subcutaneous lesions on the arms and legs. Or, he may have cutaneous oozing, hematemesis, or bleeding from incision or needle insertion sites.

◆ *Dysproteinemia.* An abnormal protein content in the blood, dysproteinemia can occur in patients with multiple myeloma as a result of an abnormal

proliferation of plasma cells that secrete protein. Petechiae and ecchymoses accompany other bleeding tendencies: hematemesis, epistaxis, gum bleeding, and excessive bleeding after surgery. Similar findings occur with cryoglobulinemia, which may also produce malignant maculopapular purpura. Hyperglobulinemia typically begins insidiously with occasional outbreaks of purpura over the lower legs and feet. These outbreaks eventually become more frequent and extensive, involving the entire lower leg and possibly the trunk.

◆ *Easy bruising syndrome.* Easy bruising syndrome is characterized by recurrent bruising on the legs, arms, and trunk, either spontaneously or following minor trauma. Bruising may be preceded by pain and is more common in women than in men, especially during menses.

◆ *Ehlers-Danlos syndrome (EDS).* Besides petechiae, EDS is marked by easy bruising, epistaxis, gum bleeding, hematuria, melena, menorrhagia, and excessive bleeding after surgery. EDS characteristically produces soft, velvety, hyperelastic skin; hyperextensible joints; and repeated dislocations of the temporomandibular joint.

◆ *Idiopathic thrombocytopenic purpura (ITP).* Chronic ITP typically begins insidiously, with scattered petechiae that are usually found on the distal arms and legs. Deep-lying ecchymoses may also occur.

◆ *Leukemia.* Leukemia produces widespread petechiae on the skin, mucous membranes, retina, and serosal surfaces that persist throughout the course of the disease. Acute leukemias also produce severe prostration and high fever and may cause dyspnea, tachycardia, palpitations, and abdominal or bone pain. Chronic leukemias begin insidiously with minor bleeding tendencies, malaise, fatigue, pallor, low-grade fever, anorexia, and weight loss.

◆ *Myeloproliferative disorders.* Myeloproliferative disorders, which include polycythemia vera, paradoxically can cause hemorrhage accompanied by ecchymoses and ruddy cyanosis. The oral mucosa takes on a deep purplish red hue, and slight trauma causes swollen gums to bleed.

◆ *Systemic lupus erythematosus (SLE).* SLE is a chronic inflammatory disorder that may produce purpura accompanied by other cutaneous findings, such as diffuse alopecia, telangiectasia, urticaria, ulceration, and scaly patches on the scalp, face, neck, and arms.

◆ *Thrombotic thrombocytopenic purpura.* Generalized purpura, hematuria, vaginal bleeding, jaundice, and pallor are among the usual presenting signs and symptoms in thrombotic thrombocytopenic purpura. Most patients have a fever, and some also experience weakness, headache, nausea, abdominal pain, arthralgia, and hepatosplenomegaly.

◆ *Trauma.* Traumatic injury can cause local or widespread purpura.

Pustular rash

A pustular rash is made up of crops of pustules—a visible collection of pus within or beneath the epidermis, commonly in a hair follicle or sweat pore. These lesions vary greatly in size and shape and can be generalized or localized. (See *Recognizing common skin lesions*, page 414.) Pustules can result from a skin or systemic disorder, the use of certain drugs, or exposure to a skin irritant. Although many pustular lesions are sterile, a pustular rash usually indicates an infection. A vesicular eruption, or even acute contact dermatitis, can become pustular if secondary infection occurs.

Assessment

Have the patient describe the appearance, location, and onset of the first pustular lesion. Did another type of skin lesion precede the pustule? Find out how the lesions spread. Ask what medications the patient takes and if he has applied a topical medication to his rash. If so, what type and when did he last apply it?

Examine the entire skin surface, noting if it's dry, oily, moist, or greasy. Record the exact location and distribution of the skin lesions and their color, shape, and size.

Causes

◆ *Acne vulgaris.* Pustules typify inflammatory lesions of acne vulgaris, which is accompanied by papules, nodules, cysts, open comedones (blackheads), and closed comedones (whiteheads).

◆ *Blastomycosis.* Blastomycosis is a fungal infection that produces small, painless, nonpruritic macules or papules that can enlarge to well-circumscribed, verrucous, crusted, or ulcerated lesions edged by pustules. Blastomycosis also produces signs of pulmonary infection.

◆ *Drugs.* Bromides and iodides commonly cause a pustular rash. Other drug causes include corticotropin (ACTH), corticosteroids, dactinomycin (Actinomycin D), lithium (Eskalith), phenytoin (Dilantin), phenobarbital (Luminal), isoniazid (INH), hormonal contraceptives, androgens, and anabolic steroids.

◆ *Folliculitis.* Folliculitis is a bacterial infection of hair follicles that produces individual pustules, each pierced by a hair and possibly accompanied by pruritus.

◆ *Furunculosis.* A furuncle is an acute, deep-seated, red, hot, tender abscess that evolves from a staphylococcal folliculitis. Furuncles usually begin as small, tender red pustules at the base of hair follicles. They're likely to occur on the face, neck, forearm, groin, axillae, buttocks, and legs or areas that are prone to repeated friction.

◆ *Impetigo contagiosa.* Impetigo contagiosa, a vesiculopustular eruptive disorder that occurs in nonbullous and bullous forms, is usually caused by streptococci or staphylococci. Vesicles form and break, and a crust forms from the exudate—a thick, yellow crust in streptococcal impetigo and a thin, clear crust in staphylococcal impetigo.

◆ *Pustular miliaria.* Pustular miliaria is an anhidrotic disorder that causes pustular lesions that begin as tiny erythematous papulovesicles located at sweat pores. Diffuse erythema may radiate from the lesion. The rash and associated burning and pruritus worsen with sweating.

◪ *Pustular psoriasis.* Small vesicles form and eventually become pustules in pustular psoriasis. The patient may report pruritus, burning, and pain. Localized pustular psoriasis usually affects the hands and feet. Generalized pustular psoriasis may erupt suddenly. Although rare, this form of psoriasis can occasionally be fatal.

◆ *Rosacea.* Rosacea is a chronic hyperemic disorder that commonly produces telangiectasia with acute episodes of pustules, papules, and edema. Characterized by persistent erythema, rosacea may begin as a flush covering the forehead, malar region, nasal creases, and chin.

◆ *Scabies.* Threadlike channels or burrows under the skin characterize scabies, which can also produce pustules, vesicles, and excoriations.

◆ *Varicella zoster.* When immunity to varicella declines, the virus reactivates along a dermatome, producing extremely painful and pruritic vesicles and pustules (herpes zoster, or shingles). Even with resolution of the rash, patients may experience chronic pain (postherpetic neuralgia) that may persist for months.

R

Raccoon eyes

Raccoon eyes are bilateral periorbital ecchymoses that don't result from facial soft-tissue trauma. This sign is usually an indicator of basilar skull fracture and develops when damage at the time of fracture tears the meninges and causes the venous sinuses to bleed into the arachnoid villi and the cranial sinuses. Raccoon eyes may be the only indicator of a basilar skull fracture, which isn't always visible on skull X-rays. Their appearance signals the need for careful assessment to detect underlying trauma because a basilar skull fracture can injure cranial nerves, blood vessels, and the brain stem. Raccoon eyes can also occur after a craniotomy if the surgery causes a meningeal tear.

Assessment

After raccoon eyes are detected, check the patient's vital signs and try to determine the nature of the head injury and when it occurred. (See *Recognizing raccoon eyes.*) Then evaluate the extent of underlying trauma.

Start by evaluating the patient's level of consciousness (LOC) using the Glasgow Coma Scale. (See *Glasgow Coma Scale,* page 342.) Next, evaluate cranial nerve (CN) function, especially CN I (olfactory), III (oculomotor), IV (trochlear), VI (abducens), and VII (facial). If the patient's condition permits, also test his visual acuity and gross hearing. Note irregularities in the facial or skull bones as well as swelling, localized pain, Battle's sign, or face or scalp lacerations. Check for ecchymoses over the mastoid bone. Inspect for hemorrhage or cerebrospinal fluid (CSF) leakage from the nose or ears.

Also, test drainage with a sterile 4″ × 4″ gauze pad, and note whether you find a halo sign—a circle of clear fluid that surrounds the drainage, indicating CSF. Also, use a glucose reagent stick to test clear drainage for glucose. An abnormal test result indicates CSF, because mucus doesn't contain glucose.

Causes

◤ *Basilar skull fracture.* A basilar skull fracture produces raccoon eyes after head trauma that doesn't involve the orbital area. Associated signs and symptoms vary with the fracture site and may include pharyngeal hemorrhage, epistaxis, rhinorrhea, otorrhea, and a bulging tympanic membrane from blood or CSF. The patient may experience difficulty hearing, head-

Recognizing raccoon eyes

It's usually easy to differentiate raccoon eyes from the "black eye" associated with facial trauma. Raccoon eyes (shown at right) are always bilateral. They develop 2 to 3 days after a closed-head injury that results in a basilar skull fracture. In contrast, the periorbital ecchymosis that occurs with facial trauma can affect one eye or both. It usually develops within hours of injury.

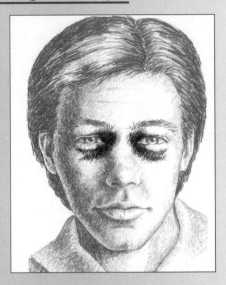

ache, nausea, vomiting, cranial nerve palsies, and an altered LOC. He may also exhibit a positive Battle's sign.

Rebound tenderness

A reliable indicator of peritonitis, rebound tenderness (also known as *Blumberg's sign*) is intense, elicited abdominal pain caused by rebound of palpated tissue. The tenderness may be localized, as in an abscess, or generalized, as in perforation of an intraabdominal organ. Rebound tenderness usually occurs with rigidity. When a patient has sudden, severe abdominal pain, this symptom is usually elicited to detect peritoneal inflammation.

Assessment

If you elicit rebound tenderness in a patient who's experiencing constant, severe abdominal pain, quickly check his vital signs. If the patient's condition permits, ask him to describe the events that led up to the tenderness. Does movement, exertion, or another activity relieve or aggravate the tenderness? Also, ask about other signs and symptoms, such as nausea and vomiting, fever, or abdominal bloating or distention. Inspect the abdomen for distention, visible peristaltic waves, and scars. Then auscultate for bowel sounds and characterize their motility. Palpate for associated rigidity or guarding, and percuss the abdomen, noting tympany. (See *Eliciting rebound tenderness,* page 470.)

Eliciting rebound tenderness

To elicit rebound tenderness, help the patient into a supine position, and push your fingers deeply and steadily into his abdomen (as shown). Then quickly release the pressure. Pain that results from the rebound of palpated tissue—rebound tenderness—indicates peritoneal inflammation or peritonitis.

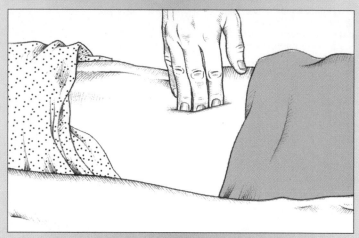

You can also elicit this symptom on a miniature scale by percussing the patient's abdomen lightly and indirectly (as shown). Better still, simply ask the patient to cough. This allows you to elicit rebound tenderness without having to touch the patient's abdomen and may also increase his cooperation because he won't associate exacerbation of his pain with your actions.

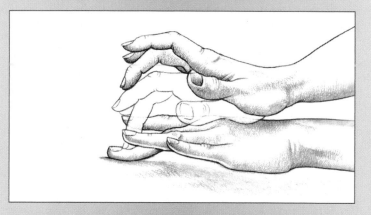

Causes

◤ *Peritonitis.* With peritonitis, rebound tenderness is accompanied by sudden and severe abdominal pain, which may be either diffuse or localized. Because movement worsens the patient's pain, he usually lies still on his back with his knees flexed or in a fetal position. Typically, he displays weakness, pallor, excessive sweating, and cold skin. He may also display abdominal distention, rigidity, and guarding and hypoactive or absent bowel sounds, tachypnea, nausea and vomiting, positive psoas and obturator signs, and a fever of 103° F (39.4° C) or higher. Inflammation of the diaphragmatic peritoneum may cause shoulder pain and hiccups.

Rectal pain

Rectal pain is a common symptom of anorectal disorders. It causes discomfort that arises in the anorectal area. Although the anal canal is separated from the rest of the rectum by the internal sphincter, the patient may refer to all local pain as rectal pain.

Because the mucocutaneous border of the anal canal and the perianal skin contains somatic nerve fibers, lesions in this area are especially painful. This pain may result from or be aggravated by diarrhea, constipation, or passage of hardened stools. It may also be aggravated by intense pruritus and continued scratching associated with drainage of mucus, blood, or fecal matter that irritates the skin and nerve endings.

Assessment

If the patient reports rectal pain, inspect the area for bleeding, abnormal drainage, or protrusions, such as skin tags or thrombosed hemorrhoids. Also check for inflammation and lesions. A rectal examination may be necessary.

After the examination, proceed with your evaluation by taking the patient's history. Ask him to describe the pain. Is it sharp or dull, burning or knifelike? How often does it occur? Ask if the pain is worse during or immediately after defecation. Does the patient avoid having bowel movements because of anticipated pain? Find out what alleviates the pain.

Be sure to ask appropriate questions about the development of associated signs and symptoms. For example, does the patient experience bleeding along with rectal pain? If so, find out how frequently it occurs and whether the blood appears on the toilet tissue, on the surface of the stool, or in the toilet bowl. Is the blood bright or dark red? Also ask whether the patient has noticed other drainage, such as mucus or pus, and whether he's experiencing constipation or diarrhea. Ask when he last had a bowel movement. Obtain a dietary history.

Causes

◆ *Abscess (perirectal).* A perirectal abscess can occur in various locations in the rectum and anus, causing pain in the perianal area. Typically, a superficial abscess produces constant, throbbing local pain that's exacerbated by sitting or walking. The local pain associated with a deeper abscess may begin insidiously, commonly high in the rectum or even in the lower abdomen, and is accompanied by an indurated anal mass. The patient may also develop associated signs and symptoms, such as a fever, malaise, anal swelling and inflammation, purulent drainage, and local tenderness.

◆ *Anal fissure.* An anal fissure is a longitudinal crack in the anal lining that causes sharp rectal pain on defecation. The patient typically experiences a burning sensation and gnawing pain that can continue for up to 4 hours after defecation. Fear of provoking this pain may lead to acute constipation. The patient may also develop anal pruritus and extreme tenderness and may report finding spots of blood on the toilet tissue after defecation.

◆ *Anorectal fistula.* An anorectal fistula is an abnormal passage between the anal canal and rectum. Pain develops when a tract formed between the anal canal and skin temporarily seals. The pain persists until drainage resumes. Other chief complaints include pruritus and drainage of pus, blood, mucus and, occasionally, stool.

◆ *Hemorrhoids.* Thrombosed or prolapsed hemorrhoids cause rectal pain that may worsen during defecation and abate after it. The patient's fear of provoking the pain may lead to constipation. Usually, rectal pain is accompanied by severe itching. Internal hemorrhoids may also produce mild, intermittent bleeding that characteristically occurs as spotting on the toilet tissue or on the stool surface. External hemorrhoids are visible outside the anal sphincter.

Respirations, grunting

Characterized by a deep, low-pitched grunting sound at the end of each breath, grunting respirations are a chief sign of respiratory distress in infants and children. They may be soft and heard only on auscultation or loud and clearly audible without a stethoscope.

Typically, the intensity of grunting respirations reflects the severity of respiratory distress. The grunting sound coincides with closure of the glottis—an effort to increase end-expiratory pressure in the lungs and prolong alveolar gas exchange—thereby enhancing ventilation and perfusion.

Grunting respirations indicate intrathoracic disease with lower respiratory involvement. Though most common in children, they sometimes occur in adults who are in severe respiratory distress. Whether they occur in children or adults, grunting respirations demand immediate medical attention.

Assessment

If the patient exhibits grunting respirations, intervene quickly. (See *Responding to grunting respirations.*)

After addressing the child's respiratory status, ask his parents when the grunting respirations began. If the patient is a premature infant, find out his gestational age. Ask the parents if anyone in the home has recently had an upper respiratory tract infection. Has the child had signs and symptoms of an infection, such as a runny nose, cough, low-grade fever, or anorexia? Does he have a history of frequent colds or upper respiratory tract infections? Does he have a history of respiratory syncytial virus? Ask the parents to describe changes in the child's activity level or feeding pattern to determine if he is lethargic or less alert than usual.

Begin the physical examination by auscultating the lungs, especially the lower lobes. Note diminished or abnormal sounds, such as crackles or sibilant rhonchi, which may indicate mucus or fluid buildup. Characterize the color, amount, and consistency of any

EMERGENCY INTERVENTIONS

Responding to grunting respirations

If the patient exhibits grunting respirations:
◆ Quickly place him in a comfortable position.
◆ Check for signs of respiratory distress, including:
– wheezing
– tachypnea—a minimum respiratory rate of 60 breaths/minute in infants, 40 breaths/minute in children ages 1 to 5, 30 breaths/minute in children older than age 5, or 20 breaths/minute in adults
– accessory muscle use
– substernal, subcostal, or intercostal retractions
– nasal flaring
– tachycardia—a minimum of 160 beats/minute in infants, 120 to 140 beats/minute in children ages 1 to 5, 120 beats/minute in children older than age 5, or 100 beats/minute in adults

– cyanotic lips or nail beds
– hypotension—less than 80/40 mm Hg in infants, less than 80/50 mm Hg in children ages 1 to 5, less than 90/55 mm Hg in children older than age 5, or less than 90/60 mm Hg in adults
– decreased level of consciousness.
If you detect any of these signs:
◆ Monitor oxygen saturation.
◆ Administer oxygen as prescribed.
◆ Administer prescribed medications such as a bronchodilator.
◆ Have emergency equipment available and prepare to intubate the patient if necessary.
◆ Obtain arterial blood gas analysis to determine oxygenation status.

---

discharge or sputum. Note the characteristics of the cough, if any.

Causes

◆ *Asthma.* Grunting respirations may be apparent during a severe asthma attack. They are usually triggered by an upper respiratory tract infection or an allergic response. As the attack progresses, dyspnea, audible wheezing, chest tightness, and coughing occur. Patients may have a silent chest if air movement is poor. Immediate bronchodilator therapy is needed.
◆ *Heart failure.* A late sign of left-sided heart failure, grunting respirations accompany increasing pulmonary edema. Associated features include a productive cough, crackles, jugular vein distention, and chest wall retractions. Cyanosis may also be evident, depending on the underlying congenital cardiac defect.
◗ *Pneumonia.* Life-threatening bacterial pneumonia is common after an upper respiratory tract infection or cold. *Pneumocystis carinii* pneumonia commonly affects children infected with human immunodeficiency virus. It causes grunting respirations accompanied by high fever, tachypnea, a productive cough, anorexia, and lethargy. Auscultation reveals diminished breath sounds, scattered crackles, and sibilant rhonchi over the affected lung. As the disorder progresses, the patient may also develop severe dyspnea, subster-

nal and subcostal retractions, nasal flaring, cyanosis, and increasing lethargy. Some infants also display GI signs, such as vomiting, diarrhea, and abdominal distention.

◆ *Respiratory distress syndrome.* Respiratory distress syndrome is the result of lung immaturity in a premature infant (less than 37 weeks' gestation), usually of low birth weight. This syndrome initially causes audible expiratory grunting along with tachycardia, tachypnea, and intercostal, subcostal, or substernal retractions. Later, as respiratory distress tires the infant, apnea or irregular respirations replace the grunting. Severe respiratory distress is characterized by cyanosis, frothy sputum, dramatic nasal flaring, lethargy, bradycardia, and hypotension. Eventually, the infant becomes unresponsive. Auscultation reveals harsh, diminished breath sounds and crackles over the base of the lungs on deep inspiration. Oliguria and peripheral edema may also occur.

Respirations, shallow

Respirations are shallow when a diminished volume of air enters the lungs during inspiration. In an effort to obtain enough air, the patient with shallow respirations usually breathes at an accelerated rate. However, as he tires or as his muscles weaken, this compensatory increase in respiratory rate diminishes, leading to inadequate gas exchange and such signs as dyspnea, cyanosis, confusion, agitation, loss of consciousness, and tachycardia.

Shallow respirations may develop suddenly or gradually and last briefly or become chronic. They're a key sign of respiratory distress and neurologic deterioration. Causes include inadequate central respiratory control over breathing, neuromuscular disorders, increased resistance to airflow into the lungs, respiratory muscle fatigue or weakness, voluntary alterations in breathing, decreased activity from prolonged bed rest, and pain.

Assessment

If you observe shallow respirations, be alert for impending respiratory failure or arrest. (See *Responding to impending respiratory failure.*) Is the patient severely dyspneic, agitated, or frightened? Look for signs of airway obstruction. If the patient is also wheezing, check for stridor, nasal flaring, and accessory muscle use. Tachycardia, increased or decreased blood pressure, poor minute volume, and deteriorating arterial blood gas levels or oxygen saturation signal the need for intubation and mechanical ventilation. (See *Measuring lung volumes,* page 476.)

If the patient isn't in severe respiratory distress, begin with the history. Ask about chronic illness and surgery or trauma. Does he have asthma, allergies, or a history of heart failure or vascular disease? Does he have a chronic respiratory disorder or respiratory tract infection, tuberculosis, or a neurologic or neuromuscular disease? Does he smoke? Obtain a drug history as well, and explore the possibility of drug abuse.

Ask about the patient's shallow respirations: When did they begin? How long do they last? What makes them subside? What aggravates them? Ask about changes in appetite, weight, activity level, and behavior.

Begin the physical examination by assessing the patient's level of consciousness (LOC) and his orientation to time, person, and place. Observe spontaneous movements, and test muscle

EMERGENCY INTERVENTIONS

Responding to impending respiratory failure

If your patient shows signs of impending respiratory failure or arrest, act quickly.
   If the patient is choking:
◆ Perform abdominal thrusts in rapid sequence.
◆ Use suction if secretions occlude the patient's airway.
   After checking for other signs:
◆ Administer oxygen via face mask or handheld resuscitation bag.
◆ Attempt to calm the patient.

◆ Administer epinephrine I.V., as ordered.
   If the patient loses consciousness:
◆ Insert an artificial airway and prepare for endotracheal intubation and ventilatory support.
◆ Measure his tidal volume and minute volume with a Wright respirometer to determine the need for mechanical ventilation.
◆ Check arterial blood gas levels, heart rate, blood pressure, and oxygen saturation.

strength and deep tendon reflexes. Next, inspect the chest for deformities or abnormal movements, such as intercostal retractions. Inspect the extremities for cyanosis and digital clubbing. Palpate for expansion and diaphragmatic tactile fremitus, and percuss for hyperresonance or dullness. Auscultate for diminished, absent, or adventitious breath sounds and for abnormal or distant heart sounds. Do you note peripheral edema? Finally, examine the abdomen for distention, tenderness, or masses.

Causes

⚑ *Acute respiratory distress syndrome (ARDS).* Initially, ARDS produces rapid, shallow respirations and dyspnea. Hypoxemia leads to intercostal and suprasternal retractions, diaphoresis, and fluid accumulation, causing rhonchi and crackles.
◆ *Amyotrophic lateral sclerosis (ALS).* Respiratory muscle weakness in ALS causes progressive shallow respira-

tions. Exertion may result in increased weakness and respiratory distress. ALS initially produces upper extremity muscle weakness and wasting, which in several years affect the trunk, neck, tongue, and muscles of the larynx, pharynx, and lower extremities.
◆ *Asthma.* With asthma, bronchospasm and hyperinflation of the lungs cause rapid, shallow respirations. In adults, mild persistent signs and symptoms may worsen during severe attacks. Related respiratory effects include wheezing, rhonchi, dyspnea, prolonged expirations, intercostal and supraclavicular retractions on inspiration, and nasal flaring.
◆ *Atelectasis.* Decreased lung expansion or pleuritic pain causes a sudden onset of rapid, shallow respirations. Other signs and symptoms include a dry cough, dyspnea, tachycardia, anxiety, cyanosis, and diaphoresis.
◆ *Bronchiectasis.* Increased secretions obstruct airflow in the lungs, leading to shallow respirations and a productive cough with copious, foul-smelling, mu-

Measuring lung volumes

Use a Wright respirometer to measure tidal volume (the amount of air inspired with each breath) and minute volume (the volume of air inspired in a minute—or tidal volume multiplied by respiratory rate). You can connect the respirometer to an intubated patient's airway via an endotracheal tube (shown here) or a tracheostomy tube. If the patient isn't intubated, connect the respirometer to a face mask, making sure the seal over the patient's mouth and nose is airtight.

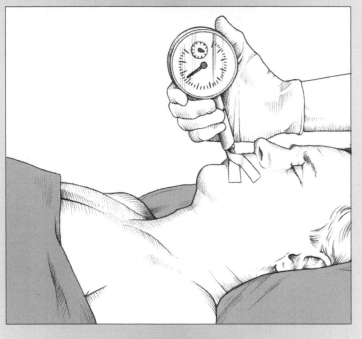

copurulent sputum. Other findings include hemoptysis, wheezing, rhonchi, coarse crackles during inspiration, and late-stage clubbing.

◆ *Coma.* Rapid, shallow respirations result from neurologic dysfunction or restricted chest movement with a coma.

◆ *Emphysema.* Increased breathing effort causes muscle fatigue, leading to chronic shallow respirations. The pa-

tient with emphysema may also display dyspnea, malaise, diminished breath sounds, cyanosis, pursed-lip breathing, and barrel chest.

◪ *Flail chest.* With flail chest, decreased air movement results in rapid, shallow respirations, paradoxical chest wall motion from rib instability, tachycardia, hypotension, ecchymoses, cyanosis, and pain over the affected area.

◤ *Guillain-Barré syndrome.* Progressive ascending paralysis causes a rapid or progressive onset of shallow respirations in this life-threatening disorder. Muscle weakness begins in the lower limbs and extends finally to the face.

◆ *Multiple sclerosis (MS).* With MS, muscle weakness causes progressive shallow respirations. Early features include diplopia, blurred vision, and paresthesia.

◆ *Myasthenia gravis.* Progression of myasthenia gravis causes respiratory muscle weakness marked by shallow respirations, dyspnea, and cyanosis.

◆ *Pleural effusion.* With pleural effusion, restricted lung expansion causes shallow respirations, beginning suddenly or gradually. Other findings include a nonproductive cough, weight loss, dyspnea, and pleuritic chest pain.

◆ *Pneumothorax.* Pneumothorax causes a sudden onset of shallow respirations and dyspnea. Related findings include tachycardia; tachypnea; sudden sharp, severe chest pain (commonly unilateral) that worsens with movement; cyanosis; accessory muscle use; restlessness; and asymmetrical chest expansion.

◤ *Pulmonary edema.* Pulmonary vascular congestion causes rapid, shallow respirations. Early findings include exertional dyspnea, paroxysmal nocturnal dyspnea, tachycardia, dependent crackles, and a ventricular gallop.

◤ *Pulmonary embolism.* Pulmonary embolism causes sudden, rapid, shallow respirations and severe dyspnea with angina or pleuritic chest pain. Other findings include tachycardia, tachypnea, diaphoresis, anxiety, restlessness, pleural friction rub, crackles, diffuse wheezing, dullness to percussion, decreased breath sounds, and signs of circulatory collapse.

Respirations, stertorous

Characterized by a harsh, rattling, or snoring sound, stertorous respirations usually result from the vibration of relaxed oropharyngeal structures during sleep or coma, causing partial airway obstruction. Less commonly, these respirations result from retained mucus in the upper airway.

This common sign occurs in about 10% of healthy adults; however, it's especially prevalent in middle-age men who are obese. It may be aggravated by a sedative before bed, which increases oropharyngeal flaccidity, the use of alcohol, or by sleeping in the supine position, which allows the relaxed tongue to slip back into the airway. The major pathologic causes of stertorous respirations are obstructive sleep apnea and life-threatening upper airway obstruction associated with an oropharyngeal tumor or with uvular or palatal edema. This obstruction may also occur during the postictal phase of a generalized seizure when mucus secretions or a relaxed tongue blocks the airway.

Occasionally, stertorous respirations are mistaken for stridor, which is another sign of upper airway obstruction. However, stridor indicates laryngeal or tracheal obstruction, whereas stertorous respirations signal higher airway obstruction.

Assessment

If you detect stertorous respirations, check the patient's mouth and throat for edema, redness, masses, or foreign objects. If edema is marked, quickly check the patient's vital signs, including oxygen saturation. Observe him for

EMERGENCY INTERVENTIONS

Responding to stertorous respirations

If your patient has stertorous respirations, and your assessment reveals marked edema:

◆ Elevate the head of the bed 30 degrees to help ease breathing and reduce edema.

◆ Administer supplemental oxygen by nasal cannula or face mask as prescribed.

◆ Prepare to assist the practitioner with intubating the patient, performing a tracheostomy, or providing mechanical ventilation.

◆ Insert an I.V. catheter for fluid and drug access.

◆ Begin cardiac monitoring.

---

signs and symptoms of respiratory distress. (See *Responding to stertorous respirations*.)

If you detect stertorous respirations while the patient is sleeping, observe his breathing pattern for 3 to 4 minutes. Do noisy respirations cease when he turns on his side and recur when he assumes a supine position? Watch carefully for periods of apnea and note their length. When possible, question the patient's partner about his snoring habits. Does the patient's snoring frequently awaken her? Does the snoring improve if the patient sleeps with the window open? Has she also observed the patient talking in his sleep or sleepwalking? Ask about signs of sleep deprivation, such as personality changes, headaches, daytime somnolence, or decreased mental acuity.

Causes

◨ *Airway obstruction.* Regardless of its cause, partial airway obstruction may lead to stertorous respirations accompanied by wheezing, dyspnea, tachypnea and, later, intercostal retractions and nasal flaring. If the obstruction be-

comes complete, the patient abruptly loses his ability to talk and displays diaphoresis, tachycardia, and inspiratory chest movement but absent breath sounds.

◆ *Obstructive sleep apnea.* Loud and disruptive snoring is a major characteristic of obstructive sleep apnea, which commonly affects people who are obese. Typically, the snoring alternates with periods of sleep apnea, which usually end with loud gasping sounds. Alternating tachycardia and bradycardia may occur. Sleep disturbances, such as somnambulism (sleep walking) and talking during sleep, may also occur. Most awaken in the morning with a generalized headache, feeling tired and unrefreshed. The most common complaint is excessive daytime sleepiness.

Retractions, costal and sternal

Retractions are visible indentations of the soft tissue covering the chest wall, a cardinal sign of respiratory distress in infants and children. Retractions may be suprasternal (directly above the sternum and clavicles), intercostal (between the ribs), subcostal (below the lower costal margin of the rib cage), or substernal (just below the xiphoid process). Retractions may be mild or severe, producing barely visible to deep indentations. (See *Observing retractions in infants and children,* page 480.)

Normally, infants and young children use abdominal muscles for breathing, unlike older children and adults, who use the diaphragm. When breathing requires extra effort, accessory muscles assist respiration, especially inspiration. Retractions typically accompany accessory muscle use.

Assessment

If you detect retractions in a child, check quickly for other signs of respiratory distress, such as cyanosis, tachypnea, tachycardia, and decreased oxygen saturation. Observe the depth and location of retractions. Also, note the rate, depth, and quality of respirations. Look for accessory muscle use, nasal flaring during inspiration, or grunting during expiration. If the child has a cough, record the amount, color, consistency, and odor of any sputum. Note whether the child appears restless or lethargic. Finally, auscultate the child's lungs to detect abnormal breath sounds.

If the child's condition permits, ask his parents about his medical history. Was he born prematurely or with a low birth weight? Was the birth complicated? Ask about recent signs of an upper respiratory tract infection, such as a runny nose, cough, and low-grade fever. How often has the child had respiratory problems during the past year? Does he participate in a day-care program or have school-age siblings? Has he been in contact with anyone who

has had a cold, the flu, or other respiratory ailments? Did he ever have respiratory syncytial virus? Could he have aspirated food, liquid, or a foreign body? Inquire about a history of allergies or asthma.

Causes

◆ *Asthma attack.* Intercostal and suprasternal retractions may accompany an asthma attack. They're preceded by dyspnea, wheezing, a hacking cough, and pallor.

◾ *Epiglottitis.* Epiglottitis is a bacterial infection that may precipitate severe respiratory distress with suprasternal, substernal, and intercostal retractions; stridor; nasal flaring; cyanosis; and tachycardia. Early features include sudden onset of a barking cough and high fever, sore throat, hoarseness, dysphagia, drooling, dyspnea, and restlessness. The child becomes panicky as edema makes breathing difficult. Total airway occlusion may occur in 2 to 5 hours.

◆ *Heart failure.* Usually linked to a congenital heart defect in children, heart failure may cause intercostal and substernal retractions along with nasal flaring, progressive tachypnea, and—in severe respiratory distress—grunting respirations, edema, and cyanosis.

◆ *Laryngotracheobronchitis (acute).* With laryngotracheobronchitis, substernal and intercostal retractions typically follow a low to moderate fever, runny nose, poor appetite, barking cough, hoarseness, and inspiratory stridor.

◆ *Pneumonia (bacterial).* Pneumonia begins with signs and symptoms of acute infection, such as high fever and lethargy, followed by subcostal and intercostal retractions, nasal flaring, dyspnea, tachypnea, grunting respirations, cyanosis, and a productive cough.

Observing retractions in infants and children

When you observe retractions in infants and children, be sure to note their exact location—an important clue to the cause and severity of respiratory distress. For example, subcostal and substernal retractions usually result from lower respiratory tract disorders; suprasternal retractions, from upper respiratory tract disorders.

Mild intercostal retractions alone may be normal. However, intercostal retractions accompanied by subcostal and substernal retractions may indicate moderate respiratory distress. Deep suprasternal retractions typically indicate severe distress.

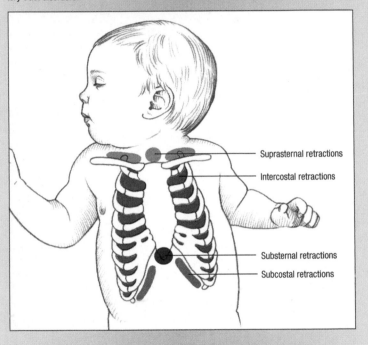

Suprasternal retractions

Intercostal retractions

Substernal retractions

Subcostal retractions

◼ *Respiratory distress syndrome.* Substernal and subcostal retractions are an early sign of respiratory distress syndrome, which affects premature neonates shortly after birth. Associated early signs include tachypnea, tachycardia, and expiratory grunting. As respiratory distress worsens, intercostal and suprasternal retractions typically occur, and apnea or irregular respirations replace grunting.

Rhinorrhea

Common but rarely serious, rhinorrhea is the free discharge of thin nasal mucus. It can be self-limiting or chronic, resulting from a nasal, sinus, or systemic disorder or from a basilar skull fracture. Rhinorrhea can also result from sinus or cranial surgery, excessive use of vasoconstricting nose drops or sprays, or inhalation of an irritant, such as tobacco smoke, dust, or fumes. Depending on the cause, the discharge may be clear, purulent, bloody, or serosanguineous.

Assessment

Begin the history by asking the patient if the discharge runs from both nostrils. Is it intermittent or persistent? Did it begin suddenly or gradually? Does the position of his head affect the discharge? Next, ask the patient to characterize the discharge. Is it watery, bloody, purulent, or foul smelling? Is it copious or scanty? Does the discharge worsen or improve with the time of day? Also, find out if the patient is using medications, especially nose drops or nasal sprays. Has he been exposed to nasal irritants at home or at work? Does he experience seasonal allergies? Did he recently experience a head injury?

Examine the patient's nose, checking airflow from each nostril. Evaluate the size, color, and condition of the turbinate mucosa (normally deep pink). Note if the mucosa is red, unusually pale, blue, or gray. Then examine the area beneath each turbinate. (See *Using a nasal speculum,* page 482.) Make sure to palpate over the frontal, ethmoid, and maxillary sinuses for tenderness.

To differentiate nasal mucus from cerebrospinal fluid (CSF), collect a small amount of drainage on a glucose test strip. If CSF (which contains glucose) is present, the test result will be abnormal.

Finally, using a familiar, nonirritating substance, such as vanilla, coffee, soap, or lemon, test for anosmia (inability to smell).

Causes

◆ *Basilar skull fracture.* A tear in the dura can lead to cerebrospinal rhinorrhea, which increases when the patient lowers his head. Other findings include Battle's sign, raccoon eyes, epistaxis, otorrhea, and a bulging tympanum from blood or fluid.

◆ *Common cold.* An initially watery nasal discharge may become thicker and mucopurulent. Related findings include sneezing, nasal congestion, a dry and hacking cough, sore throat, mouth breathing, and a transient loss of smell and taste.

◆ *Nasal or sinus tumors.* Nasal tumors can produce an intermittent, unilateral bloody or serosanguineous discharge that may be purulent and foul smelling. Nasal congestion, postnasal drip, and headache may also occur.

◆ *Rhinitis. Allergic rhinitis* produces an episodic, profuse watery discharge. (A mucopurulent discharge indicates infection.) Typical associated signs and symptoms include increased lacrimation, nasal congestion, recurrent sneezing, and itchy eyes, nose, and throat. The turbinates are pale and engorged; the mucosa, pale and boggy.

With *atrophic rhinitis,* the nasal discharge is scanty, purulent, and foul smelling. Nasal obstruction is common, and the crusts may bleed on removal. The mucosa is pale pink and shiny.

Using a nasal speculum

To visualize the interior of the nares, use a nasal speculum and a good light source such as a penlight. Hold the speculum in the palm of one hand and the penlight in the other hand. Have the patient tilt her head back slightly and rest it against a wall or other firm support, if possible. Insert the speculum blades about ½" (1.3 cm) into the nasal vestibule, as shown.

Place your index finger on the tip of the patient's nose for stability. Carefully open the speculum blades. Shine the light source in the direction of the nares. Now, inspect the nares. The mucosa should be deep pink. Note any discharge, masses, lesions, or mucosal swelling. Check the nasal septum for perforation, bleeding, or crusting. Bluish turbinates suggest allergy. A rounded, elongated projection suggests a polyp.

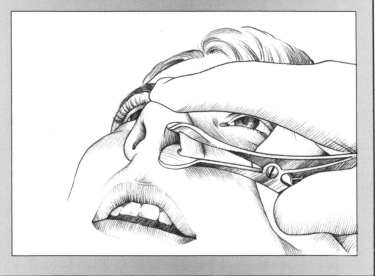

With *vasomotor rhinitis,* a profuse and watery nasal discharge accompanies chronic nasal obstruction, sneezing, recurrent postnasal drip, and pale, swollen turbinates. The nasal septum is pink; the mucosa, blue.

◆ *Sinusitis.* With *acute sinusitis,* a thick and purulent nasal discharge leads to a purulent postnasal drip that results in throat pain and halitosis. The patient may also experience nasal congestion, severe pain and tenderness over the involved sinuses, fever, headache, and malaise.

With *chronic sinusitis,* the nasal discharge is usually scanty, thick, and intermittently purulent. Nasal congestion and low-grade discomfort or pressure over the involved sinuses can be persistent or recurrent. The patient may also be suffering from chronic sore throat and nasal polyps.

Chronic fungal sinusitis may progress rapidly to exophthalmos, blindness, intracranial extension and, eventually, death—especially in patients who are immunocompromised.

Rhonchi

Rhonchi are continuous adventitious breath sounds detected by auscultation. They're usually louder and lower-pitched than crackles—more like a hoarse moan or a deep snore—though they may be described as rattling, sonorous, bubbling, rumbling, or musical. However, sibilant rhonchi, or wheezes, are high pitched.

Rhonchi are heard over large airways such as the trachea. They can occur in a patient with a pulmonary disorder when air flows through passages that have been narrowed by secretions, a tumor or foreign body, bronchospasm, or mucosal thickening. The resulting vibration of airway walls produces the rhonchi.

Assessment

If you auscultate rhonchi, check the patient's vital signs, including oxygen saturation, and be alert for signs of respiratory distress. Characterize the patient's respirations as rapid or slow, shallow or deep, and regular or irregular. Inspect the chest, noting accessory muscle use. Is the patient audibly wheezing or gurgling? Auscultate for other abnormal breath sounds, such as crackles and a pleural friction rub. If you detect these sounds, note their location. Are breath sounds diminished or absent? Next, percuss the chest. If the patient has a cough, note its frequency and characterize its sound. If

it's productive, examine the sputum for color, odor, consistency, and blood.

Ask related questions: Does the patient smoke? If so, obtain a history in pack-years. Has he recently lost weight or felt tired or weak? Does he have asthma or another pulmonary disorder? Is he taking any prescribed or over-the-counter medication?

During the examination, keep in mind that thick or excessive secretions, bronchospasm, or inflammation of mucous membranes may lead to airway obstruction. If necessary, suction the patient and keep equipment available for inserting an artificial airway. Keep a bronchodilator available to treat bronchospasm.

Causes

◆ *Asthma.* An asthma attack can cause rhonchi, crackles and, commonly, wheezing. Other features include apprehension, a dry cough that later becomes productive, prolonged expirations, and intercostal and supraclavicular retractions on inspiration.
◆ *Bronchiectasis.* Bronchiectasis causes lower-lobe rhonchi and crackles, which coughing may help relieve. Its classic sign is a cough that produces mucopurulent, foul-smelling and, possibly, bloody sputum.
◆ *Bronchitis.* Acute tracheobronchitis produces sonorous rhonchi and wheezing due to bronchospasm or increased mucus in the airways. Related findings include sore throat, low-grade fever, muscle and back pain, and substernal tightness. With chronic bronchitis, auscultation may reveal scattered rhonchi, coarse crackles, wheezing, high-pitched piping sounds, and prolonged expirations. An early hacking cough later becomes productive.

◆ *Pneumonia.* Bacterial pneumonia can cause rhonchi and a dry cough that later becomes productive. Related findings develop suddenly and include shaking chills, high fever, myalgia, pleuritic chest pain, tachypnea, tachycardia, dyspnea, cyanosis, diaphoresis, decreased breath sounds, and fine crackles.

◆ *Pulmonary coccidioidomycosis.* Pulmonary coccidioidomycosis causes rhonchi and wheezing. Other findings include cough, fever, pleuritic chest pain, sore throat, headache, and an itchy macular rash.

S

Scotoma

A scotoma is an area of partial or complete blindness within an otherwise normal or slightly impaired visual field. Usually located within the central 30-degree area, the defect ranges from absolute blindness to a barely detectable loss of visual acuity. Typically, the patient can pinpoint the scotoma's location in the visual field. (See *Locating scotomas*, page 486.)

A scotoma can result from a retinal, choroid, or optic nerve disorder. It can be classified as absolute, relative, or scintillating. An absolute scotoma refers to the total inability to see all sizes of test objects used in mapping the visual field. A relative scotoma, in contrast, refers to the ability to see only large test objects. A scintillating scotoma refers to the flashes or bursts of light commonly seen during a migraine headache.

Assessment

Begin by identifying and characterizing the scotoma, using such visual field tests as the tangent screen examination, the Goldmann perimeter test, and the automated perimetry test. Two other visual field tests—confrontation testing and the Amsler grid—may also help in identifying a scotoma. Explore the patient's medical history, noting especially eye disorders, vision problems, or chronic systemic disorders. Ask the patient if he takes medications or uses eye drops.

Next, test the patient's visual acuity and inspect his pupils for size, equality, and reaction to light. An ophthalmoscopic examination and measurement of intraocular pressure are necessary.

Causes

◆ *Chorioretinitis.* Inflammation of the choroid and retina produces a paracentral scotoma. Ophthalmoscopic examination reveals clouding and cells in the vitreous humour, subretinal hemorrhage, and neovascularization. The patient may have photophobia along with blurred vision.

◆ *Macular degeneration.* Any degenerative process or disorder affecting the fovea centralis results in a central scotoma. Ophthalmoscopic examination reveals changes in the macular area. The patient may notice subtle changes in visual acuity, in color perception, and in the size and shape of objects.

◆ *Optic neuritis.* Inflammation, degeneration, or demyelination of the optic

Locating scotomas

Scotomas, or "blind spots," are classified according to the affected area of the visual field. The normal scotoma—shown in the temporal region of the right eye—appears in black in all the illustrations.

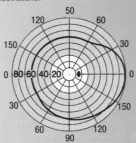

The *normally present scotoma* represents the position of the optic nerve head in the visual field. It appears between 10 and 20 degrees on this chart of the normal visual field.

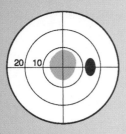

A *central scotoma* involves the point of central fixation. It's always associated with decreased visual acuity.

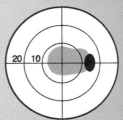

A *centrocecal scotoma* involves the point of central fixation and the area between the blind spot and the fixation point.

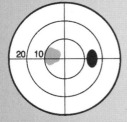

A *paracentral scotoma* affects an area of the visual field that's nasal or temporal to the point of central fixation.

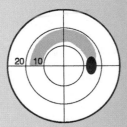

An *arcuate scotoma* arches around the fixation point, usually ending on the nasal side of the visual field.

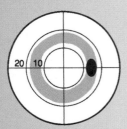

An *annular scotoma* forms a circular defect around the fixation point. It's common with retinal pigmentary degeneration.

nerve produces a central, circular, or centrocecal scotoma. The scotoma may be unilateral or bilateral, with involvement of one or both nerves. The patient may report severe vision loss or blurring, lasting up to 3 weeks, and pain—especially with eye movement. Common ophthalmoscopic findings include hyperemia of the optic disk, retinal vein distention, blurred disk margins, and filling of the physiologic cup.

◆ *Retinal pigmentary degeneration.* Retinal pigmentary degeneration causes premature retinal cell changes leading to cell death. One disorder, retinitis pigmentosa, initially involves loss of peripheral rods; the resulting annular scotoma progresses concentrically until only a central field of vision (tunnel vision) remains. The earliest symptom— impaired night vision—appears during adolescence. Associated signs include narrowing of the retinal blood vessels and pallor of the optic disk. Eventually, with invasion of the macula, blindness may occur.

Scrotal swelling

Scrotal swelling occurs when a condition affecting the testicles, epididymis, or scrotal skin produces edema or a mass; the penis may be involved. Scrotal swelling can affect males of any age.

The sudden onset of painful scrotal swelling suggests torsion of a testicle or testicular appendages, especially in a prepubescent male. This emergency requires immediate surgery to untwist and stabilize the spermatic cord or to remove the appendage.

Assessment

If severe pain accompanies scrotal swelling, ask the patient when the swelling began. Using a Doppler stethoscope, evaluate blood flow to the testicle. If it's decreased or absent, suspect testicular torsion and prepare the patient for surgery. If the patient isn't in distress, proceed with the history. Ask about injury to the scrotum, urethral discharge, cloudy urine, increased urinary frequency, and dysuria. Is the patient sexually active? When was his last sexual contact? Does he have a history of sexually transmitted disease? Find out about recent illnesses, particularly mumps. Does he have a history of prostate surgery or prolonged catheterization? Does changing his body position or level of activity affect the swelling?

Check the patient's vital signs, especially noting fever, and palpate his abdomen for tenderness. Then examine the entire genital area. Assess the scrotum with the patient supine and standing. Note its size and color. Is the swelling unilateral or bilateral? Do you see signs of trauma or bruising? Are there rashes or lesions present? Gently palpate the scrotum for a cyst or lump. Note any tenderness or increased firmness. Check the testicles' position in the scrotum. Finally, transilluminate the scrotum to distinguish a fluid-filled cyst from a solid mass. (A solid mass can't be transilluminated.)

Causes

◆ *Epididymal cysts.* Located in the head of the epididymis, epididymal cysts produce painless scrotal swelling.
◆ *Epididymitis.* With epididymitis, other key findings are pain, extreme tenderness, and swelling in the groin and scrotum. While walking, the patient waddles to avoid pressure on the groin and scrotum. He may have a high temperature, malaise, urethral discharge and cloudy urine, and lower ab-

dominal pain on the affected side. His scrotal skin may be hot, red, dry, flaky, and thin.

◆ *Hydrocele.* An accumulation of serous fluid in the scrotum produces gradual scrotal swelling that's usually painless. The scrotum may be soft and cystic or firm and tense. Palpation reveals a round, nontender scrotal mass.

◆ *Idiopathic scrotal edema.* Swelling occurs quickly with idiopathic scrotal edema and usually disappears within 24 hours. The affected testicle is pink.

◆ *Orchitis (acute).* Mumps, syphilis, or tuberculosis may precipitate orchitis, which causes sudden painful swelling of one or, at times, both testicles. Related findings include extreme weakness, fever, chills, lower abdominal pain, and a hot, reddened scrotum. Urinary signs are usually absent.

◆ *Scrotal trauma.* Blunt trauma causes scrotal swelling with bruising and severe pain. The scrotum may appear dark or bluish.

◆ *Spermatocele.* Spermatocele is a small, movable, painless cystic mass that lies above and behind the testicle. It contains opaque fluid and sperm, and it can be transilluminated. Its onset may be acute or gradual.

◆ *Testicular torsion.* Most common before puberty, testicular torsion is a urologic emergency that causes scrotal swelling; sudden, severe pain; and, possibly, elevation of the affected testicle within the scrotum.

◆ *Testicular tumor.* Typically painless, smooth, and firm, a testicular tumor produces swelling and a sensation of excessive weight in the scrotum.

◆ *Torsion of a hydatid of Morgagni.* Torsion of this small, pea-sized cyst severs its blood supply, causing a hard, painful swelling on the testicle's upper pole.

Seizures, absence

Absence seizures are benign, generalized seizures thought to originate subcortically. These brief episodes of unconsciousness usually last 3 to 20 seconds and can occur 100 or more times per day, causing periods of inattention. Absence seizures usually begin between ages 4 and 12. Their first sign may be deteriorating schoolwork and behavior. The cause of these seizures is unknown.

Absence seizures occur without warning. The patient suddenly stops all purposeful activity and stares blankly ahead, as if he were daydreaming. They may produce automatisms, such as repetitive lip smacking, or mild clonic or myoclonic movements, including mild jerking of the eyelids. The patient may drop an object that he's holding, and muscle relaxation may cause him to drop his head or arms or to slump. After the attack, the patient resumes activity, typically unaware of the episode.

Absence status, a rare form of absence seizure, occurs as a prolonged absence seizure or as repeated episodes of these seizures. Usually not life threatening, absence status occurs most commonly in patients who have previously experienced absence seizures.

Assessment

If you suspect a patient is having an absence seizure, evaluate its occurrence and duration by reciting a series of numbers and then asking him to repeat them after the attack ends. If the patient has had an absence seizure, he can't do this. Alternatively, if the seizures are occurring within minutes of each other, ask the patient to count for about 5 minutes. He'll stop counting during a seizure and resume when it's over. Look for accompanying automatisms. Ask family members if they have noticed a change in the patient's behavior or deterioration in his schoolwork.

Causes

♦ *Drugs.* Various drugs that lower the seizure threshold include alcohol, cocaine, high-dose penicillin, isoniazid overdose, and neuroleptics. These are most likely to cause absence seizures in patients with epilepsy. Withdrawal of alcohol, benzodiazepines, and other sedatives also cause absence seizures.
♦ *Idiopathic epilepsy.* With idiopathic epilepsy, absence seizures may be accompanied by learning disabilities.
♦ *Lack of sleep.* This is the most frequent cause of seizure exacerbation in children with epilepsy.

Seizures, complex partial

A complex partial seizure occurs when a focal seizure begins in the temporal lobe and causes a partial alteration of consciousness—usually confusion. Psychomotor seizures can occur at any age, but their incidence usually increases during adolescence and adulthood. Two-thirds of patients also have generalized seizures.

An aura—usually a complex hallucination, illusion, or sensation—typically precedes a psychomotor seizure. The hallucination may be audiovisual, auditory, or olfactory. Other types of auras include sensations of déjà vu, unfamiliarity with surroundings, or depersonalization. The patient may become fearful or anxious, experience lip smacking, or have an unpleasant feeling in the epigastric region that rises toward the chest and throat. In most cases, the patient will recognize the aura and lie down before losing consciousness.

A period of unresponsiveness follows the aura. The patient may experience automatisms, appear dazed and wander aimlessly, perform inappropriate acts (such as undressing in public), be unresponsive, utter incoherent phrases, or (rarely) go into a rage or tantrum. After the seizure, the patient is confused, drowsy, and doesn't remember the seizure. Behavioral automatisms rarely last longer than 5 minutes, but postseizure confusion, agitation, and amnesia may persist.

Between attacks, the patient may exhibit slow and rigid thinking, outbursts of anger and aggressiveness, tedious conversation, a preoccupation with naive philosophical ideas, a diminished libido, mood swings, and paranoia.

Assessment

If you witness a complex partial seizure, never attempt to restrain the patient. Instead, lead him gently to a safe area. *(Exception:* Don't approach him if he's angry or violent.) Calmly encourage him to sit down, and remain with him until he's fully alert. After the seizure, ask him if he experienced an aura. Ask the patient whether he has a history of seizure activity or a history of head trauma (recent or remote). Also ask if he has had a recent fever or headache. Record all observations and findings.

Causes

♦ *Brain abscess.* If the brain abscess is in the temporal lobe, complex partial seizures commonly occur after the abscess disappears. Related problems may include a headache, generalized seizures, and a decreased level of consciousness.

◆ *Head trauma.* Severe trauma to the temporal lobe (especially from a penetrating injury) can produce complex partial seizures months or years later. The seizures may decrease in frequency and eventually stop. Head trauma also causes generalized seizures.

◼ *Herpes simplex encephalitis.* The herpes simplex virus commonly attacks the temporal lobe, resulting in complex partial seizures. Other features include fever, headache, coma, and generalized seizures.

◆ *Temporal lobe tumor.* Complex partial seizures may be the first sign of a temporal lobe tumor. Other signs and symptoms include headache, pupillary changes, and mental dullness.

Seizures, generalized tonic-clonic

Generalized tonic-clonic seizures are caused by the paroxysmal, uncontrolled discharge of central nervous system neurons, leading to neurologic dysfunction. Unlike most other types of seizures, this cerebral hyperactivity isn't confined to the original focus or to a localized area but extends to the entire brain.

Generalized tonic-clonic seizures may begin with or without an aura and usually last from 2 to 5 minutes. They typically occur singly. (See *What happens during a generalized tonic-clonic seizure.*) Possible complications include respiratory arrest due to airway obstruction from secretions, status epilepticus, head or spinal injuries and bruises, Todd's paralysis and, rarely, cardiac arrest. Status epilepticus is marked by prolonged seizure activity or by rapidly recurring seizures with no intervening periods of recovery. It's most commonly triggered by the abrupt discontinuation of anticonvulsant therapy.

Generalized seizures may be caused by a physiologic disorder, exposure to toxins, or a genetic defect. They may also result from a focal seizure. With recurring seizures, or epilepsy, the cause may be unknown.

Assessment

If you witness the beginning of the seizure, first check the patient's airway, breathing, and circulation, and ensure that the cause isn't asystole or a blocked airway. Stay with the patient and ensure a patent airway. If the seizure lasts longer than 4 minutes or if a second seizure occurs before full recovery from the first, suspect status epilepticus. (See *Generalized seizures: What you can do,* page 492.) If you didn't witness the seizure, obtain a description from the patient's companion, if one is available. Ask when the seizure started and how long it lasted. Did the patient report unusual sensations before the seizure began? Did the seizure start in one area of the body and spread, or did it affect the entire body right away? Did the patient fall on a hard surface? Did he turn blue? Did he lose bladder control? Did he have other seizures before recovering?

If the patient may have sustained a head injury, observe him closely for loss of consciousness, unequal or nonreactive pupils, and focal neurologic signs. Is he increasingly difficult to arouse when you check on him at 15-minute intervals? Examine his arms, legs, and face (including tongue) for injury, residual paralysis, or limb weakness.

What happens during a generalized tonic-clonic seizure

Before the seizure

Prodromal signs and symptoms, such as myoclonic jerks, a throbbing headache, and mood changes, may occur over several hours or days. The patient may have premonitions of the seizure. For example, he may report an *aura,* such as seeing a flashing light or smelling a characteristic odor.

During the seizure

If a generalized seizure begins with an aura, this indicates that irritability in a specific area of the brain quickly became widespread. Common auras include palpitations, epigastric distress rapidly rising to the throat, head or eye turning, and sensory hallucinations.

Next, *loss of consciousness* occurs as a sudden discharge of intense electrical activity overwhelms the brain's subcortical center. The patient falls and experiences brief, bilateral myoclonic contractures. Air forced through spasmodic vocal cords may produce a birdlike, piercing cry.

During the *tonic phase,* skeletal muscles contract for 10 to 20 seconds. The patient's eyelids are drawn up, his arms are flexed, and his legs are extended. His mouth opens wide, then snaps shut; he may bite his tongue. His respirations cease because of respiratory muscle spasm, and initial pallor of the skin and mucous membranes (the result of impaired venous return) changes to cyanosis secondary to apnea. The patient

arches his back and slowly lowers his arms (as shown below). Other effects include dilated, nonreactive pupils; greatly increased heart rate and blood pressure; increased salivation and tracheobronchial secretions; and profuse diaphoresis.

During the *clonic phase,* lasting about 60 seconds, mild trembling progresses to violent contractures or jerks. Other motor activity includes facial grimaces (with possible tongue biting) and violent expiration of bloody, foamy saliva from clonic contractures of thoracic cage muscles. Clonic jerks slowly decrease in intensity and frequency. The patient is still apneic.

After the seizure

The patient's movements gradually cease, and he becomes unresponsive to external stimuli. Other postseizure features include stertorous respirations from increased tracheobronchial secretions, equal or unequal pupils (but becoming reactive), and urinary incontinence resulting from brief muscle relaxation. After about 5 minutes, the patient's level of consciousness increases, and he appears confused and disoriented. His muscle tone, heart rate, and blood pressure return to normal.

After several hours' sleep, the patient awakens exhausted and may have a headache, sore muscles, and amnesia about the seizure.

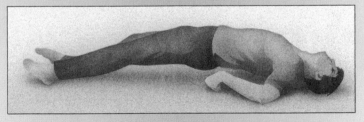

EMERGENCY INTERVENTIONS

Generalized seizures: What you can do

If you witness the beginning of a seizure, focus your care on observing the seizure and protecting the patient. Follow these steps:
◆ Place a towel under his head to prevent injury.
◆ Loosen his clothing.
◆ Remove sharp or hard objects from the area.
◆ Don't restrain him or force a hard object into his mouth.
◆ If possible, turn him to one side to allow secretions to drain and to prevent aspiration.
◆ Continuously check his airway, breathing, and circulation.
◆ If necessary, suction his airway, perform cardiopulmonary resuscitation, and prepare for intubation or mechanical ventilation as indicated.

After the seizure:
◆ Provide a safe area where he can rest.
◆ Reassure and reorient him.
◆ Check his vital signs and neurologic status.
◆ Carefully record these data and your observations during the seizure.

If you suspect status epilepticus:
◆ Establish an airway.
◆ Insert an I.V. catheter.
◆ Give supplemental oxygen.
◆ Begin cardiac monitoring.
◆ Draw blood for appropriate studies.
◆ Turn the patient on his side, with his head in a semi-dependent position, to drain secretions and prevent aspiration.
◆ Check his arterial blood gas levels.
◆ Administer diazepam (Valium) or lorazepam (Ativan)—by slow I.V. push—and other medications, as ordered.
◆ Expect to insert a nasogastric tube to prevent vomiting and aspiration.

Next, obtain a history. Has the patient ever had generalized or focal seizures before? If so, do they occur frequently? Is he receiving drug therapy? Is he compliant? Also, ask about sleep deprivation and emotional or physical stress at the time the seizure occurred.

Causes

◪ *Arsenic poisoning.* Arsenic poisoning may cause a garlicky breath odor, increased salivation, and generalized pruritus in addition to generalized seizures.

◆ *Barbiturate withdrawal.* In chronically intoxicated patients, barbiturate withdrawal may produce generalized seizures 2 to 4 days after the last dose. Status epilepticus is possible.
◆ *Brain abscess.* Generalized seizures may occur in the acute stage of abscess formation or after the abscess disappears.
◆ *Brain tumor.* Generalized seizures may occur, depending on the tumor's location and type.
◆ *Chronic renal failure.* End-stage renal disease may produce the rapid onset of twitching, trembling, myoclonic jerks, and generalized seizures. Other

findings include anuria or oliguria, fatigue, malaise, irritability, and muscle cramps.

◆ *Drugs.* Toxic blood levels of some drugs, such as theophylline (Theo-Dur), meperidine (Demerol), penicillins, and cimetidine (Tagamet) may cause generalized seizures. Phenothiazines, tricyclic antidepressants, amphetamines, isoniazid (INH), and vincristine (Oncovin) may cause seizures in patients with preexisting epilepsy.

▧ *Eclampsia.* Generalized seizures are a hallmark of eclampsia. Other findings include increased blood pressure, peripheral edema, and sudden weight gain.

▧ *Encephalitis.* Seizures are an early sign of encephalitis, indicating a poor prognosis; they may also occur after recovery as a result of residual damage.

◆ *Epilepsy (idiopathic).* In most cases of epilepsy, the cause of recurrent seizures is unknown.

▧ *Head trauma.* In severe cases of head trauma, generalized seizures may occur at the time of injury. (Months later, focal seizures may occur.)

▧ *Hepatic encephalopathy.* Generalized seizures may occur late in hepatic encephalopathy. Associated late-stage findings in the comatose patient include fetor hepaticus, asterixis, and a positive Babinski's sign.

▧ *Hypoglycemia.* Generalized seizures usually occur with severe hypoglycemia. They may be accompanied by blurred or double vision, motor weakness, trembling, excessive diaphoresis, tachycardia, and a decreased level of consciousness.

▧ *Hyponatremia.* Seizures may develop when serum sodium levels fall below 125 mEq/L, especially if the decrease is rapid. Severe hyponatremia may also cause cyanosis and vasomotor collapse, with a thready pulse.

◆ *Hypoparathyroidism.* Worsening tetany causes generalized seizures. Chronic hypoparathyroidism produces neuromuscular irritability and hyperactive deep tendon reflexes.

▧ *Hypoxic encephalopathy.* Along with generalized seizures, hypoxic encephalopathy may produce myoclonic jerks and coma. Later, if the patient recovers, dementia, visual agnosia, choreoathetosis, and ataxia may occur.

◆ *Neurofibromatosis.* Multiple brain lesions from neurofibromatosis cause focal and generalized seizures. Inspection reveals café-au-lait spots, multiple skin tumors, scoliosis, and kyphoscoliosis.

▧ *Stroke.* Seizures (focal more commonly than generalized) may occur within 6 months of an ischemic stroke. Associated signs and symptoms vary with the location and extent of brain damage.

Seizures, simple partial

Resulting from an irritable focus in the cerebral cortex, simple partial seizures typically last about 30 seconds and don't alter the patient's level of consciousness (LOC). The type and pattern reflect the location of the irritable focus. Simple partial seizures may be classified as motor (including Jacksonian seizures and epilepsia partialis continua) or somatosensory (including visual, olfactory, and auditory seizures).

A *focal motor seizure* is a series of unilateral clonic (muscle jerking) and tonic (muscle stiffening) movements of one part of the body. The patient's head and eyes characteristically turn away from the hemispheric focus—usually the frontal lobe near the motor strip. A tonic-clonic contraction of the trunk or extremities may follow.

Body functions affected by focal seizures

The site of the irritable focus determines which body functions are affected by a focal seizure, as shown in the illustration below.

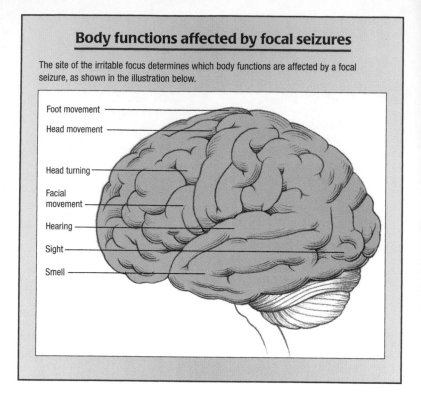

A *Jacksonian motor seizure* typically begins with a tonic contraction of a finger, the corner of the mouth, or one foot. Clonic movements follow, spreading to other muscles on the same side of the body, moving up the arm or leg, and eventually involving the whole side. Alternatively, clonic movements may spread to the opposite side, becoming generalized and leading to loss of consciousness. In the postictal phase, the patient may experience paralysis in the affected limbs, usually resolving within 24 hours.

Epilepsia partialis continua causes clonic twitching of one muscle group, usually in the face, arm, or leg. Twitching occurs every few seconds and persists for hours, days, or months without spreading. Spasms usually affect the distal arm and leg muscles more than the proximal ones; in the face, they affect the corner of the mouth, one or both eyelids and, occasionally, the neck or trunk muscles unilaterally.

A *focal somatosensory seizure* affects a localized body area on one side. Usually, this type of seizure initially causes numbness, tingling, or crawling or "electric" sensations; occasionally, it causes pain or burning sensations in the lips, fingers, or toes.

A *visual seizure* involves sensations of darkness or of stationary or moving lights or spots, usually red at first, then blue, green, and yellow. It can affect both visual fields or the visual field on the side opposite the lesion. The irritable focus is in the occipital lobe. In contrast, the irritable focus in an *auditory* or *olfactory seizure* is in the temporal lobe. (See *Body functions affected by focal seizures.*)

Assessment

Record the patient's seizure activity in detail; your data may be critical in locating the lesion in the brain. Does the patient turn his head and eyes? Where does movement first start? Because a partial seizure may become generalized, you'll need to watch closely for loss of consciousness, bilateral tonicity and clonicity, cyanosis, tongue biting, and urinary incontinence. (See "Seizures, generalized tonic-clonic," page 490.)

After the seizure, ask the patient to describe exactly what he remembers about the seizure. Check the patient's LOC, and test for residual deficits and sensory disturbances.

Then obtain a history. Ask the patient what happened before the seizure. Can he describe an aura or did he recognize its onset? If so, how? How does this seizure compare with others he has had? Also, explore any history—recent or remote—of head trauma. Check for a history of stroke or recent infection.

Causes

◆ *Brain abscess.* Seizures can occur in the acute stage of abscess formation or after resolution of the abscess. A decreased LOC varies from drowsiness to deep stupor.
◆ *Brain tumor.* Focal seizures are commonly the earliest indicators of a brain tumor. The patient may report a morning headache, dizziness, confusion, vision loss, and motor and sensory disturbances.
◆ *Head trauma.* Any head injury can cause seizures, but penetrating wounds are characteristically associated with focal seizures. The seizures usually begin 3 to 15 months after injury and decrease in frequency after several years.
◼ *Stroke.* A major cause of seizures in patients older than age 50, a stroke may induce focal seizures up to 6 months after its onset. Related effects depend on the type and extent of the stroke.

Setting-sun sign

Setting-sun sign (also known as *sunset eyes*) refers to the downward deviation of an infant's or a young child's eyes as a result of pressure on cranial nerves III, IV, and VI. With this late and ominous sign of increased intracranial pressure (ICP), both eyes are rotated downward, typically revealing an area of sclera above the irises; occasionally, the irises appear to be forced outward. Pupils are sluggish, responding to light unequally. (See *Identifying setting-sun sign,* page 496.) Increased ICP typically results from space-occupying lesions—such as tumors—or from an accumulation of fluid in the brain's ventricular system, as occurs with hydrocephalus. It also results from intracranial bleeding or cerebral edema.

Setting-sun sign may be intermittent—for example, it may disappear when the infant is upright because this position slightly reduces ICP. The sign may be elicited in a healthy infant younger than age 4 weeks by suddenly changing his head position, and in a healthy infant up to age 9 months by

Identifying setting-sun sign

With this late sign of increased intracranial pressure in an infant or a young child, pressure on cranial nerves III, IV, and VI forces the eyes downward, revealing a rim of sclera above the irises.

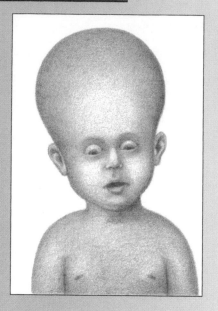

shining a bright light into his eyes and removing it quickly.

Assessment

If you observe the setting-sun sign in an infant, evaluate his neurologic status. Then obtain a brief history from his parents. Has the infant experienced a fall or even a minor trauma? When did this sign appear? Ask about early nonspecific signs of increasing ICP: Has the infant's sucking reflex diminished? Is he irritable, restless, or unusually tired? Does he cry when moved? Is his cry high pitched? Has he vomited recently?

Next, perform a physical examination, keeping in mind that neurologic responses are primarily reflexive during early infancy. Assess the infant's level of consciousness (LOC). Is he awake, irritable, or lethargic? Keeping in mind his age and level of development, try to determine his ability to reach for a bright object or turn toward the sound of music. Observe his posture for normal flexion and extension or opisthotonos. Examine muscle tone, and observe for seizure automatisms. Also examine for a globular appearance of the head, a loss of upgaze, distended scalp veins, and the anterior fontanel for bulging. Measure his head circumference and compare it to previous results, and observe his breathing pattern. Also, check his pupillary response to light. Finally, elicit reflexes that are diminished in increased ICP, especially Moro reflex. Keep endotracheal intubation equipment available.

Causes

◪ *Increased ICP.* Transient or intermittent setting-sun sign usually occurs late in the infant with increased ICP. He may have bulging, widened fontanels, an increased head circumference, and widened sutures. He may also exhibit a decreased LOC, behavioral changes, a high-pitched cry, pupillary abnormalities, and impaired motor movement as ICP increases.

Skin, clammy

Clammy skin—moist, cool, and usually pale—is a sympathetic response to stress, which triggers release of the hormones epinephrine and norepinephrine. These hormones cause cutaneous vasoconstriction and secretion of cold sweat from eccrine glands, particularly on the palms, forehead, and soles.

Clammy skin typically accompanies shock, acute hypoglycemia, anxiety reactions, arrhythmias, and heat exhaustion. It also occurs as a vasovagal reaction to severe pain associated with nausea, anorexia, epigastric distress, hyperpnea, tachypnea, weakness, confusion, tachycardia, and pupillary dilation or a combination of these findings. Marked bradycardia and syncope may follow.

Assessment

If you detect clammy skin, remember that rapid evaluation and intervention are paramount. (See *Clammy skin: A key finding,* page 498.) Ask the patient if he has a history of type 1 diabetes mellitus or a cardiac disorder. Is he taking medications, especially an antiarrhythmic? Is he experiencing pain, chest pressure, nausea, or epigastric distress? Does he feel weak? Does he have a dry mouth? Does he have diarrhea or increased urination?

Next, examine the pupils for dilation. Also, check for abdominal distention and increased muscle tension.

Causes

◆ *Anxiety.* An acute anxiety attack commonly produces cold, clammy skin on the forehead, palms, and soles.
◪ *Cardiac arrhythmias.* Cardiac arrhythmias may produce generalized cool, clammy skin along with mental status changes, dizziness, and hypotension.
◪ *Cardiogenic shock.* Generalized cool, moist, pale skin accompanies confusion, restlessness, hypotension, tachycardia, tachypnea, narrowing pulse pressure, cyanosis, and oliguria.
◆ *Heat exhaustion.* In the acute stage of heat exhaustion, generalized cold, clammy skin accompanies an ashen appearance, a headache, confusion, and syncope.
◪ *Hypoglycemia (acute).* With hypoglycemia, generalized cool, clammy skin or diaphoresis may accompany irritability, tremors, palpitations, hunger, headache, tachycardia, and anxiety.
◪ *Hypovolemic shock.* With hypovolemic shock, generalized pale, cold, clammy skin accompanies a subnormal body temperature, hypotension with narrowing pulse pressure, tachycardia, tachypnea, and a rapid, thready pulse.
◪ *Septic shock.* The cold shock stage causes generalized cold, clammy skin. Associated findings include a rapid and thready pulse, severe hypotension, per-

EMERGENCY INTERVENTIONS

Clammy skin: A key finding

Be alert for clammy skin because it commonly accompanies emergency conditions, such as shock, acute hypoglycemia, and arrhythmias. To know what to do, review these typical clinical situations.

You detect clammy skin in a patient who appears anxious and restless.

↓

Quickly check his vital signs, noting tachypnea, hypotension, and a weak, irregular pulse. If present:

↓

Suspect *shock*.

↓

Place the patient in a supine position in bed. Elevate his legs 20 to 30 degrees to promote perfusion to vital organs.

↓

Insert an I.V. catheter for administration of drugs, fluids, or blood. Also, give supplemental oxygen and begin cardiac monitoring.

You detect clammy skin and possible tremors in a patient who appears irritable, anxious, and confused. He may also be difficult to arouse and report persistent hunger.

↓

Quickly check his vital signs, which will typically be normal. A vagal reaction to the stress of hypoglycemia may cause hypotension and tachycardia. If present:

↓

Suspect *acute hypoglycemia*.

↓

Immediately draw blood for glucose studies and test a drop with a glucose reagent strip. Insert an I.V. catheter, and give a 50-ml bolus of dextrose 50%, as ordered. Also, begin cardiac monitoring.

You detect clammy skin in a patient with changes in mental status such as confusion.

↓

Quickly check his vital signs, which will typically be normal. A vagal reaction to the stress of hypoglycemia may cause hypotension and tachycardia. If present:

↓

Suspect an *arrhythmia*.

↓

Insert an I.V. catheter. Expect to administer an antiarrhythmic. Also, give supplemental oxygen and begin cardiac monitoring.

sistent oliguria or anuria, and respiratory failure.

Skin, mottled

Mottled skin is patchy discoloration indicating primary or secondary changes of the deep, middle, or superficial dermal blood vessels. It can result from a hematologic, immune, or connective tissue disorder; chronic occlusive arterial disease; dysproteinemia; immobility; exposure to heat or cold; or shock. Mottled skin can be a normal reaction such as the diffuse mottling that occurs when exposure to cold causes venous stasis in cutaneous blood vessels.

Mottling that occurs with other signs and symptoms usually affects the extremities, typically indicating restricted blood flow. For example, livedo reticularis, a characteristic network pattern of reddish blue discoloration, occurs when vasospasm of the mid-dermal blood vessels slows local blood flow in dilated superficial capillaries and small veins. Shock causes mottling from systemic vasoconstriction.

Assessment

If the patient's skin is pale, cool, clammy, and mottled at the elbows and knees or all over, he may be developing hypovolemic shock. Quickly check his vital signs, noting tachycardia or a weak, thready pulse. Observe the neck for flattened veins. These findings may indicate an emergency condition requiring rapid intervention. (See *Mottled skin: Knowing what to do.*) However, if the patient isn't in distress, obtain a history. Ask if the mottling began suddenly or gradually. What precipitated it? How long has he had it? Does any-

---

EMERGENCY INTERVENTIONS

Mottled skin: Knowing what to do

If your patient has mottled skin and you detect other signs and symptoms of hypovolemia, respond quickly:
◆ Place the patient in a supine position in bed with his legs elevated 20 to 30 degrees.
◆ Administer oxygen by nasal cannula or face mask.
◆ Begin cardiac monitoring.
◆ Insert a large-bore I.V. catheter for rapid fluid or blood product administration, as prescribed.
◆ Prepare to assist with central venous catheter or pulmonary artery catheter insertion.

◆ Prepare to catheterize the patient to monitor urine output if ordered.

Localized mottling in a pale, cool extremity that the patient says feels painful, numb, and tingling may signal acute arterial occlusion. Take these nursing actions:
◆ Immediately check the patient's distal pulses.
◆ Prepare to insert an I.V. catheter in an unaffected extremity.
◆ Prepare the patient for arteriography or immediate surgery.

thing make it go away? Does the patient have other symptoms, such as pain, numbness, or tingling in an extremity? If so, do they disappear with temperature changes?

Observe the patient's skin color, and palpate his arms and legs for skin texture, swelling, and temperature differences between extremities. Check capillary refill time and palpate for the presence and quality of pulses. Note breaks in the skin, muscle appearance, and hair distribution. Also, assess motor and sensory function.

Causes

◼ *Arterial occlusion (acute).* Initial signs of acute arterial occlusion include temperature and color changes. Pallor may change to blotchy cyanosis and livedo reticularis. Color and temperature demarcation develop at the level of obstruction. Examination reveals diminished or absent pulses, cool extremities, and increased capillary refill time.

◆ *Arteriosclerosis obliterans.* Atherosclerotic buildup narrows intra-arterial lumina, resulting in reduced blood flow through the affected artery. Obstructed blood flow to the extremities (most commonly the legs) produces such peripheral signs and symptoms as leg pallor, cyanosis, blotchy erythema, and livedo reticularis.

◆ *Buerger's disease.* Buerger's disease produces unilateral or asymmetrical color changes and mottling, particularly livedo networking in the lower extremities. It also typically causes intermittent claudication and erythema along extremity blood vessels.

◆ *Cryoglobulinemia.* Cryoglobulinemia is a necrotizing disorder that causes patchy livedo reticularis, petechiae, and ecchymoses.

◼ *Hypovolemic shock.* Vasoconstriction from shock commonly produces skin mottling, initially in the knees and elbows. As shock worsens, mottling becomes generalized. As shock progresses the skin becomes cool and clammy.

◆ *Livedo reticularis (idiopathic or primary).* With this condition, symmetrical, diffuse skin mottling can involve the hands, feet, arms, legs, buttocks, and trunk. Initially, networking is intermittent and most pronounced on exposure to cold or stress; eventually, mottling persists even with warming.

◆ *Periarteritis nodosa.* Skin findings in periarteritis nodosa include palpable nodules along the path of medium-sized arteries, erythema, purpura, muscle wasting, ulcers, and asymmetrical, patchy livedo reticularis.

◆ *Polycythemia vera.* Polycythemia vera is a hematologic disorder that produces livedo reticularis, hemangiomas, purpura, rubor, ulcerative nodules, and scleroderma-like lesions.

◆ *Systemic lupus erythematosus (SLE).* SLE is a connective tissue disorder that can cause livedo reticularis, most commonly on the outer arms.

Skin, scaly

Scaly skin results when cells of the uppermost skin layer (stratum corneum) desiccate and shed, causing excessive accumulation of loosely adherent flakes of normal or abnormal keratin. Normally, skin cell loss is imperceptible; the appearance of scale indicates increased cell proliferation secondary to altered keratinization.

Scaly skin varies in texture from fine and delicate to branlike, coarse, or stratified. Scales are typically dry, brittle, and shiny, but they can be greasy and dull. Their color ranges from whitish gray, yellow, or brown to a silvery sheen.

Usually benign, scaly skin occurs with fungal, bacterial, and viral infections, lymphomas, and lupus erythematosus; it's also common in those with inflammatory skin disease. A form of scaly skin—generalized fine desquamation—commonly follows prolonged febrile illness, sunburn, and thermal burns. Red patches of scaly skin that appear or worsen in winter may result from dry skin or from actinic keratosis, common in elderly patients. Certain drugs also cause scaly skin. Aggravating factors include cold, heat, immobility, and frequent bathing.

Assessment

Begin the history by asking how long the patient has had scaly skin and whether he has had it before. Where did it first appear? Did a lesion or skin eruption, such as erythema, precede it? Has the patient used a new or different topical skin product recently? How often does he bathe? Has he had recent joint pain, illness, or malaise? Ask the patient about work exposure to chemicals, use of prescribed drugs, and a family history of skin disorders. Find out what kinds of soap, detergent, dryer sheets, cosmetics, skin lotion, and hair preparations he uses.

Next, examine the entire skin surface. Is it dry, oily, moist, or greasy? Observe the general pattern of skin lesions, and record their location. Note their color, shape, and size. Are they thick or fine? Do they itch? Does the patient have other lesions? Examine the mucous membranes of his mouth, lips, and nose, and inspect his ears, hair, and nails.

Causes

◆ *Bowen's disease.* Bowen's disease is a common form of intraepidermal carcinoma that causes painless, erythematous plaques that are raised and indurated with a thick, hyperkeratotic scale and, possibly, ulcerated centers.
◼ *Dermatitis. Exfoliative dermatitis* begins with rapidly developing generalized erythema. Desquamation with fine scales or thick sheets of all or most of the skin surface may cause life-threatening hypothermia. Other possible complications include cardiac output failure and septicemia.

With *nummular dermatitis,* round, pustular lesions commonly ooze purulent exudate, itch severely, and rapidly become encrusted and scaly. Lesions appear on the extensor surfaces of the limbs, posterior trunk, and buttocks.

Seborrheic dermatitis begins with erythematous, scaly papules that progress to larger, dry or moist, greasy scales with yellowish crusts. This disorder primarily involves the center of the face, the chest and scalp. Pruritus occurs with scaling.
◆ *Dermatophytosis. Tinea capitis* produces lesions with reddened, slightly elevated borders and a central area of dense scaling; these lesions may become inflamed and pus-filled. *Tinea pedis* causes scaling and blisters between the toes. The squamous type produces diffuse, fine, branlike scales. Adherent and silvery white, they're most prominent in skin creases and may affect the entire dorsum of the foot. *Tinea corporis* produces crusty lesions. As they enlarge, their centers heal, causing the classic ringworm shape. *Tinea versicolor* is a benign fungal skin infection that typically produces macular hypopigmented, fawn-colored, or brown patches of varying

sizes and shapes. All are slightly scaly. Lesions commonly affect the upper trunk, arms, and lower abdomen; sometimes the neck; and, rarely, the face.

◆ *Eczema.* Eczema can occur on any part of the body and is most commonly characterized by inflammation and scaly, red, extremely itchy patches on the skin. Scratching these patches results in the appearance of a rash.

◆ *Lymphoma.* Hodgkin's disease and non-Hodgkin's lymphoma commonly cause scaly rashes. Hodgkin's disease may cause pruritic scaling dermatitis that begins in the legs and spreads to the entire body. Small nodules and diffuse pigmentation are related signs. Non-Hodgkin's lymphoma initially produces erythematous patches with some scaling that later become interspersed with nodules. Pruritus and discomfort are common.

◆ *Parapsoriasis (chronic).* Parapsoriasis produces small or moderate-sized maculopapular, erythematous eruptions, with a thin, adherent scale on the trunk, hands, and feet. Removal of the scale reveals a shiny brown surface.

◆ *Pityriasis.* Pityriasis rosea produces widespread scales. It begins with an erythematous, raised, oval herald patch anywhere on the body. A few days or weeks later, yellow-tan or erythematous patches with scaly edges erupt on the trunk and limbs and sometimes on the face, hands, and feet. Pruritus also occurs. Pityriasis rubra pilaris, an uncommon disorder, initially produces seborrheic scaling on the scalp, progressing to the face and ears.

◆ *Psoriasis.* Silvery white, micaceous scales cover erythematous plaques that have sharply defined borders. Psoriasis usually appears on the scalp, chest, elbows, knees, back, buttocks, and genitalia.

◆ *Systemic lupus erythematosus (SLE).* SLE produces a bright-red maculopapular eruption, sometimes with scaling. Patches are sharply defined and involve the nose and malar regions of the face in a butterfly pattern.

Skin turgor, decreased

Skin turgor—the skin's elasticity—is determined by observing the time required for the skin to return to its normal position after being stretched or pinched. With decreased turgor, pinched skin "holds" for up to 30 seconds, and then slowly returns to its normal contour. Skin turgor is commonly assessed over the arm or sternum—areas normally free from wrinkles and with wide variations in tissue thickness. (See *Evaluating skin turgor.*)

Decreased skin turgor results from dehydration, or volume depletion, which moves interstitial fluid into the vascular bed to maintain circulating blood volume, leading to slackness in the skin's dermal layer. It's a normal finding in elderly patients and in people who have lost weight rapidly; it also occurs with disorders affecting the GI, renal, endocrine, and other systems.

Assessment

If your examination reveals decreased skin turgor, ask the patient about food and fluid intake and fluid loss. Has he recently experienced prolonged fluid loss from vomiting, diarrhea, draining wounds, or increased urination? Has he recently had a fever with sweating? Is

Evaluating skin turgor

To evaluate skin turgor in an adult, pick up a fold of skin over the sternum or the arm, as shown below left. (In an infant, roll a fold of loosely adherent skin on the abdomen between your thumb and forefinger.) Then release it. Normal skin will immediately return to its previous contour. In decreased skin turgor, the skin fold will "hold," or "tent," as shown below right, for up to 30 seconds.

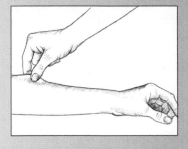
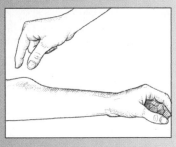

the patient taking a diuretic? Does he drink alcohol, if so, how much and how often?

Next, check the patient's vital signs. Note if his systolic blood pressure is abnormally low (90 mm Hg or less) when he's in a supine position, if it drops 15 to 20 mm Hg or more when he stands, or if his pulse increases by 10 beats/minute when he sits or stands. If you detect these signs of orthostatic hypotension or resting tachycardia, insert an I.V. catheter for fluids. Evaluate the patient for confusion, disorientation, and signs of profound dehydration. Inspect his oral mucosa, the furrows of his tongue (especially under the tongue), and his axillae for dryness. Also, check his jugular veins for flatness, and monitor his urine output.

Causes

◾ *Cholera.* Cholera is characterized by abrupt watery diarrhea and vomiting, which leads to severe water and electrolyte loss. Without treatment, death can occur within hours.

◆ *Dehydration.* Decreased skin turgor commonly occurs with moderate to severe dehydration. Associated findings include dry oral mucosa, decreased perspiration, resting tachycardia, orthostatic hypotension, a dry and furrowed tongue, increased thirst, weight loss, oliguria, fever, and fatigue.

Splenomegaly

Because it occurs with various disorders and in up to 5% of normal adults, splenomegaly—an enlarged spleen—isn't a diagnostic sign by itself. Usually, however, it points to infection, trauma, or a hepatic, autoimmune, neoplastic, or hematologic disorder.

Because the spleen functions as the body's largest lymph node, splenomegaly can result from any process that triggers lymphadenopathy. For example, it may reflect reactive hyperplasia (a response to infection or inflammation), proliferation or infiltration of neoplastic cells, extramedullary hemopoiesis, phagocytic cell proliferation, increased blood cell destruction, or vascular congestion associated with portal hypertension.

Splenomegaly may be detected by light palpation under the left costal margin. (See *How to palpate for splenomegaly*.) However, because this technique isn't always advisable or effective, splenomegaly may need to be confirmed by a computed tomography or radionuclide scan.

Assessment

If the patient has a history of abdominal or thoracic trauma, don't palpate the abdomen because this may aggravate internal bleeding. Instead, examine him for left-upper-quadrant pain and signs of shock. If you detect these signs, suspect splenic rupture and prepare the patient for possible surgery. If you detect splenomegaly during a routine physical examination, begin by exploring associated signs and symptoms. Ask the patient if he has been unusually tired lately. Does he frequently have colds, sore throats, or other infections? Does he bruise easily? Ask about left-upper-quadrant pain, abdominal fullness, and early satiety. Finally, examine the patient's skin for pallor and ecchymoses, and palpate his axillae, groin, and neck for lymphadenopathy.

Causes

◆ *Cirrhosis.* About one-third of patients with advanced cirrhosis develop moderate to marked splenomegaly. Among other late findings are jaundice, hepatomegaly, leg edema, hematemesis, and ascites.

◆ *Felty's syndrome.* Splenomegaly is characteristic in Felty's syndrome, which occurs with chronic rheumatoid arthritis. Associated findings are joint pain and deformity, sensory or motor loss, rheumatoid nodules, palmar erythema, lymphadenopathy, and leg ulcers.

◆ *Histoplasmosis.* Acute disseminated histoplasmosis commonly produces splenomegaly and hepatomegaly. It may also cause lymphadenopathy, jaundice, fever, anorexia, emaciation, and signs and symptoms of anemia.

◆ *Leukemia.* Moderate to severe splenomegaly is an early sign of acute and chronic leukemia. With chronic granulocytic leukemia, splenomegaly is sometimes painful.

◆ *Mononucleosis (infectious).* A common sign of mononucleosis, splenomegaly is most pronounced during the second and third weeks of illness. Typically, it's accompanied by a triad of signs and symptoms: sore throat, cervical lymphadenopathy, and fluctuating temperature with an evening peak of 101° to 102° F (38.3° to 38.9° C).

◼ *Pancreatic cancer.* Pancreatic cancer may cause moderate to severe splenomegaly if tumor growth compresses the splenic vein. Other findings include abdominal or back pain, jaundice, pruritus, skin lesions, and fatigue.

◆ *Polycythemia vera.* Late in polycythemia vera, the spleen may become markedly enlarged, resulting in easy satiety, abdominal fullness, and left-upper-quadrant or pleuritic chest pain. Accompanying signs and symptoms are widespread and numerous.

◆ *Sarcoidosis.* Sarcoidosis is a granulomatous disorder that may produce splenomegaly and hepatomegaly, possibly accompanied by vague abdominal

How to palpate for splenomegaly

Detecting splenomegaly requires skillful and gentle palpation to avoid rupturing the enlarged spleen. Follow these steps carefully:

◆ Place the patient in the supine position, and stand at her right side. Place your left hand under the left costovertebral angle and push lightly to move the spleen forward. Then press your right hand gently under the left front costal margin.

◆ Have the patient take a deep breath and then exhale. As she exhales, move your right hand along the tissue contours under the border of the ribs, feeling for the spleen's edge. The enlarged spleen should feel like a firm mass that bumps against your fingers. Remember to begin palpation low enough in the abdomen to catch the edge of a massive spleen.

◆ Grade the splenomegaly as slight (½″ to 1½″ [1 to 4 cm] below the costal margin), moderate (1½ to 3″ [4 to 8 cm] below the costal margin), or great (greater than or equal to 3″ [8 cm] below the costal margin).

◆ Reposition the patient on her right side with her hips and knees flexed slightly to move the spleen forward. Then repeat the palpation procedure.

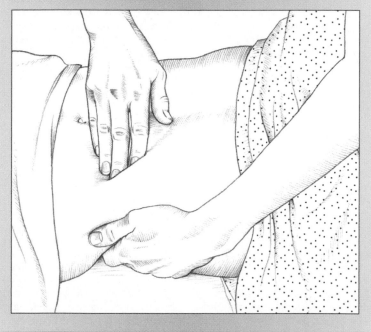

discomfort. Other signs and symptoms vary with the affected body system.

◼ *Splenic rupture.* Splenomegaly may result from massive hemorrhage with splenic rupture. The patient may also experience left-upper-quadrant pain, abdominal rigidity, and Kehr's sign.

◆ *Thrombotic thrombocytopenic purpura.* This disorder may produce splenomegaly and hepatomegaly accompanied by fever, generalized purpura, jaundice, pallor, vaginal bleeding, and hematuria.

Stools, clay-colored

Pale, putty-colored stools usually result from hepatic, gallbladder, or pancreatic disorders. Normally, bile pigments give the stool its characteristic brown color. However, hepatocellular degeneration or biliary obstruction may interfere with the formation or release of these pigments into the intestine, resulting in clay-colored stools. These stools are commonly associated with jaundice and dark "cola-colored" urine.

Assessment

After documenting when the patient first noticed clay-colored stools, explore associated signs and symptoms, such as abdominal pain, nausea and vomiting, fatigue, anorexia, weight loss, and dark urine. Does the patient have trouble digesting fatty foods or heavy meals? Does he bruise easily?

Next, review the patient's medical history for gallbladder, hepatic, or pancreatic disorders. Has he ever had biliary surgery? Has he recently undergone barium studies? (Barium lightens stool color for several days.) Also, ask about antacid use because large amounts may lighten stool color. Note a history of alcoholism or exposure to other hepatotoxic substances.

After assessing the patient's general appearance, check his vital signs. Check his skin and eyes for jaundice. Then examine the abdomen: inspect for distention and ascites and auscultate for hypoactive bowel sounds. Percuss and palpate for masses and rebound tenderness. Finally, obtain urine and stool specimens for laboratory analysis.

Causes

◆ *Bile duct cancer.* Clay-colored stools are a common presenting sign of bile duct cancer. They may be accompanied by jaundice, pruritus, anorexia and weight loss, upper abdominal pain, bleeding tendencies, and a palpable mass.

◆ *Biliary cirrhosis.* Clay-colored stools typically follow unexplained pruritus that worsens at bedtime, weakness, fatigue, weight loss, and vague abdominal pain; these features may be present for years with biliary cirrhosis.

◆ *Cholangitis (sclerosing).* Characterized by fibrosis of the bile ducts, cholangitis may cause clay-colored stools, chronic or intermittent jaundice, pruritus, right upper quadrant pain, chills, and fever.

◆ *Cholelithiasis.* Stones in the biliary tract may cause clay-colored stools when they obstruct the common bile duct. However, if the obstruction is intermittent, the stools may alternate between normal and clay colored. Associated symptoms include dyspepsia and—in sudden, severe obstruction— characteristic biliary colic.

◼ *Hepatic cancer.* Before clay-colored stools develop, the patient usually experiences weight loss, weakness, and anorexia. Later, he may develop jaundice, right upper quadrant pain, ascites, dependent edema, and fever.

◆ *Hepatitis.* With viral hepatitis, clay-colored stools signal the start of the icteric phase and are typically followed by jaundice within 1 to 5 days. Cholestatic nonviral hepatitis produces clay-colored stools along with other signs of viral hepatitis.

◪ *Pancreatic cancer.* Common bile duct obstruction associated with pancreatic cancer may cause clay-colored stools. Classic associated features include abdominal or back pain, jaundice, pruritus, nausea and vomiting, anorexia, weight loss, fatigue, weakness, and fever.

◪ *Pancreatitis (acute).* Pancreatitis is an inflammatory disorder that may cause clay-colored stools, dark urine, and jaundice. Typically, it also causes severe epigastric pain that radiates to the back and is aggravated by lying down. With severe pancreatitis, findings include marked restlessness, tachycardia, mottled skin, and cold, sweaty extremities.

Stridor

A loud, harsh, musical respiratory sound, stridor results from an obstruction in the trachea or larynx. Usually heard during inspiration, this sign may also occur during expiration in severe upper airway obstruction. It may begin as low-pitched "croaking" and progress to high-pitched "crowing" as respirations become more vigorous.

Life-threatening upper airway obstruction can stem from foreign-body aspiration, increased secretions, an intraluminal tumor, localized edema or muscle spasms, and external compression by a tumor or aneurysm.

Assessment

If you hear stridor, quickly check the patient's vital signs, including oxygen saturation, and examine him for other signs of partial airway obstruction. Be aware that abrupt cessation of stridor signals complete obstruction in which the patient has inspiratory chest movement but absent breath sounds. Unable to talk, he quickly becomes lethargic and loses consciousness. (See *Responding to airway obstruction* and *Emergency endotracheal intubation,* pages 508 and 509.)

If the patient's condition permits, obtain a medical history from him or his family members. First, find out when the stridor began. Has he had it before? Does he have an upper respiratory tract infection? If so, how long has he had it? Ask about a history of aller-

---

EMERGENCY INTERVENTIONS

Responding to airway obstruction

If you detect stridor and signs of airway obstruction in your patient, take immediate action:

◆ Attempt to clear his airway with abdominal thrusts.

◆ Administer oxygen by nasal cannula or face mask.

◆ Prepare him for emergency endotracheal (ET) intubation or tracheostomy and mechanical ventilation.

◆ Be ready to suction aspirated vomitus or blood through the ET or tracheostomy tube.

◆ Connect him to a cardiac monitor.

◆ Position him in Fowler's position to ease his breathing.

EMERGENCY INTERVENTIONS

Emergency endotracheal intubation

For a patient with stridor, you may have to perform emergency endotracheal (ET) intubation to establish a patent airway and administer mechanical ventilation. Follow these essential steps:

◆ Gather the necessary equipment.

◆ Explain the procedure to the patient.

◆ Place the patient flat on his back with a small blanket or pillow under his head if cervical spine injury isn't suspected. This position aligns the axis of the oropharynx, posterior pharynx, and trachea.

◆ Check the cuff on the ET tube for leaks.

◆ After intubation (see illustration), inflate the cuff, using the minimal leak technique.

◆ Check tube placement by auscultating for bilateral breath sounds and using a capnometer; observe the patient for chest expansion and feel for warm exhalations at the ET tube's opening.

◆ Insert an oral airway or bite block, if necessary.

◆ Secure the tube and airway with an ET tube holder or tape.

◆ Suction secretions from the patient's mouth and the ET tube as needed.

◆ Administer oxygen or initiate mechanical ventilation (or both).

◆ Suction secretions as needed.

◆ Check cuff pressure once every shift (correcting any air leaks with the minimal leak technique).

◆ Provide mouth care every 2 hours and as needed.

◆ Prepare the patient for chest X-rays to check tube placement.

◆ Restrain and reassure the patient as needed.

gies, tumors, and respiratory and vascular disorders. Note recent exposure to smoke or noxious fumes or gases. Next, explore associated signs and symptoms. Does stridor occur with pain or a cough?

Then examine the patient's mouth for excessive secretions, foreign matter, inflammation, and swelling. Assess his neck for swelling, masses, subcutaneous crepitation, and scars. Observe the patient's chest for delayed, decreased, or asymmetrical chest expansion. Auscultate for wheezes, rhonchi, crackles, rubs, and other abnormal breath sounds. Percuss for dullness, tympany, or flatness. Finally, note burns or signs of trauma, such as ecchymoses and lacerations.

Causes

◣ *Airway trauma.* Local trauma to the upper airway commonly causes acute obstruction, resulting in the sudden onset of stridor. Other findings include dysphonia, dysphagia, cyanosis, intercostal retractions, nasal flaring, progressive dyspnea, and shallow respirations. Palpation may reveal subcutaneous crepitation in the neck or upper chest.

◣ *Anaphylaxis.* With a severe allergic reaction, upper airway edema and laryngospasm cause stridor and other

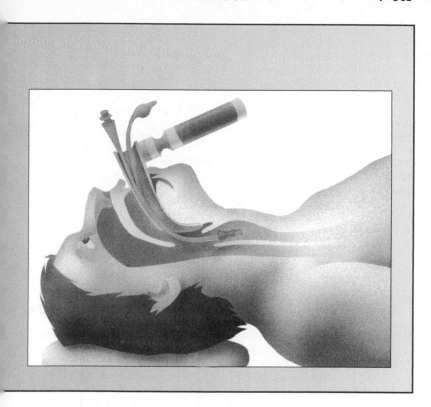

signs and symptoms of respiratory distress: nasal flaring, wheezing, accessory muscle use, intercostal retractions, and dyspnea.

◤ *Aspiration of a foreign body.* Sudden stridor is characteristic in foreign body aspiration. Related findings include an abrupt onset of dry, paroxysmal coughing; gagging or choking; hoarseness; tachycardia; wheezing; dyspnea; tachypnea; intercostal muscle retractions; diminished breath sounds; cyanosis; and shallow respirations.

◤ *Hypocalcemia.* With hypocalcemia, laryngospasm can cause stridor. Other findings include paresthesia, carpopedal spasm, and positive Chvostek's and Trousseau's signs.

◤ *Inhalation injury.* Within 48 hours after inhalation of smoke or noxious fumes, the patient may develop laryngeal edema and bronchospasm, resulting in stridor. Other findings include singed nasal hairs, orofacial burns, coughing, hoarseness, sooty sputum, crackles, rhonchi, wheezes, and other signs and symptoms of respiratory distress.

◤ *Mediastinal tumor.* Commonly producing no symptoms at first, a mediastinal tumor may eventually compress the trachea and bronchi, resulting in stridor. Other findings include hoarseness, brassy cough, tracheal shift or tug, swelling of the face and neck, stertorous respirations, and suprasternal retractions on inspiration.

◆ *Retrosternal thyroid.* Retrosternal thyroid is an anatomic abnormality that causes stridor, dysphagia, cough, hoarseness, and tracheal deviation. It can also cause signs of thyrotoxicosis.

Syncope

A common neurologic sign, syncope (or fainting) refers to a transient loss of consciousness associated with impaired cerebral blood supply or cerebral hypoxia. It usually occurs abruptly and lasts for seconds to minutes. An episode of syncope usually starts as a feeling of light-headedness. A patient can usually prevent an episode of syncope by lying down with his legs elevated or sitting with his head between his knees. Typically, the patient lies motionless with his skeletal muscles relaxed but sphincter muscles controlled. However, the depth of unconsciousness varies—some patients can hear voices or see blurred outlines; others are unaware of their surroundings.

In many ways, syncope simulates death: The patient is strikingly pale with a slow, weak pulse, hypotension, and almost imperceptible breathing. If severe hypotension lasts for 20 seconds or longer, the patient may also develop tonic-clonic seizures.

Syncope may result from cardiac and cerebrovascular disorders, hypoxemia, and orthostatic changes in the presence of autonomic dysfunction. It may also follow vigorous coughing, injury, shock, or pain. Hysterical syncope may also follow emotional stress but isn't accompanied by other vasodepressor effects.

Assessment

If you see a patient faint, ensure a patent airway and the patient's safety. Check his vital signs. Be alert for tachycardia, bradycardia, or an irregular pulse. Base your response on your assessment findings.

If the patient reports a fainting episode, gather information about the episode from him and his family. Did he feel weak, light-headed, nauseous, or sweaty just before he fainted? Did he get up quickly from a chair or from lying down? During the fainting episode, did he have muscle spasms or incontinence? How long was he unconscious? When he regained consciousness, was he alert or confused? Did he have a headache? Has he fainted before? If so, how often does it occur?

Examine the patient for any injuries that may have occurred during his fall.

Causes

◆ *Aortic arch syndrome.* With aortic arch syndrome, the patient experiences syncope and may exhibit weak or abruptly absent carotid pulses and unequal or absent radial pulses.

◆ *Aortic stenosis.* A late sign of aortic stenosis, syncope is accompanied by exertional dyspnea and angina. Typically, auscultation reveals atrial and ventricular gallops as well as a harsh, crescendo-decrescendo systolic ejection murmur that's loudest at the right sternal border of the second intercostal space.

▨ *Cardiac arrhythmias.* Any arrhythmia that decreases cardiac output and impairs cerebral circulation may cause syncope. Other findings, such as palpitations, diaphoresis, dyspnea, and hypotension, usually develop first. However, with Adams-Stokes syndrome, syncope may occur without warning. During syncope, the patient develops asystole, which may precipitate spasm and myoclonic jerks if prolonged.

◣ *Hypoxemia.* Regardless of its cause, severe hypoxemia may produce syncope. Common related effects include confusion, tachycardia, restlessness, and incoordination.

◆ *Orthostatic hypotension.* Syncope occurs when the patient rises quickly from a recumbent position. Look for a drop of 10 to 20 mm Hg or more in systolic or diastolic blood pressure as well as tachycardia, pallor, dizziness, blurred vision, and diaphoresis.

◆ *Transient ischemic attack (TIA).* Marked by transient neurologic deficits, TIAs may produce syncope and a decreased level of consciousness. Other findings vary with the affected artery.

T

Tachycardia

Tachycardia is a heart rate greater than 100 beats/minute. It's easily detected by counting the apical, carotid, or radial pulse. The patient with tachycardia usually complains of palpitations or of a "racing" heart. This common sign normally occurs in response to emotional or physical stress, such as excitement, exercise, pain, anxiety, and fever. It may also result from the use of stimulants, such as caffeine and tobacco. However, tachycardia may be an early sign of a life-threatening disorder, such as cardiogenic, hypovolemic, or septic shock. It may also result from a cardiovascular, respiratory, or metabolic disorder or from the effects of certain drugs, tests, or treatments. (See *What happens in tachycardia.*)

Assessment

If you detect tachycardia in your patient, check his other vital signs and determine his level of consciousness (LOC). If he has increased or decreased blood pressure and is drowsy or confused, administer oxygen and begin cardiac monitoring. Perform electrocardiography to examine for reduced cardiac output, which may initiate or result from tachycardia. If the patient's condition permits, take a focused history. Find out if he has had palpitations. If so, how were they treated? Explore associated symptoms. Is the patient dizzy or short of breath? Is he weak or fatigued? Is he experiencing episodes of syncope or chest pain? Next, ask about a history of trauma, diabetes, or cardiac, pulmonary, or thyroid disorders. Also, obtain an alcohol and drug history, including prescription, over-the-counter, and illicit drugs.

Inspect the patient's skin for pallor or cyanosis. Assess pulses, noting peripheral edema. Finally, auscultate the heart and lungs for abnormal sounds or rhythms.

When examining a child for tachycardia, recognize that normal heart rates for children are higher than those for adults. (See *Normal pediatric vital signs,* pages 514 and 515.) In children, tachycardia may result from many of the same causes for adults.

Causes

◾ *Acute respiratory distress syndrome (ARDS).* Besides tachycardia, ARDS causes crackles, rhonchi, dyspnea, tachypnea, nasal flaring, and grunting respirations.

◆ *Adrenocortical insufficiency.* With adrenocortical insufficiency, tachycardia commonly occurs with a weak pulse as well as progressive weakness and fatigue, which may become so severe that the patient requires bed rest.

◘ *Anaphylactic shock.* With anaphylactic shock, tachycardia and hypotension develop within minutes after exposure to an allergen, such as penicillin or an insect sting. Typically, the patient is visibly anxious and has severe pruritus, perhaps with urticaria and a pounding headache.

◆ *Anemia.* Tachycardia and bounding pulse are characteristic with anemia. Other findings include fatigue, pallor, and dyspnea. Auscultation may reveal an atrial gallop, a systolic bruit over the carotid arteries, and crackles.

◆ *Aortic insufficiency.* Accompanying tachycardia with aortic insufficiency are a "water-hammer" bounding pulse and a large, diffuse apical heave. With severe insufficiency, widened pulse pressure occurs. Auscultation reveals a diastolic murmur that starts with the second heart sound and is heard best at the left sternal border of the second and third intercostal spaces. The murmur is decrescendo, high-pitched, and blowing.

◆ *Aortic stenosis.* Typically, aortic stenosis causes tachycardia, a weak, thready pulse, and an atrial gallop. Its chief findings, however, are exertional dyspnea, angina, dizziness, and syncope.

◘ *Cardiac arrhythmias.* Tachycardia may occur with an irregular heart rhythm. The patient may be hypotensive and report dizziness, palpitations, weakness, and fatigue. He may also exhibit tachypnea, decreased LOC, and pale, cool, clammy skin.

◆ *Cardiac contusion.* The result of blunt chest trauma, cardiac contusion

What happens in tachycardia

Tachycardia represents the heart's effort to deliver more oxygen to body tissues by increasing the rate at which blood passes through the vessels. This sign can reflect overstimulation within the sinoatrial node, the atrium, the atrioventricular node, or the ventricles.

Because heart rate affects cardiac output (cardiac output = heart rate × stroke volume), tachycardia can lower cardiac output by reducing ventricular filling time and stroke volume (the output of each ventricle at every contraction). As cardiac output plummets, arterial pressure and peripheral perfusion decrease. Tachycardia further aggravates myocardial ischemia by increasing the heart's demand for oxygen while reducing the duration of diastole—the period of greatest coronary flow.

may cause tachycardia, substernal pain, dyspnea, and palpitations. Assessment may detect sternal ecchymoses and a pericardial friction rub.

◘ *Cardiac tamponade.* With cardiac tamponade, tachycardia is commonly accompanied by paradoxical pulse, dyspnea, and tachypnea. The patient is visibly anxious and restless and has cyanotic, clammy skin and distended jugular veins.

◘ *Cardiogenic shock.* With cardiogenic shock, tachycardia is accompanied by a weak, thready pulse and narrowing pulse pressure. Other signs include hypotension, tachypnea, oliguria, restlessness, altered LOC, and cold, pale, clammy, and cyanotic skin.

Normal pediatric vital signs

This chart lists the average normal resting respiratory rate, blood pressure, and pulse rate for girls and boys to age 16.

VITAL SIGNS	NEONATE	2 YEARS	4 YEARS	6 YEARS
Respiratory rate				
Girls	28	26	25	24
Boys	30	28	25	24
Blood pressure (mm Hg)				
Girls	80/50	98/60	98/60	98/64
Boys	80/50	96/60	98/60	98/62
Pulse rate (beats/minute)				
Girls	130	110	100	100
Boys	130	110	100	100

◼ *Diabetic ketoacidosis.* Diabetic ketoacidosis commonly produces tachycardia and a thready pulse. Its cardinal sign, however, is Kussmaul's respirations—abnormally rapid, deep breathing.

◆ *Drugs.* Various drugs affect the nervous system, circulatory system, or heart muscle, resulting in tachycardia.

◆ *Heart failure.* Especially common with left-sided heart failure, tachycardia may be accompanied by ventricular gallop, fatigue, dyspnea (exertional and paroxysmal nocturnal), orthopnea, and leg edema.

◼ *Hyperosmolar hyperglycemic nonketotic syndrome (HHNS).* With HHNS, tachycardia, hypotension, tachypnea, seizures, oliguria, and severe dehydration with poor skin turgor and dry mucous membranes commonly accompany a rapidly deteriorating LOC.

◼ *Hypertensive crisis.* Hypertensive crisis is characterized by tachycardia, tachypnea, diastolic blood pressure that exceeds 120 mm Hg, and systolic blood pressure that may exceed 200 mm Hg.

◼ *Hypoglycemia.* A common sign of hypoglycemia, tachycardia accompanies hypothermia, nervousness, trembling, fatigue, malaise, weakness, headache, hunger, nausea, diaphoresis, and moist, clammy skin.

◆ *Hypovolemia.* Tachycardia may occur with hypovolemia. Associated findings include hypotension, decreased

8 YEARS	10 YEARS	12 YEARS	14 YEARS	16 YEARS
24	22	20	18	16
22	23	20	16	16
104/68	110/72	114/74	118/76	120/78
102/68	110/72	112/74	120/76	120/78
90	90	90	85	80
90	90	85	80	75

skin turgor, sunken eyeballs, thirst, syncope, and dry skin and tongue.

◤ *Hypovolemic shock.* Mild tachycardia, an early sign of hypovolemic shock, may be accompanied by tachypnea, restlessness, thirst, and pale, cool skin.

◤ *Neurogenic shock.* Tachycardia or bradycardia may accompany tachypnea, apprehension, oliguria, variable body temperature, decreased LOC, and warm, dry skin.

◆ *Orthostatic hypotension.* Tachycardia accompanies the characteristic signs and symptoms of orthostatic hypotension, which include dizziness, syncope, pallor, blurred vision, diaphoresis, and nausea.

◤ *Pneumothorax.* Pneumothorax causes tachycardia and other signs and symptoms of distress, such as severe dyspnea and chest pain, tachypnea, and cyanosis.

◤ *Pulmonary embolism.* With pulmonary embolism, sudden dyspnea, angina, or pleuritic chest pain usually precedes tachycardia.

◆ *Thyrotoxicosis.* Tachycardia is a classic finding in thyrotoxicosis. Because thyrotoxicosis affects virtually every body system, its associated findings are diverse and numerous.

Tachypnea

Tachypnea is a common sign of cardiopulmonary disorders. It's an abnormally fast respiratory rate—greater than 20 breaths/minute. Tachypnea may reflect the need to increase minute volume—the amount of air breathed each minute. Under these circumstances, it may be accompanied by an increase in tidal volume—the volume of air inhaled or exhaled per breath—resulting in hyperventilation. Tachypnea, however, may also reflect stiff lungs or overloaded ventilatory muscles, in which case tidal volume may actually be reduced.

Tachypnea may result from reduced arterial oxygen tension or arterial oxygen content, decreased perfusion, or increased oxygen demand. Heightened oxygen demand, for example, may result from fever, exertion, anxiety, and pain. It may also occur as a compensatory response to metabolic acidosis or may result from pulmonary irritation, stretch receptor stimulation, or a neurologic disorder that upsets medullary respiratory control. Generally, respirations increase by 4 breaths/minute for every 1° F (0.6° C) increase in body temperature.

Assessment

After detecting tachypnea, quickly evaluate cardiopulmonary status. Check the patient's vital signs and oxygen saturation level, and then check for cyanosis, chest pain, dyspnea, tachycardia, and hypotension. If the patient has paradoxical chest movement, suspect flail chest. (See *Flail chest: Reducing respiratory distress.*) Be alert for signs of respiratory failure.

If the patient's condition permits, obtain a medical history. Find out when the tachypnea began. Did it follow activity? Has he had it before? Does the patient have a history of asthma, chronic obstructive pulmonary disease (COPD), or any other pulmonary or cardiac conditions? Have him describe other signs and symptoms, such as diaphoresis, chest pain, and recent weight loss. Is he anxious about anything, or does he have a history of anxiety attacks? Note whether he takes any drugs for pain relief. If so, how effective are they?

Begin the physical examination by obtaining the patient's vital signs, including oxygen saturation, and by observing his overall behavior. Does he seem restless, confused, or fatigued? Then auscultate the chest for abnormal heart and breath sounds. If the patient has a productive cough, record the color, amount, and consistency of sputum. Finally, check for jugular vein distention, and examine the skin for pallor, cyanosis, edema, and warmth or coolness.

Causes

◪ *Acute respiratory distress syndrome (ARDS).* With ARDS, tachypnea and apprehension may be the earliest findings. Tachypnea gradually worsens as fluid accumulates in the patient's lungs, causing them to stiffen. Eventually, ARDS produces hypoxemia, resulting in tachycardia, dyspnea, cyanosis, respiratory failure, and shock.

◪ *Anaphylactic shock.* With anaphylactic shock, tachypnea develops within minutes after exposure to an allergen, such as penicillin or insect venom.

◆ *Asthma.* Tachypnea is common with asthma attacks, which commonly oc-

EMERGENCY INTERVENTIONS

Flail chest:
Reducing respiratory distress

If you suspect flail chest in a patient with tachypnea, follow these steps:
◆ Immediately splint his chest with your hands or with sandbags.
◆ Administer supplemental oxygen.
◆ Place the patient in semi-Fowler's position to help ease his breathing, if possible.

◆ Insert an I.V. catheter for fluid and drug administration.
◆ Begin cardiac monitoring.
◆ Understand that intubation and mechanical ventilation may be necessary if respiratory failure occurs.

cur at night. These attacks usually begin with mild wheezing and a dry cough that progresses to mucus expectoration.

◆ *Cardiac arrhythmias.* Depending on the patient's heart rate, tachypnea may occur along with hypotension, dizziness, palpitations, weakness, and fatigue. The patient's level of consciousness (LOC) may be decreased.

◆ *Cardiac tamponade.* With cardiac tamponade, tachypnea may accompany tachycardia, dyspnea, and paradoxical pulse. Related findings include muffled heart sounds, pericardial friction rub, chest pain, hypotension, narrowed pulse pressure, and hepatomegaly.

◆ *Cardiogenic shock.* With cardiogenic shock, tachypnea is accompanied by a weak, thready pulse; narrowing pulse pressure; hypotension; tachycardia; cold, pale, clammy, and cyanotic skin; oliguria; restlessness; and altered LOC.

◆ *Emphysema.* Emphysema commonly produces tachypnea accompanied by exertional dyspnea. It may also cause anorexia, malaise, peripheral cyanosis, pursed-lip breathing, accessory muscle use, and chronic productive cough.

◆ *Flail chest.* Tachypnea usually appears early in flail chest. Other findings include paradoxical chest wall movement, rib bruises and palpable fractures, localized chest pain, hypotension, and diminished breath sounds.

◆ *Hyperosmolar hyperglycemic nonketotic syndrome.* Rapidly deteriorating LOC occurs with tachypnea, tachycardia, hypotension, seizures, oliguria, and signs of dehydration.

◆ *Hypovolemic shock.* An early sign of hypovolemic shock, tachypnea is accompanied by mild tachycardia, hypotension, restlessness, thirst, and cool, pale skin. As shock progresses, the patient's skin becomes clammy and his pulse increasingly rapid and thready.

◆ *Hypoxia.* Lack of oxygen from any cause increases the rate (and commonly the depth) of breathing. Associated symptoms are related to the cause of the hypoxia.

◆ *Interstitial fibrosis.* With interstitial fibrosis, tachypnea develops gradually and may become severe. Associated findings include exertional dyspnea, pleuritic chest pain, a paroxysmal dry cough, crackles, late inspiratory wheezing, cyanosis, fatigue, and weight loss.

◆ *Lung abscess.* With lung abscess, tachypnea is usually paired with dyspnea and accentuated by fever. However, the chief sign is a productive cough with copious amounts of purulent, foul-smelling, usually bloody sputum.

◆ *Mesothelioma (malignant).* Commonly related to asbestos exposure, this pleural mass initially produces tachypnea and dyspnea on mild exertion.

◼ *Neurogenic shock.* Tachypnea is characteristic in neurogenic shock. It's commonly accompanied by apprehension, bradycardia or tachycardia, oliguria, fluctuating body temperature, and decreased LOC that may progress to coma.

◆ *Pneumonia (bacterial).* A common sign of pneumonia, tachypnea is usually preceded by a painful, hacking, dry cough that rapidly becomes productive.

◼ *Pneumothorax.* Tachypnea, a common sign of pneumothorax, is typically accompanied by severe, sharp, and commonly unilateral chest pain that's aggravated by chest movement. Examination of the affected lung reveals hyperresonance or tympany, subcutaneous crepitation, decreased vocal fremitus, and diminished or absent breath sounds on the affected side. The patient with tension pneumothorax also develops a deviated trachea.

◼ *Pulmonary edema.* An early sign of pulmonary edema, tachypnea is accompanied by exertional dyspnea, paroxysmal nocturnal dyspnea and, later, orthopnea. With severe pulmonary edema, respirations become increasingly rapid and labored, tachycardia worsens, and crackles become more diffuse.

◼ *Pulmonary embolism (acute).* Tachypnea occurs suddenly with pulmonary embolism and is usually accompanied by dyspnea. The patient may complain of angina or pleuritic chest pain.

◼ *Septic shock.* Early in septic shock, the patient usually experiences tachypnea, sudden fever, chills, and flushed, warm, yet dry skin. Nausea, vomiting, and diarrhea may accompany these symptoms. The patient may also develop tachycardia and normal or slightly decreased blood pressure.

Throat pain

Throat pain—commonly known as *sore throat*—refers to discomfort in any part of the pharynx: the nasopharynx, the oropharynx, or the hypopharynx. This common symptom ranges from a sensation of scratchiness to severe pain. In many cases, it may be accompanied by ear pain because cranial nerves IX and X innervate the pharynx as well as the middle and external ear. (See *Anatomy of the throat.*)

Throat pain may result from infection, trauma, allergy, cancer, or a systemic disorder. It may also follow surgery and endotracheal intubation. Nonpathologic causes include dry mucous membranes associated with mouth breathing and laryngeal irritation associated with alcohol consumption, inhaling smoke or chemicals like ammonia, and vocal strain.

Assessment

Ask the patient when he first noticed the pain, and have him describe it. Has he had throat pain before? Is it accompanied by fever, ear pain, or dysphagia? Review the patient's medical history for throat problems, allergies, and systemic disorders.

Next, carefully examine the pharynx, noting redness, exudate, or

Anatomy of the throat

The throat, or pharynx, is divided into three areas: the nasopharynx (the soft palate and the posterior nasal cavity), the oropharynx (the area between the soft palate and the upper edge of the epiglottis), and the hypopharynx (the area between the epiglottis and the level of the cricoid cartilage). A disorder affecting any of these areas may cause throat pain. Pinpointing the causative disorder begins with accurate assessment of the throat structures illustrated here.

FRONTAL VIEW

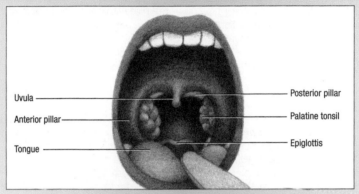

Uvula
Anterior pillar
Tongue
Posterior pillar
Palatine tonsil
Epiglottis

CROSS-SECTIONAL VIEW

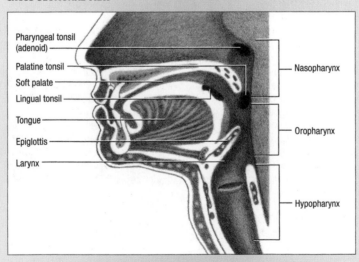

Pharyngeal tonsil (adenoid)
Palatine tonsil
Soft palate
Lingual tonsil
Tongue
Epiglottis
Larynx
Nasopharynx
Oropharynx
Hypopharynx

swelling. Examine the oropharynx, using a warmed metal spatula or tongue blade, and the nasopharynx, using a warmed laryngeal mirror or a fiber-optic nasopharyngoscope. Laryngoscopic examination of the hypopharynx may be required. Observe the tonsils for redness, swelling, or exudate. Obtain an exudate specimen for culture. Then examine the nose, using a nasal speculum. Also, check the patient's ears, especially if he reports ear pain. Finally, palpate the neck and oropharynx for nodules or lymph node enlargement.

Causes

◆ *Agranulocytosis.* With agranulocytosis, sore throat may accompany other signs and symptoms of infection, such as fever, chills, and headache. Typically, it follows progressive fatigue and weakness.

◆ *Bronchitis (acute).* Acute bronchitis may produce lower throat pain associated with fever, chills, cough, and muscle and back pain. Auscultation reveals rhonchi, wheezing and, at times, crackles.

◆ *Chronic fatigue syndrome.* Chronic fatigue syndrome is a nonspecific symptom complex that's characterized by incapacitating fatigue. Associated findings include sore throat, myalgia, and cognitive dysfunction.

◆ *Common cold.* A sore throat that occurs with a cold may accompany cough, sneezing, nasal congestion, rhinorrhea, fatigue, headache, myalgia, and arthralgia.

◆ *Contact ulcers.* Common in men with stressful jobs, contact ulcers appear symmetrically on the posterior vocal cords, resulting in sore throat. The pain is aggravated by talking and may be accompanied by referred ear pain.

◆ *Foreign body.* A foreign body lodged in the palatine or lingual tonsil and pyriform sinus may produce localized throat pain. The pain may persist after the foreign body is dislodged until mucosal irritation resolves.

◆ *Gastroesophageal reflux disease (GERD).* With GERD, an incompetent gastroesophageal sphincter allows gastric juices to enter the hypopharynx and irritate the larynx, causing chronic sore throat and hoarseness. The arytenoids may also appear red and swollen, resulting in a sensation of a lump in the throat.

◆ *Influenza.* Patients with the flu commonly complain of sore throat, fever with chills, headache, weakness, malaise, muscle aches, cough and, occasionally, hoarseness and rhinorrhea.

◆ *Laryngeal cancer.* With extrinsic laryngeal cancer, the chief symptom is pain or burning in the throat when drinking citrus juice or hot liquids or a lump in the throat; with intrinsic laryngeal cancer, the chief symptom is hoarseness that persists for longer than 3 weeks.

◆ *Mononucleosis (infectious).* Sore throat is one of the three classic findings in this infection. The other two classic signs are cervical lymphadenopathy and fluctuating temperature with an evening peak of 101° to 102° F (38.3° to 38.9° C).

◆ *Necrotizing ulcerative gingivitis (acute).* Also known as *trench mouth,* necrotizing ulcerative gingivitis usually begins abruptly with sore throat and tender gums that ulcerate and bleed. A gray exudate may cover the gums and pharyngeal tonsils.

◆ *Peritonsillar abscess.* A complication of bacterial tonsillitis, this abscess typically causes severe throat pain that radiates to the ear. Accompanying the pain may be dysphagia, drooling, dysarthria, halitosis, and fever with chills.

◆ *Pharyngitis.* Whether bacterial, fungal, or viral, pharyngitis may cause sore throat and localized erythema and edema. *Bacterial pharyngitis* begins abruptly with a unilateral sore throat. Also known as *thrush, fungal pharyngitis* causes diffuse sore throat—commonly described as a burning sensation—accompanied by pharyngeal erythema and edema. White plaque marks the pharynx, tonsil, tonsillar pillars, base of the tongue, and oral mucosa. With *viral pharyngitis,* findings include diffuse sore throat, malaise, fever, and mild erythema and edema of the posterior oropharyngeal wall.

◆ *Sinusitis (acute).* Sinusitis may cause sore throat with purulent nasal discharge and postnasal drip, resulting in halitosis.

◆ *Tongue cancer.* With tongue cancer, the patient experiences localized throat pain that may occur around a raised white lesion or ulcer. The pain may radiate to the ear and be accompanied by dysphagia.

◆ *Tonsillar cancer.* Sore throat is the presenting symptom in tonsillar cancer. Unfortunately, the cancer is usually quite advanced before the appearance of this symptom. The pain may radiate to the ear and is accompanied by a superficial ulcer on the tonsil or one that extends to the base of the tongue.

◆ *Tonsillitis.* With *acute tonsillitis,* mild to severe sore throat is usually the first symptom. The pain may radiate to the ears and be accompanied by dysphagia and headache. *Chronic tonsillitis* causes mild sore throat, malaise, and tender cervical lymph nodes. The tonsils appear smooth, pink and, possibly, enlarged, with purulent debris in the crypts. Unilateral or bilateral throat pain just above the hyoid bone occurs

with lingual tonsillitis. The lingual tonsils appear red and swollen and are covered with exudate.

◆ *Uvulitis.* Uvulitis may cause throat pain or a sensation of something in the throat. The uvula is usually swollen and red but, in allergic uvulitis, it's pale.

Thyroid enlargement

An enlarged thyroid can result from inflammation, physiologic changes, iodine deficiency, thyroid tumors, and drugs. Depending on the medical cause, hyperfunction or hypofunction may occur with resulting excess or deficiency, respectively, of the hormone thyroxine. If no infection is present, enlargement is usually slow and progressive. An enlarged thyroid that causes visible swelling in the front of the neck is called a *goiter.*

Assessment

The patient's history commonly reveals the cause of thyroid enlargement. Important data includes a family history of thyroid disease, onset of thyroid enlargement, a previous irradiation of the thyroid or neck, recent infections, and the use of thyroid replacement drugs.

Begin the physical examination by inspecting the patient's trachea for midline deviation. Although you can usually see the enlarged gland, you should always palpate it. To palpate the thyroid gland, you'll need to stand behind the patient. Give the patient a cup of water, and have him extend his neck slightly. Place the fingers of both hands on the patient's neck, just below the cricoid cartilage and just lateral to the trachea. Tell the patient to take a sip of water and swallow. The thyroid gland should rise as he swallows. Use your fingers to palpate laterally and downward to feel the whole thyroid gland. Palpate over the midline to feel the isthmus of the thyroid.

During palpation, note the size, shape, and consistency of the gland and the presence or absence of nodules. Using the bell of a stethoscope, listen over the lateral lobes for a bruit. The bruit is often continuous.

Causes

◆ *Hypothyroidism.* Signs and symptoms of hypothyroidism include an enlarged thyroid, weight gain despite anorexia, fatigue, cold intolerance, menorrhagia, slowed intellectual and motor activity, and dry, pale, cool skin.
◆ *Iodine deficiency.* A goiter may result from a lack of iodine in the diet. If the goiter arises from a deficiency of iodine in the food or water of a particular area, it's called an *endemic goiter.* Associated signs and symptoms of an endemic goiter include dysphagia, dyspnea, and tracheal deviation.
◆ *Thyroiditis.* Thyroiditis may be classified as acute or subacute. It may be due to bacterial or viral infections, in which case associated findings include fever and thyroid tenderness.
◆ *Thyrotoxicosis.* Overproduction of thyroid hormone causes thyrotoxicosis. The most common form is Graves' disease, which may result from genetic or immunologic factors.
◆ *Tumors.* An enlarged thyroid may result from a malignant or nonmalignant tumor. A malignant tumor usually appears as a single nodule in the neck; a nonmalignant tumor may appear as multiple nodules in the neck. Thyroid tissue contained in ovarian dermoid tumors can function autonomously or in combination with thyrotoxicosis.

Tics

A tic is an involuntary, repetitive movement of a specific group of muscles—usually those of the face, neck, shoulders, trunk, and hands. This sign typically occurs suddenly and intermittently. It may involve a single isolated movement, such as lip smacking, grimacing, blinking, sniffing, tongue thrusting, throat clearing, hitching up one shoulder, or protruding the chin. Or, it may involve a complex set of movements. Mild tics, such as twitching of an eyelid, are especially common. Tics differ from minor seizures in that they aren't associated with transient loss of consciousness or amnesia.

Tics are usually psychogenic and may be aggravated by stress or anxiety. Psychogenic tics often begin between ages 5 and 10 as voluntary, coordinated, and purposeful actions that the child feels compelled to perform to decrease anxiety. Unless they are severe, the child may be unaware of them. Tics may subside as the child matures, or they may persist into adulthood. However, tics are also associated with one rare affliction—Tourette syndrome, which typically begins during childhood.

Assessment

Begin by asking the parents how long and how often the child has had the tic. Can they identify any precipitating or exacerbating factors? Can the patient control the tics with conscious effort? Ask about stress in the child's life such as difficult schoolwork. Carefully observe the tic. Is it a purposeful or involuntary movement? Note whether it's localized or generalized, and describe it in detail.

Causes

◆ *Stress.* Stress can increase the severity of the presence of established tics.

◆ *Tourette syndrome.* Tourette syndrome, which is thought to be largely a genetic disorder, typically begins between ages 2 and 15 with a tic that involves the face or neck. Indications include both motor and vocal tics that may involve the muscles of the shoulders, arms, trunk, and legs. The tics may be associated with violent movements and outbursts of obscenities. The patient snorts, barks, and grunts and may emit explosive sounds, such as hissing, when he speaks. He may involuntarily repeat another person's words or movements. At times, this syndrome subsides spontaneously or undergoes a prolonged remission, but it may persist throughout life.

Tinnitus

Tinnitus literally means ringing in the ears, although many other abnormal sounds fall under this term. For example, tinnitus may be described as the sound of escaping air, running water, the inside of a seashell, or as a sizzling, buzzing, or humming noise. Occasionally, it's described as a roaring or musical sound. This common symptom may be unilateral or bilateral and constant or intermittent. Although the brain may adjust to or suppress constant tinnitus, tinnitus may be so disturbing that some patients contemplate suicide as their only source of relief.

Tinnitus can be classified in several ways. Subjective tinnitus is heard only by the patient; objective tinnitus is also heard by the observer who places a stethoscope near the patient's affected ear. Tinnitus aurium refers to noise that the patient hears in his ears; tinnitus cerebri to noise that he hears in his head.

Tinnitus is usually associated with neural injury within the auditory pathway, resulting in altered, spontaneous firing of sensory auditory neurons. Commonly resulting from an ear disorder, tinnitus may also stem from a cardiovascular or systemic disorder or from the effects of drugs. Nonpathologic causes of tinnitus include acute anxiety and presbycusis. (See *Common causes of tinnitus,* page 524.)

Assessment

Ask the patient to describe the sound he hears, including its onset, pattern, pitch, location, and intensity. Ask whether it's accompanied by other symptoms, such as vertigo, headache, or hearing loss. Next, take a health history, including a complete drug history.

Using an otoscope, inspect the patient's ears and examine the tympanic membrane. To check for hearing loss, perform Weber's test and the Rinne test. (See *Differentiating conductive from sensorineural hearing loss,* page 294.)

Also, auscultate for bruits in the neck. Then compress the jugular or carotid artery to see if this affects the tinnitus. Finally, examine the nasopharynx for masses that might cause eustachian tube dysfunction and tinnitus.

Causes

◆ *Acoustic neuroma.* Unilateral tinnitus is an early symptom of acoustic neuroma and precedes unilateral sensorineural hearing loss and vertigo. Facial paralysis, headache, nausea, vomiting, and papilledema may also occur.

Common causes of tinnitus

Tinnitus usually results from a disorder that affects the external, middle, or inner ear. Below are some of its more common causes and their locations.

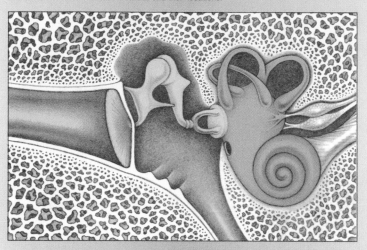

External ear
◆ Ear canal obstruction by cerumen or a foreign body
◆ Otitis externa
◆ Tympanic membrane perforation

Middle ear
◆ Ossicle dislocation
◆ Otitis media
◆ Otosclerosis

Inner ear
◆ Acoustic neuroma
◆ Atherosclerosis of the carotid artery
◆ Labyrinthitis
◆ Ménière's disease

◆ *Atherosclerosis of the carotid artery.* With atherosclerosis of the carotid artery, the patient has constant tinnitus that can be stopped by applying pressure over the carotid artery.

◆ *Cervical spondylosis.* With degenerative cervical spondylosis, osteophytic growths may compress the vertebral arteries, resulting in tinnitus. Typically, a stiff neck and pain aggravated by activity accompany tinnitus.

◆ *Eustachian tube patency.* Normally, the eustachian tube remains closed, except during swallowing. However, persistent patency of this tube can cause tinnitus, audible breath sounds, loud and distorted voice sounds, and a sense of fullness in the ear.

◆ *Glomus jugulare (tympanicum tumor).* A pulsating sound is usually the first symptom of this tumor. Other early findings include a reddish blue mass behind the tympanic membrane and progressive conductive hearing loss.

◆ *Hypertension.* Bilateral, high-pitched tinnitus may occur with severe hypertension.

◆ *Labyrinthitis (suppurative)*. With labyrinthitis, tinnitus may accompany sudden, severe attacks of vertigo, unilateral or bilateral sensorineural hearing loss, nystagmus, dizziness, nausea, and vomiting.

◆ *Ménière's disease*. Ménière's disease is characterized by attacks of tinnitus, vertigo, a feeling of fullness or blockage in the ear, and fluctuating sensorineural hearing loss.

◆ *Ossicle dislocation*. Acoustic trauma, such as a slap on the ear, may dislocate the ossicle, resulting in tinnitus and sensorineural hearing loss. Bleeding from the middle ear may also occur.

◆ *Otosclerosis*. With otosclerosis, the patient may describe ringing, roaring, or whistling tinnitus or a combination of these sounds. He may also report progressive hearing loss, which may lead to bilateral deafness, and vertigo.

◆ *Presbycusis*. Presbycusis is an otologic effect of aging that produces tinnitus and a progressive, symmetrical, bilateral sensorineural hearing loss, usually of high-frequency tones.

◆ *Tympanic membrane perforation*. With tympanic membrane perforation, tinnitus and hearing loss go hand-in-hand. Tinnitus is usually the chief complaint in a small perforation; hearing loss is usually the chief complaint in a larger perforation.

Tracheal deviation

Normally, the trachea is located at the midline of the neck—except at the bifurcation, where it shifts slightly toward the right. Visible deviation from its normal position signals an underlying condition that can compromise pulmonary function and possibly cause respiratory distress. A hallmark of life-threatening tension pneumothorax, tracheal deviation occurs with disorders that produce mediastinal shift due to asymmetrical thoracic volume or pressure. A nonlesion pneumothorax can produce tracheal deviation to the ipsilateral side. (See *Detecting slight tracheal deviation*, page 526.)

Assessment

If you detect tracheal deviation, be alert for signs and symptoms of respiratory distress. In addition, palpate for subcutaneous crepitation in the neck and chest, a sign of tension pneumothorax. (See *Responding to tracheal deviation*, page 527.)

If the patient doesn't display signs of distress, ask about a history of pulmonary or cardiac disorders, surgery, trauma, or infection. If he smokes, determine how much. Ask about associated signs and symptoms, especially breathing difficulty, pain, and cough.

Causes

◆ *Atelectasis*. Extensive lung collapse can produce tracheal deviation toward the affected side. Respiratory findings include dyspnea, tachypnea, pleuritic chest pain, dullness on percussion, decreased breath sounds, inspiratory lag, and substernal or intercostal retraction.

◆ *Hiatal hernia*. Intrusion of abdominal viscera into the pleural space causes tracheal deviation toward the unaffected side. The degree of attendant respiratory distress depends on the extent of herniation.

◆ *Kyphoscoliosis*. Kyphoscoliosis can cause rib cage distortion and mediastinal shift, producing tracheal deviation toward the compressed lung. Respiratory findings include dyspnea and asymmetrical chest expansion.

Detecting slight tracheal deviation

Although gross tracheal deviation is visible, detection of slight deviation requires palpation and perhaps even an X-ray. Try palpation first.

With the tip of your index finger, locate the patient's trachea by palpating between the sternocleidomastoid muscles as shown below. Then, compare the trachea's position to an imaginary line drawn vertically through the suprasternal notch. Any deviation from midline is usually considered abnormal.

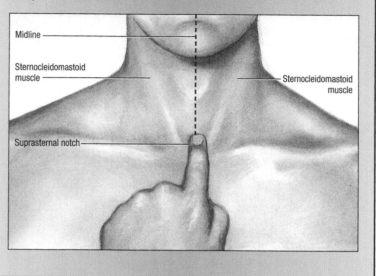

Midline

Sternocleidomastoid
muscle

Sternocleidomastoid
muscle

Suprasternal notch

◆ *Mediastinal tumor.* Often producing no symptoms in its early stages, a mediastinal tumor, when large, can press against the trachea and nearby structures, causing tracheal deviation and dysphagia.

◆ *Retrosternal thyroid.* Retrosternal thyroid—an anatomic abnormality—can displace the trachea. The gland is felt as a movable neck mass above the suprasternal notch.

◪ *Tension pneumothorax.* Tension pneumothorax is an acute condition that produces tracheal deviation. It's marked by a sudden onset of respiratory distress with sharp chest pain, dry cough, severe dyspnea, tachycardia, wheezing, cyanosis, accessory muscle use, nasal flaring, air hunger, and asymmetrical chest movement.

◪ *Thoracic aortic aneurysm.* Thoracic aortic aneurysm usually causes the trachea to deviate to the right. Highly variable associated findings may include stridor, dyspnea, wheezing, brassy cough, hoarseness, and dysphagia.

EMERGENCY INTERVENTIONS

Responding to tracheal deviation

If you detect tracheal deviation in a patient, check for signs and symptoms of respiratory distress, and then proceed with these steps:
◆ Place the patient in semi-Fowler's position to aid respiratory excursion and improve oxygenation, if possible.
◆ Give supplemental oxygen.

◆ Palpate for subcutaneous crepitation in the neck and chest.
◆ Insert an I.V. catheter for fluid and drug administration.
◆ Prepare for intubation as necessary.
◆ Be aware that chest tube insertion may be necessary to release trapped air or fluid and to restore normal intrapleural and intrathoracic pressure gradients.

Tracheal tugging

A visible recession of the larynx and trachea that occurs in synchrony with cardiac systole, tracheal tugging (also known as *Cardarelli's sign* or *Oliver's sign*) commonly results from an aneurysm or a tumor near the aortic arch and may signal dangerous compression or obstruction of major airways. The tugging movement, best observed with the patient's neck hyperextended, reflects abnormal transmission of aortic pulsations because of compression and distortion of the heart, esophagus, great vessels, airways, and nerves.

Assessment

If you observe tracheal tugging, examine the patient for signs of respiratory distress. If the patient is in distress, check airway patency. If the patient isn't in distress, obtain a pertinent history. Ask about associated symptoms, especially pain, and about any history of cardiovascular disease, cancer, chest surgery, or trauma.

Then examine the patient's neck and chest for abnormalities. Palpate the neck for masses, enlarged lymph nodes, abnormal arterial pulsations, and tracheal deviation. Percuss and auscultate the lung fields for abnormal sounds, auscultate the heart for murmurs, and auscultate the neck and chest for bruits. Palpate the chest for a thrill.

Causes

◣ *Aortic arch aneurysm.* A large aneurysm can distort and compress surrounding tissues and structures, producing tracheal tugging. The cardinal sign of this aneurysm is severe pain in the substernal area, sometimes radiating to the back or side of the chest. A sudden increase in pain may herald impending rupture.
◆ *Hodgkin's disease.* A tumor that develops adjacent to the aortic arch can cause tracheal tugging. Initial signs and symptoms include usually painless cervical lymphadenopathy, sustained or remittent fever, fatigue, malaise, pruritus, night sweats, and weight loss.

◆ *Thymoma.* Thymoma is a rare tumor that can cause tracheal tugging if it develops in the anterior mediastinum. Cough, chest pain, dysphagia, dyspnea, hoarseness, a palpable neck mass, jugular vein distention, and edema of the face, neck, or upper arm are common findings.

Tremors

Tremors are regular rhythmic oscillations that result from alternating contraction of opposing muscle groups. They are the most common type of involuntary muscle movement. Tremors are typical signs of extrapyramidal or cerebellar disorders and can also result from certain drugs.

Tremors can be characterized by their location, amplitude, and frequency. They're classified as resting, intention, or postural. Resting tremors occur when an extremity is at rest and subside with movement. They include the classic pill-rolling tremor of Parkinson's disease. Conversely, intention tremors occur only with movement and subside with rest. Postural tremors appear when an extremity or the trunk is actively held in a particular posture or position. A common type of postural tremor is called an *essential tremor.* Tremorlike movements may also be elicited, such as asterixis—the characteristic flapping tremor seen in hepatic failure. (See "Asterixis," page 109.) Stress or emotional upset tends to aggravate a tremor. Alcohol commonly diminishes postural tremors.

Assessment

Begin the patient history by asking the patient about the tremor's onset (sudden or gradual) and about its duration, progression, and any aggravating or alleviating factors. Does the tremor interfere with the patient's normal activities? Does he have other symptoms? Ask about behavioral changes or memory loss. Explore the patient's personal and family medical history for a neurologic, endocrine, or metabolic disorder. Obtain a complete drug history, noting especially the use of phenothiazines. Also, ask about alcohol use.

Assess the patient's overall appearance and demeanor, noting mental status. Test range of motion and strength in all major muscle groups while observing for chorea, athetosis, dystonia, and other involuntary movements. Check deep tendon reflexes and, if possible, observe the patient's gait.

Causes

◆ *Alcohol withdrawal syndrome.* Acute alcohol withdrawal after long-term dependence may first be manifested by resting and intention tremors that appear as soon as 7 hours after the last drink and progressively worsen. Severe withdrawal may produce profound tremors, agitation, confusion, hallucinations and, possibly, seizures.

◆ *Alkalosis.* Severe alkalosis may produce a severe intention tremor along with twitching, carpopedal spasms, agitation, diaphoresis, and hyperventilation.

◆ *Benign familial essential tremor.* Benign familial essential tremor, a tremor of early adulthood, produces a bilateral essential tremor that typically begins in the fingers and hands and may spread to the head, jaw, lips, and tongue. Laryngeal involvement may result in a quavering voice.

◆ *Cerebellar tumor.* An intention tremor is a cardinal sign of cerebellar tumor; related findings may include ataxia, nystagmus, incoordination, muscle weakness and atrophy, and hypoactive or absent deep tendon reflexes.

◆ *Graves' disease.* Fine tremors of the hand, nervousness, weight loss, palpitations, dyspnea, and increased heat intolerance are some of the typical signs of Graves' disease.

◼ *Hypercapnia.* Elevated partial pressure of carbon dioxide may result in a rapid, fine intention tremor. Other findings include headache, fatigue, blurred vision, weakness, lethargy, and decreasing level of consciousness.

◼ *Hypoglycemia.* Acute hypoglycemia may produce a rapid, fine intention tremor accompanied by confusion, weakness, tachycardia, diaphoresis, and cold, clammy skin. The tremor may disappear as hypoglycemia worsens.

◆ *Multiple sclerosis (MS).* An intention tremor that waxes and wanes may be an early sign of MS. Commonly, visual and sensory impairments are the earliest findings. Associated findings vary greatly.

◆ *Parkinson's disease.* Tremors, a classic early sign of Parkinson's disease, usually begin in the fingers. The slow, regular, rhythmic resting tremor takes the form of flexion-extension or abduction-adduction of the fingers or hand, or pronation-supination of the hand. Flexion-extension of the fingers combined with abduction-adduction of the thumb yields the characteristic pill-rolling tremor.

◆ *Thalamic syndrome.* Central midbrain syndromes are heralded by contralateral ataxic tremors, other abnormal movements, oculomotor palsy with contralateral hemiplegia, paralysis of vertical gaze, and stupor or coma. Anteromedial-inferior thalamic syndrome produces varying combinations of tremor, deep sensory loss, and hemiataxia. However, the main effect of this syndrome may be an extrapyramidal dysfunction.

◆ *Thyrotoxicosis.* Neuromuscular findings of thyrotoxicosis include a rapid, fine intention tremor of the hands and tongue, along with clonus, hyperreflexia, and Babinski's reflex.

◆ *Wernicke's disease.* An intention tremor is an early sign of Wernicke's disease—a thiamine deficiency. Other findings include ocular abnormalities, ataxia, apathy, and confusion.

Tunnel vision

Tunnel vision results from severe constriction of the visual field that leaves only a small central area of sight. It is typically described as the sensation of looking through a tunnel or gun barrel. It may be unilateral or bilateral and usually develops gradually. (See *Comparing tunnel vision with normal vision*, page 530.)

This abnormality results from chronic open-angle glaucoma and advanced retinal degeneration. Tunnel vision may also result from laser photocoagulation therapy, which aims to correct retinal detachment. Also a common complaint of malingerers, tunnel vision can be verified or discounted by visual field examination performed by an ophthalmologist.

Assessment

Ask the patient when he first noticed a loss of peripheral vision and to describe the progression of vision loss. Ask him to describe in detail exactly what and how far he can see peripherally. Explore the patient's personal and family history for ocular problems, es-

Comparing tunnel vision with normal vision

The patient with tunnel vision experiences drastic constriction of his peripheral visual field. The illustrations here convey the extent of this constriction, comparing test findings for normal and tunnel vision.

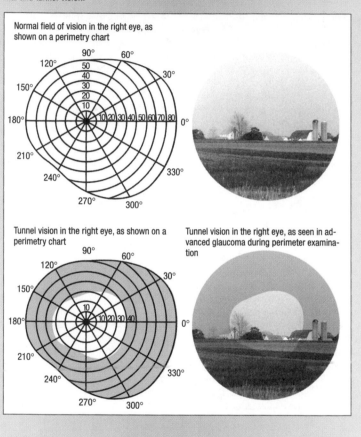

Normal field of vision in the right eye, as shown on a perimetry chart

Tunnel vision in the right eye, as shown on a perimetry chart

Tunnel vision in the right eye, as seen in advanced glaucoma during perimeter examination

pecially progressive blindness that began at an early age.

To rule out malingering, observe the patient as he walks. A patient with severely limited peripheral vision typically bumps into objects (and may even have bruises), whereas the malingerer manages to avoid them.

If your examination findings suggest tunnel vision, refer the patient to an ophthalmologist for further evaluation.

Causes

◆ *Chronic open-angle glaucoma.* With chronic open-angle glaucoma, bilateral tunnel vision occurs late and progresses slowly to complete blindness. Other late findings include mild eye pain, halo vision, and reduced visual acuity (especially at night) that isn't correctable with glasses.

◆ *Retinal pigmentary degeneration.* Retinal pigmentary degeneration disorders, a group of hereditary disorders such as retinitis pigmentosa, produces an annular scotoma that progresses concentrically, causing tunnel vision and eventually resulting in complete blindness, usually by age 50. Impaired night vision, the earliest symptom, typically appears during the first or second decade of life.

U

Urethral discharge

This excretion from the urinary meatus may be purulent, mucoid, or thin; sanguineous or clear; and scant or profuse. It usually develops suddenly, most commonly in men with a prostate infection.

Assessment

Ask the patient when he first noticed the discharge and have him describe its color, consistency, and quantity. Does he experience pain or burning on urination? Does he have difficulty initiating a urine stream? Does he experience urinary frequency? Ask the patient about other associated signs and symptoms, such as fever, chills, and perineal fullness. Explore his history for prostate problems, sexually transmitted disease, and urinary tract infection. Ask the patient if he has had recent sexual contacts or a new sexual partner.

Inspect the patient's urethral meatus for inflammation and swelling. Using proper technique, obtain a culture specimen. (See *Collecting a urethral discharge specimen*.) Then obtain a urine specimen for urinalysis, culture, and possibly a three-glass urine sample. (See *Performing the three-glass urine test*, page 534.) In the male patient, the prostate gland may have to be palpated.

Causes

◆ *Prostatitis.* Acute prostatitis is characterized by purulent urethral discharge. Initial signs and symptoms include sudden fever, chills, low back pain, myalgia, perineal fullness, and arthralgia. Urination becomes increasingly frequent and urgent, and the urine may appear cloudy. Chronic prostatitis may produce a persistent urethral discharge that's thin, milky, or clear and sometimes sticky. The discharge appears at the meatus after a long interval between voidings, as in the morning. Other findings include a dull aching in the prostate or rectum, sexual dysfunction such as ejaculatory pain, and urinary disturbances.
◆ *Reiter's syndrome.* In Reiter's syndrome, urethral discharge and other signs of acute urethritis occur 1 to 2 weeks after sexual contact. Asymmetrical arthritis, conjunctivitis, and ulcerations on the oral mucosa, glans penis, palms, and soles may also occur with Reiter's syndrome.
◆ *Urethritis.* Urethritis, which is usually sexually transmitted, commonly

◆

Collecting a urethral discharge specimen

To obtain a urethral specimen from a male patient, follow these steps:

To obtain a urethral specimen from a female patient, follow these steps:

Instruct the patient not to void for 1 hour before specimen collection to prevent flushing of secretions from the urethra.

Instruct the patient not to void for 1 hour before specimen collection to prevent flushing of secretions from the urethra.

Provide privacy for the patient. Help him onto an examination table and into a supine position, and expose his penis. Have him grasp and raise his penis to allow visualization of the urethra.

Provide privacy for the patient. Help her onto an examination table and into the lithotomy position.

Wash your hands, and put on sterile gloves. Then insert a thin, sterile urogenital alginate swab no more than $3/4''$ (2 cm) into the urethra. Rotate the swab, and leave it in place for 10 to 30 seconds to absorb organisms.

Wash your hands, and put on sterile gloves. Then insert a thin, sterile urogenital alginate swab into the urethral meatus. Gently rotate the swab, and leave it in place for 10 to 30 seconds to absorb organisms. Take care not to touch the swab to the area around the urethral meatus.

Remove the swab, allow it to dry, and then send it to the laboratory. Help the patient off the examination table, and tell him to dress.

Remove the swab, allow it to dry, and then send it to the laboratory. Assist the patient off the examination table, and tell her to dress.

Performing the three-glass urine test

If your male patient complains of urinary frequency and urgency, dysuria, flank or low back pain, or other signs or symptoms of urethritis, and if his urine specimen is cloudy, perform the three-glass urine test.

First, ask him to void into three conical glasses labeled with numbers 1, 2, and 3. First-voided urine goes into glass #1, midstream urine into glass #2, and the remainder into glass #3. Tell the patient to avoid interrupting the stream of urine when shifting glasses, if possible.

Next, observe each glass for pus and mucus shreds. Also, note urine color and odor. Glass #1 will contain matter from the anterior urethra; glass #2, matter from the bladder; and glass #3, sediment from the prostate and seminal vesicles.

Some common findings are shown here. However, confirming diagnosis requires microscopic examination and a bacteriology report.

	SPECIMEN 1	SPECIMEN 2	SPECIMEN 3
Acute or subacute urethritis	Cloudy	Clear	Clear
Acute posterior urethritis	Cloudy	Clear or cloudy	Cloudy
Chronic anterior urethritis	Small shreds	Clear	Clear
Chronic posterior urethritis	Large shreds	Clear	Clear
Chronic urethritis (anterior and posterior)	Small and large shreds	Clear	Clear
Prostatitis	Clear or large shreds	Clear	Cloudy or large shreds
Cystitis and pyelonephritis	Cloudy	Cloudy	Cloudy

produces urethral discharge. Other effects include urinary hesitancy, urgency, and frequency; dysuria; and itching and burning around the meatus.

Urinary frequency

Urinary frequency refers to increased incidence of the urge to void without an increase in the total volume of urine produced. Usually resulting from decreased bladder capacity, frequency is a cardinal sign of urinary tract infection. However, it can also stem from another urologic disorder, neurologic dysfunction, or pressure on the bladder from a nearby tumor or from organ enlargement (as with pregnancy).

Assessment

Ask the patient how many times per day he voids. How does this compare to his previous pattern of voiding? Ask about the onset and duration of the abnormal frequency and about any associated urinary signs or symptoms.

Ask also about neurologic symptoms, such as muscle weakness, numbness, or tingling. Explore his medical history for urinary tract infection, other urologic problems or recent urologic procedures, and neurologic disorders. With a male patient, ask about a history of prostatic enlargement. If the patient is a female of childbearing age, ask whether she is or could be pregnant.

Obtain a clean-catch midstream specimen for urinalysis and culture and sensitivity tests. Then palpate the patient's suprapubic area, abdomen, and flanks, noting any tenderness. Examine his urethral meatus for redness, discharge, or swelling. In a male patient, the practitioner may palpate the prostate gland.

If the patient's medical history reveals symptoms or a history of neurologic disorders, perform a neurologic examination.

Causes

◆ *Benign prostatic hyperplasia.* Prostatic enlargement causes urinary frequency, along with nocturia and possibly

incontinence and hematuria. Initial effects are those of prostatism: reduced caliber and force of the urine stream, urinary hesitancy and tenesmus, inability to stop the urine stream, and a feeling of incomplete voiding.
◆ *Bladder calculus.* Bladder irritation may lead to urinary frequency and urgency, dysuria, terminal hematuria, and suprapubic pain from bladder spasms. The patient may have overflow incontinence if the calculus lodges in the bladder neck. Greatest discomfort usually occurs at the end of micturition if the stone lodges in the bladder neck. This may also cause overflow incontinence and referred pain to the lower back or heel.
◆ *Prostate cancer.* In advanced stages of prostate cancer, urinary frequency may occur, along with hesitancy, dribbling, nocturia, dysuria, bladder distention, perineal pain, constipation, and a hard, irregularly shaped prostate.
◆ *Prostatitis.* Acute prostatitis commonly produces urinary frequency, along with urgency, dysuria, nocturia, and purulent urethral discharge.
◆ *Rectal tumor.* The pressure exerted by a rectal tumor on the bladder may cause urinary frequency. Early findings include changed bowel habits, commonly starting with an urgent need to defecate on arising or obstipation alternating with diarrhea, blood or mucus in the stool, and a sense of incomplete evacuation.
◆ *Reiter's syndrome (reactive arthritis).* In Reiter's syndrome, urinary frequency occurs with symptoms of acute urethritis 1 to 2 weeks after sexual contact. Asymmetrical arthritis, conjunctivitis, and ulcerations on the oral mucosa, glans penis, palms, and soles may also occur with Reiter's syndrome.
◆ *Reproductive tract tumor.* A tumor in the female reproductive tract may com-

press the bladder, causing urinary frequency. Other findings vary but may include abdominal distention, menstrual disturbances, and vaginal bleeding.

◆ *Spinal cord lesion.* Incomplete cord transection results in urinary frequency, continuous overflow dribbling, urgency, urinary hesitancy, and bladder distention.

◆ *Urethral stricture.* Bladder decompensation produces urinary frequency, along with urgency and nocturia. Early signs include hesitancy, tenesmus, and reduced caliber and force of the urine stream.

◆ *Urinary tract infection.* Affecting the urethra, bladder, or kidneys, this common cause of urinary frequency may also produce urgency, dysuria, hematuria, cloudy urine and, in males, urethral discharge.

Urinary hesitancy

Urinary hesitancy—difficulty starting a urine stream generally followed by a decrease in the force of the stream—can result from a urinary tract infection, a partial lower urinary tract obstruction, a neuromuscular disorder, or use of certain drugs. It's most common in older men with prostatic enlargement. It also occurs in women with a gravid uterus, tumors in the reproductive system, or ovarian, uterine, or vaginal cancer. Hesitancy usually arises gradually, commonly going unnoticed until urine retention causes bladder distention and discomfort.

Assessment

Ask the patient when he first noticed hesitancy and if he's ever had the problem before. Ask about other urinary problems, especially reduced force

or interruption of the urine stream. Ask if he's ever been treated for a prostate problem or urinary tract infection or obstruction. Obtain a drug history.

Inspect the patient's urethral meatus for inflammation, discharge, and other abnormalities. Examine the anal sphincter and test sensation in the perineum. Obtain a clean-catch specimen for urinalysis and culture. In a male patient, the prostate gland requires palpation. A female patient requires a gynecologic examination.

Causes

◆ *Benign prostatic hyperplasia (BPH).* Signs and symptoms of BPH depend on the extent of prostatic enlargement and the lobes affected. Characteristic early findings include urinary hesitancy, reduced caliber and force of urine stream, perineal pain, a feeling of incomplete voiding, and inability to stop the urine stream.

◆ *Prostatic cancer.* Urinary hesitancy may occur in patients with advanced cancer, accompanied by frequency, dribbling, nocturia, dysuria, bladder distention, perineal pain, and constipation.

◆ *Spinal cord lesion.* A lesion below the micturition center that has destroyed the sacral nerve roots causes urinary hesitancy, tenesmus, and constant dribbling from retention and overflow incontinence.

◆ *Urethral stricture.* Partial obstruction of the lower urinary tract secondary to trauma or infection produces urinary hesitancy, tenesmus, and decreased force and caliber of the urine stream.

◆ *Urinary tract infection.* Urinary hesitancy may be associated with urinary tract infection. Characteristic urinary changes include urinary frequency, possible hematuria, dysuria, nocturia, and cloudy urine.

Urinary incontinence

Incontinence, the uncontrollable passage of urine, can result from a bladder abnormality, a neurologic disorder, or an alteration in pelvic muscle strength. It can be classified as neurogenic, stress, overflow, urge, or total incontinence. *Neurogenic incontinence* occurs when there's damage to the spinal nerves controlling bladder relaxation and contraction. *Stress incontinence* refers to intermittent leakage resulting from a sudden physical strain, such as a cough, sneeze, laugh, or quick movement. *Overflow incontinence* is a dribble resulting from urine retention, which fills the bladder and prevents it from contracting with sufficient force to expel a urine stream. *Urge incontinence* refers to the inability to suppress a sudden urge to urinate. *Total incontinence* is continuous leakage resulting from the bladder's inability to retain urine.

Incontinence can sometimes be corrected by implementing a bladder-retraining program. (See *Correcting incontinence with bladder retraining,* page 538.)

Assessment

Ask the patient when he first noticed the incontinence and whether it began suddenly or gradually. Have him describe his typical urinary pattern: Does incontinence usually occur during the day or at night? Does he have any urinary control, or is he totally incontinent? If he's occasionally able to control urination, ask him the usual times and amounts voided. Determine his normal fluid intake. Ask about other urinary problems, such as hesitancy, frequency, urgency, nocturia, and decreased force or interruption of the urine stream. Also ask if he's ever sought treatment for incontinence or found a way to deal with it himself.

Obtain a medical history, especially noting urinary tract infection, prostate conditions, spinal injury or tumor, stroke, or surgery involving the bladder, prostate, or pelvic floor. Ask a woman how many pregnancies she has had and how many childbirths.

After completing the history, have the patient empty his bladder. Inspect the urethral meatus for obvious inflammation or anatomic defect. Have female patients bear down; note any urine leakage. Gently palpate the abdomen for bladder distention, which signals urine retention. Perform a complete neurologic assessment, noting motor and sensory function and obvious muscle atrophy.

Causes

◆ *Benign prostatic hyperplasia (BPH).* Overflow incontinence is common with BPH as a result of urethral obstruction and urine retention. BPH begins with a group of signs and symptoms known as prostatism: reduced caliber and force of urine stream, urinary hesitancy, and a feeling of incomplete voiding.
◆ *Bladder cancer.* Obstruction by a tumor may produce overflow incontinence. The patient commonly also presents with urge incontinence and hematuria. A mass may be palpable on bimanual examination.
◆ *Diabetic neuropathy.* Diabetic neuropathy may cause painless bladder distention with overflow incontinence.

Correcting incontinence with bladder retraining

The incontinent patient typically feels frustrated, embarrassed and, sometimes, hopeless. Fortunately, though, his problem may be corrected by bladder retraining—a program that aims to establish a regular voiding pattern. Here are some guidelines for establishing such a program:

◆ Before you start the program, assess the patient's intake pattern, voiding pattern, and behavior (for example, restlessness or talkativeness) before each voiding episode.

◆ Encourage the patient to use the toilet 30 minutes before he's usually incontinent. If this isn't successful, readjust the schedule. Once he's able to stay dry for 2 hours, increase the time between voidings by 30 minutes each day until he achieves a 3- to 4-hour voiding schedule.

◆ When your patient voids, make sure that the sequence of conditioning stimuli is always the same.

◆ Make sure that the patient has privacy while voiding—any inhibiting stimuli should be avoided.

◆ Keep a record of continence and incontinence for 5 days—this may reinforce your patient's efforts to remain continent.

Clues to success

Remember that the positive attitudes of you and your patient are crucial to successful bladder retraining. Here are some additional tips that may help your patient succeed:

◆ Make sure the patient is close to a bathroom or portable toilet. Leave a light on at night, and make sure there's a clear pathway to the bathroom.

◆ If your patient needs assistance getting out of his bed or chair, promptly answer his call for help.

◆ Encourage the patient to wear his usual clothing as an indication that you're confident he can remain continent. Acceptable alternatives to diapers include condoms for the male patient and incontinence pads, or panties, for the female patient.

◆ Encourage the patient to drink 2 to 2½ qt (2 to 2.5 L) of fluid each day. Less fluid doesn't prevent incontinence but does promote bladder infection. Limiting his intake after 5 P.M., however, will help him remain continent during the night.

◆ Reassure your patient that episodes of incontinence don't signal a failure of the program. Encourage him to maintain a persistent, tolerant attitude.

◆ Teach the patient how to perform Kegel exercises.

Related findings include episodic constipation or diarrhea (which is commonly nocturnal), syncope, and dysphagia.

◆ *Multiple sclerosis (MS).* Urinary incontinence, urgency, and frequency are common urologic findings in MS.

◆ *Prostatitis (chronic).* Urinary incontinence may occur as a result of urethral obstruction from an enlarged prostate. Other findings include urinary frequency and urgency, dysuria, hematuria, bladder distention, persistent urethral discharge, dull perineal pain that may radiate, ejaculatory pain, and decreased libido.

◆ *Spinal cord injury.* Complete cord transection above the sacral level causes flaccid paralysis of the bladder. Overflow incontinence follows rapid bladder distention.

◤ *Stroke.* Urinary incontinence may be transient or permanent. Associated findings reflect the site and extent of the lesion and may include impaired mentation, altered level of consciousness, and seizures.

◆ *Urethral stricture.* Eventually, overflow incontinence may occur with urethral stricture. As obstruction increases, urine extravasation may lead to formation of urinomas and urosepsis.

◆ *Urinary tract infection (UTI).* Besides incontinence, UTI may produce urinary urgency, dysuria, hematuria, cloudy urine and, in males, urethral discharge. Bladder spasms or a feeling of warmth during urination may occur.

Urinary urgency

A sudden compelling urge to urinate accompanied by bladder pain is a classic symptom of urinary tract infection (UTI). As inflammation decreases bladder capacity, discomfort results from the accumulation of even small amounts of urine. Repeated, frequent voiding in an effort to alleviate this discomfort produces urine output of only a few milliliters at each voiding.

Urgency without bladder pain may point to an upper-motor-neuron lesion that has disrupted bladder control.

Assessment

Ask the patient about the onset of urinary urgency and whether he has ever experienced it before. Ask about other urologic symptoms, such as dysuria and cloudy urine. Also ask about neurologic symptoms, such as paresthesia. Examine his medical history for recurrent or chronic UTIs or for surgery or procedures involving the urinary tract.

Obtain a clean-catch specimen for urinalysis and culture. Note urine character, color, and odor, and use a reagent strip to test for pH, glucose, and blood. Then palpate the suprapubic area and both flanks for distention and tenderness. If the patient's history or symptoms suggest neurologic dysfunction, perform a neurologic examination.

Causes

◆ *Bladder calculus.* Bladder irritation can lead to urinary urgency and frequency, dysuria, terminal hematuria, and suprapubic pain from bladder spasms.

◆ *Multiple sclerosis (MS).* Urinary urgency can occur with or without the frequent UTIs that can accompany MS. Like MS's other variable effects, urinary urgency may wax and wane.

◆ *Reiter's syndrome.* In Reiter's syndrome, urgency occurs with other symptoms of acute urethritis 1 to 2 weeks after sexual contact. Arthritic and ocular symptoms and skin lesions usually develop within several weeks after sexual contact.

◆ *Spinal cord lesion.* Urinary urgency can result from incomplete cord transection when voluntary control of sphincter function weakens. Urinary frequency, difficulty initiating and inhibiting a urine stream, and bladder distention and discomfort may also occur.

◆ *Urethral stricture.* Bladder decompensation produces urinary urgency, frequency, and nocturia. Early signs and symptoms include hesitancy, tenesmus, and reduced caliber and force of the urine stream.

◆ *Urinary tract infection.* Urinary urgency is often associated with UTI. Other characteristic urinary changes include frequency, hematuria, dysuria, nocturia, and cloudy urine. Urinary hesitancy may also occur.

Urine cloudiness

Cloudy, murky, or turbid urine reflects the presence of bacteria, mucus, leukocytes or erythrocytes, epithelial cells, fat, or phosphates (in alkaline urine). It's characteristic of urinary tract infection (UTI) but can also result from prolonged storage of a urine specimen at room temperature.

Assessment

Ask about symptoms of UTI, such as dysuria, urinary urgency or frequency, or pain in the flank, lower back, or suprapubic area. Also ask about recurrent UTIs or recent surgery or treatment involving the urinary tract.

Obtain a urine specimen to check for pus or mucus. (See *Performing the three-glass urine test,* page 534.) Using a reagent strip, test for blood, glucose, and pH. Palpate the suprapubic area and flanks for tenderness.

If you note cloudy urine in a patient with an indwelling urinary catheter, especially with concurrent fever, remove the catheter immediately (or change it if the patient must have one in place).

Causes

◆ *UTI.* Cloudy urine is common with UTI. Other urinary changes include urgency, frequency, hematuria, dysuria, nocturia and, in males, urethral discharge. Urinary hesitancy, bladder spasms, costovertebral angle tenderness, and suprapubic, lower back, or flank pain may occur. Other findings

include fever, chills, malaise, nausea, and vomiting.

Urticaria

Urticaria, or hives, is a vascular skin reaction characterized by the eruption of transient pruritic wheals—smooth, slightly elevated patches with well-defined erythematous margins and pale centers of various shapes and sizes. Urticaria is produced by the local release of histamine or other vasoactive substances as part of a hypersensitivity reaction. (See *Recognizing common skin lesions,* page 414.)

Acute urticaria evolves rapidly and usually has a detectable cause, commonly hypersensitivity to certain drugs, foods, insect bites, inhalants, or contactants; emotional stress; or environmental factors. Although individual lesions usually subside within 12 to 24 hours, new crops of lesions may erupt continuously, thus prolonging the attack.

Urticaria lasting longer than 6 weeks is classified as chronic. The lesions may recur for months or years, and the underlying cause is usually unknown. Occasionally, a diagnosis of psychogenic urticaria is made.

Angioedema, or *giant urticaria,* is characterized by the acute eruption of wheals involving the mucous membranes and, occasionally, the arms, legs, or genitals.

Assessment

In an acute case of urticaria, quickly evaluate the patient's respiratory status, and check his vital signs. Observe him for respiratory difficulty or signs of impending anaphylactic shock. (See *Responding to acute urticaria.*)

EMERGENCY INTERVENTIONS

Responding to acute urticaria

If your patient has acute urticaria, quickly evaluate his respiratory status and vital signs. If you observe signs of distress, take these steps:

◆ Ensure patent I.V. access.

◆ Give local epinephrine or apply ice to the affected site, as ordered, to decrease absorption through vasoconstriction.

◆ Clear and maintain his airway.

◆ Give oxygen as needed.

◆ Institute cardiac monitoring.

◆ Have resuscitation equipment at hand, and be prepared to begin cardiopulmonary resuscitation.

◆ Prepare for possible intubation or tracheostomy.

If the patient isn't in distress, obtain a complete history. Does he have any known allergies? Does the urticaria follow a seasonal pattern? Do certain foods or drugs seem to aggravate it? Is there a relationship to physical exertion? Is the patient routinely exposed to chemicals on the job or at home? Has the patient recently changed or used new skin products or detergents? Obtain a detailed drug history, including prescription and over-the-counter drugs. Note any history of chronic or parasitic infection, skin disease, or a GI disorder.

Causes

◼ *Anaphylaxis.* Anaphylaxis is marked by the rapid eruption of diffuse urticaria and angioedema, with wheals ranging from pinpoint to palm-size or larger. Lesions are usually pruritic and stinging; paresthesia commonly precedes their eruption.

◆ *Drugs.* Drugs that can produce urticaria include aspirin, codeine, dextrans, immune serums, insulin, morphine, penicillin, quinine, sulfonamides, and vaccines.

◆ *Hereditary angioedema.* With hereditary angioedema, cutaneous involvement is manifested by nonpitting, nonpruritic edema of an extremity or the face. Respiratory mucosal involvement can produce life-threatening acute laryngeal edema.

◆ *Lyme disease.* Although not diagnostic of Lyme disease, urticaria may result from the characteristic skin lesion (erythema chronicum migrans).

V

Vaginal bleeding, postmenopausal

Postmenopausal vaginal bleeding—bleeding that occurs 6 or more months after menopause—is an important indicator of gynecologic cancer. However, it can also result from infection, a local pelvic disorder, estrogenic stimulation, atrophy of the endometrium, and physiologic thinning and drying of the vaginal mucous membranes. Vaginal bleeding may be indicative of bleeding from the vagina or another gynecological location, such as the ovaries, fallopian tubes, uterus, or cervix because bleeding from these areas also exits the body through the vagina.

Vaginal bleeding usually occurs as slight, brown or red spotting developing either spontaneously or following coitus or douching, but it may also occur as oozing of fresh blood or as bright red hemorrhage. Many patients—especially those with a history of heavy menstrual flow—minimize the importance of this bleeding, delaying diagnosis.

Assessment

Determine the patient's age and her age at menopause. Ask when she first noticed the abnormal bleeding. Then obtain a thorough obstetric and gynecologic history. When did she begin menstruating? Were her periods regular? If not, ask her to describe any menstrual irregularities. How old was she when she first had intercourse? How many sexual partners has she had? Has she had children? Has she had fertility problems? If possible, obtain an obstetric and gynecologic history of the patient's mother, and ask about a family history of gynecologic cancer. Determine if the patient has any associated symptoms and if she's taking estrogen.

Observe the external genitalia, noting the character of any vaginal discharge and the appearance of the labia, vaginal rugae, and clitoris. Carefully palpate the patient's breasts and lymph nodes for nodules or enlargement. The patient will require pelvic and rectal examinations.

Causes

◆ *Atrophic vaginitis.* When bloody staining occurs, it usually follows coitus or douching. A characteristic white, watery discharge may be accompanied by pruritus, dyspareunia, and a burning sensation in the vagina and labia.

◆

◆ *Cervical cancer.* Early invasive cervical cancer causes vaginal spotting or heavier bleeding, usually after coitus or douching but occasionally spontaneously. Related findings include persistent, watery, pink-tinged, and foul-smelling vaginal discharge and postcoital pain. As the cancer spreads, the drainage becomes dark and malodorous.

◆ *Cervical or endometrial polyps.* Cervical or endometrial polyps are small, pedunculated growths that may cause spotting (possibly as a mucopurulent, pink discharge) after coitus, douching, or straining to defecate.

◆ *Endometrial hyperplasia or cancer.* Bleeding occurs early and can be brownish and scant or bright red and profuse. It usually follows coitus or douching. Later, it becomes heavier and more frequent, leading to clotting and anemia.

◆ *Ovarian tumors (feminizing).* Estrogen-producing ovarian tumors can stimulate endometrial shedding and cause heavy bleeding unassociated with coitus or douching.

◆ *Vaginal cancer.* Characteristic spotting or bleeding may be preceded by a thin, watery vaginal discharge. Bleeding may be spontaneous but usually follows coitus or douching.

Vaginal discharge

Common in women of childbearing age, physiologic vaginal discharge is mucoid, clear or white, nonbloody, and odorless. Produced by the cervical mucosa and, to a lesser degree, by the vulvar glands, this discharge may occasionally be scant or profuse due to estrogenic stimulation and changes during the patient's menstrual cycle. However, a marked increase in discharge or a change in discharge color, odor, or consistency can signal disease. The discharge may result from infection, sexually transmitted disease, reproductive tract disease, fistulas, and certain drugs. In addition, the prolonged presence of a foreign body, such as a tampon or diaphragm, in the patient's vagina can cause irritation and an inflammatory exudate, as can frequent douching, feminine hygiene products, contraceptive products, bubble baths, and colored or perfumed toilet tissues.

Assessment

Ask the patient to describe the onset, color, consistency, odor, and texture of her vaginal discharge. How does the discharge differ from her usual vaginal secretions? Is the onset related to her menstrual cycle? Also, ask about associated symptoms. Does she have spotting after coitus or douching? Ask about recent changes in her sexual habits and hygiene practices. Is she or could she be pregnant? Next, ask if she has had vaginal discharge before or has ever been treated for a vaginal infection or sexually transmitted disease. Ask about her current use of medications, especially antibiotics, oral estrogens, and hormonal contraceptives.

Examine the external genitalia and note the character of the discharge. (See *Identifying causes of vaginal discharge,* page 544.) Observe vulvar and vaginal tissues for redness, edema, and excoriation. Palpate the inguinal lymph nodes to detect tenderness or enlargement, and palpate the abdomen for tenderness. A pelvic examination may be required. Obtain vaginal discharge specimens for testing.

Identifying causes of vaginal discharge

The color, consistency, amount, and odor of your patient's vaginal discharge provide important clues about the underlying disorder. For quick reference, use this chart to match common characteristics of vaginal discharge and their possible causes.

CHARACTERISTICS	POSSIBLE CAUSES
Thin, scant, watery white discharge	Atrophic vaginitis
Thin, green or gray-white, foul-smelling discharge	*Bacterial* vaginosis
White, curdlike, profuse discharge with yeasty, sweet odor	Candidiasis
Mucopurulent, foul-smelling discharge	Chancroid
Yellow, mucopurulent, odorless, or acrid discharge	*Chlamydial* infection
Scant, serosanguineous, or purulent discharge with foul odor	Endometritis
Copious mucoid discharge	Genital herpes
Profuse, mucopurulent discharge, possibly foul-smelling	Genital warts
Yellow or green, foul-smelling discharge from the cervix or occasionally from Bartholin's or Skene's ducts	Gonorrhea
Chronic, watery, bloody, or purulent discharge, possibly foul-smelling	Gynecologic cancer
Frothy, green-yellow, and profuse (or thin, white, and scant) foul-smelling discharge	Trichomoniasis

Causes

◆ *Atrophic vaginitis.* With atrophic vaginitis, a thin, scant, watery white vaginal discharge may be accompanied by pruritus, burning, tenderness, and bloody spotting after coitus or douching.

◆ *Bacterial vaginosis.* Bacterial vaginosis results when the normal balance of bacteria in the vagina is disrupted, resulting in an overgrowth of a certain type of bacterium. It causes a thin, foul-smelling, green or gray-white discharge that adheres to the vaginal walls and can be easily wiped away, leaving healthy-looking tissue.

◆ *Candidiasis.* Infection with *Candida albicans* causes a profuse, white, curdlike discharge with a yeasty, sweet odor. Onset is abrupt, usually just before menses or during a course of antibiotics. Intense labial itching and burning may also occur.

◆ *Chancroid.* Chancroid produces a mucopurulent, foul-smelling discharge and vulvar lesions that are initially erythematous and later ulcerated.

◆ *Chlamydial infection.* Chlamydial infection causes a yellow, mucopurulent, odorless, or acrid vaginal discharge.

◆ *Endometritis.* A scant, serosanguineous discharge with a foul odor can result from bacterial invasion of the endometrium.

◆ *Genital warts.* Genital warts are mosaic, papular vulvar lesions that can cause a profuse, mucopurulent vaginal discharge, which may be foul-smelling if the warts are infected.

◆ *Gonorrhea.* Although 80% of women with gonorrhea are asymptomatic, others have a yellow or green, foul-smelling discharge that can be expressed from Bartholin's or Skene's ducts.

◆ *Gynecologic cancer.* Endometrial or cervical cancer produces a chronic, watery, bloody or purulent vaginal discharge that may be foul-smelling.

◆ *Herpes simplex (genital).* A copious mucoid discharge results from herpes simplex, but the initial complaint is painful, indurated vesicles and ulcerations on the labia, vagina, cervix, anus, thighs, or mouth.

◆ *Trichomoniasis.* Trichomoniasis can cause a foul-smelling discharge, which may be frothy, green-yellow, and profuse or thin, white, and scant.

Vertigo

Vertigo is an illusion of movement in which the patient feels that he's revolving in space (subjective vertigo) or that his surroundings are revolving around him (objective vertigo). He may complain of feeling pulled sideways, as though drawn by a magnet.

A common symptom, vertigo usually begins abruptly. It may worsen when the patient moves and subside when he lies down. It's commonly confused with dizziness—a nonspecific sensation of imbalance and light-headedness. However, unlike dizziness, vertigo can be accompanied by nausea, vomiting, nystagmus, and tinnitus or hearing loss. Although the patient's limb coordination is unaffected, vertiginous gait may occur.

Vertigo may result from a neurologic or otologic disorder that affects the equilibratory apparatus. However, this symptom may also result from alcohol intoxication, hyperventilation, and postural changes (benign postural vertigo). It may also be an adverse effect of certain drugs, tests, or procedures.

Assessment

Ask your patient to describe the onset and duration of his vertigo, being careful to distinguish this symptom from dizziness. Does he feel that he's moving or that his surroundings are moving around him? How often do the attacks occur? Do they follow position changes or are they unpredictable? Find out if the patient can walk during an attack, if he leans to one side, and if he's ever fallen. Ask if he experiences motion sickness and if he prefers one position during an attack. Obtain a recent drug history, and note any evidence of alcohol abuse.

Perform a neurologic assessment, focusing particularly on eighth cranial nerve function. Observe the patient's gait and posture for abnormalities.

Causes

◆ *Acoustic neuroma.* Acoustic neuroma is a tumor of the eighth cranial nerve that causes mild, intermittent vertigo and unilateral sensorineural hearing loss.

◆ *Benign positional vertigo.* With benign positional vertigo, debris in a semicircular canal produces vertigo on head position change, which lasts a few minutes. It's usually temporary and can be effectively treated with positional maneuvers.

◆ *Brain stem ischemia.* Brain stem ischemia produces sudden, severe vertigo that may become episodic and later persistent.

◆ *Head trauma.* Persistent vertigo, occurring soon after injury, accompanies spontaneous or positional nystagmus and, if the temporal bone is fractured, hearing loss.

◆ *Herpes zoster.* Infection of the eighth cranial nerve produces sudden onset of vertigo accompanied by facial paralysis, hearing loss in the affected ear, and herpetic vesicular lesions in the auditory canal.

◆ *Labyrinthitis.* Severe vertigo begins abruptly with labyrinthitis, an inner ear infection. Vertigo may occur in a single episode or may recur over months or years.

◆ *Ménière's disease.* With Ménière's disease, labyrinthine dysfunction causes abrupt onset of vertigo, lasting minutes, hours, or days. Unpredictable episodes of severe vertigo and unsteady gait may cause the patient to fall. During an attack, any sudden motion of the head or eyes can precipitate nausea and vomiting.

◆ *Multiple sclerosis (MS).* Episodic vertigo may occur early and become persistent with MS. Other early findings include diplopia, visual blurring, and paresthesia.

◆ *Seizures.* Temporal lobe seizures may produce vertigo, usually associated with other symptoms of partial complex seizures.

◆ *Vestibular neuritis.* With vestibular neuritis, severe vertigo usually begins abruptly and lasts several days, without tinnitus or hearing loss. Other findings include nausea, vomiting, and nystagmus.

Vesicular rash

A vesicular rash is a scattered or linear distribution of blisterlike lesions— sharply circumscribed and filled with clear, cloudy, or bloody fluid. The lesions, which are usually less than 0.5 cm in diameter, may occur singly or may occur in groups. (See *Recognizing common skin lesions,* page 414.) They sometimes occur with bullae— fluid-filled lesions that are larger than 0.5 cm in diameter.

A vesicular rash may be mild or severe, temporary or permanent. It can result from infection, inflammation, or allergic reactions.

Assessment

Ask your patient when the rash began, how it spread, and whether it has appeared before. Did other skin lesions precede eruption of the vesicles? Obtain a thorough drug history. If the patient has used a topical medication, what type did he use and when was it last applied? Also, ask about associated signs and symptoms. Ask about allergies, recent infections, insect bites, and exposure to allergens.

Examine the patient's skin, noting if it's dry, oily, or moist. Observe the general distribution of the lesions and record their exact location. Note the color, shape, and size of the lesions, and check for crusts, scales, scars, macules, papules, or wheals. Palpate the vesicles or bullae to determine if they're flaccid or tense. Slide your finger across the skin to see if the outer layer of epidermis separates easily from the basal layer.

Causes

◆ *Burns (second degree).* Thermal burns that affect the epidermis and part of the dermis cause vesicles and bullae, with erythema, swelling, pain, and moistness.

◆ *Dermatitis.* With *contact dermatitis,* a hypersensitivity reaction produces an eruption of small vesicles surrounded by redness and marked edema. The vesicles may ooze, scale, and cause severe pruritus.

Dermatitis herpetiformis produces a chronic inflammatory eruption marked by vesicular, papular, bullous, pustular, or erythematous lesions. Usually, the rash is symmetrically distributed on the buttocks, shoulders, extensor surfaces of the elbows and knees, and sometimes the face, scalp, and neck.

With *nummular dermatitis,* groups of pinpoint vesicles and papules appear on erythematous or pustular lesions that are nummular or annular. Commonly, the pustular lesions ooze a purulent exudate, itch severely, and rapidly become crusted and scaly.

◆ *Herpes simplex.* Herpes simplex is a common viral infection that produces groups of vesicles on an inflamed base, most commonly on the lips and lower face. The vesicles are preceded by itching, tingling, burning, or pain.

◆ *Herpes zoster.* With herpes zoster, a vesicular rash is preceded by erythema and, occasionally, by a nodular skin eruption and unilateral, sharp, pain along a dermatome. The rash follows a regional linear pattern.

◆ *Insect bites.* With insect bites, vesicles appear on red hivelike papules and may become hemorrhagic.

◆ *Pompholyx (dyshidrosis or dyshidrosis eczema).* Pompholyx is a common, recurrent disorder that produces symmetrical vesicular lesions that can become pustular. The pruritic lesions are more common on the palms than on

---

Drugs that cause toxic epidermal necrolysis

Various drugs can trigger toxic epidermal necrolysis—a rare but potentially fatal immune reaction characterized by a vesicular rash. This type of necrolysis produces large, flaccid bullae that rupture easily, exposing extensive areas of denuded skin. The resulting loss of fluid and electrolytes—along with widespread systemic involvement—can lead to such life-threatening complications as pulmonary edema, shock, renal failure, sepsis, and disseminated intravascular coagulation.

Here's a list of some drugs that can cause toxic epidermal necrolysis:
◆ allopurinol (Zyloprim)
◆ aspirin
◆ barbiturates
◆ chloramphenicol (Chloromycetin)
◆ chlorpropamide (Diabinese)
◆ gold salts
◆ nitrofurantoin (Macrodantin)
◆ penicillin
◆ phenytoin (Dilantin)
◆ primidone (Mysoline)
◆ sulfonamides
◆ tetracycline.

the soles and may be accompanied by minimal erythema.

◆ *Scabies.* Small vesicles erupt on an erythematous base and may be at the end of a threadlike burrow. Burrows are a few millimeters long, with a swollen nodule or red papule that contains a mite.

◆ *Tinea pedis.* Tinea pedis is a fungal infection that causes vesicles and scaling between the toes and, possibly, scaling over the entire sole. Severe infection causes inflammation, pruritus, and difficulty walking.

◆ *Toxic epidermal necrolysis.* Toxic epidermal necrolysis is an immune reaction to drugs or other toxins, in which vesicles and bullae are preceded by a diffuse, erythematous rash and followed by large-scale epidermal necrolysis and desquamation. (See *Drugs that cause toxic epidermal necrolysis,* page 547.)

Violent behavior

Marked by sudden loss of self-control, violent behavior refers to the use of physical force to violate, injure, or abuse an object or person. This behavior may also be self-directed. It may result from an organic or psychiatric disorder or from the use of certain drugs.

Assessment

During your evaluation, determine if the patient has a history of violent behavior. Is he intoxicated or suffering symptoms of alcohol or drug withdrawal? Does he have a history of family violence, including corporal punishment and child or spouse abuse? (See *Understanding family violence.*)

Watch for clues indicating that the patient is losing control and may become violent. Has he exhibited abrupt behavioral changes? Is he unable to sit still? Increased activity may indicate an attempt to discharge aggression. Does he suddenly cease activity (suggesting the calm before the storm)? Does he make verbal threats or angry gestures? Is he jumpy, extremely tense, or laughing? Such intensifying of emotion may herald loss of control.

Understanding family violence

Effectively managing the violent patient requires an understanding of the roots of his behavior. For example, his behavior may be spawned by a family history of corporal punishment or child or spouse abuse. His violent behavior may also be associated with drug or alcohol abuse and fixed family roles that stifle growth and individuality.

Causes of family violence

Social scientists suggest that family violence stems from cultural attitudes fostering violence and from the frustration and stress associated with overcrowded living conditions and poverty. Albert Bandura, a social learning theorist, believes that individuals learn violent behavior by observing and imitating other family members who vent their aggressive feelings through verbal abuse and physical force. (They also learn from television and the movies, especially when the violent hero gains power and recognition.) Members of families with these characteristics may have an increased potential for violent behavior, thus initiating a cycle of violence that passes from generation to generation.

If your patient's violent behavior is a new development, he may have an organic disorder. Obtain a medical history and perform a physical examination. Watch for a sudden change in his level of consciousness. Disorientation, failure to recall recent events, and the display of tics, jerks, tremors, and asterixis all suggest an organic disorder.

Causes

◆ *Drugs and alcohol.* Violent behavior is an adverse effect of some drugs, such as lidocaine and penicillin G. Alcohol abuse or withdrawal, hallucinogens, amphetamines, and barbiturate withdrawal may also cause violent behavior.
◆ *Organic disorders.* Disorders resulting from metabolic or neurologic dysfunction can cause violent behavior. Common causes include epilepsy, brain tumor, encephalitis, head injury, endocrine disorders, metabolic disorders (such as uremia and calcium imbalance), and severe physical trauma.
◆ *Psychiatric disorders.* Violent behavior occurs as a protective mechanism in response to a perceived threat in psychotic disorders such as schizophrenia. A similar response may occur in personality disorders, such as antisocial or borderline personality.

Vision loss

Vision loss—the inability to perceive visual stimuli—can be sudden or gradual, temporary or permanent. The deficit can range from a slight impairment of vision to total blindness. It can result from an ocular, a neurologic, or a systemic disorder or from trauma or the use of certain drugs. The ultimate visual outcome may depend on early, accurate diagnosis and treatment.

Assessment

Sudden vision loss can signal an ocular emergency. (See *Managing sudden vision loss,* page 550.) Don't touch the eye if the patient has perforating or penetrating ocular trauma.

If the patient's vision loss occurred gradually, ask him if it affects one eye or both and all or only part of the visual field. Is the vision loss transient or persistent? Did the vision loss occur abruptly, or did it develop over hours, days, or weeks? What is the patient's age? Ask the patient if he has experienced photosensitivity, and ask him about the location, intensity, and duration of any eye pain. You should also obtain an ocular history and a family history of eye problems or systemic diseases that may lead to eye problems, such as hypertension, diabetes mellitus, infections, cancer, and thyroid, rheumatic, or vascular disease.

The first step in performing the eye examination is to assess visual acuity, with best available correction in each eye. (See *Testing visual acuity,* page 551.)

Carefully inspect both eyes, noting edema, foreign bodies, drainage, or conjunctival or scleral redness. Observe whether lid closure is complete or incomplete, and check for ptosis. Using a flashlight, examine the cornea and iris for scars, irregularities, and foreign bodies. Observe the size, shape, and color of the pupils, and test the direct and consensual light reflex (See "Pupils, nonreactive," page 460.) and the effect of accommodation. Evaluate extraocular muscle function by testing the six cardinal fields of gaze. (See *Testing extraocular muscles,* page 217.)

EMERGENCY INTERVENTIONS

Managing sudden vision loss

Sudden vision loss can signal central retinal artery occlusion or acute angle-closure glaucoma—ocular emergencies that require immediate intervention. If your patient reports sudden vision loss, immediately notify an ophthalmologist for an emergency examination, and perform these interventions:

For a patient with suspected central retinal artery occlusion, perform light massage over his closed eyelid. Increase his carbon dioxide level by administering a set flow of oxygen and carbon dioxide through a Venturi mask, or have the patient rebreathe in a paper bag to retain exhaled carbon dioxide. These steps will dilate the artery and, possibly, restore blood flow to the retina.

For a patient with suspected acute angle-closure glaucoma, measure intraocular pressure (IOP) with a tonometer. (You can also estimate IOP without a tonometer by placing your fingers over the patient's closed eyelid. A rock-hard eyeball usually indicates increased IOP.) Expect to instill timolol (Timoptic) drops and administer I.V. acetazolamide (Diamox) to help decrease IOP.

SUSPECTED CENTRAL RETINAL ARTERY OCCLUSION

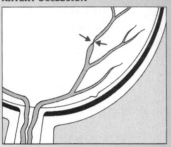

SUSPECTED ACUTE ANGLE-CLOSURE GLAUCOMA

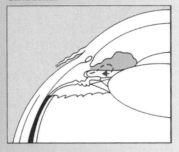

Causes

◆ *Amaurosis fugax.* With amaurosis fugax, recurrent attacks of unilateral vision loss may last from a few seconds to a few minutes. Vision is normal at other times. Elevated intraocular pressure (IOP) in the affected eye may also occur.
◆ *Cataract.* Typically, painless and gradual visual blurring precedes vision loss. As the cataract progresses, the pupil turns milky white.
◆ *Concussion.* Immediately or shortly after blunt head trauma, vision may be blurred, double, or lost. Generally, vision loss is temporary.
◆ *Diabetic retinopathy.* Retinal edema and hemorrhage lead to visual blurring, which may progress to blindness.
◆ *Endophthalmitis.* Typically, endophthalmitis follows penetrating trauma, I.V. drug use, or intraocular surgery,

Testing visual acuity

Use a Snellen letter chart to test visual acuity in the literate patient older than age 6. Have the patient sit or stand 20′ (6 m) from the chart. Then, tell him to cover his left eye and read aloud the smallest line of letters that he can see. Record the fraction assigned to that line on the chart (the numerator indicates distance from the chart; the denominator indicates the distance at which a normal eye can read the chart). Normal vision is 20/20. Repeat the test with the patient's right eye covered.

If your patient can't read the largest letter from a distance of 20′, have him approach the chart until he can read it. Then, record the distance between him and the chart as the numerator of the fraction. For example, if he can see the top line of the chart at a distance of 3′ (1 m), record the test result as 3/20.

Use a Snellen symbol chart to test children ages 3 to 6 and patients who are illiterate. Follow the same procedure as for the Snellen letter chart, but ask the patient to indicate the direction of the E's fingers as you point to each symbol.

SNELLEN LETTER CHART   **SNELLEN SYMBOL CHART**

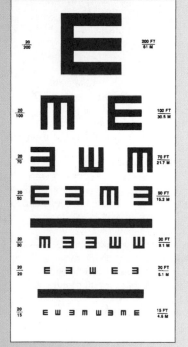

causing possibly permanent unilateral vision loss; a sympathetic inflammation may affect the other eye.

◆ *Glaucoma.* Glaucoma produces gradual visual blurring that may progress to total blindness. *Acute angle-closure glaucoma* is an ocular emergency that may produce blindness within 3 to 5 days. *Chronic angle-closure glaucoma* has a gradual onset and usually produces no symptoms, although blurred or halo vision may occur. If untreated, it progresses to blindness and extreme pain. *Chronic open-angle glaucoma* is usually bilateral, with an insidious onset and a slowly progressive course. It causes peripheral vision loss, aching eyes, halo vision, and reduced visual acuity (especially at night).

◆ *Ocular trauma.* Following eye injury, sudden unilateral or bilateral vision loss may occur. Vision loss may be total or partial and permanent or temporary. The eyelids may be reddened, edematous, and lacerated.

◆ *Optic atrophy.* Degeneration of the optic nerve, optic atrophy can develop spontaneously or follow inflammation or edema of the nerve head, causing irreversible loss of the visual field with changes in color vision.

◆ *Optic neuritis.* An umbrella term for inflammation, degeneration, or demyelinization of the optic nerve, optic neuritis usually produces temporary but severe unilateral vision loss. Pain around the eye occurs, especially with movement of the globe.

◆ *Paget's disease.* Bilateral vision loss may develop as a result of bony impingements on the cranial nerves. This occurs with hearing loss, tinnitus, vertigo, and severe, persistent bone pain.

◆ *Pituitary tumor.* As a pituitary adenoma grows, blurred vision progresses to hemianopia and, possibly, unilateral

blindness. Double vision, nystagmus, ptosis, limited eye movement, and headaches may also occur.

◆ *Retinal artery occlusion (central).* Retinal artery occlusion is a painless ocular emergency that causes sudden unilateral vision loss, which may be partial or complete. Pupil examination reveals a sluggish direct pupillary response and a normal consensual response. Permanent blindness may occur within hours.

◆ *Retinal detachment.* Depending on the degree and location of detachment, painless vision loss may be gradual or sudden and total or partial. Macular involvement causes total blindness.

◆ *Retinal vein occlusion (central).* Most common in geriatric patients, retinal vein occlusion—a painless disorder—causes a unilateral decrease in visual acuity with variable vision loss. IOP may be elevated in both eyes.

◆ *Senile macular degeneration.* Senile macular degeneration causes painless blurring or loss of central vision. Vision loss may proceed slowly or rapidly, eventually affecting both eyes. Visual acuity may be worse at night.

◆ *Stevens-Johnson syndrome.* Corneal scarring from associated conjunctival lesions produces marked vision loss in this syndrome. Purulent conjunctivitis, eye pain, and difficulty opening the eyes can occur.

◆ *Temporal arteritis.* Vision loss and visual blurring with a throbbing, unilateral headache characterize this disorder.

◆ *Vitreous hemorrhage.* With vitreous hemorrhage, sudden unilateral vision loss may result from intraocular trauma, ocular tumors, or systemic disease. Visual floaters and partial vision with a reddish haze may occur.

Visual blurring

Visual blurring is a common symptom that refers to the loss of visual acuity with indistinct visual details. It may result from eye injury, a neurologic or eye disorder, or a disorder with vascular complications such as diabetes mellitus. Visual blurring may also result from mucus passing over the cornea, a refractive error, improperly fitted contact lenses, or certain drugs.

Assessment

If your patient has visual blurring accompanied by sudden, severe eye pain, a history of trauma, or sudden vision loss, request an ophthalmologic examination. (See *Managing sudden vision loss,* page 550.) If the patient has a penetrating or perforating eye injury, don't touch the eye.

If the patient isn't in distress, ask him how long he has had the visual blurring. Does it occur only at certain times? Ask about associated signs and symptoms, such as pain or discharge. If visual blurring followed injury, obtain details of the accident, and ask if vision was impaired immediately after the injury. Obtain a medical and drug history.

Inspect the patient's eye, noting lid edema, drainage, or conjunctival or scleral redness. Also note an irregularly shaped iris, which may indicate previous trauma, and excessive blinking, which may indicate corneal damage. Assess the patient for pupillary changes, and test visual acuity in both eyes. (See *Testing visual acuity,* page 551.)

Causes

◆ *Brain tumor.* Visual blurring may occur with a brain tumor.
◆ *Cataract.* Cataract is a painless disorder that causes gradual visual blurring. Other effects include halo vision (an early sign), visual glare in bright light, progressive vision loss, and a gray pupil that later turns milky white.
◆ *Concussion.* Immediately or shortly after blunt head trauma, vision may be blurred, double, or temporarily lost.
◆ *Corneal abrasions.* Visual blurring may occur with severe eye pain, photophobia, redness, and excessive tearing.
◆ *Corneal foreign bodies.* Visual blurring may accompany a foreign-body sensation, excessive tearing, photophobia, intense eye pain, miosis, conjunctival injection, and a dark corneal speck.
◆ *Diabetic retinopathy.* Retinal edema and hemorrhage produce gradual blurring, which may progress to blindness.
◆ *Dislocated lens.* Dislocation of the lens, especially beyond the line of vision, causes visual blurring.
◆ *Eye tumor.* If the tumor involves the macula, visual blurring may be the presenting symptom. Related findings include varying visual field losses.
◆ *Glaucoma.* With *acute angle-closure glaucoma,* an ocular emergency, unilateral visual blurring and severe pain begin suddenly. With *chronic angle-closure glaucoma,* transient visual blurring and halo vision may precede pain and blindness.
◆ *Hereditary corneal dystrophies.* Visual blurring may remain stable or may progressively worsen throughout life. Some dystrophies cause associated pain, vision loss, photophobia, tearing, and corneal opacities.
◆ *Hypertension.* Hypertension may cause visual blurring and a constant

morning headache that decreases in severity during the day.

◆ *Hyphema.* Blunt eye trauma with hemorrhage into the anterior chamber causes visual blurring in this disorder. Other effects include moderate pain, diffuse conjunctival injection, visible blood in the anterior chamber, ecchymoses, eyelid edema, and a hard eye.

◆ *Iritis.* Acute iritis causes sudden visual blurring, moderate to severe eye pain, photophobia, conjunctival injection, and a constricted pupil.

◆ *Optic neuritis.* Inflammation, degeneration, or demyelinization of the optic nerve usually causes an acute attack of visual blurring and vision loss. Related findings include scotomas and eye pain.

◆ *Retinal detachment.* Sudden visual blurring may be the initial symptom of retinal detachment. Blurring worsens, accompanied by visual floaters and recurring flashes of light. Progressive detachment increases vision loss.

◆ *Retinal vein occlusion (central).* Retinal vein occlusion causes gradual unilateral visual blurring and varying degrees of vision loss.

◆ *Senile macular degeneration.* Senile macular degeneration may cause visual blurring (initially worse at night) and slowly or rapidly progressive vision loss.

◆ *Stroke.* Brief attacks of bilateral visual blurring may precede or accompany a stroke.

◆ *Temporal arteritis.* Temporal arteritis causes sudden blurred vision accompanied by vision loss and a throbbing unilateral headache in the temporal or frontotemporal region.

◆ *Vitreous hemorrhage.* Sudden unilateral visual blurring and varying vision loss occur with this condition. Visual floaters or dark streaks may also occur.

Visual floaters

Visual floaters are particles of blood or cellular debris that move about in the vitreous humour. As these enter the visual field, they appear as spots or dots. Chronic floaters may occur normally in elderly or myopic patients. However, the sudden onset of visual floaters commonly signals retinal detachment, an ocular emergency.

Assessment

Ask the patient if he also sees flashing lights or spots in the affected eye. Is he experiencing a curtainlike loss of vision? If so, notify an ophthalmologist immediately—he may have a retinal detachment. Restrict his eye movements until the diagnosis is made. If the patient's condition permits, obtain a drug and allergy history. Ask about nearsightedness (a predisposing factor), use of corrective lenses, eye trauma, or other eye disorders. Also ask about a history of granulomatous disease, diabetes mellitus, or hypertension, which may have predisposed him to retinal detachment, vitreous hemorrhage, or uveitis. If appropriate, inspect his eyes for signs of injury, such as bruising or edema, and determine his visual acuity. (See *Testing visual acuity*, page 551.)

Causes

◆ *Retinal detachment.* Floaters and light flashes appear suddenly in the portion of the visual field where the retina is detached from the choroid. As the retina detaches further (a painless process), gradual vision loss occurs, likened to a cloud or curtain falling in front of the eyes. Ophthalmoscopic examination reveals a gray, opaque, detached retina with an indefinite margin. Retinal vessels appear almost black.

◆ *Uveitis (posterior).* Uveitis may cause visual floaters accompanied by gradual eye pain, photophobia, blurred vision, and conjunctival injection.

◆ *Vitreous hemorrhage.* Rupture of retinal vessels produces a shower of red or black dots or a red haze across the visual field. Vision is suddenly blurred in the affected eye. Visual acuity may be greatly reduced.

Vomiting

Vomiting is the forceful expulsion of gastric contents through the mouth. Characteristically preceded by nausea, vomiting results from a coordinated sequence of abdominal muscle contractions and reverse esophageal peristalsis.

A common sign of GI disorders, vomiting also occurs with fluid and electrolyte imbalances, infections, and metabolic, endocrine, labyrinthine, central nervous system (CNS), and cardiac disorders. It can also result from drug therapy, surgery, or radiation.

Vomiting occurs normally during the first trimester of pregnancy, but its subsequent development may signal complications. It can also result from stress, anxiety, pain, alcohol intoxication, overeating, or ingestion of distasteful foods or liquids.

Assessment

Ask your patient to describe the onset, duration, and intensity of his vomiting. What started it? What makes it subside? If possible, collect, measure, and inspect the character of the vomitus. (See *Vomitus: Characteristics and causes.*) Explore

Vomitus: Characteristics and causes

When you collect a sample of the patient's vomitus, observe it carefully for clues to the underlying disorder. Here's what vomitus may indicate:

Bile-stained (greenish) vomitus
Obstruction below the pylorus, as from a duodenal lesion

Bloody vomitus
Upper GI bleeding (if bright red, may result from gastritis or a peptic ulcer; if dark red, from esophageal or gastric varices)

Brown vomitus with a fecal odor
Intestinal obstruction or infarction

Burning, bitter-tasting vomitus
Excessive hydrochloric acid in gastric contents

Coffee-ground vomitus
Digested blood from slowly bleeding gastric or duodenal lesion

Undigested food
Gastric outlet obstruction, as from gastric tumor or ulcer

any associated complaints, particularly nausea, abdominal pain, anorexia and weight loss, changes in bowel habits or stools, excessive belching or flatus, and bloating or fullness.

Then obtain a medical history, noting GI, endocrine, and metabolic disorders; recent infections; and cancer, including chemotherapy or radiation therapy. Ask about current medication use and alcohol consumption. If the patient is a female of childbearing age, ask if she is or could be pregnant.

Inspect the abdomen for distention and localized bulging, and auscultate for bowel sounds and bruits. Palpate for rigidity and tenderness, and test for rebound tenderness. Next, palpate and percuss the liver for enlargement. Assess other body systems as appropriate.

◆ **ALERT** Projectile vomiting unaccompanied by nausea may indicate increased intracranial pressure (ICP), a life-threatening emergency. If this occurs in a patient with CNS injury, you should quickly check his vital signs. Be alert for widened pulse pressure or bradycardia.

Causes

◆ *Adrenal insufficiency.* Common GI findings with this disorder include vomiting, nausea, anorexia, and diarrhea.
◆ *Appendicitis.* Vomiting and nausea may follow or accompany abdominal pain. Pain typically begins as vague epigastric or periumbilical discomfort and rapidly progresses to severe, stabbing pain in the right lower quadrant.
◆ *Cholecystitis (acute).* With cholecystitis, nausea and mild vomiting commonly follow severe right-upper-quadrant pain that may radiate to the back or shoulders.
◆ *Cholelithiasis.* Nausea and vomiting accompany severe unlocalized right-upper-quadrant or epigastric pain after ingestion of fatty foods.
◪ *Cholera.* Signs and symptoms include vomiting and abrupt watery diarrhea. Severe water and electrolyte loss leads to muscle cramps, decreased skin turgor, and hypotension. Without treatment, death can occur within hours.

◆ *Cirrhosis.* Insidious early signs and symptoms of cirrhosis typically include nausea and vomiting, anorexia, aching abdominal pain, and constipation or diarrhea.
◆ *Electrolyte imbalances.* Such disturbances as hyponatremia, hypernatremia, hypokalemia, and hypercalcemia frequently cause nausea and vomiting.
◆ Escherichia coli *O157:H7.* The signs and symptoms of *E. coli* include vomiting, watery or bloody diarrhea, nausea, fever, and abdominal cramps.
◆ *Food poisoning.* Vomiting is a common finding of food poisoning, caused by preformed toxins produced by bacteria typically found in foods. Diarrhea and fever also usually occur.
◆ *Gastritis.* Nausea and vomiting of mucus or blood are common with gastritis, especially after ingestion of alcohol, aspirin, spicy foods, or caffeine. Epigastric pain, belching, and fever may occur.
◆ *Gastroenteritis.* Gastroenteritis causes nausea, vomiting (commonly of undigested food), diarrhea, and abdominal cramping.
◆ *Heart failure.* Nausea and vomiting may occur, especially with right-sided heart failure.
◆ *Hepatitis.* Vomiting commonly follows nausea as an early sign of viral hepatitis.
◆ *Hyperemesis gravidarum.* Unremitting nausea and vomiting that last beyond the first trimester characterize this disorder of pregnancy. Vomitus contains undigested food, mucus, and small amounts of bile early in the disorder; later, it has a coffee-ground appearance.
◪ *Increased ICP.* Projectile vomiting that isn't preceded by nausea is a sign of increased ICP. The patient may exhibit Cushing's triad (bradycardia,

hypertension, and widened pulse pressure).

◆ *Intestinal obstruction.* Nausea and vomiting (bilious or fecal) are common with intestinal obstruction, especially of the upper small intestine. Abdominal pain is usually episodic and colicky but can become severe and steady.

◆ *Labyrinthitis.* Nausea and vomiting commonly occur with this acute inner ear inflammation.

◪ *Listeriosis.* After the ingestion of food contaminated with the bacterium *Listeria monocytogenes*, vomiting, fever, myalgias, abdominal pain, nausea, and diarrhea occur. If the infection spreads to the nervous system, meningitis may develop.

◆ *Mesenteric venous thrombosis.* Insidious or acute onset of nausea, vomiting, and abdominal pain occurs with mesenteric venous thrombosis.

◆ *Migraine headache.* Nausea and vomiting are prodromal signs and symptoms, with fatigue, photophobia, light flashes, increased noise sensitivity, and possibly partial vision loss and paresthesia.

◆ *Motion sickness.* Nausea and vomiting may be accompanied by headache, vertigo, dizziness, fatigue, diaphoresis, and dyspnea.

◪ *Pancreatitis (acute).* Vomiting, usually preceded by nausea, is an early sign of pancreatitis.

◆ *Peritonitis.* Nausea and vomiting usually accompany acute abdominal pain in the area of inflammation.

◆ *Preeclampsia.* Nausea and vomiting are common with preeclampsia, a disorder of pregnancy. Rapid weight gain, generalized edema, elevated blood pressure, severe frontal headache, and blurred or double vision also occur.

◆ *Renal and urologic disorders.* Cystitis, pyelonephritis, calculi, and other disorders of this system can cause vomiting. Accompanying findings reflect the specific disorder.

◆ *Rhabdomyolysis.* Signs and symptoms of this disorder include vomiting, muscle weakness or pain, fever, nausea, malaise, and dark urine.

◆ *Typhus.* Typhus is a rickettsial disease transmitted to humans by fleas, mites, or body lice. Initial symptoms include headache, myalgia, arthralgia, and malaise, followed by an abrupt onset of vomiting, nausea, chills, and fever.

Vulvar lesions

Vulvar lesions are cutaneous lumps, nodules, papules, vesicles, or ulcers that result from benign or malignant tumors, dystrophies, dermatoses, or infection. They can appear anywhere on the vulva and may go undetected until a gynecologic examination. Usually, however, the patient notices lesions because of associated symptoms, such as pruritus, dysuria, or dyspareunia.

Assessment

Begin by asking the patient when she first noticed the vulvar lesion and then ask about associated features, such as swelling, pain, tenderness, itching, or discharge. Does she have lesions elsewhere on her body? Ask about signs and symptoms of systemic illness, such as malaise, fever, or rash on other body areas. Is the patient sexually active? Could she have been exposed to sexually transmitted disease?

Also, examine the lesion, do a pelvic examination, and obtain cultures. (See *Recognizing common vulvar lesions*, pages 558 and 559.)

Recognizing common vulvar lesions

Various disorders can cause vulvar lesions. For example, sexually transmitted diseases account for most vulvar lesions in premenopausal women, whereas vulvar tumors and cysts account for most lesions in women ages 50 to 70. The illustrations below will help you recognize some of the most common lesions.

Primary genital herpes produces multiple ulcerated lesions surrounded by red halos.

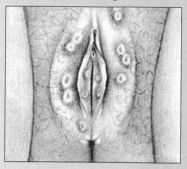

Primary syphilis produces chancres that appear as ulcerated lesions with raised borders.

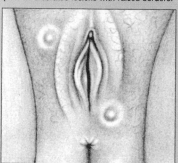

Basal cell carcinoma can produce an ulcerated lesion with raised, poorly rolled edges.

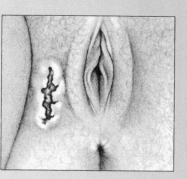

Epidermal inclusion cysts produce a round lump that usually appears on the labia majora.

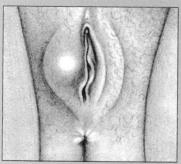

Causes

◆ *Basal cell carcinoma.* Most common in postmenopausal women, this nodular tumor has a central ulcer and a raised, poorly rolled border.

◆ *Benign cysts.* Epidermal inclusion cysts, the most common vulvar cysts, appear primarily on the labia majora, are usually round, and produce no symptoms. Occasionally, they become

Squamous cell carcinoma can produce a large, granulomatous-appearing ulcer.

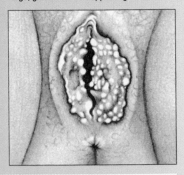

Bartholin's duct cysts produce a tense, nontender, palpable lump that usually appears on the labia minora.

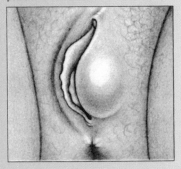

erythematous and tender. Bartholin's duct cysts are usually unilateral, tense, nontender, and palpable; they appear on the posterior labia minora and may cause minor discomfort during inter-course or, when large, difficulty with intercourse or even walking. Bartholin's abscess, infection of a Bartholin's duct cyst, causes gradual pain and tenderness and possibly vulvar swelling, redness, and deformity.

◆ *Benign vulvar tumors.* Cystic or solid benign vulvar tumors usually produce no symptoms.

◆ *Chancroid.* Chancroid, a rare, sexually transmitted disease, causes painful vulvar lesions. Headache, malaise, and fever may occur, with enlarged, tender inguinal lymph nodes.

◆ *Genital warts.* Genital warts are painless warts on the vulva, vagina, and cervix. Warts start as tiny red or pink swellings that grow and become pedunculated. Multiple swellings with a cauliflower appearance are common. Other findings include pruritus, erythema, and a profuse, mucopurulent vaginal discharge.

◆ *Gonorrhea.* Vulvar lesions, which are usually confined to Bartholin's glands, may develop in a patient with gonorrhea along with pruritus, a burning sensation, pain, and a green-yellow vaginal discharge; however, most patients are asymptomatic.

◆ *Granuloma inguinale.* Initially, a single painless macule or papule appears on the vulva, ulcerating into a raised, beefy-red lesion with a granulated, friable border.

◆ *Herpes simplex (genital).* With herpes simplex, fluid-filled vesicles appear on the cervix, vulva, labia, perianal skin, vagina, or mouth.

◆ *Lymphogranuloma venereum.* Patients with lymphogranuloma venereum commonly present with a single, painless papule or ulcer on the posterior vulva that heals in a few days. Painful, swollen lymph nodes, usually unilateral, develop 2 to 6 weeks later.

◆ *Squamous cell carcinoma.* Invasive carcinoma occurs primarily in post-menopausal women and may produce vulvar pruritus, pain, and a vulvar lump. As the tumor enlarges, it may encroach on the vagina, anus, and urethra, causing bleeding, discharge, or dysuria. Carcinoma in situ is most common in premenopausal women, producing a vulvar lesion that may be white or red, raised, well defined, moist, crusted, and isolated.

◆ *Squamous cell hyperplasia.* These vulvar lesions may be well delineated or poorly defined; localized or extensive; and red, brown, white, or both red and white. Intense pruritus, possibly with vulvar pain, intense burning, and dyspareunia, is the cardinal symptom.

◆ *Syphilis.* Chancres, the primary vulvar lesions of syphilis, may appear on the vulva, vagina, or cervix 10 to 90 days after initial contact. Usually painless, they start as papules that then erode, with indurated, raised edges and clear bases. Condylomata lata, highly contagious secondary vulvar lesions, are raised, gray, flat-topped, and commonly ulcerated.

◆ *Viral disease (systemic).* Varicella, measles, and other systemic viral diseases may produce vulvar lesions.

WXYZ

Weight gain, excessive

Weight gain occurs when ingested calories exceed body requirements for energy, causing increased adipose tissue storage. It can also occur when fluid retention causes edema. When weight gain results from overeating, emotional factors—most commonly anxiety, guilt, and depression—and social factors may be the primary causes.

Among the elderly, weight gain commonly reflects a sustained food intake in the presence of the normal, progressive fall in basal metabolic rate. Among women, a progressive weight gain occurs with pregnancy, whereas a periodic weight gain usually occurs with menstruation.

Weight gain, a primary sign of many endocrine disorders, also occurs with conditions that limit activity, especially cardiovascular and pulmonary disorders. It can also result from drug therapy that increases appetite or causes fluid retention or from cardiovascular, hepatic, and renal disorders that cause edema.

Assessment

Determine your patient's previous patterns of weight gain and loss. Does he have a family history of obesity, thyroid disease, or diabetes mellitus? Assess his eating and activity patterns. Has his appetite increased? Does he exercise regularly? Next, ask about associated symptoms. Has he experienced vision disturbances, hoarseness, paresthesia, or increased urination and thirst? Has he become impotent? If the patient is female, has she had menstrual irregularities or experienced weight gain during menstruation?

Form an impression of the patient's mental status. Is he anxious or depressed? Does he respond slowly? Is his memory poor? What medications is he using?

During your physical examination, measure skin-fold thickness to estimate fat reserves. (See *Evaluating nutritional status,* pages 562 and 563.) Note fat distribution and the presence of localized or generalized edema and overall nutritional status. Inspect for other abnormalities, such as abnormal body hair distribution or hair loss and dry skin. Take and record the patient's vital signs.

(*Text continues on page 564.*)

Evaluating nutritional status

If your patient exhibits excessive weight loss or gain, you can help assess his nutritional status by measuring his skin-fold thickness and midarm circumference and by calculating his midarm muscle circumference. Skin-fold measurements reflect adipose tissue mass (subcutaneous fat accounts for about 50% of the body's adipose tissue). Midarm measurements reflect skeletal muscle and adipose tissue mass.

Use the steps described here to gather these measurements. Then express them as a percentage of standard by using this formula:

$$\frac{\text{Actual measurement}}{\text{Standard measurement}} \times 100 = \underline{\qquad} \%$$

Standard anthropometric measurements vary according to the patient's age and sex and can be found in a chart of normal anthropometric values. The abridged chart below lists standard arm measurements for adult men and women.

A triceps or subscapular skin-fold measurement below 60% of the standard value indicates severe depletion of fat reserves; measurement between 60% and 90% indicates moderate to mild depletion; and above 90% indicates significant fat reserves. A midarm circumference of less than 90% of the standard value indicates caloric deprivation; greater than 90% indicates adequate or ample muscle and fat. A midarm muscle circumference of less than 90% indicates protein depletion; greater than 90% indicates adequate or ample protein reserves.

TEST	STANDARD	
Triceps skin fold	Men	12.5 mm
	Women	16.5 mm
Midarm circumference	Men	29.3 mm
	Women	28.5 mm
Midarm muscle circumference	Men	25.3 mm
	Women	23.2 mm

To measure the triceps skin fold, locate the midpoint of the patient's upper arm, using a nonstretch tape measure. Mark the midpoint with a felt-tip pen. Then grasp the skin with your thumb and forefinger about 1 cm above the midpoint. Place the calipers at the midpoint and squeeze them for about 3 seconds. Record the measurement registered on the handle gauge to the nearest 0.5 mm. Take two more readings and average all three to compensate for any measurement error.

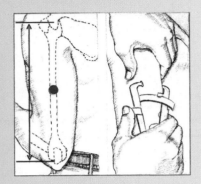

To measure the subscapular skin fold, use your thumb and forefinger to grasp the skin just below the angle of the scapula, in line with the natural cleavage of the skin. Apply the calipers and proceed as you would when measuring the triceps skin fold. Both subscapular and triceps skin-fold measurements are reliable measurements of fat loss or gain during hospitalization.

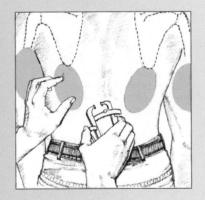

To measure midarm circumference, return to the midpoint you marked on the patient's upper arm. Then use a tape measure to determine the arm circumference at this point. This measurement reflects skeletal muscle and adipose tissue mass and helps evaluate protein and calorie reserves. To calculate midarm muscle circumference, multiply the triceps skin-fold thickness (in centimeters) by 3.143, and subtract this figure from the midarm circumference. Midarm muscle circumference reflects muscle mass alone, providing a more sensitive index of protein reserves.

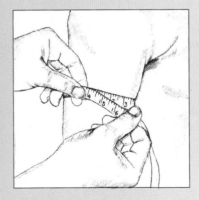

Causes

◆ *Acromegaly.* Acromegaly causes moderate weight gain. Other findings include coarsened facial features, prognathism, enlarged hands and feet, increased sweating, back and joint pain, sleepiness, and heat intolerance.

◆ *Diabetes mellitus.* The increased appetite associated with diabetes mellitus may lead to weight gain, although weight loss sometimes occurs instead. Other findings include fatigue, polydipsia, polyuria, and polyphagia.

◆ *Drugs.* Corticosteroids, phenothiazines, and tricyclic antidepressants cause weight gain from fluid retention and increased appetite. Other drugs that can lead to weight gain include hormonal contraceptives, which cause fluid retention, and lithium (Eskalith), which can induce hypothyroidism.

◆ *Hypercortisolism.* Excessive weight gain, usually over the trunk and the back of the neck (buffalo hump), occurs in hypercortisolism. Other cushingoid features include moon face, purple striae, and increased susceptibility to infection. Gynecomastia may occur in men; hirsutism, acne, and menstrual irregularities may occur in women.

◆ *Hyperinsulinism.* Hyperinsulinism increases appetite, leading to weight gain. Emotional lability, indigestion, weakness, diaphoresis, tachycardia, vision disturbances, and syncope also occur.

◆ *Hypogonadism.* Weight gain is common in hypogonadism. Prepubertal hypogonadism causes eunuchoid body proportions with relatively sparse facial and body hair and a high-pitched voice. Postpubertal hypogonadism causes loss of libido, impotence, and infertility.

◆ *Hypothalamic dysfunction.* Conditions such as Laurence-Moon-Biedl syndrome cause a voracious appetite with subsequent weight gain, along with altered body temperature and sleep rhythms.

◆ *Hypothyroidism.* With hypothyroidism, weight gain occurs despite anorexia. Other findings include fatigue; cold intolerance; constipation; menorrhagia; dry, pale, cool skin; dry, sparse hair; and thick, brittle nails.

◆ *Nephrotic syndrome.* With nephrotic syndrome, weight gain results from edema. In severe cases, anasarca develops—increasing body weight up to 50%. Other findings include abdominal distention and orthostatic hypotension.

◆ *Pancreatic islet cell tumor.* Pancreatic islet cell tumor causes excessive hunger, which leads to weight gain. Other findings include emotional lability, malaise, fatigue, diaphoresis, palpitations, tachycardia, vision disturbances, and syncope.

◆ *Preeclampsia.* With preeclampsia, rapid weight gain (exceeding the normal weight gain of pregnancy) may accompany nausea and vomiting, epigastric pain, elevated blood pressure, and visual blurring or double vision.

◆ *Sheehan's syndrome.* Most common in women who experience severe obstetric hemorrhage, Sheehan's syndrome may cause weight gain.

Weight loss, excessive

Weight loss can reflect decreased food intake, decreased food absorption, increased metabolic requirements, or a combination of the three. Its causes include endocrine, neoplastic, GI, and psychiatric disorders; nutritional deficiencies; infections; and neurologic lesions that cause paralysis and dysphagia. However, weight loss may accompany conditions that prevent sufficient food intake, such as painful oral lesions, ill-fitting dentures, and loss of teeth. It may be the metabolic effect of poverty, fad diets, excessive exercise, or certain drugs.

Weight loss may occur as a late sign of chronic diseases such as heart failure and renal disease. In these diseases, however, weight loss is the result of anorexia. (See "Anorexia," page 94.)

Assessment

Begin with a thorough diet history because weight loss almost always is caused by inadequate caloric intake. If the patient hasn't been eating properly, try to determine why. Ask him about previous weight and if the recent loss was intentional. Be alert to lifestyle or occupational changes that may be a source of anxiety or depression. Inquire about recent changes in bowel habits, such as diarrhea or bulky, floating stools. Has the patient experienced nausea, vomiting, or abdominal pain? Has he had excessive thirst, excessive urination, or heat intolerance? Take a careful drug history, noting especially any use of diet pills and laxatives.

Carefully check the patient's height and weight. Check his vital signs and note his general appearance: Is he well nourished? Do his clothes fit? Is muscle wasting evident? Ask about exact weight changes (with approximate dates).

Next, examine the patient's skin for turgor and abnormal pigmentation, especially around the joints. (Hyperpigmentation around the joints may signal adrenal insufficiency.) Does he have pallor or jaundice? Examine his mouth, including the condition of his teeth or dentures. Look for signs of infection or irritation on the roof of the mouth, and note any hyperpigmentation of the buccal mucosa. Also check the patient's eyes for exophthalmos and his neck for swelling; evaluate his lungs for adventitious sounds. Then inspect his abdomen for signs of wasting and palpate for masses, tenderness, and an enlarged liver.

Conventional laboratory and radiologic investigations, such as complete blood count, serum albumin levels, urinalysis, chest X-ray, and upper GI series, usually reveal the cause. Cancer, GI disorders, and depression are the most common pathologic causes.

Causes

◆ *Adrenal insufficiency.* Weight loss occurs with adrenal insufficiency, along with anorexia, weakness, fatigue, irritability, syncope, nausea, vomiting, abdominal pain, and diarrhea or constipation. Hyperpigmentation may occur at the joints, belt line, palmar creases, lips, gums, tongue, and buccal mucosa.
◆ *Anorexia nervosa.* Anorexia nervosa is a psychogenic disorder that's characterized by a severe, self-imposed weight loss ranging from 10% to 50% of premorbid weight, which typically was normal or not more than 5 lb (2.3 kg) over ideal weight. Related findings include skeletal muscle atrophy, hypotension, dental caries, blotchy or sallow skin, cold intolerance, and amenorrhea. Self-induced vomiting or use of laxatives or diuretics may lead to dehydration or to metabolic alkalosis or acidosis.
◆ *Cancer.* Weight loss is commonly a sign of cancer. Other findings reflect the type, location, and stage of the tumor.
◆ *Crohn's disease.* With Crohn's disease, weight loss occurs with chronic cramping, abdominal pain, and anorexia. Other findings include diarrhea, nausea, tachycardia, hyperactive bowel

sounds, abdominal distention, and pain.

◆ *Cryptosporidiosis.* Weight loss may occur with cryptosporidiosis, an opportunistic protozoan infection. Other findings include profuse watery diarrhea, abdominal cramping, flatulence, anorexia, nausea, vomiting, and myalgia.

◆ *Depression.* Weight loss or weight gain may occur with severe depression, along with insomnia or hypersomnia, anorexia, apathy, fatigue, and feelings of worthlessness.

◆ *Diabetes mellitus.* Weight loss may occur with diabetes mellitus, despite increased appetite. Other findings include polydipsia, weakness, fatigue, and polyuria with nocturia.

◆ *Esophagitis.* Painful inflammation of the esophagus leads to temporary avoidance of eating and subsequent weight loss. Intense pain in the mouth and anterior chest occurs, along with hypersalivation, dysphagia, and tachypnea.

◆ *Gastroenteritis.* Malabsorption and dehydration cause weight loss in gastroenteritis. The loss may be sudden in acute viral infections or gradual in parasitic infection.

◆ *Leukemia.* Acute leukemia causes progressive weight loss accompanied by severe prostration and swollen, bleeding gums. Dyspnea, tachycardia, palpitations, and abdominal or bone pain may occur. Chronic leukemia, which occurs insidiously in adults, causes progressive weight loss with malaise, fatigue, pallor, enlarged spleen, bleeding tendencies, anemia, skin eruptions, anorexia, and fever.

◆ *Lymphoma.* Hodgkin's disease and non-Hodgkin's lymphoma cause gradual weight loss. Associated findings include fever, fatigue, night sweats, malaise, hepatosplenomegaly, and lymphadenopathy.

◆ *Pulmonary tuberculosis (TB).* Pulmonary TB causes gradual weight loss, along with fatigue, weakness, anorexia, night sweats, and low-grade fever.

◆ *Stomatitis.* With stomatitis, an inflamed and ulcerated oral mucosa causes weight loss due to decreased eating.

◆ *Thyrotoxicosis.* With thyrotoxicosis, increased metabolism causes weight loss. Other findings include nervousness, heat intolerance, diarrhea, increased appetite, palpitations, tachycardia, diaphoresis, and fine tremors.

Wheezing

Wheezes are adventitious breath sounds with a high-pitched, musical, squealing, creaking, or groaning quality. They are caused by air flowing at a high velocity through a narrowed airway. When they originate in the large airways, they can be heard by placing an unaided ear over the chest wall or at the mouth. When they originate in smaller airways, they can be heard by placing a stethoscope over the anterior or posterior chest. Unlike crackles and rhonchi, wheezes can't be cleared by coughing.

Usually, prolonged wheezing occurs during expiration when bronchi are shortened and narrowed. Causes of airway narrowing include bronchospasm; mucosal thickening or edema; partial obstruction from a tumor, a foreign body, or secretions; and extrinsic pressure, as in tension pneumothorax or goiter. With airway obstruction, wheezing occurs during inspiration.

Assessment

Begin your assessment by determining if the patient is in respiratory distress. Is he responsive, restless, confused, anxious, or afraid? Are his respirations abnormally fast, slow, shallow, or deep? Are they irregular? Can you hear wheezing through his mouth? Does he exhibit increased use of accessory muscles; increased chest wall motion; intercostal, suprasternal, or supraclavicular retractions; stridor; or nasal flaring? Check his other vital signs, noting hypotension or hypertension, decreased oxygen saturation, or an irregular, weak, rapid, or slow pulse.

Ask the patient about chest pain. If he reports pain, determine its quality, onset, duration, intensity, and radiation. Does it increase with breathing, coughing, or certain positions? If the patient isn't in distress, obtain a history. What provokes his wheezing? Does he have asthma or allergies? Does he smoke or have a history of a pulmonary, cardiac, or circulatory disorder? Does he have cancer? Ask about recent surgery, illness, or trauma or changes in appetite, weight, exercise tolerance, or sleep patterns. Obtain a drug history. Ask about exposure to toxic fumes or any respiratory irritants. If he has a cough, ask how it sounds, when it starts, and how often it occurs. Does he have paroxysms of coughing? Ask him to describe his sputum.

Examine the patient's nose and mouth for congestion, drainage, or signs of infection, such as halitosis. If he produces sputum, obtain a sample for examination. Check for cyanosis, pallor, clamminess, masses, tenderness, swelling, distended jugular veins, and enlarged lymph nodes. Inspect his chest for abnormal configuration and asymmetrical motion, and determine if the trachea is midline. (See *Detecting slight tracheal deviation,* page 526.) Percuss for dullness or hyperresonance, and auscultate for crackles, rhonchi, or pleural friction rubs. Note absent or hypoactive breath sounds, abnormal heart sounds, gallops, or murmurs. Also note arrhythmias, bradycardia, or tachycardia. (See *Evaluating breath sounds,* pages 568 and 569.)

Causes

◼ *Anaphylaxis.* Anaphylaxis can cause tracheal edema or bronchospasm, resulting in severe wheezing and stridor. Respiratory distress occurs with nasal flaring, accessory muscle use, and intercostal retractions.

◼ *Aspiration of a foreign body.* Partial obstruction by a foreign body produces sudden onset of wheezing and possibly stridor, gagging, hoarseness, and a dry, paroxysmal cough.

◆ *Aspiration pneumonitis.* With aspiration pneumonitis, wheezing may accompany tachypnea, marked dyspnea, cyanosis, tachycardia, fever, productive (eventually purulent) cough, and pink, frothy sputum.

◆ *Asthma.* Wheezing is an initial and cardinal sign of asthma. It's heard at the mouth during expiration. An initially dry cough later becomes productive with thick mucus.

◆ *Bronchial adenoma.* Bronchial adenoma produces unilateral and, possibly, severe wheezing. Common findings include chronic cough and recurring hemoptysis. Symptoms of airway obstruction may occur later.

◆ *Bronchiectasis.* Excessive mucus commonly causes intermittent and localized or diffuse wheezing. A copious, foul-smelling, mucopurulent cough is classic. It's accompanied by hemoptysis, rhonchi, and coarse crackles.

Evaluating breath sounds

Diminished or absent breath sounds indicate some interference with airflow. If pus, fluid, or air fills the pleural space, breath sounds will be quieter than normal. If a foreign body or secretions obstruct a bronchus, breath sounds will be diminished or absent over distal lung tissue. Increased thickness of the chest wall, such as with a patient who is obese or extremely muscular, may cause breath sounds to be decreased, distant, or inaudible. Absent breath sounds typically indicate loss of ventilation power.

Adventitious breath sounds will be heard when air passes through narrowed airways or

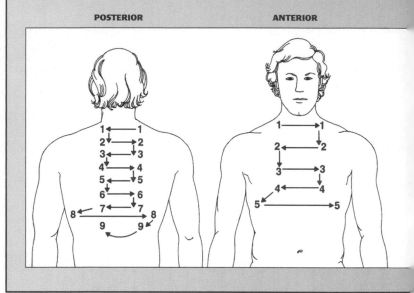

POSTERIOR   ANTERIOR

◆ *Bronchitis (chronic).* Bronchitis causes wheezing that varies in severity, location, and intensity. Other findings include prolonged expiration, coarse crackles, scattered rhonchi, and a hacking cough that later becomes productive.

◆ *Bronchogenic carcinoma.* Obstruction from a tumor may cause localized wheezing. Typical findings include a cough, dyspnea, hemoptysis (initially blood-tinged sputum, possibly leading to massive hemorrhage), anorexia, and weight loss.

◆ *Emphysema.* Mild to moderate wheezing may occur with emphysema. Related findings include dyspnea, malaise, tachypnea, diminished breath sounds, peripheral cyanosis, pursed-lip breathing, anorexia, and malaise.

◆ *Pulmonary coccidioidomycosis.* Pulmonary coccidioidomycosis may cause wheezing and rhonchi along with cough, fever, chills, pleuritic chest through moisture, or when the membranes lining the chest cavity become inflamed. These sounds include crackles, rhonchi, wheezes, and pleural friction rubs. Usually, these sounds indicate pulmonary disease.

Follow the auscultation sequences shown to assess the patient's breath sounds. Have the patient take full, deep breaths, and compare sound variations from one side to the other. Note the location, timing, and character of any abnormal breath sounds.

LEFT LATERAL   RIGHT LATERAL

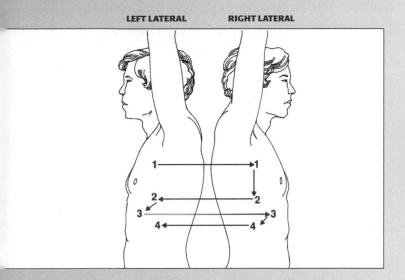

pain, headache, weakness, malaise, anorexia, and macular rash.

◆ *Pulmonary edema.* Wheezing may occur with pulmonary edema. Other findings include coughing, exertional and paroxysmal nocturnal dyspnea, tachycardia, tachypnea, dependent crackles, and a diastolic gallop.

◆ *Tracheobronchitis.* Auscultation may detect wheezing, rhonchi, and crackles. The patient also has a cough, slight fever, sudden chills, muscle and back pain, and substernal tightness.

Less common
signs and symptoms

A

Aaron's sign Pain in the chest or abdominal (precordial or epigastric) area that's elicited by applying gentle but steadily increasing pressure over McBurney's point. A positive sign indicates appendicitis.

Abadie's sign Spasm of the levator muscle of the upper eyelid. This sign may be slight or pronounced and may affect one eye or both eyes. It reflects an exophthalmic goiter in Graves' disease.

adipsia Abnormal absence of thirst. This symptom commonly occurs in hypothalamic injury or tumor, head injury, bronchial tumor, and cirrhosis.

agnosia Inability to recognize and interpret sensory stimuli, even though the principal sensation of the stimulus is known. Auditory agnosia refers to the inability to recognize familiar sounds. Astereognosis, or tactile agnosia, is the inability to recognize objects by touch or feel. Anosmia is the inability to recognize familiar smells; gustatory agnosia, the inability to recognize familiar tastes. Visual agnosia refers to the inability to recognize familiar objects by sight. Autotopagnosia is the inability to recognize body parts. Anosognosia refers to the denial or lack of awareness of a disease or defect (especially paralysis).

Agnosias stem from lesions that affect the association areas of the parietal sensory cortex. They're a common sequelae of stroke.

agraphia Inability to express thoughts in writing. Aphasic agraphia is associated with spelling and grammatical errors, whereas constructional agraphia refers to the reversal or incorrect ordering of correctly spelled words. Apraxic agraphia refers to the inability to form letters in the absence of significant motor impairment.

Agraphia commonly results from a stroke.

Amoss' sign A sparing maneuver to avoid pain upon flexion of the spine. To detect this sign, ask the patient to rise from a supine to a sitting position. If he supports himself by placing his hands far behind him on the examination table, you've observed this sign.

anesthesia Absence of cutaneous sensation of touch, temperature, and pain. This sensory loss may be partial or total, unilateral or bilateral. To detect anesthesia, ask the patient to close his eyes. Then touch him and ask him to specify the location. If the patient's verbal skills are immature or poor, watch for movement or changes in facial expression in response to your touch.

anisocoria A difference of 0.5 to 2 mm in pupil size. Anisocoria occurs normally in about 2% of people, in whom the pupillary inequality remains constant over time and despite changes in light. However, if anisocoria results from fixed dilation or constriction of one pupil or from slowed or impaired constriction of one pupil in response to light, it may indicate neurologic disease. Determining whether the abnormal pupil is dilated or constricted aids diagnosis.

aphonia Inability to produce speech sounds. This sign may result from overuse of the vocal cords, disorders of the larynx or laryngeal nerves, psychological disorders, or muscle spasm.

Argyll Robertson pupil A small, irregular pupil that constricts normally in accommodation for near vision, but poorly or not at all in response to light. Response to mydriatics also is poor or absent. This condition may be unilateral, bilateral, or asymmetrical and most commonly results from chronic syphilitic meningitis or other forms of late syphilis.

arthralgia Joint pain. This symptom may have no pathologic importance or may indicate such disorders as arthritis or systemic lupus erythematosus.

asthenocoria Slow dilation or constriction of the pupils in response to light changes. Photophobia may be present if constriction occurs slowly. Asthenocoria occurs in adrenal insufficiency. It's also known as *Arroyo's sign.*

asynergy Impaired coordination of muscles or organs that normally function harmoniously.

◆

571

This extrapyramidal symptom stems from disorders of the basal ganglia and cerebellum.

atrophy Shrinkage or wasting away of a tissue or organ due to a reduction in the size or number of its cells. Its etiology may be physiologic, as can be seen in ovary, brain, and skin atrophy, or pathologic, such as atrophy commonly associated with neurologic disorders or spleen, liver, and thyroid abnormalities. This symptom is normally observed using inspection and palpation techniques.

B

Barlow's sign An indicator of congenital dislocation of the hip, detected during the first 6 weeks of life. To elicit this sign, place the infant in a supine position with the hips flexed 90 degrees and the knees fully flexed. Place your palm over the infant's knee, your thumb in the femoral triangle opposite the lesser trochanter, and your index finger over the greater trochanter. Bring the hip into midabduction while gently exerting posterior and lateral pressure with your thumb, and posterior and medial pressure with your palm. If you detect a click of the femoral head as it dislocates across the posterior lip of the acetabular socket, you've elicited this sign.

Barré's sign Delayed contraction of the iris, seen in mental deterioration.

Beau's lines Transverse white linear depressions on the fingernails. These lines may develop after any severe illness or toxic reaction. Other common causes include malnutrition, nail bed trauma, and coronary artery occlusion.

Beevor's sign Upward movement of the umbilicus upon contraction of the abdominal muscles. To detect this sign, help the patient into a supine position and then ask him to sit up. If the umbilicus moves upward, you've observed this sign—an indicator of paralysis of the lower recti abdominis muscles associated with lesions at T10.

Bell's sign Reflexive upward and outward deviation of the eyes that occurs when the patient attempts to close his eyelid. It occurs on the affected side in Bell's palsy and indicates that the defect is supranuclear. Also known as *Bell's phenomenon.*

Bezold's sign Swelling and tenderness of the mastoid area. Resulting from formation of an abscess beneath the sternocleidomastoid muscle, Bezold's sign indicates mastoiditis.

Bitot's spots Triangular white or foamy gray spots, varying from a few bubbles to a frothy white coating. Appearing on the conjunctiva at the lateral margin of the cornea, they're associated with vitamin A deficiency.

blepharoclonus Excessive blinking of the eyes. This extrapyramidal sign occurs with disorders of the basal ganglia and cerebellum.

blocking A cognitive disturbance resulting in interruption of a stream of speech or thought. It usually occurs in midsentence or before completion of a thought. Generally, the patient is unable to explain the interruption. Blocking may occur in normal individuals but most commonly occurs in schizophrenics.

Bonnet's sign Pain on adduction of the thigh, seen in sciatica.

Bozzolo's sign Pulsation of arteries in the nasal mucous membrane, seen occasionally with thoracic aortic aneurysms. To detect this sign, examine both nostrils, using a speculum and light.

bradykinesia Slowness of all voluntary movement and speech, believed to be due to a reduced level of dopamine to the neurons in the brain stem region. Normal function within the central nervous system is inhibited. Bradykinesia is most frequently associated with parkinsonism, or extrapyramidal or cerebellar disorders. It can also result from certain drugs. Patients displaying bradykinesia are usually older than age 50, but it may also occur in children who have suffered hypoxic accidents. Associated findings include tremor and muscle rigidity.

Braunwald sign Occurrence of a weak pulse rather than a strong pulse immediately after a premature ventricular contraction (PVC). To detect this sign, watch for a PVC during cardiac monitoring and check the quality of the pulse after it. Braunwald sign may indicate idiopathic hypertrophic subaortic stenosis.

breath sounds, absent or decreased Diminished loudness of breath sounds—or their absence—detected by auscultation. This may reflect reduced airflow to a lung segment caused by a tumor, foreign body, mucous plug, or mucosal edema. It may also reflect hyperinflation of the lungs in emphysema or an asthma attack. Or, it may indicate air or fluid in the pleural cavity from a pneumothorax, hemothorax, pleural effusion, atelectasis, or empyema. In an obese or extremely muscular patient, breath sounds may be diminished or inaudible because of increased thickness of the chest wall.

C

catatonia Marked inhibition or excitation in motor behavior, occurring in psychotic disorders. Catatonic stupor refers to extreme inhibition of spontaneous activity or movement. Catatonic excitement refers to extreme psychomotor agitation.

Chaddock's sign Chaddock's toe sign: extension (dorsiflexion) of the great toe and fanning of the other toes. To elicit this sign, firmly stroke the side of the patient's foot just distal to the lateral malleolus. A positive sign indicates pyramidal tract disorders.

Chaddock's wrist sign: flexion of the wrist and extension of the fingers. To elicit this sign, stroke the ulnar surface of the patient's forearm near the wrist. A positive sign occurs on the affected side in hemiplegia. Although Chaddock's sign signals disease in children and adults, it's a normal finding in infants up to age 7 months.

cherry red spot The choroid appearing as a red circular area surrounded by an abnormal gray-white retina. It's viewed through the fovea centralis of the eye with an ophthalmoscope. A cherry red spot appears in infantile cerebral sphingolipidosis; for example, this spot is detected in more than 90% of patients with Tay-Sachs disease.

clicks Extra, brief, high-frequency heart sounds auscultated during systole or diastole. Ejection clicks occur soon after the first heart sound. Presumably, they result from sudden distention of a dilated pulmonary artery or the aorta, or from forceful opening of the pulmonic or aortic valves. Associated with increased pulmonary resistance and hypertension, they usually occur with septal defects or patent ductus arteriosus. To detect ejection clicks best, have the patient sit upright or lie down, then auscultate the heart with the diaphragm of the stethoscope.

Systolic clicks occur most commonly in mid-to-late systole. They're characteristic of mitral valve prolapse. A click is heard most distinctly at or medial to the heart's apex, but it may also be heard at the lower left sternal border. Clicks are heard best using the diaphragm of the stethoscope.

clonus Abnormal response of a muscle to stretching. It's a sign of damage to nerve fibers that carry impulses to a particular muscle from the motor cortex. Usually, a muscle that's stretched responds by contracting once and then relaxing. In clonus, stretching sets off a series of contractions of the muscle or muscles in rapid succession. Clonuslike, or clonic, muscle contractions are also a feature of generalized tonic-clonic seizures.

Codman's sign Pain resulting from rupture of the supraspinatus tendon. To elicit this sign, have the patient relax the arm on the affected side while you abduct it. If the patient reports no pain until you remove your support and the deltoid muscle contracts, you've detected Codman's sign.

cognitive dysfunction Inability to perceive, organize, and interpret sensory stimuli, and to think and solve problems. It may arise from various causes, including central nervous system disturbances, extrapyramidal conditions, systemic illness, endocrine diseases, deficiency states, or from unknown etiology, as in chronic fatigue syndrome.

compulsion Stereotyped, repetitive behavior in which the individual recognizes the irrationality of his actions but is unable to stop them. An example is constant hand washing. Compulsion occurs in obsessive-compulsive disorders and occasionally in schizophrenia.

confabulation Fabrication to cover gaps in memory. The recounts are generally plausible and detailed. Confabulation is most commonly seen in alcoholism and Korsakoff's syndrome and in those with dementia, lead poisoning, or head injuries.

conjunctival paleness Lack of color in the tissues inside the eyelid. Although the conjunctiva is a transparent mucous membrane, the portion lining the eyelids normally appears pink or red because it overlies the vasculature of the inner lid. Pale conjunctiva indicates anemia. To detect this sign, separate the eyelids widely by applying gentle pressure against the orbit of the eye. Ask the patient to look up, down, and to each side.

conversion An alteration in physical activity or function that resembles an organic disorder but lacks an organic cause. Occurring without voluntary control, conversion is generally considered symbolic of psychological conflict and usually occurs in conversion disorders.

Coopernail's sign Ecchymoses on the perineum, scrotum, or labia. This sign indicates pelvic fracture.

Corrigan's pulse A jerky pulse in which a strong surge precedes an abrupt collapse. To detect this sign, hold the patient's hand above his head and palpate the carotid artery. Corrigan's pulse occurs in aortic insufficiency. It may also occur in severe anemia, patent ductus arteriosus, coarctation of the aorta, and systemic arteriosclerosis.

Cowen's sign A jerky consensual pupillary light reflex. To detect this sign, observe for constriction and dilation of one pupil while the other is stimulated by increased and decreased light. This sign occurs in Graves' disease.

crossed extensor reflex Extension of one leg in response to stimulation of the opposite leg; a normal reflex in neonates. It's mediated at the spinal cord level and should disappear after age 6 months. To elicit this sign, place the infant in a supine position with his legs extended. Tap the medial aspect of the thigh just above the patella. The infant should respond by extending and adducting the opposite leg and fanning the toes of that foot. Persistence of this reflex beyond 6 months of age indicates anoxic brain damage. Its appearance in a child signals a central nervous system lesion or injury.

crowing respirations Slow, deep inspirations accompanied by a high-pitched crowing sound—the characteristic whoop of the paroxysmal stage of pertussis.

Cruveilhier's sign Swelling in the groin associated with inguinal hernia. To detect this sign, ask the patient to flex one knee slightly while you insert your index finger in the inguinal canal on the same side. When your finger is inserted as deeply as possible, ask the patient to cough. If a hernia is present, you'll feel a mass of tissue that meets your finger and then withdraws.

Cullen's sign Irregular, bluish hemorrhagic patches on the skin around the umbilicus and occasionally around abdominal scars. Cullen's sign indicates massive hemorrhage after trauma or rupture in such disorders as duodenal ulcer, ectopic pregnancy, abdominal aneurysm, gallbladder or common bile duct obstruction, or acute hemorrhagic pancreatitis. Usually, Cullen's sign appears gradually; blood travels from a retroperitoneal organ or structure to the periumbilical area, where it diffuses through subcutaneous tissues. It may be difficult to detect in a dark-skinned patient. The extent of discoloration depends on the extent of bleeding. In time, the bluish discoloration fades to greenish yellow and then yellow before disappearing.

D

Delbet's sign Adequate collateral circulation to the distal portion of a limb associated with aneurysmal occlusion of the main artery. To detect this sign, check pulses, color, and temperature in the affected limb. If you find absent pulses but normal color and temperature, you've detected Delbet's sign.

delirium Acute confusion characterized by restlessness, agitation, incoherence, and usually hallucinations. Typically, delirium develops suddenly and lasts for a short period. It's a common effect of drug and alcohol abuse, metabolic disorders, and high fever. Delirium may also follow head trauma or seizure.

delusion A persistent false belief held despite invalidating evidence. A delusion of grandeur, which may occur in schizophrenia and bipolar disorders, refers to an exaggerated belief in one's importance, wealth, or talent. The patient may take a powerful figure, such as Napoleon, as his persona. In a paranoid delusion, which may occur in schizophrenia and paranoid disorders, the patient believes that he or someone close to him is the victim of an attack, harassment, or conspiracy. In a somatic delusion, which may occur in psychotic disorders, the patient believes that his body is diseased or distorted.

Demianoff's sign Lumbar pain caused by stretching the sacrolumbalis muscle. To elicit this sign, help the patient into a supine position on the examination table and raise his extended leg. Lumbar pain that prevents lifting the leg high enough to form a 10-degree angle to the table—a positive Demianoff's sign—occurs in lumbago.

denial An unconscious defense mechanism used to ward off distressing feelings, thoughts, wishes, or needs. Denial occurs in normal and pathologic mental states. In terminal illness, it represents the first stage of the response to dying.

depersonalization Perception of the self as strange or unreal. For example, a person may report feeling as if he's observing himself from a distance. This symptom occurs in patients with schizophrenia and depersonalization disorders, and in normal individuals during periods of great stress, fatigue, or anxiety.

Dorendorf's sign Fullness at the supraclavicular groove. This sign may occur in an aneurysm of the aortic arch.

Duchenne's sign Inward movement of the epigastrium during inspiration. This may indicate diaphragmatic paralysis or accumulation of fluid in the pericardium.

Dugas' sign An indicator of a dislocated shoulder. To detect this sign, ask the patient to place the hand of the affected side on his opposite shoulder and to move his elbow toward his chest. The inability to perform this maneuver—a positive Dugas' sign—indicates dislocation.

Duroziez's sign A double murmur heard over a large peripheral artery. To detect this sign, auscultate over the femoral artery, alternately compressing the vessel proximally and then distally. If you hear a systolic murmur with proximal compression and a diastolic murmur with distal compression, you've detected Duroziez's sign—an indicator of aortic insufficiency. It's also known as *Duroziez's murmur.*

dysphonia Hoarseness or difficulty in producing voice sounds. This sign may reflect disorders of the larynx or laryngeal nerves, overuse or spasm of the vocal cords, or central nervous system disorders, such as Parkinson's disease. Pubertal changes are termed dysphonia puberum.

E

echolalia In an adult: repetition of another's words or phrases with no comprehension of their meaning. This sign occurs in schizophrenia and frontal lobe disorders.

In a child: an imitation of sounds or words produced by others.

echopraxia Repetition of another's movements with no comprehension of their meaning. This sign may occur in catatonic schizophrenia and certain neurologic disorders.

ectropion Eversion of the eyelid. It may affect the lower eyelid or both lids, exposing the palpebral conjunctiva. If the lacrimal puncta are everted, the eye can't drain properly, and tearing occurs. Ectropion may occur gradually as part of aging but may also occur with injury or paralysis of the facial nerve.

entropion Inversion of the eyelid. It typically affects the lower lid but may also affect the upper lid. The eyelashes may touch and irritate the cornea. Usually associated with aging, entropion may also stem from chemical burns, mechanical injuries, spasm of the orbicularis muscle, pemphigoid, Stevens-Johnson syndrome, and trachoma.

epicanthal folds Vertical skin folds that partially or fully obscure the inner canthus of the eye. These folds may make the eyes appear crossed because the pupil lies closer to the inner canthus than to the outer canthus. Epicanthal folds are a normal characteristic in many young children and Asians. They also occur as a familial trait in other ethnic groups and as an acquired trait in aging. However, the presence of epicanthal folds along with oblique palpebral fissures in non-Asian children indicates Down syndrome.

Erben's reflex Slowing of the pulse when the head and trunk are forcibly bent forward. It may indicate vagal excitability.

Erb's sign In tetany, increased irritability of motor nerves, detected by electromyography. Erb's sign also refers to dullness on percussion over the sternum's manubrium in acromegaly.

Escherich's sign Contraction of the lips, tongue, and masseters, occurring in tetany. To elicit Escherich's sign, percuss the inner surface of the lips or the tongue.

euphoria A feeling of great happiness or well-being. When euphoria doesn't accompany enlightening experiences or superb achievements, it may reflect bipolar disorder, organic brain disease, or use of such drugs as heroin, cocaine, and amphetamines.

Ewart's sign Bronchial breathing heard on auscultation of the lungs and dullness heard on percussion below the angle of the left scapula. These compression signs commonly occur in pericardial effusion. They also occur beneath the prominence of the sternal end of the first rib in some cases of pericardial effusion.

F

Fajersztajn's crossed sciatic sign In sciatica, pain on the affected side caused by lifting the extended opposite leg. To elicit this sign, place the patient in a supine position and have him flex his unaffected hip, keeping his knee extended. Flexion at the hip will produce pain on the affected side caused by stretching of the irritated sciatic nerve.

flexor withdrawal reflex Flexion of the knee upon stimulation of the sole; a normal reflex in neonates. This reflex is mediated at the spinal cord level and should disappear after age 6 months.

To elicit this reflex, place the infant in a supine position, extend his legs, and pinch the sole. Normally, an infant younger than age 6 months will respond with slow, uncontrolled flexion of the knee. This reflex may be weak in premature neonates. Its persistence beyond age 6 months may indicate anoxic brain damage. Its recurrence signals a central nervous system lesion or injury.

flight of ideas Continuous, often seemingly pressured speech with abrupt changes of topic. In contrast with loose association, a listener can discern the connection between topics based on word similarities or sounds. This sign characteristically occurs in the manic phase of a bipolar disorder.

foot malposition, congenital Anomalous positioning of the foot, present at birth in roughly 0.4% of infants. It may reflect the fetal position of comfort, neuromuscular disease, or malformation of a joint or connective tissue. To assess this sign, observe the resting infant's foot to determine the position of comfort. Then observe the foot during spontaneous activity. Using gentle passive maneuvers, determine the full range of motion of the foot and ankle.

Fränkel's sign In tabes dorsalis, the excessive range of passive motion at the hip joint. This excessive motion stems from decreased tone in the surrounding muscles.

G

Galant's reflex Movement of the pelvis toward the stimulated side when the back is stroked laterally to the spinal column. Normally present at birth, this reflex disappears by age 2 months. To elicit this reflex, place the infant in a prone position on the examination table or on your hand. Then, using a pin or your finger, stroke the back laterally to the midline. Normally, the infant responds by moving the pelvis toward the stimulated side, indicating integrity of the spinal cord from T1 to S1. The absence, irregularity, or asymmetry of this reflex may indicate a spinal cord lesion.

Galeazzi sign Unequal leg lengths in an infant, seen in congenital dislocation of the hip. To detect this sign, place the infant in a supine position on a flat, hard surface. Flex the knees and hips 90 degrees and compare the heights of the knees. With dislocation of the hip, the knee will be lower and the femur will appear shortened on the affected side.

Gifford's sign Resistance to everting the upper eyelid, seen in thyrotoxicosis. To detect this sign, attempt to raise the eyelid and evert it over a blunt object.

Gowers' sign In an adult: irregular contraction of the iris, occurring when the eye is illuminated. This sign can be detected in certain stages of tabes dorsalis.

In a child: the characteristic maneuver used to rise from the floor or a low sitting position to compensate for proximal muscle weakness in Duchenne's or Becker's muscular dystrophy.

Grasset's phenomenon Inability to raise both legs simultaneously, even though each can be raised separately. In an adult: this phenomenon occurs in complete organic hemiplegia. To elicit it, help the patient into a supine position and lift and support the affected leg; then attempt to lift the opposite leg. In Grasset's phenomenon, the unaffected leg will drop—the result of an upper-motor-neuron lesion.

In an infant: this sign is normally present until age 5 to 7 months.

grief Deep anguish or sorrow typically felt upon separation, bereavement or loss. In patients with terminal illness, grief may precede acceptance of dying. Unlike depression, grief proceeds in stages and usually resolves with the passage of time.

Griffith's sign Lagging motion of the lower eyelids during upward rotation of the eyes, seen in thyrotoxicosis. To detect this sign, ask the patient to focus on a steadily rising point, such as your moving finger. If the lower lid doesn't follow eye motion smoothly, you've observed this sign.

Guilland's sign Quick, energetic flexion of the hip and knee in response to pinching of the contralateral quadriceps muscle. This sign indicates meningeal irritation.

H

hallucination A sensory perception without corresponding external stimuli that occurs while awake. Hallucinations may occur in depression, schizophrenia, bipolar disorder, organic brain disorders, and drug-induced and toxic conditions.

An *auditory hallucination* refers to the perception of nonexistent sounds—typically voices but occasionally music or other sounds. Occurring in schizophrenia, this is the most common type of hallucination.

An *olfactory hallucination*—a perception of nonexistent odors from the patient's own body or from some other person or object—is typically associated with somatic delusions. It occurs most commonly in temporal lobe lesions and may also occur in schizophrenia.

A *tactile hallucination* refers to the perception of nonexistent tactile stimuli, generally described as something crawling on or under the skin. It occurs mainly in toxic conditions and with addiction to certain drugs. Formication—the sensation of insects crawling on the skin—most commonly occurs in alcohol withdrawal syndrome and cocaine abuse.

A *visual hallucination* is a perception of images of nonexistent people, flashes of light, or other scenes. It occurs most commonly in acute, reversible organic brain disorders but may also occur in drug and alcohol intoxication, schizophrenia, febrile illness, and encephalopathy.

A *gustatory hallucination* refers to the perception of nonexistent, usually unpleasant tastes.

Hamman's sign A loud, crushing, crunching sound synchronous with the heartbeat. Auscultated over the precordium, it reflects mediastinal emphysema, which occurs in such life-threatening conditions as pneumothorax or rupture of the trachea or bronchi. To detect this sign, help the patient into a left lateral recumbent position and gently auscultate over the precordium.

harlequin sign A benign, erythematous color change occurring especially in low-birth-weight infants. This reddening of one longitudinal half of the body appears when the infant is placed on either side for a few minutes. When he's placed on his back, the sign usually disappears immediately but may persist up to 20 minutes.

hemorrhage, subungual Bleeding under the nail plate. Hemorrhagic lines, called *splinter hemorrhages*, run proximally from the distal edge and serve as an indicator of subacute bacterial endocarditis and trichinosis. Large hemorrhagic areas generally reflect nail bed injury.

Hill's sign A femoral systolic pulse pressure 60 to 100 mm Hg higher in the right leg than in the right arm. Hill's sign may indicate severe aortic insufficiency. To detect this sign, help the patient into a supine position and take blood pressure readings, first in the right arm and then in the right leg, noting the difference.

hyperacusis Abnormally acute hearing caused by increased irritability of the auditory neural mechanism. It results in an unusually low hearing threshold.

hyperesthesia Increased or altered cutaneous sensitivity to touch, temperature, or pain.

hypernasality A voice quality reflecting excessive expiration of air through the nose during speech. It's commonly associated with symptoms of dysarthria and possibly with swallowing defects. The sudden onset of hypernasality may indicate a neuromuscular disorder. This sign may also accompany cleft palate, a short soft and hard palate, abnormal nasopharyngeal size, and partial or complete velar paralysis. To detect this sign, ask the patient to extend vowel sounds first with the nostrils open, then closed (pinched). A significant shift in tone may indicate hypernasality.

hypoesthesia Decreased cutaneous sensitivity to touch, temperature, or pain.

I

idea of reference A delusion that other people, statements, actions, or events have a meaning specific to oneself. This delusion occurs in schizophrenia and paranoid states. Also known as *delusion of reference*.

illusion A misperception of external stimuli—usually visual or auditory, for example, the sound of the wind being perceived as a voice. Illusions occur normally as well as in schizophrenia and toxic states.

J

Jellinek's sign Also known as *Rasin's sign*, brownish pigmentation on the eyelids, usually more prominent on the upper lid than on the lower one. This sign appears in Graves' disease.

Joffroy's sign Immobility of the facial muscles with upward rotation of the eyes, associated with exophthalmos in Graves' disease. To detect this sign, observe the patient's forehead as he quickly rotates his eyes upward.

Joffroy's sign also refers to the inability to perform simple mathematics—a possible early sign of organic brain disorder.

K

Kanavel's sign An area of tenderness in the palm, caused by inflammation of the tendon sheath of the little finger. To detect this sign, apply pressure to the palm proximal to the metacarpophalangeal joint of the little finger.

Keen's sign Increased ankle circumference in Pott's fracture of the fibula. To detect this sign, measure the ankles at the malleoli and compare their circumferences.

Kleist's sign Flexion, or hooking, of the fingers when passively raised, associated with frontal lobe and thalamic lesions. To elicit this sign, have the patient turn his palms down, then gently raise his fingers. If his fingers hook onto yours, you've detected this sign.

Koplik's spots Also known as *Koplik's sign*. Small red spots with bluish white centers on the lingual and buccal mucosa characteristic of measles. After this sign appears, the measles rash usually erupts in 1 to 2 days.

Kussmaul's respirations An abnormal breathing pattern characterized by deep, rapid sighing respirations, generally associated with diabetic ketoacidosis.

Kussmaul's sign Distention of the jugular veins on inspiration, occurring in constrictive pericarditis and mediastinal tumor.

Kussmaul's sign also refers to a paradoxical pulse and to seizures and coma that result from absorption of toxins.

L

large for gestational age Neonatal weight that exceeds the 90th percentile for the gestational age of the infant. The high-birth-weight neonate is at increased risk for birth trauma, respiratory distress, hypocalcemia, hypoglycemia, and polycythemia.

Lasègue's sign Pain upon passive movement of the leg that distinguishes hip joint disease from sciatica. To elicit this sign, help the patient into a supine position, raise one of his legs, and bend the knee to flex the hip joint. Pain with this movement indicates hip joint disease. With the hip still flexed, slowly extend the knee. Pain with this movement results from stretching an irritated sciatic nerve, indicating sciatica.

lead-pipe rigidity Diffuse muscle stiffness occurring, for example, in Parkinson's disease.

Leichtenstern's sign Pain upon gentle tapping of the bones of an extremity. This sign occurs in cerebrospinal meningitis. The patient may wince, draw back suddenly, or cry out loudly.

Lhermitte's sign Sensations of sudden, transient, electric-like shocks spreading down the back and into the extremities, precipitated by forward flexion of the head. This sign occurs in multiple sclerosis, spinal cord degeneration, and cervical spinal cord injury.

Linder's sign Pain upon neck flexion, indicating sciatica. To elicit this sign, help the patient into a supine or sitting position with his legs fully extended. Then passively flex his neck, noting if he experiences pain in the lower back or the affected leg, resulting from stretching of the irritated sciatic nerve.

Lloyd's sign Referred loin pain elicited by deep percussion over the kidney. This sign is associated with renal calculi.

loose association A cognitive disturbance marked by absence of a logical link between spoken statements. It occurs in schizophrenia, bipolar disorders, and other psychotic disorders.

low-set ears A position of the ears in which the superior helix lies lower than the eyes. This sign appears in several genetic syndromes, including Down, Apert's, Turner's, Noonan's, and Potter's, and may also appear in other congenital abnormalities.

Ludloff's sign Inability to raise the thigh while sitting, along with edema and ecchymosis at the base of Scarpa's triangle (the depressed area just below the fold of the groin). Occurring in children, this sign indicates traumatic separation of the epiphyseal growth plate of the greater trochanter.

lumbosacral hair tuft Abnormal growth of hair over the lower spine, possibly accompanied by skin depression or discoloration. This may mark the site of spina bifida occulta or spina bifida cystica.

M

malaise Listlessness, weariness, or absence of the sense of well-being. This nonspecific symptom may begin suddenly or gradually and may precede characteristic signs of an illness by several days or weeks. Malaise may reflect the metabolic alterations that precede or accompany infectious, endocrine, or neurologic disorders.

malingering Exaggeration or simulation of symptoms to avoid an unpleasant situation or to gain attention or some other goal.

mania An alteration in mood characterized by increased psychomotor activity, euphoria, flight of ideas, and pressured speech. It occurs most commonly in the manic phase of a bipolar disorder.

Mannkopf's sign Elevated pulse rate upon application of pressure over a painful area. It can help distinguish real pain from simulated pain—the sign doesn't occur in the latter.

Mean's sign Lagging eye motion when the patient looks upward. In this sign of Graves' disease, the globe of the eye moves more slowly than the upper lid.

meconium staining of amniotic fluid The presence of greenish brown or yellow meconium in the amniotic fluid during labor. Although not necessarily indicative of distress, this sign signals the need for close fetal monitoring to detect decreased variability, or deceleration, of heart rate. It may also signal the need for infant intubation and resuscitation at delivery to prevent meconium aspiration into the lungs.

menorrhagia Abnormally heavy menstrual flow occurring at the normal time but abnormally prolonged, saturating a pad or tampon in less than an hour.

metrorrhagia Vaginal bleeding or spotting between menses.

Möbius' sign Inability to maintain convergence of the eyes. To detect this sign of Graves' disease, observe the patient's attempt to focus on any small object, such as a pencil, as you move it toward him in line with his nose.

Murphy's sign The arrest of inspiratory effort when gentle finger pressure beneath the right subcostal arch and below the margin of the liver causes pain during deep inspiration. This classic (but not always present) sign of acute cholecystitis may also occur in hepatitis.

muscle rigidity Muscle tension, stiffness, and resistance to passive movement. This extrapyramidal symptom occurs in disorders affecting the basal ganglia and cerebellum, such as Parkinson's disease, Wilson's disease, Hallervorden-Spatz disease in adults, and kernicterus in infants.

myalgia Diffuse muscle pain, usually accompanied by malaise, occurring in many infectious diseases. These diseases include brucellosis, dengue, influenza, leptospirosis, measles, and poliomyelitis. Myalgia also occurs in arteriosclerosis obliterans, fibrositis, fibromyositis, Guillain-Barré syndrome, hyperparathyroidism, hypoglycemia, hypothyroidism, muscle tumor, myoglobinuria, myositis, and renal tubular acidosis. In addition, various drugs may cause myalgia, including amphotericin B, chloroquine, clofibrate, and corticosteroids.

N

nail dystrophy Changes in the nail plate, such as pitting, furrowing, splitting, or fraying. It usually results from injury, chronic nail infection, neurovascular disorders affecting the extremities, or collagen disorders. It also occurs secondary to repeated wetting and drying of the nails associated with frequent immersion in water.

nail plate discoloration A change in the color of the nail plate, resulting from infection or drugs. Blue-green discoloration may occur with Pseudomonas infection; brown or black, with fungal infection or fluorosis; and bluish gray, with excessive use of silver salts.

nail plate hypertrophy Thickening of the nail plate resulting from the accumulation of irregular keratin layers. This condition is commonly associated with fungal infection of the nails, although it can be hereditary.

nail separation The separation of the nail plate from the nail bed. This occurs primarily in injury or infection of the nail, and in thyrotoxicosis.

neologism A new word or condensation of several words with special meaning for the patient but not readily understood by others. This coining occurs in schizophrenia and organic brain disorders.

neuralgia Severe, paroxysmal pain over an area innervated by specific nerve fibers. The cause is typically unknown, but it may be precipitated by pressure, cold, movement, or stimulation of a trigger zone. Usually brief, neuralgia may be accompanied by vasomotor symptoms, such as sweating or tearing.

nodules Small, solid, circumscribed masses of differentiated tissue, detected on palpation.

O

obsession A persistent, usually disturbing thought or image that can't be eliminated by reason or logic. It's associated with an obsessive-compulsive disorder and, occasionally, schizophrenia.

obturator sign Pain in the right hypogastric region, occurring with flexion of the right leg at the hip with the knee bent and internally rotated. It indicates irritation of the obturator muscle.

In children, this sign may signal acute appendicitis because the appendix lies rectocecally over the obturator muscle.

oculocardiac reflex Also known as *Aschner's phenomenon.* Refers to bradycardia in response to vagal stimulation, caused by application of pressure to the eyeball or carotid sinus. This reflex can aid in the diagnosis of angina or it can relieve it. *Caution:* Repeated application of pressure to the eye to elicit this response may precipitate retinal detachment.

orbicularis sign Inability to close one eye at a time, occurring in hemiplegia.

orthotonos A form of tetanic spasm producing a rigid, straight line of the neck, limbs, and body.

ostealgia Bone pain associated with such disorders as osteomyelitis.

otorrhagia Bleeding from the ear occurring with a tumor, severe infection, or injury affecting the auricle, external canal, tympanic membrane, or temporal bone.

PQ

palmar crease abnormalities An abnormal line pattern on the palms, resulting from faulty embryonic development during the second and fourth months of gestation. This pattern may occur normally but usually appears in Down syndrome (called the *simian crease*) as a single transverse crease formed by fusion of the proximal and distal palmar creases. It also appears in Turner's syndrome and congenital rubella syndrome.

paradoxical respirations An abnormal breathing pattern marked by paradoxical movement of an injured portion of the chest wall—it contracts on inspiration and bulges on expiration. This ominous sign is characteristic of flail chest—a thoracic injury involving multiple free-floating, fractured ribs.

paranoia Extreme suspiciousness related to delusions of persecution by another person, group, or institution. This may occur in schizophrenia, drug-induced or toxic states, or paranoid disorders.

Pastia's sign Petechiae or hemorrhagic lines appearing along skin creases in such areas as the antecubital fossa, the groin, and the wrists. They accompany the rash of scarlet fever as a response to the erythrogenic toxin produced by scarlatinal strains of group A streptococci.

peroneal sign Dorsiflexion and abduction of the foot upon tapping over the common peroneal nerve. To elicit this sign of latent tetany, tap over the lateral neck of the fibula with the patient's knee relaxed and slightly flexed.

phobia An irrational and persistent fear of an object, situation, or activity. Occurring in phobic disorders, it may interfere with normal functioning. Typical manifestations include faintness, fatigue, palpitations, diaphoresis, nausea, tremor, and panic.

Potain's sign Dullness on percussion over the aortic arch, extending from the manubrium to the third costal cartilage on the right. This occurs in aortic dilation.

Prehn's sign Relief of pain with elevation and support of the scrotum, occurring in epididymitis. This sign differentiates epididymitis from testicular torsion. Both disorders produce severe pain, tenderness, and scrotal swelling.

pressured speech Verbal expression that's accelerated, difficult to interrupt, and at times unintelligible. This may accompany flight of ideas in the manic phase of a bipolar disorder.

Prévost's sign Conjugate deviation of the head and eyes in hemiplegia. Typically, the eyes gaze toward the affected hemisphere.

prognathism An enlarged, protuberant jaw associated with normal mandible condyles and temporomandibular joints. This sign usually appears in acromegaly.

R

rectal tenesmus Spasmodic contraction of the anal sphincter with a persistent urge to defecate and involuntary, ineffective straining. This occurs in inflammatory bowel disorders, such as ulcerative colitis and Crohn's disease, and in rectal tumors. Typically painful, rectal tenesmus usually accompanies passage of small amounts of blood, pus, or mucus.

regression Return to a behavioral level appropriate to an earlier developmental age. This defense mechanism may occur in various psychiatric and organic disorders. It may also result from worsening of symptoms, or of a disease process.

repression The unconscious retreat or thrusting back from awareness of unacceptable ideas or impulses. This defense mechanism may occur normally or may accompany psychiatric disorders.

Rosenbach's sign Absence of the abdominal skin reflex, associated with intestinal inflammation and hemiplegia. This sign also refers to the fine, rapid tremor of gently closed eyelids in Graves' disease; and to the inability to close the eyes immediately on command, as is seen in neurasthenia.

Rotch's sign Dullness on percussion over the right lung at the fifth intercostal space. This sign occurs in pericardial effusion.

Rovsing's sign Pain in the right lower quadrant upon palpation and quick withdrawal of the fingers in the left lower quadrant. This referred rebound tenderness suggests appendicitis.

S

Seeligmüller's sign Pupillary dilation on the affected side, in facial neuralgia.

spine sign Resistance to anterior flexion of the spine, resulting from pain in poliomyelitis.

spoon nails Malformation of the nails characterized by a concave instead of the normal convex outer surface. The nail is also abnormally thin. This commonly occurs in severe hypochromic anemia but occasionally may be hereditary.

Stellwag's sign Incomplete and infrequent blinking, usually related to exophthalmos in Graves' disease.

stepping reflex In the neonate, spontaneous stepping movements that simulate walking. This reciprocal flexion and extension of the legs disappears after about age 4 weeks. To elicit this sign, hold the infant erect with the soles touching a hard surface. However, scissoring movements with persistent extension and crossing of the legs or asymmetrical stepping is abnormal, possibly indicating central nervous system damage.

Strunsky's sign Pain on plantar flexion of the toes and forefoot, caused by inflammatory disorders of the anterior arch. To detect this sign, have the patient assume a relaxed position with his foot exposed, then grasp his toes and quickly plantarflex his toes and forefoot.

succussion splash A splashing sound heard over a hollow organ or body cavity, such as the stomach or thorax, after rocking or shaking the patient's body. Indicating the presence of fluid or air and gas, this sound may be auscultated in pyloric or intestinal obstruction, a large hiatal hernia, or hydropneumothorax.

However, it may also be auscultated over a normal, empty stomach.

sucking reflex Involuntary circumoral sucking movements in response to stimulation. Present at about 26 weeks', this reflex is initially weak and isn't synchronized with swallowing. It persists through infancy, becoming more discriminating during the first few months and disappearing by age 1. To elicit this response, place your finger in the infant's mouth. Rhythmic sucking movements are normal. Weakness or absence of these movements may indicate elevated intracranial pressure.

T

tangentiality Speech characterized by tedious detail that prevents ever reaching the point of the statement. This occurs in schizophrenia and organic brain disorders.

Terry's nails A white, opaque surface over more than 80% of the nail and a normal pink distal edge. This sign is commonly associated with cirrhosis.

testicular pain Unilateral or bilateral pain localized in or around the testicle and possibly radiating along the spermatic cord and into the lower abdomen. It usually results from trauma, infection, or torsion. Typically, its onset is sudden and severe; however, its intensity can vary from sharp pain accompanied by nausea and vomiting to a chronic, dull ache. In a child, sudden onset of severe testicular pain is a urologic emergency. Assume torsion is the cause until disproven. If a young male complains of abdominal pain, always carefully examine the scrotum because abdominal pain commonly precedes testicular pain in testicular torsion.

Thornton's sign Severe flank pain resulting from nephrolithiasis.

thrill A palpable sensation resulting from the vibration of a loud murmur or from turbulent blood flow in an aneurysm. Thrills are associated with heart murmurs of grades IV to VI and may be palpable over major arteries.

Tinel's sign Distal paresthesia on percussion over an injured nerve in an extremity, as in carpal tunnel syndrome. To elicit this sign in the patient's wrist, tap over the median nerve on the wrist's flexor surface. This sign indicates a partial lesion or the early regeneration of the nerve.

tongue, hairy Hypertrophy and elongation of the tongue's filiform papillae. Normally white, the papillae may turn yellow, brown, or black from bacteria, food, tobacco, coffee, or dyes in drugs and food. Hairy tongue may also result from antibiotic therapy, irradiation of the head and neck, chronic debilitating disorders, and habitual use of mouthwashes containing oxidizing or astringent agents.

tongue, red Patchy or uniform redness (ranging from pink to magenta) of the tongue, which may be swollen and smooth, rough, or fissured. It usually indicates glossitis, resulting from emotional stress or nutritional disorders, such as pernicious anemia, Plummer-Vinson syndrome, pellagra, sprue, and folic acid and vitamin B deficiency.

tongue, smooth Absence or atrophy of the filiform papillae, causing a smooth (patchy or uniform), glossy, red tongue. This primary sign of malnutrition results from anemia and vitamin B deficiency.

tongue, white A uniform white coating or plaques on the tongue. Lesions associated with a white tongue may be premalignant or malignant and may require a biopsy. Necrotic white lesions—collections of cells, bacteria, and debris—are painful and can be scraped from the tongue. They commonly appear in children, typically resulting from candidiasis and thermal burns. Keratotic white lesions—thickened, keratinized patches—are usually asymptomatic and can't be scraped from the tongue. These lesions commonly result from alcohol use and local irritation from tobacco smoke or other substances.

tongue enlargement An increase in the tongue's size, causing it to protrude from the mouth. Its causes include Down syndrome, acromegaly, lymphangioma, Beckwith's syndrome, and congenital micrognathia. An enlarged tongue can also result from cancer of the tongue, amyloidosis, and neurofibromatosis.

tongue fissures Shallow or deep grooving of the dorsum of the tongue. Usually a congenital defect, tongue fissures occur normally in about 10% of the population. However, deep fissures may promote collection of food particles, leading to chronic inflammation and tenderness.

tongue swelling Edema of the tongue, usually associated with pernicious anemia, pellagra, hypothyroidism, and allergic angioneurotic edema.

tongue ulcers Circumscribed necrotic lesions of the dorsum, margin, tip, and inferior surface of the tongue. Ulcers usually result from biting, chewing, or burning of the tongue. They may also stem from Type I herpes simplex virus, tuberculosis, histoplasmosis, and cancer of the tongue.

tooth discoloration Bluish yellow or gray teeth may result from hypoplasia of the dentin and pulp, nerve damage, or caries. Yellow teeth may indicate caries. Mottling and staining suggest fluorine excess and may also be associated with the effects of certain drugs, such as tetracycline. Tooth discoloration (and small tooth size) may occur in osteogenesis imperfecta.

tophi Deposits of sodium urate crystals in cartilage, soft tissue, synovial membranes, and tendon sheaths, producing painless nodular swellings, a classic symptom of gout. Tophi commonly appear on the ears, hands, and feet. They may erode the skin, producing open lesions, and cause gross deformity, limiting joint mobility. Inflammatory flare-ups may occur.

transference Unconscious process of transferring feelings and attitudes originally associated with important figures, such as parents, to another. Used therapeutically in psychoanalysis, transference can also occur in other settings and relationships.

Troisier's sign Enlargement of a single lymph node, usually in the left supraclavicular group. It indicates metastasis from a primary carcinoma in the upper abdomen, commonly the stomach. To detect this sign, have the patient sit erect facing you. Palpate the region behind the sternocleidomastoid muscle as the patient performs Valsalva's maneuver. Although the enlarged node usually lies so deep that it escapes detection, it may rise and become palpable with this maneuver.

Turner's sign A bruiselike discoloration of the skin of the flanks. This sign appears 6 to 24 hours after onset of retroperitoneal hemorrhage in acute pancreatitis.

twitching Nonspecific intermittent contraction of muscles or muscle bundles.

U

urinary tenesmus Persistent, ineffective, painful straining to empty the bladder. This results from irritation of nerve endings in the bladder mucosa, caused by infection or an indwelling catheter.

V

vaginal bleeding abnormalities Passage of blood from the vagina at times other than menses. It may indicate abnormalities of the uterus, cervix, ovaries, fallopian tubes, or vagina. It may also indicate an abnormal pregnancy.

vein sign A palpable, bluish, cordlike swelling along the line formed in the axilla by the junction of the thoracic and superficial epigastric veins. This sign appears in tuberculosis and obstruction of the superior vena cava.

WX

Weill's sign In infantile pneumonia, absence of expansion in the subclavicular area of the affected side on inspiration.

Westphal's sign Absence of the knee jerk reflex, occurring in tabes dorsalis.

Wilder's sign Subtle twitching of the eyeball on medial or lateral gaze. This early sign of Graves' disease is discernible as a slight jerk of the eyeball when the patient changes his direction of gaze.

YZ

yawning, excessive Persistent involuntary opening of the mouth, accompanied by attempted deep inspiration. In the absence of sleepiness, excessive yawning may indicate cerebral hypoxia.

Selected references

Anatomy & Physiology Made Incredibly Easy, 2nd ed. Philadelphia: Lippincott Williams & Wilkins, 2005.

Baranoski, S., and Ayello, E.A. *Wound Care Essentials: Practice Principles*. Philadelphia: Lippincott Williams & Wilkins, 2004.

Bender, K., and Thompson, F. E., Jr. "West Nile Virus: A Growing Challenge," *AJN* 103(6): 32-40, June 2003.

Bickley, L., and Szilagyi, P. *Bates' Guide to Physical Examination and History Taking*, 9th ed. Philadelphia: Lippincott Williams & Wilkins, 2007.

Craven R., and Hirnle, C. *Fundamentals of Nursing Human Health and Function*, 5th ed. Philadelphia: Lippincott Williams & Wilkins, 2007.

Dinwiddie, L., et al. "Stage 4 Chronic Kidney Disease," *AJN* 106(9):40-52, September 2006.

ECG Interpretation Made Incredibly Easy, 3rd ed. Philadelphia: Lippincott Williams & Wilkins, 2005.

Ferri, F. *Ferri's Clinical Advisor: Instant Diagnosis and Treatment*. St. Louis: Mosby–Year Book, Inc., 2004.

Handbook of Signs & Symptoms, 3rd ed. Philadelphia: Lippincott Williams & Wilkins, 2006.

Hickey, J. *The Clinical Practice of Neurological and Neurosurgical Nursing*, 5th ed. Philadelphia: Lippincott Williams & Wilkins, 2003.

Kasper, D.L., et al., eds. *Harrison's Principles of Internal Medicine*, 16th ed. New York: McGraw-Hill Book Co., 2005.

Kozier, B., et al. *Fundamentals of Nursing Concepts, Process, and Practice*, 7th ed. Upper Saddle River, N.J.: Prentice Hall Health, 2004.

Legg, V. "Complications of Chronic Kidney Disease," *AJN* 105(6):40-49, June 2005.

Nurse's Quick Check: Diseases. Philadelphia: Lippincott Williams & Wilkins, 2005.

Nurse's Quick Check: Signs & Symptoms. Philadelphia: Lippincott Williams & Wilkins, 2006.

Nursing2007 Drug Handbook, 27th ed. Philadelphia: Lippincott Williams & Wilkins, 2007.

Nutrition Made Incredibly Easy, 2nd ed. Philadelphia: Lippincott Williams & Wilkins, 2007.

Porth, C.M. *Pathophysiology Concepts of Altered Health States*, 7th ed. Philadelphia: Lippincott Williams & Wilkins, 2005.

Rubin, E. *Rubin's Pathophysiology: Clinicopathologic Foundations of Medicine*, 4th ed. Philadelphia: Lippincott Williams & Wilkins, 2005.

Shives, L. *Basic Concepts of Psychiatric-Mental Health Nursing*, 6th ed. Philadelphia: Lippincott Williams & Wilkins, 2005.

Smeltzer, S.C., and Bare, B.G. *Brunner and Suddarth's Textbook of Medical-Surgical Nursing*, 10th ed. Philadelphia: Lippincott Williams & Wilkins, 2004.

Supplement to Circulation: Journal of the American Heart Association. Philadelphia: Lippincott Williams & Wilkins, December 2005.

Tierney, L., et al. *Current Medical Diagnosis and Treatment*, 45th ed. New York: McGraw-Hill Book Co., 2006.

Woods, S.L., et al. *Cardiac Nursing*, 5th ed. Philadelphia: Lippincott Williams & Wilkins, 2005.

Index

i refers to an illustration; t refers to a table.

◆

---

i refers to an illustration; t refers to a table.

---

i refers to an illustration; t refers to a table.

---

i refers to an illustration; t refers to a table.

i refers to an illustration; t refers to a table.

---

i refers to an illustration; t refers to a table.

---

i refers to an illustration; t refers to a table.

---

i refers to an illustration; t refers to a table.

---

i refers to an illustration; t refers to a table.